The Research Process
in Nursing

The Research Process in Nursing

SIXTH EDITION

Edited by

Kate Gerrish
PhD, MSc, BNurs, RN, RM, NDN Cert
*Professor of Nursing, Sheffield Hallam University and
Sheffield Teaching Hospitals NHS Foundation Trust*

Anne Lacey
DPhil, MSc, BSc Hons, RGN, CertEd (FE)
*Diocesan Health Coordinator,
Diocese of Madi and West Nile, Uganda,
Honorary Senior Research Fellow, University of Sheffield*

WILEY-BLACKWELL

A John Wiley & Sons, Ltd., Publication

This edition first published 2010
© 2010 Blackwell Publishing Ltd

Blackwell Publishing was acquired by John Wiley & Sons in February 2007. Blackwell's publishing programme has been merged with Wiley's global Scientific, Technical, and Medical business to form Wiley-Blackwell.

Registered office
John Wiley & Sons Ltd, The Atrium, Southern Gate, Chichester, West Sussex PO19 8SQ, United Kingdom

Editorial offices
9600 Garsington Road, Oxford OX4 2DQ, United Kingdom
2121 State Avenue, Ames, Iowa 50014-8300, USA

For details of our global editorial offices, for customer services and for information about how to apply for permission to reuse the copyright material in this book please see our website at www.wiley.com/wiley-blackwell.

Library of Congress Cataloging-in-Publication Data

The research process in nursing. – 6th ed. / edited by Kate Gerrish, Anne Lacey.
p. ; cm.
Includes bibliographical references and index.
ISBN 978-1-4051-9048-0 (pbk. : alk. paper)   1. Nursing–Research.   I. Gerrish, Kate, 1955–   II. Lacey, Anne.
[DNLM: 1. Nursing Research–methods.   2. Data Collection–methods.   3. Research Design. WY 20.5 R4324 2010]
RT81.5.R465 2010
610.73072–dc22
2009048118

A catalogue record for this book is available from the British Library.

Set in 10 on 12 pt Times by Toppan Best-set Premedia Limited
Printed and bound in Singapore by Fabulous Printers Pte Ltd

2   2011

Contents

Section 2 Preparing the Ground

Section 3 Choosing the Right Approach

Section 5 Making Sense of the Data

Section 6 Putting Research into Practice

Contributors

Leanne M Aitken
PhD, BHSc(Nurs) Hons, RN, Int Care Cert,
   GCertMgt, GDipScMed(ClinEpi)
Professor of Critical Care Nursing, Research Centre
   for Clinical and Community Practice Innovation,
   Griffith University & Princess Alexandra
   Hospital, Australia

Teresa Allan
MSc, BA Hons
Senior Lecturer in Health and Care Statistics,
   School of Community and Health Sciences, City
   University London, UK

Claire Beecroft
MA, BA Hons, DPS
Information Specialist, School of Health and
   Related Research (ScHARR), University of
   Sheffield, UK

Andrew Booth
MSc, BA, Dip Lib, MCLIP
Reader in Evidence Based Information Practice,
   School of Health and Related Research
   (ScHARR), University of Sheffield, UK

Jo Booth
PhD, BSc(Hons), BA, RGN, RNT
Reader, School of Nursing, Midwifery and
   Community Health, Glasgow Caledonian
   University, UK

Tracey Bucknall
PhD, RN, Int Care Cert, GDACN
Professor of Nursing, Deakin University, Head,
   Cabrini-Deakin Centre for Nursing Research,
   Cabrini Health, Australia

Charlotte L Clarke
DSocSc, PhD, MSc, PGCE, BA, RN
Associate Dean (Research) and Professor of
   Nursing Practice Development Research,
   Northumbria University, UK

Kara DeCorby
MSc
Research Coordinator, Faculty of Health Sciences,
   McMaster University, Ontario, Canada

Jo Dumville
PhD, MSc
Research Fellow, York Trials Unit, University of
   York, UK

George Ellison
PhD, MSc (Med), BSc Hons
Professor of Interdisciplinary Studies and Director
   of the Graduate School & Research Office,
   London Metropolitan University, UK

Catherine Evans
PhD, MSc, BSc, RN, RHV, DN
Research Fellow, Centre for Research in Primary
   and Community Care, University of
   Hertfordshire, UK

Jenny Freeman
PhD, MSc, BSc, CSTAT
Senior Lecturer in Medical Statistics, School of
  Health and Related Research (ScHARR),
  University of Sheffield, UK

Dawn Freshwater
PhD, BA Hons, RN RNT, FRCN
Professor of Mental Health and Dean of School of
  Health Care, University of Leeds, UK

Leslie Gelling
PhD, MA, BSc Hons, RN MICR FRSA
Senior Research Fellow, Faculty of Health and
  Social Care, Anglia Ruskin University, UK

Kate Gerrish
PhD, MSc, BNurs, RN, RM, NDN Cert
Professor of Nursing, Centre for Health & Social
  Care Research, Sheffield Hallam University and
  Sheffield Teaching Hospitals NHS Foundation
  Trust, UK

Claire Goodman
PhD, MSc, BSc, RN, DN
Professor of Health Care Research, Centre for
  Research in Primary and Community Care,
  University of Hertfordshire, UK

Gordon Grant
PhD, MSc, BSc Hons
Emeritus Professor, Centre for Health and Social
  Care Research, Sheffield Hallam University, UK

Peter Griffiths
PhD, BA Hons, RN
Professor and Director National Nursing Research
  Unit, King's College London, UK

Carol Haigh
PhD, MSc, BSc Hons, RGN
Professor in Nursing, Faculty of Health, Psychology
  and Social Care, Manchester Metropolitan
  University, UK

Felicity Hasson
MSc, PgDip, BA Hons
Research Fellow, Institute of Nursing Research,
  School of Nursing, University of Ulster, UK

Immy Holloway
PhD, MA, Bed, Cert Ed
Visiting Professor, School of Health and Social
  Care, Bournemouth University, UK

Alison Hutchinson
PhD, MBioeth, BAppSc, RN, Certificate in
  Nursing, Certificate in Midwifery
Postdoctoral Fellow, Faculty of Nursing, University
  of Alberta, Canada, Honorary Senior Fellow,
  School of Nursing and Social Work, The
  University of Melbourne, Australia

Martin Johnson
PhD, MSc, RN, RNT
Professor in Nursing, School of Nursing, University
  of Salford, UK

Martyn Jones
PhD, CPsychol, BSc Hons, RNMH, Dip Ed
Reader, School of Nursing and Midwifery,
  University of Dundee, UK

Sinead Keeney
PhD, MRes, BA Hons
Senior Lecturer, Institute of Nursing Research,
  School of Nursing, University of Ulster, UK

Anne Lacey
DPhil, MSc, BSc Hons, RGN, RNT, DipN(Lond)
Diocesan Health Coordinator, Diocese of Madi and
  West Nile, Uganda, Honorary Senior Research
  Fellow, School of Health and Related Research
  (ScHARR), University of Sheffield, UK

Judith Lathlean
DPhil (Oxon), MA; BSc(Econ) Hons
Professor of Health Research, School of Health
  Sciences, University of Southampton, UK

Tony Long
PhD, MA, BSc Hons, SRN, RSCN
Professor of Child and Family Health, School of
    Nursing, University of Salford, UK

Brendan McCormack
DPhil, BSc Hons, DPSN, PGCEA, RNT, RGN,
    RMN
Professor of Nursing Research, University of
    Ulster, UK

Hugh McKenna
CBE, PhD, BSc Hons, RMN, RGN, RNT,
    DipN(Lond), AdvDipEd, FFN RCSI FEANS,
    FRCN, FAAN
Dean, Faculty of Life and Health Sciences,
    University of Ulster, UK

Ann McMahon
PhD, MSc, BSc, PGDip, CMS, RMN, RGN
RCN Research and Development Adviser/Manager,
    RCN Research & Development Co-ordinating
    Centre, Royal College of Nursing, UK

Julienne Meyer
PhD, MSc, BSc, Cert Ed(FE), RN, RNT
Professor of Nursing, Care for Older People, City
    University London, UK

Andrea Nelson
PhD, BSc Hons, RN
Professor of Wound Healing, School of Healthcare,
    University of Leeds, UK

Susan Procter
PhD, BSc Hons, RGN, Cert Ed
Professor of Public Health and Primary Care,
    School of Community and Health Sciences, City
    University London, UK

Anne Marie Rafferty
CBE, DPhil, MPhil, BSc, RGN, DN, FRCN, FQNI
Dean and Head of School, Florence Nightingale
    School of Nursing and Midwifery, King's
    College London, UK

Paul Ramcharan
PhD, BSc Hons, Grad Dip Ed
Coordinator Research and Public Policy, Australian
    Centre for Human Rights Education, RMIT
    University, Melbourne, Australia

Janice Rattray
PhD, MN, Cert Ed, RGN, SCM
Senior Lecturer, School of Nursing and Midwifery,
    University of Dundee, UK

Jan Reed
PhD, BA, Cert Ed
Professor of Health Care for Older People, School
    of Health, Social Care and Education,
    Northumbria University, UK

Angie Rees
MA, BA Hons, DPS, MCLIP
Information Specialist, School of Health and
    Related Research (ScHARR), University of
    Sheffield, UK

Colin Robson
PhD, BSc Hons, BSc Hons, PGCE
Emeritus Professor, School of Human and Health
    Sciences, University of Huddersfield, UK

Jo Rycroft-Malone
PhD, MSc, BSc Hons, RN
Professor of Implementation Research, Bangor
    University, UK

Sarah Salway
PhD, MSc, BSc Hons
Reader in Public Health, Centre for Health & Social
    Care Research, Sheffield Hallam University, UK

Lucy Simons
PhD, MA Hons, RGN
Senior Research Fellow, School of Health Sciences,
    University of Southampton, UK

Julie Taylor
PhD, MSc, BSc Hons, RN, FEANS
Professor of Family Health and Research Dean,
  School of Nursing and Midwifery, University of
  Dundee, UK

Angela Tod
PhD, MSc, MMedSci, BA Hons, RN
Principal Research Fellow, Centre for Health and
  Social Care Research, Sheffield Hallam
  University, UK

Les Todres
PhD, MSocSc (Clin Psych), BSocSc Hons,
  CPsychol
Professor of Qualitative Research, Centre for
  Qualitative Research, School of Health and
  Social Care, Bournemouth University, UK

Annie Topping
PhD, PGCE, BSc Hons, RGN
Professor of Health & Social Care, Centre for
  Health and Social Care Research, University of
  Huddersfield, UK

David Torgerson
PhD, MSc
Director York Trials Unit, University of York, UK

Rosemary Wall
PhD, MSc, BA
History of Nursing Postdoctoral Research
  Associate, Florence Nightingale School of
  Nursing and Midwifery, King's College London,
  UK

Stephen Walters
PhD, MSc, PGCE, BSc Hons, CStat
Professor of Medical Statistics, School of Health
  and Related Research (ScHARR), University of
  Sheffield, UK

Hazel Watson
PhD, MN, RGN, RMN, RNT
Visiting Professor of Health Sciences, School of
  Nursing, Health and Culture, University West,
  Sweden, (formerly) Professor of Nursing, School
  of Nursing, Midwifery and Community Health,
  Glasgow Caledonian University, UK

Rosemary Whyte
PhD, BA Hons, RGN, RCNT, RNT
(Formerly) Research Fellow, School of Nursing,
  Midwifery and Community Health, Glasgow
  Caledonian University, UK

Introduction

Since the 5th edition of *The Research Process in Nursing* was published in 2006, there have been some significant developments in nursing research in the UK. A framework for clinical academic careers in nursing has been developed, creating for the first time the opportunity for nurses to progress through masters preparation, doctoral and post-doctoral research fellowships while combining research activity with clinical practice. The results of the 2008 Research Assessment Exercise, an appraisal of the quality of research in UK higher education institutions, showed marked improvement in the quality of nursing research, with a significant proportion of the research undertaken by nurses judged to be of world-class standard. At the same time, the pace of change in nursing research has been rapid, with a broader range of research approaches and methods being used to answer research questions arising from nursing practice. Finally, the drive to ensure that research evidence is used to inform practice has continued to gain momentum in both policy and the everyday work of practising nurses. Patients expect to receive high quality healthcare informed by the very best evidence. Nursing research is central to this endeavour.

As editors, we have felt it necessary to ensure that this well-established research text reflects these developments in nursing research. In compiling the 6th edition of *The Research Process in Nursing*, we have made some significant changes to the content of the book, although the overall structure remains unchanged. There are 10 completely new chapters,

and several other chapters have been substantially revised or written by new authors. The remaining chapters have been revised and updated to ensure that the reader is provided with the very latest information on research processes and methods. The 6th edition is also the first to include a website associated with the book (www.wiley.com/go/gerrish), enabling readers to complement their studies by accessing the many web resources that are available in the field of healthcare research, and highlighting work being undertaken by some of the chapter authors.

We, the editors, have been privileged to continue to work with chapter authors who are leaders in nursing research and other disciplines across the four countries of the UK, and, in this new edition, in Australia and Canada. We are indebted to our team of authors for their wide-ranging and authoritative contributions to the research methodology literature. We have continued to target the book at novice researchers, be they pre-registration students or those embarking on a postgraduate research degree, but the book should also be of value to many who are further on in their research careers. We have encouraged the authors to write in an accessible style, but not to shrink away from complex debates and technical issues.

The book is structured into six sections.

Section 1, *Setting the Scene*, deals with the background issues of nursing research in the current policy context in the UK, the nature of the research process, and ethics. This section also includes two chapters encouraging inclusive approaches to the research process. The previous edition included a chapter on user involvement, and in this edition a new chapter on research in a multi-ethnic society has been added. Readers new to the context in which nursing research takes place will find that this section orients them to the subject and, we hope, will enthuse them to engage with an activity that has the potential to change and improve the provision of healthcare.

Section 2, *Preparing the Ground*, includes chapters that take the reader through the steps that are essential before a research project can begin. Regulatory frameworks governing research in the UK have continued to evolve, and the chapter on this issue has therefore been rewritten by a new author. Chapters dealing with the preparation of a research proposal and management of a project have also been completely rewritten.

Section 3, *Choosing the Right Approach*, is the longest section and in many ways the heart of the book. It has been expanded considerably from the 5th edition. After an introduction to the philosophical debates underlying the different research approaches available to nurses, and a chapter on sampling, 15 research approaches used in nursing research are explored in detail. New chapters for this edition include narrative research, Delphi approach, practitioner research, realist synthesis and mixed methods. Although some of these approaches are less common in nursing research than surveys and grounded theory, for example, they are now appearing in the literature and represent new ways of thinking about carrying out research. They are commended to the reader as possible ways into difficult-to-research areas, particularly those related closely to nursing practice. A chapter on historical research included in earlier editions of the book has been rewritten for this 6th edition.

Section 4, *Collecting Data*, and Section 5, *Making Sense of Data*, are both practical sections dealing with the skills required for data collection and analysis. Here the emphasis is on research tools, such as interviewing and statistical analysis, common to many different research approaches. Two new chapters have been included in Section 4 – on 'think aloud' techniques, and on outcome measures. The chapter on outcome measures replaces the chapter on

physiological measurement in the previous edition, but includes some of the same content.

Section 6, *Putting Research into Practice*, concludes the book by taking the reader through the process of disseminating research findings and getting them implemented into policy and practice. As well as addressing active researchers, these chapters will be of use to nurses who, though not wanting to engage themselves in research, want to incorporate it into their professional lives through evidence-based practice. The chapter on translating research into practice has been completely rewritten by the author of the evidence-based practice chapter, which makes for a more coherent central theme in this section. The final chapter has undergone major revision, and now includes a policy review and up-to-date analysis of the state of nursing research and its aspirations for the future.

Although the book is designed in a logical fashion, as outlined above, each chapter is also intended to be complete in itself. Many readers will dip in and out of different sections as necessary. For this reason, wherever possible we have included cross-references to other chapters that may be helpful, and have provided key point summaries at the beginning of each chapter. We have also compiled a glossary of research terms to help the reader with new language with which they may be unfamiliar.

Throughout the book we have adopted certain generic terms to assist readability and reduce repetition. Foremost among these is the term 'nursing'. By this we mean all the professions of nursing, midwifery, health visiting and related specialisms. We hope that members of these professions will forgive our shorthand, but we have tried to ensure that examples given are taken from a wide range of healthcare settings. We have also used the terms 'evidence' and 'evidence-based practice' to denote the plethora of resources and implementation activities that have become so important in healthcare today.

This book is intended to be used primarily by nurses, midwives and health visitors, but it has much wider application to any health and social care practitioner who wishes to learn about research. Members of the allied health professions in particular face many of the same debates and dilemmas as nurses in developing research capacity. The contributors to the book are not all nurses, but include statisticians, social scientists, information specialists, academic researchers and psychologists.

We trust that this 6th edition of a well-established book will continue to make a valuable contribution to research capacity building in nursing and healthcare.

Kate Gerrish and Anne Lacey
Editors to the 6th edition,
2010

Setting the Scene

Nursing research does not exist in a vacuum, but is an applied discipline set in the context of a dynamic academic community and relating to a complex healthcare system. This section explores this context and introduces the reader to the nature of nursing research.

Chapter 1 presents the fundamental concepts of the discipline, reviews the current context of nursing research, and emphasises the essential connection between nursing research and the practice of the profession. Even those who do not see themselves as active researchers should be users of the knowledge generated by research, and so need to understand much of what follows in the sections of this book. Chapter 2 then takes the reader through the essential steps in the research process, each of which will be dealt with in much more depth in later sections, but with the aim of giving an overview of the entire undertaking that is research. Recent examples from the literature are used to illustrate the varied nature of nursing research.

Research in nursing, as in healthcare generally, is complicated by the fact that it is involved with vulnerable human beings, and ethical principles need to be observed from the outset of any research project. Chapter 3, therefore, tackles this moral obligation on the researcher, drawing out the practical implications for the researcher and setting the context for the more specific ethical regulations dealt with in Section 2 of the book.

The final two chapters in this section deal with the need for nursing research to be inclusive in scope. User involvement in research has been advocated from within and outside the profession for more than a decade now, and Chapter 4 argues for the full inclusion in the research process of those to whom the outcomes might apply. New to this edition of the book is Chapter 5 on research in a multi-ethnic society. Although there are many minority groups that deserve special consideration when designing nursing research, ethnicity perhaps merits particular consideration as a major factor impacting on healthcare in UK society.

1 Research and Development in Nursing

Kate Gerrish and Anne Lacey

Key points

- Research is concerned with generating new knowledge through a process of systematic scientific enquiry, the research process.

- Research in nursing can provide new insights into nursing practice, develop and improve methods of caring, and test the effectiveness of care.

- Whereas comparatively few nurses may undertake research, all nurses should develop research awareness and use research findings in their practice.

- Evidence-based practice involves the integration of the best available research evidence with expert clinical opinion while taking account of the preferences of patients.

INTRODUCTION

Significant changes in healthcare have taken place in the 26 years since the first edition of this book was published and these changes are set to continue. Technological developments have led to improved health outcomes and at the same time have raised public expectations of healthcare services. Increased life expectancy and lower birth rates mean that the United Kingdom (UK) population is ageing. An older population is more likely to experience complex health needs, especially in regard to chronic disease, and this places additional demands on an already pressurised health service. At the same time, the escalating cost of healthcare is leading to a shift from expensive resource-intensive hospital care to more services being provided in the primary and community care sectors. In response to these changes, government health policy is increasingly focused on improving the clinical and cost-effectiveness of healthcare, while at the same time reducing the burden of ill health through active public health and health promotion strategies. For example, the recent review of the NHS in England undertaken by Lord Darzi has identified a number of priorities that need to be progressed in order to provide high quality care for patients and the wider public (DoH 2008). The review stresses the importance of improving health outcomes by preventing illness, as well as enhancing the quality of care provided to people with particular needs, for example patients with common long-term conditions such as diabetes, or those in need of palliative and end-of-life care.

To achieve the outcomes for enhancing quality set out in the review, there is a need to change the way healthcare professionals work and the way health services fit together, and to ensure that patients have access to the best available treatments. However, achieving quality in healthcare is a moving target.

What was considered high quality care in 1948 when the NHS was first founded is no longer considered to be the case 60 years on. Knowledge about effective healthcare interventions has increased enormously, and this is certainly the case with nursing interventions. In the past, custom and practice, often based on the ward sister's or doctor's likes and dislikes, dictated what nurses did to patients, but nursing research has provided a new evidence base to inform the care that nurses provide. One clear example is in the field of pressure area care. It is not that long ago that nurses applied various techniques in an attempt to reduce the risk of a patient developing a pressure sore, these included egg white and oxygen, methylated spirits and vigorously rubbing the area at risk. Yet research by Doreen Norton more than 30 years ago clearly identified that moving patients regularly, keeping their skin clean and dry, and using the right equipment was the most effective way to reduce the risk (Norton *et al.* 1975).

It is essential that nurses respond proactively to the developments outlined above in order to provide high quality care in response to the needs of the individuals and communities with whom they work. To do this, they need up-to-date knowledge to inform their practice. Such knowledge is generated through research. This chapter introduces the concept of nursing research and considers how research contributes to the development of nursing knowledge. In recognising that nursing is a practice-based profession the relevance of research to nursing policy and practice is examined within the context of evidence-based practice and the responsibilities of nurses is explored in respect of research awareness, research utilisation and research activity.

NURSING RESEARCH AND DEVELOPMENT

The definition of research provided by Hockey (1984) in the first edition of this book is still pertinent today:

> 'Research is an attempt to increase the sum of what is known, usually referred to as a "body of knowledge" by the discovery of new facts or relationships through a process of systematic scientific enquiry, the research process' (Hockey 1984: 4)

Other definitions of research emphasise the importance of the knowledge generated through research being applicable beyond the research setting in which it was undertaken, i.e. that it is generalisable to other similar populations or settings. The Department of Health, for example, defines research as:

> 'the attempt to derive generalisable new knowledge by addressing clearly defined questions with systematic and rigorous methods' (DoH 2005: 3, section 1.10)

Research is designed to investigate explicit questions. In the case of nursing research these questions relate to those aspects of professional activity that are predominantly and appropriately the concern and responsibility of nurses (Hockey 1996). The International Council of Nursing's (ICN) definition of nursing research captures the broad areas of interest that are relevant to nurse researchers.

> 'Nursing research is a systematic enquiry that seeks to add new nursing knowledge to benefit patients, families and communities. It encompasses all aspects of health that are of interest to nursing, including promotion of health, prevention of illness, care of people of all ages during illness and recovery or towards a peaceful and dignified death' (ICN 2009)

The ICN has identified nursing research priorities in two broad areas, namely health and illness, and the delivery of care services. These priority areas are outlined in Box 1.1. In addition, research in the field of nursing education is important, for unless nurses are prepared appropriately for their role, they will not be able to respond to the needs of patients, families and communities. Priorities for research in nursing education are broad ranging as illustrated in Box 1.2. Most nursing research investigates contemporary issues; however, some studies may take an historical perspective in order to examine the development of nursing by studying documentary sources and other artefacts (see Chapter 26).

The questions that nursing research may address vary in terms of their focus. More than 20 years ago, Crow (1982) identified four approaches that research could take; these remain pertinent today:

Box 1.1 Priorities for nursing research identified by the International Council of Nurses

Health and illness

Nursing research priorities in health and illness focus on:

- health promotion
- prevention of illness
- control of symptoms
- living with chronic conditions and enhancing quality of life
- caring for clients experiencing changes in their health and illness
- assessing and monitoring client problems
- providing and testing nursing care interventions
- measuring the outcomes of care.

Delivery of care services

Nursing research priorities in delivery of care services focus on:

- quality and cost-effectiveness of care
- impact of nursing interventions on client outcomes
- evidence-based nursing practice
- community and primary healthcare
- nursing workforce to include quality of nurses' work life, retention, satisfaction with work
- impact of healthcare reform on health policy, programme planning and evaluation
- impact on equity and access to nursing care and its effects on nursing
- financing of healthcare.

Source: ICN (2009)

Box 1.2 Priorities for research in nursing education

- Curriculum design and evaluation, including community-driven models for curriculum development
- New pedagogies
- Innovation in teaching and learning
- Use of instructional technology, including new approaches to simulated learning
- Student/teacher learning partnerships
- Clinical teaching models
- Assessment of student learning in classroom and practice settings
- New models for teacher preparation and faculty development
- Quality improvement processes
- Educational systems and infrastructures

Adapted from National League for Nursing (2008)

- research that will provide new insights into nursing practice
- research that will deepen an understanding of the concepts central to nursing care
- research that is concerned with the development of new and improved methods of caring
- research that is designed to test the effectiveness of care.

Nursing research does not necessarily need to be undertaken by nurses. Indeed, some seminal studies into nursing practice and nurse education have been undertaken by sociologists. For example, in the 1970s, Robert Dingwall, a sociologist, undertook an influential study of health visitor training (Dingwall 1977). Likewise, nurses who engage in research may not confine their area of enquiry to nursing research. The growing emphasis on multidisciplinary, multi-agency working means that nurse researchers may choose to examine questions that extend beyond the scope of nursing into other areas of health and social care. Nurse researchers may find themselves working in multidisciplinary teams including statisticians, health economists, sociologists and other health professionals, working on research areas such as rehabilitation, which encompass a wide range of disciplines. Nurse researchers work appropriately in university departments such as social science, health services research and complementary medicine, as well as in departments of nursing and midwifery.

Whereas the generation of new knowledge is valuable in its own right, the application and utilisation of knowledge gained through research is essential to a practice-based profession such as nursing. This latter activity is known as 'development'. Thus research and development, 'R&D', go hand in hand.

Research and development can be divided into three types of activity.

Basic research is original, experimental or theoretical work, primarily for the purpose of obtaining new knowledge rather than focusing on the specific use of the findings. For example, biomedical laboratory-based research falls within this category.

Applied research is also original investigation with a view to obtaining new knowledge, but it is undertaken primarily for practical purposes. Much nursing research falls within this category and is undertaken with the intention of generating knowledge that can be used to inform nursing practice and can involve both clinical and non-clinical methods.

Development activity involves the systematic use of knowledge obtained through research and/or practical experience for the purpose of producing new or improved products, processes, systems or services.

Development activity that focuses on the utilisation of knowledge generated through research can take different forms. The most common activities include clinical audit, practice development and service evaluation (see Box 1.3). Like research, these activities often employ systematic methods to address questions arising from practice. Research, however, is undertaken with the explicit purpose of generating new knowledge, which has applicability beyond the immediate setting. By contrast, clinical audit, practice development and service evaluation are primarily concerned with generating information that can inform local decision making (NPSA 2008). Yet, the boundaries between some forms of research, for example action research (see Chapter 22) and practice development, and evaluation research (see Chapter 21) and service evaluation, are often blurred (Gerrish & Mawson 2005). It is, however, important to be able to differentiate between these activities as they require very different approval processes before the work can begin (see Chapter 10).

DEVELOPING NURSING KNOWLEDGE

Nursing research is concerned with developing new knowledge about the discipline and practice of nursing. Nursing knowledge, like any other knowledge, is never absolute. As the external world changes, nursing develops and adapts in response. In parallel, nursing knowledge develops and changes. This year's 'best available evidence' has the potential of being superseded by new insights and discoveries. Therefore nursing knowledge is temporal, and will always be partial and hence imperfect. This does not mean, however, that nurses should not continually strive to develop new knowledge to inform nursing and healthcare policy and practice.

Box 1.3 Definitions of research, clinical audit and practice development

Research involves the attempt to extend the available knowledge by means of a systematically and scientifically defensible process of inquiry (Clamp *et al.* 2004).

Clinical audit is a professional-led initiative that seeks to improve the quality and outcome of patient care through practitioners examining their practices and results and modifying practice where indicated (NHSE 1996: 16). Clinical audit measures care against predetermined standards.

Practice development encompasses a broad range of innovations that are initiated to improve practice and the services in which that practice takes place. It involves a continuous process of improvement towards increased effectiveness in patient-centred care. This is brought about by helping healthcare teams to develop their knowledge and skills, and transform the culture and context of care (Garbett & McCormack 2002).

Service evaluation seeks to assess how well a service is achieving its intended aims. It is undertaken to benefit those who use a particular service and is designed and conducted solely to define or judge current service (NPSA 2008).

Whereas the focus of this book is on the generation of knowledge through research, it is important to recognise that nursing knowledge may take different forms. In addition to empirical knowledge derived through research, nurses use other forms of knowledge, such as practical knowledge derived from experience, and aesthetic or intuitive knowledge derived from nursing practice (Thompson 2000). Nurses use these different forms of knowledge to varying degrees to inform their practice (Gerrish *et al.* 2008). It is beyond the scope of this book to examine in detail the various forms of nursing knowledge; however, Chapter 38 introduces the reader to some of these within the context of promoting evidence-based practice.

The definitions of research given earlier in this chapter emphasise the role of systematic scientific enquiry – the research process – in generating new knowledge. The research process comprises a series of logical steps that have to be undertaken to develop knowledge. Different disciplines may interpret the research process in different ways, depending on the specific paradigms (ways of interpreting the world)

and theories that underpin the discipline. A biological scientist's approach to generating new knowledge will be different from that of a sociologist. However, the basic principles of the systematic research process will be followed by all disciplines. Nursing, as a discipline in its own right, is relatively young in comparison to more established professional groups such as medicine, and is in the process of generating theories that are unique to describing, explaining or predicting the outcomes of nursing actions. Nursing theories are generated through the process of undertaking research and may also be tested and refined through further research. However, nursing also draws on a unique mix of several disciplines, such as physiology, psychology and sociology, and any of these disciplines may be appropriate for research in nursing. For example, the management of pain can be studied from a psychological or physiological perspective; whichever approach is chosen will be influenced by the theories relevant to the particular discipline.

The research process in nursing is no different from that of other disciplines and the same rules of scientific method apply. Chapter 2 sets out a systematic approach to research – the scientific method in action – and subsequent chapters consider the various components of the research process in detail. At this stage, it is worth noting that in some texts, the 'scientific method' is taken to reflect a particular view of the world which values the notion that we can be totally objective in our research endeavours. Here, the term is not restricted in this way and we use the term 'scientific method' to mean a rigorous approach to a systematic form of enquiry. Chapter 11 introduces the reader to the different ways in which the scientific method can be interpreted, depending on the assumptions that the researcher holds about the nature of the social world and reality. These can be broadly classified as quantitative and qualitative approaches to research. Quantitative research is designed to test a hypothesis and generally involves evaluating or comparing interventions, particularly new ones, whereas qualitative research usually involves seeking to understand how interventions and relationships are experienced by patients and nurses (NPSA 2008).

RESEARCH AWARENESS, UTILISATION AND ACTIVITY

Research-based practice is arguably the hallmark of professional nursing and is essential for high quality clinical and cost-effective nursing care (ICN 2009). It is now more than 35 years since the Report of the Committee on Nursing (Committee on Nursing/Briggs report 1972) stressed the need for nursing to become research based to the extent that research should become part of the mental equipment of every practising nurse. Although considerable progress has been made in the intervening period, this objective still remains a challenge. For nursing to establish its research base, nurses need to develop an awareness of research in relation to practice, they need to be able to utilise research findings and some nurses need to undertake research activity.

Research awareness implies recognition of the importance of research to the profession and to patient care. It requires nurses to develop a critical and ques-

tioning approach to their work and in so doing identify problems or questions that can be answered through research. Nurses who are research aware will be able find out about the latest research in their area and have the ability to evaluate its relevance to practice. They will also be open to changing their practice when new knowledge becomes available. Research awareness implies a willingness to share the task of keeping abreast of new developments by sharing information with colleagues. It also entails supporting and co-operating with researchers in an informed way. Nurses need to understand the implications for patients that arise from research being undertaken in the clinical area in which they work. For example, nurses may need to provide care according to an agreed research protocol, and deviating from the protocol may jeopardise the research. However, they must ensure that the wellbeing of patients remains paramount and report promptly any concerns they may have about the research to more senior clinicians/managers as well as researchers. Arguably, all nurses should develop research awareness as part of pre-registration nurse education programmes and continue to develop their knowledge and skills following registration.

Research utilisation is concerned with incorporating research findings into practice so that care is based on research evidence. Not all research, even that which is published in reputable journals, is necessarily of high quality. Before findings can be applied a research study needs to be evaluated critically to judge the quality of the research. All nurses should be able to appraise a research report, although specialist advice may be needed to help judge the appropriateness of complex research designs or unusual statistical tests. Chapter 7 provides guidance on how to appraise research reports.

Research studies do not always provide conclusive findings that can be used to guide practice. Different studies examining the same phenomenon may produce contradictory results. Wherever possible a systematic review of a number of studies examining a particular phenomenon should be undertaken to provide more robust guidance for practice than the findings of a single study would allow. Chapter 24 outlines the procedures for undertaking a systematic review. It is a time-consuming process and requires a good understanding of research designs and methods together with knowledge of techniques for analysis, including statistical tests. Whereas some nurses may develop the skills to undertake a systematic review as part of a postgraduate course, many systematic reviews are undertaken by people who are experts in the technique. For example, the Centre for Reviews and Dissemination at the University of York has been set up specifically for the purpose of undertaking systematic reviews on a range of health-related topics.

The findings from a systematic review then need to be incorporated into clinical guidelines or care protocols that can be applied to practice. Whereas some guidelines may be developed at a national level, nurses may need to adapt national guidelines for application at a local level or develop their own guidelines where no national ones are available (see Chapters 38 and 39 for more information).

All nurses should be research aware and use research findings in their practice; however, not all nurses need to undertake research. To carry out rigorous research, nurses need to be equipped with appropriate knowledge and skills. Pre-registration and undergraduate post-registration nursing programmes tend to focus on developing research awareness and research utilisation. It is generally not until nurses embark on a master's programme or a specialist research course that they will learn how to undertake a small-scale research study under the supervision of a more experienced researcher. This represents the first step in acquiring the skills to become a competent researcher. Comparatively few nurses progress to develop a career in nursing research in which they undertake large-scale studies funded by external agencies. The ability to lead a large-scale study generally requires study at doctoral level, followed by an 'apprenticeship' working within a research team with supervision and support from experienced researchers. A recently published report on clinical academic careers for nurses provides a framework to enable nurses to develop their competence as researchers while still maintaining and developing their clinical role. The new clinical academic training pathway creates opportunities for nurses to progress from master's programmes in clinical research, through doctoral and post-doctoral clinical research opportunities with the ultimate aim of holding a senior clinical academic appointment between a university and an NHS trust (UKCRC 2007).

Although relatively few nurses progress to lead large research studies, many more nurses participate in research led by nurse researchers, doctors and other health professionals. Nurses working in clinical practice may be asked to undertake data collection for other researchers, and their clinical nursing experience can be valuable to the research enterprise. Even if they are not leading a study, nurses who assist other researchers should have a sound understanding of the research process in order to collect valid and reliable data and to adhere to the research governance and ethical requirements outlined in Chapter 10.

RESEARCH AND NURSING PRACTICE

Current policy initiatives seek to promote a culture of evidence-based practice. There are generally considered to be three components to evidence-based practice, namely the best available evidence derived from research, clinical expertise and patient preferences (Sackett *et al*. 1996). In recognising that knowledge derived from research is never absolute, nurses should draw on their own expertise and that of other more experienced nurses when deciding on an appropriate intervention. Equally, clinical expertise should not be seen as a substitute for research evidence, but rather as contributing to the decision about the most appropriate intervention for a particular patient. The third component of evidence-based practice involves taking account of patient perspectives. Nurses have a responsibility to share their knowledge of the best available evidence with patients to help them make informed choices about the care they receive. This is particularly important where there are alternative courses of action that can be selected. These issues are examined in more detail in Chapters 38 and 39.

Nursing's progress towards becoming evidence based needs to be viewed within the context of wider influences on healthcare. The UK (England, Northern Ireland, Scotland and Wales) governments are each seeking to modernise the NHS through major policy reforms. Central among these initiatives has been the introduction of the concept of clinical governance, a process whereby healthcare organisations are accountable for continually improving the quality of their services and safeguarding high standards of care by creating an environment that promotes excellence (Currie *et al.* 2003). It is, however, difficult to achieve the aspiration of 'excellence' in healthcare because of financial constraints and pressure on resources (Maynard 1999). Nevertheless, the objective of seeking to develop the quality of healthcare, together with recognition of the importance of healthcare organisations and the individuals who work in them being accountable for the quality of services, is laudable. Research is essential for making progress towards achieving this objective. As outlined earlier in this chapter, the knowledge generated through nursing research should be used to develop evidence-based practice, improve the quality of care and maximise health outcomes (ICN 2009).

In order to enhance the quality of nursing care it is important to ensure that care is clinically effective. Often referred to as 'doing the right thing right', clinical effectiveness involves providing the most appropriate intervention in the correct manner at the most expedient time, in order to achieve the best outcomes for the patient. Nurses need to draw on knowledge generated through research to decide which intervention is most appropriate and how and when to deliver it. Research may also highlight reasons for non-compliance. For example, a particular dressing may have been shown through research to be effective in promoting wound healing, but if it is unacceptable to the patient problems with compliance may arise.

As mentioned earlier, the findings from a single study may not provide sufficient evidence to direct practice, and wherever possible nurses should rely on knowledge generated through systematic reviews of research evidence drawn from several research studies. There are a number of national initiatives to assist nurses and other health professionals, to provide clinically effective care. These include the development of clinical guidelines based on the best research evidence by, for example, the National Institute for Health and Clinical Excellence (NICE) and the Scottish Intercollegiate Guideline Network (SIGN). In addition, the recently launched NHS Evidence portal provides healthcare professionals with access to a comprehensive evidence base to inform clinical practice. It is intended to provide a 'one-stop shop' for a range of information types, including primary research literature, practical implementation tools, guidelines and policy documents (see the list of websites at the end of the chapter).

Increasing demands on the finite resources within the NHS have resulted in the need to ensure that healthcare interventions are not only clinically effective but also cost-effective. There is little point pursuing a costly intervention if a cheaper one is seen to be equally as effective. The field of health economics is concerned with examining the financial and wider resource implications of providing a specific intervention or service. Economic evaluations can be undertaken to evaluate different treatments or alternative ways of providing services from an economic perspective and providing information that can be used to inform judgements about the clinical and cost-effectiveness of a particular intervention or service (Chambers & Boath 2001). NICE and SIGN guidelines take account of both clinical and cost-effectiveness when making recommendations for best practice.

CONCLUSIONS

Research is necessary to develop the knowledge base to inform nursing policy and practice. In an era of evidence-based practice, nurses are constantly challenged to identify new and better ways of delivering care that is grounded in knowledge derived from research (ICN 2009). They have a professional obligation to their patients and to wider society to provide care that is based on the best available evidence. Whereas relatively few nurses will develop a career in nursing research, all nurses should become research aware. This means developing a critical and questioning approach in order to identify areas where practice could be improved on the basis of research findings or areas where research evidence is lacking and new knowledge needs to be generated through research. Nurses also need to utilise research findings in their day-to-day practice. However, in order to provide evidence-based care nurses need to be able to evaluate the quality of published research reports. This requires a sound understanding of the research process, together with knowledge of different research designs and the methods that can be used to collect and analyse data. The following chapters of this book examine the research process, designs and methods in detail in order to equip nurses with the knowledge base to critically appraise research reports and to engage in the process of undertaking research under the supervision of a more experienced researcher.

References

Chambers R, Boath E (2001) *Clinical Effectiveness and Clinical Governance Made Easy*, 2nd edition. Abingdon, Radcliffe Medical Press.

Clamp C, Gough S, Land L (2004) *Resources for Nursing Research: an annotated bibliography*, 4th edition. London, Sage.

Committee on Nursing (1972) *Report of the Committee on Nursing*. London, HMSO.

Crow R (1982) How nursing and the community can benefit from nursing research. *International Journal of Nursing Studies* **19**(1): 37–45.

Currie L, Morrell CJ, Scrivener R (2003) *Clinical Governance: an RCN resource guide*. London, Royal College of Nursing.

Department of Health (2008) *High Quality Care for All: NHS next stage review final report*. Cm. 7432. London, The Stationery Office.

Department of Health (2005) *Research Governance Framework for Health and Social Care*, 2nd edition. London, Department of Health.

Dingwall R (1977) *The Social Organisation of Health Visitor Training*. London, Croom Helm.

Garbett R, McCormack B (2002) A concept analysis of practice development. *Nursing Times Research* **7**(2): 87–100.

Gerrish K, Ashworth P, Lacey A, Bailey J (2008) Developing evidence-based practice: experiences of senior and junior clinical nurses. *Journal of Advanced Nursing* **62**: 62–73.

Gerrish K, Mawson S (2005) Research, audit, practice development and service evaluation: implications for research and clinical governance. *Practice Development in Health Care* **4**(1): 33–39.

Hockey L (1996) The nature and purpose of research. In: Cormack DFS (ed) *The Research Process in Nursing*, 3rd edition. London, Blackwell Science, pp 3–13.

Hockey L (1984) The nature and purpose of research. In: Cormack DFS (ed) *The Research Process in Nursing*, 1st edition. London, Blackwell Science, pp 1–10.

International Council of Nurses (2009) Nursing research: a tool kit. Geneva, International Council of Nurses. www.icn.ch/matters_research.htm (accessed July 2009).

Maynard A (1999) Clinical governance: the unavoidable economic challenges. *NT Research* **4**: 188–191.

National Health Service Executive (1996) *Promoting clinical effectiveness: a framework for action*. London, NHSE.

National League for Nursing (2008) *Research Priorities for Nursing Education*. New York, National League for Nursing. www.nln.org/research/priorities.htm (accessed July 2009).

National Patient Safety Agency (2008) *Defining Research*. London, National Patient Safety Agency.

Norton D, McLaren R, Exton-Smith A (1975) *An Investigation of Geriatric Nursing in Hospital*. London, Churchill Livingstone.

Sackett DL, Rosenburg WM, Muir Gray JA, Haynes RB, Richardson WS (1996) Evidence-based medicine: what it is and what it isn't. *British Medical Journal* **312**: 71–72.

Thompson DR (2000) An exploration of knowledge development in nursing – a personal perspective. *NT Research* **5**(5): 391–394.

UKCRC Subcommittee for Nurses in Clinical Research (Workforce) (2007) *Developing the Best Research Professionals. Qualified Graduate Nurses: recommendations for preparing and supporting clinical academic nurses of the future*. London, UKCRC.

Websites

www.evidence.nhs.uk – NHS Evidence website provides access to a comprehensive evidence base to inform clinical practice. It provides a 'one-stop shop' for a range of information types, including primary research literature, practical implementation tools, guidelines and policy documents.

www.nice.org.uk – National Institute for Health and Clinical Excellence (NICE) publishes recommendations on treatments and care using the best available evidence of clinical and cost-effectiveness.

www.rcn.org.uk/development/researchanddevelopment – RCN Research and Development Co-ordinating Centre website provides links to a range of resources to support nursing research and evidence-based practice.

www.sign.ac.uk – Scottish Intercollegiate Guidelines Network (SIGN) publishes national clinical guidelines containing recommendations for effective practice based on current evidence.

www.york.ac.uk/inst/crd – Centre for Reviews and Dissemination (CRD) undertakes and publishes reviews of research about the effects of interventions used in health and social care.

2 The Research Process

Anne Lacey

Key points

- The research process is a series of steps that need to be undertaken to carry out any piece of research.

- The precise stages of the research process, and the order in which they are undertaken, will vary depending on the nature of the research, but will always follow a systematic pattern from initial ideas through to dissemination and implementation.

- Rigour in research is essential if the work is to be trustworthy and free from bias.

INTRODUCTION

The process of undertaking research is essentially the same whether the subject matter of the research is pure science, medicine, history or nursing. The following rather expansive definition from Graziano and Raulin (2004) sums up the breadth of scope of the research process:

> 'Research is a systematic search for information, a process of inquiry. It can be carried out in libraries, laboratories, schoolrooms, hospitals, factories, in the pages of the Bible, on street corners, or in the wild watching a herd of elephants' (Graziano & Raulin 2004: 31)

In all cases the researcher must ascertain the extent of existing knowledge, define their own area of enquiry, collect data and analyse it, and draw conclusions. For the pure scientist, however, the research might take place in the context of a laboratory, where experimentation is relatively straightforward as the researcher is in control of the environment and can eliminate potential confounding factors that might invalidate the research. Unless using animals or human tissue, there are few ethical considerations to take into account.

For the student of nursing research, or any research in a social context, the process is complicated by practical and ethical constraints of working in the 'real world' (Robson 2002). There is no single, universally accepted way of carrying out research in the social world, but a plethora of different designs and methodologies ranging from phenomenology to randomised controlled trials, from epidemiology to action research. The range of approaches derives from different paradigms, or ways of seeing the world. However, all are valid ways of conducting research, provided the methodology used is appropriate for the research question and is applied in a rigorous, systematic fashion.

In this chapter the research process that is common to all nursing research will be explored, and subsequent chapters in Section 2 will look at each of the stages of research in more detail. Different methodologies or research designs are discussed in turn, and in detail, in Section 3.

Although the research process will be presented as a linear, sequential process, the stages are often revisited several times during the process. In qualitative research, in particular, it is likely that the 'stages' of the research process will be modified to take account of the emergent nature of the enterprise. Qualitative researchers sometimes find it difficult or even inappropriate to formulate a precise research question until they have begun to collect, and possibly even analyse, data.

However, it is helpful in the first instance to think through the entire research process in a systematic way. Many authors (Hek *et al.* 2006, Parahoo 2006, Moule & Goodman 2009) have described the research process, and each comes up with a different number of stages, but essentially they contain the same elements. Table 2.1 illustrates the process as it will be described in this chapter, and indicates the principal chapters in the book that deal with each stage. This chapter gives a brief overview of the various stages to enable readers to see the whole before looking at each stage in more detail.

DEVELOPING THE RESEARCH QUESTION

Most research questions begin with a 'hunch' or initial idea that is not precisely defined. The idea might arise from clinical practice, from professional discussion among colleagues, from an issue in the media, or from reading an article or book. Alternatively the question may be derived from a 'call for proposals' from a funding body that asks researchers to develop a proposal on a specific topic. Box 2.1 provides an example of such a call, in this case from the National Institute for Health Research Service Delivery and Organisation (SDO) Programme. The call is specifically about the research areas to be investigated, indicates the methods to be used, the funding available and timescale required. Full details are available from the SDO website, together with a standard application form and a deadline by which proposals have to be submitted.

But most nurse researchers begin with an initial idea that is not yet well defined. Let us consider how research questions might be developed, using some real examples from the nursing literature to illustrate our discussion (see Research Examples 2.1, 2.2 and 2.3).

Question 1

Perhaps a research team has a 'hunch' that the use of pelvic floor exercises might help women in the

Table 2.1 The research process

Stages in the research process	Chapters in this book
Developing the research question	2
Searching and evaluating the literature	6, 7
Choice of methodology, research design	11, 13–27
Preparing a research proposal	8
Gaining access to the data	10
Sampling	12
Pilot study	2
Data collection	28–33
Data analysis	34–36
Dissemination of the results	37
Implementation of research	38, 39

Box 2.1 SDO call Patient and carer-centred services/technology adoption

NIHR Service Delivery and Organisation programme

NHS
National Institute for Health Research

Call for Research Proposals

The NIHR Service Delivery and Organisation (SDO) programme improves health outcomes for people by: commissioning research evidence that improves practice in relation to the organisation and delivery of healthcare; and building research capability and capacity to carry out research amongst those who manage, organise and deliver services and to improve their understanding of the research literature and how to use research evidence.

Promising Innovations in Healthcare Delivery in the NHS
(Ref: EV2001)

The SDO programme is seeking innovations which are likely to have the following four characteristics:

▶ Promising innovations in healthcare delivery which have a substantial potential benefit and could be applied more widely in the NHS.

▶ Being piloted, tested or implemented in a number of healthcare organisations.

▶ Involving the application of ideas or technologies introduced or transferred from other countries, sectors or settings.

▶ Have not already been well explored and tested through research.

Application process
Applicants are asked to submit full proposals for the above call by **Thursday 5 November 2009 by 1pm**. Please note that applications received after this deadline will not be considered. Proposals will be considered by the NHS Evaluations Panel at its December meeting. The commissioning brief and application form are available on the NIHR SDO programme website at **www.sdo.nihr.ac.uk/ev2001**.
Please quote advert reference **HSJ06b**.

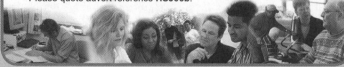

Reproduced by permission of the NIHR Service Delivery and Organisation programme Call EV2001. © Queen's Printer and Controller of HMSO 2009.

second stage of labour. This hunch is probably based on knowledge of the anatomy of the pelvic muscles and the process of delivery. It might also be supported by personal or professional experience of midwives. There are several ways in which the question could be developed. The following are examples of research questions derived from this area of interest.

2.1 A Quantitative Experimental Study

Salvesen KA, Morkved S (2004) Randomised controlled trial of pelvic floor muscle training during pregnancy. *British Medical Journal* **329**: 378–380.

This study used a quantitative experimental approach to assess the effectiveness of using a structured training programme of pelvic floor exercises in reducing time spent in the second stage of labour during childbirth. Researchers in Norway recruited 301 first-time mothers during pregnancy, and randomly allocated them to either a training group (who were given an exercise programme delivered by a physiotherapist) or a control group (who had normal care). Time spent in the second stage of labour was measured for the two groups. Results showed that women in the training group had a lower rate of prolonged second stage labour than women in the control group (25% compared to 33%).

2.2 A Quantitative Questionnaire Survey

Chevalier I, Benoit G, Gauthier M, Phan V, Bonnin A, Lebel M (2008) Antibiotic prophylaxis for childhood urinary tract infection: a national survey. *Journal of Paediatrics and Child Health* **44**: 572–578.

A national survey of Canadian paediatricians was conducted to assess their practice in prescribing prophylactic antibiotics for children with urinary tract infections, with and without vesicoureteral reflux. A self-completion questionnaire was mailed to a sample of 1136 paediatricians and 42 paediatric nephrologists. A response rate of 58.1% was obtained. Although a majority of respondents prescribed prophylaxis for children with reflux, only 15% felt that this practice was evidence based. A quarter of respondents also prescribed prophylaxis for children under one year with a first febrile urinary tract infection without evidence of reflux. Again, only 19% felt that this practice was evidence based. The overall conclusion was that practice in this area varies widely in Canada because of a lack of solid evidence about prophylaxis.

2.3 A Qualitative Study

Hasson F, Kernohan W, Waldron M, Whittaker E, McLaughlin D (2008) The palliative care link nurse role in nursing homes: barriers and facilitators. *Journal of Advanced Nursing* **64**: 233–242.

This descriptive qualitative study explored the views and experiences of link nurses for palliative care working in nursing homes in Northern Ireland. A purposive sample of 14 link nurses from 10 nursing homes was selected and interviewed using focus groups. Data from the focus groups were recorded, transcribed and analysed. Link nurses identified a number of barriers to their role as educators and facilitators of palliative care, including lack of management support, a transient workforce and lack of adequate preparation for the role. Facilitators included external support, peer support and access to a resource file. The researchers concluded that the link nurse role had considerable potential to improve care in this area, but managers needed to be aware of the sustained support needed for the role, and more work needs to be done to find ways of developing the role further.

Q1(a) Are pelvic floor exercises taught to women during antenatal classes?

Q1(b) Do pregnant women understand what pelvic floor exercises are, and are they willing to learn the skills of doing them?

Q1(c) Does the use of pelvic floor exercises reduce the length of labour?

Obviously, each of these research questions will give us very different kinds of information and will require different research methods to be employed. They would also need to be refined further – the precise pelvic floor exercises to be taught needs to be clarified, for example, and the stage of pregnancy at which they are taught needs to be defined. Q1(b) suggests the need to measure understanding and willingness to learn – neither of these concepts is straightforward and tools to measure them would need to be developed. Perhaps a qualitative study needs to be undertaken to explore the concepts first. Research Example 2.1 (Salveson & Morkved 2004) describes an experimental study related to Q1(c). In this case the outcome measure was defined as time taken in second stage of labour, and only first-time mothers were recruited to the study.

Question 2

Alternatively, a research team might be interested in the evidence base used by doctors in their prescribing practice. Overuse of antibiotics in children, for instance, is known to cause problems with the development of drug resistance, and it is important that clinical practice is based on sound clinical evidence. Again, a number of research questions could be asked.

Q2(a) How reliable is the research evidence about prophylactic antibiotic prescription in children with urinary disease?

Q2(b) How effective are prophylactic antibiotics in preventing urinary tract infections in children at risk?

Q2(c) What is the prescribing practice of paediatric doctors regarding antibiotic prophylaxis?

Again, these three questions lead to very different types of study, and again, each question needs further clarification and refinement. What is meant by 'urinary disease'? How do we decide that research evidence is reliable? What age children are concerned? Which children are 'at risk'? Research Example 2.2 (Chevalier *et al.* 2008) is an example of a survey to answer Q2(c), but it was undertaken with a specific group of paediatric doctors in Canada. Is it appropriate to apply the answers gained from this study to doctors in Europe or China?

Question 3

In our last example, research questions might be generated concerning the best way to deliver palliative care in nursing homes. This setting is known to be a common one in which palliative care is delivered, but formal training and facilities are not always available. Three questions could be constructed to investigate this.

Q3(a) Is patient satisfaction with palliative care delivered in nursing homes lower or higher than that delivered in a hospital setting?

Q3(b) What is the level of knowledge about palliative care among nurses working in nursing homes?

Q3(c) What is the experience of link nurses for palliative care working in nursing homes?

Before setting out with any of these questions the researcher would need to be clear how 'nursing home' was to be defined, and for Q3(b) a validated tool to measure knowledge would need to be available. Q3(a) suggests a comparative survey of samples of nursing homes and hospitals, but would the underlying question be answered by asking patients' views alone? Palliative care is needed up to and after the point of death, and so it might be necessary to extend the survey to satisfaction of next of kin, who can give a full picture of care given. Q3(c) suggests a research design that needs a more in-depth approach, and the answer will be contained in words rather than numbers – Research Example 2.3 (Hasson *et al.* 2008) describes a study to answer this question using a qualitative approach.

USING A HYPOTHESIS

A hypothesis is a statement that can be tested, and is used mostly in experimental research. Qualitative designs and surveys do not usually have a hypothesis, although sometimes surveys do test for differences between groups and so might use one. Statistics are required to test the hypothesis, which has to be very precisely written. The hypothesis expresses the predicted outcome of the experiment, either in positive or negative terms. As an example, Q2(b) above could be answered by testing a hypothesis, which would be something like the following.

Children under five years of age with reflux given prophylactic antibiotics will experience fewer episodes of urinary tract infection in one year than children with reflux not given prophylactic antibiotics.

The hypothesis might even express the magnitude of the expected difference – in this case, it might be predicted that children given antibiotics will experience, on average, at least 50% fewer infections than those not given antibiotics. But for the purpose of statistical testing, the hypothesis is more often expressed in negative terms, or as a null hypothesis, such as the following example.

Children under five years of age with reflux given prophylactic antibiotics will experience the same number of urinary tract infections in one year as those not given prophylactic antibiotics.

In this case, the experiment would aim to find the null hypothesis false, assuming that prophylactic antibiotics are effective in such cases. Chapter 36 gives more information about how such hypotheses are tested for statistical significance.

SEARCHING AND EVALUATING THE LITERATURE

The next stage is to find out what evidence already exists in the chosen research area. It is a waste of time and money to conduct research where the answer to the question is already known. What is already known about a subject can be found from a variety of sources. Books may be a starting point, but quickly become out of date if the subject matter is topical. Academic journals are a better place to start, and access to online databases such as CINAHL (Cumulative Index of Nursing and Allied Health Literature; see Chapter 6 for more details) make this task speedy and relatively simple. If anything, the problem is that there will be too much information, and Chapter 6 discusses how to refine the search. Beyond written sources, evidence may be found on the internet and various online resources. As well as locating the evidence, it must be appraised and evaluated. Not all that is written is of good quality, and evidence from one country or in one population may not necessarily generalise to other cultures or situations. Chapters 6 and 7 of this book discuss this stage in considerable detail.

Sometimes the research process may consist entirely of a review of the literature. A well-designed systematic review is an accepted research approach in its own right, systematically searching out and evaluating all the research that has been published on a particular topic. In an increasingly complex and fragmented world of information it is important to develop an evidence base that is well validated, and on which practice can be based. Q2(a) above would suggest the need for a systematic literature review, and Chapter 24 deals with this specialised form of research. Research Example 2.4 gives an example of a systematic review.

Most of the questions in the examples above would require a literature review before being able to refine the question further. It might be, for example, that a study has already been conducted testing the effectiveness of pelvic floor exercises in first-time mothers, and found them to be ineffective in reducing time taken in second stage. But can this be applied to women having their second or subsequent child? And can a study conducted in, say, the USA be applied in the UK? A literature search on palliative care in nursing homes might show that nurses in this setting have very low levels of knowledge or interest in palliative care. But the studies are few, out of date and somewhat contradictory. Is it justifiable to conduct a further piece of research in the area?

Q RESEARCH EXAMPLE

2.4 Systematic Review

Frasure J (2008) Analysis of instruments measuring nurses' attitudes towards research utilization: a systematic review. *Journal of Advanced Nursing* **61**: 5–8.

This research study used established methods of systematic review to assess instruments that have been developed to measure nurses' attitudes towards research utilisation. Four electronic databases were searched for relevant articles published during the period 1982 to 2007, and 186 sources were identified. Of these, 25 met the criteria for review, but only 14 were developed with sound psychometric properties. Only one, that by Estabrooks, was found to have been rigorously tested. This instrument was recommended for use, but further work was suggested to develop this area of research.

CHOICE OF METHODOLOGY, RESEARCH DESIGN

The majority of this book (Section 3) is devoted to a description of different research designs. In many ways, the choice of research design is the most important stage of the research process, for it affects all the others. Some questions are more appropriate for an experimental approach; others are entirely suited to an in-depth ethnographic study. Researchers often make explicit a *conceptual framework* within which they are working, which will determine the overall research approach. A conceptual framework makes clear the researcher's 'world view' – their assumptions and preconceptions about the subject under consideration. In Question 1 above, for example, the researchers may have a conceptual framework that emphasises womens' right to autonomy in decisions and policies relating to labour. Consequently any research study would be concerned with gathering the experiences and feelings of women about their labour, rather than purely objective clinical data. The kind of data collected, the types of analysis that are possible and the way in which the results can be applied to practice will all depend on the research design.

Some research designs are *quantitative*. This means they ultimately collect numerical data and are amenable to statistical analysis. Such research designs may or may not have a hypothesis, but experimental studies always require such a statement to be tested statistically. Research Example 2.1 (Salvesen & Morkved 2004) and Research Example 2.2 (Chevalier *et al.* 2008) both describe quantitative studies. Quantitative designs may be experimental, such as Salveson and Morkved's design, but may also be observational, such as Chevalier *et al.*'s survey using a questionnaire. In the latter, structured answers such as ticked boxes enable the data to be coded and translated into numerical form. Surveys may also use medical records or laboratory tests as their data source to estimate the numbers of patients in a community who have measles, for example. Epidemiological studies of the incidence and distribution of diseases also use quantitative methods.

Other research designs are *qualitative*. These designs use narrative, words, documents or graphical material as their data source, and analyse material to identify themes, relationships, concepts and, in some cases, to develop theory. Such research approaches explore an experience, culture or situation in depth, taking account of context and complexity. Qualitative designs may be used where comparatively little is known about a subject, so no hypothesis can be formulated. The purpose is exploratory rather than explanatory, although qualitative studies may certainly contribute much to our understanding of phenomena and many also develop theory. An example of a qualitative study is given in Research Example 2.3 (Hasson *et al.* 2008).

Both approaches are valid ways of advancing nursing knowledge. A quantitative study may be very good at finding out the extent of compliance with diabetic therapy, for instance, by measuring levels of the blood glucose in a sample of diabetic patients. A qualitative study, on the other hand, may tell us why it is that certain diabetic patients do not take their insulin as prescribed, by observing and talking to them, and gaining understanding of the context in which the insulin is (or is not) taken.

More than this, qualitative and quantitative methodologies are based on different philosophical assumptions and derive from different historical traditions. Chapter 11 discusses these issues in much more detail, and the reader is encouraged to get to grips with this academic debate. Nursing needs to embrace all research methodologies in order to engage with the breadth of questions that need to be asked. Ours is a discipline drawing on many different traditions of academic enquiry.

The research design (or *methodology*) is distinct from the *methods* used for data collection. A single data collection method, for example interview or observation, may be used for many different research designs.

So we can return to our hypothetical questions generated in questions 1–3 above, and consider the research methodology that might be appropriate to answer each one. In the example relating to pelvic floor exercises for pregnant women, Q1(a) and Q1(b) are both essentially asking for information that can be gathered in a quantitative survey, but Q1(a) might also be answered by observation of antenatal classes, or examination of the women's records. Q1(c) will require an experimental design to compare outcomes in two groups (Research Example 2.1). With regard to a potential study examining the prescribing of prophylactic antibiotics, Q2(a) suggests a literature review as described above, but Q2(b) would require a rigorous experimental design to answer the question about effectiveness. Q2(c) requires a survey, as described in Research Example 2.2. Finally, in relation to examining the best way to deliver palliative care in nursing homes, Q3(a) and Q3(b) both suggest a quantitative survey design, but Q3(a) will require a comparative survey, measuring satisfaction in the two types of care setting. It might also be answered using qualitative methods, asking in-depth questions of palliative care patients and their relatives in two

types of setting. Indeed, this question might require mixed methods, as discussed in Chapter 27. Q3(c) certainly needs a qualitative approach (Research Example 2.3).

PREPARING A RESEARCH PROPOSAL

Whether a large-scale, multi-centre study costing many thousands of pounds or a small, unfunded study for an educational degree is planned, a formal research proposal is likely to be needed.

Such a proposal is a written statement of *what* the researcher intends to do, *why*, *how*, *when* and, often, *how much it will cost*. It is used to gain approval for the research, secure funding if it is required, and then to guide the research process during its execution. It will often be modified in the light of pilot studies or practical difficulties, but it is important that the detailed intentions are clear at the outset. It has been said that if you don't know where you are going you are unlikely to get there!

Chapter 8 sets out the content of a research proposal in detail, but the precise form of the proposal will vary according to the nature of the research and the purpose of the written proposal. A proposal written in response to a funding call from the National Institute of Health Research or the Medical Research Council is likely to be a substantial document of many pages, written by a team of experienced researchers. One written for the purpose of outlining a small study for a master's degree may be only a few pages, written by the postgraduate student themself with some guidance from their supervisor.

Whatever the context, however, the proposal will certainly include a section on each of the stages of the research process outlined in Table 2.1. It will also include a section detailing the ethical issues raised by the research, and how the researcher will ensure that confidentiality, informed consent and other ethical principles are respected. Chapter 3 discusses these issues in more detail. It is usual to include a table or Gantt chart showing the timescale of the project. Table 2.2 shows such a chart for a complex evaluation study involving a survey, documentary analysis, case studies and focus groups. It is also helpful to

Table 2.2 Example of a Gantt chart for a mixed method piece of research

Timetable	Year One July 2008 – June 2009						Year Two July 2009 – June 2010					
Months of evaluation	2	4	6	8	10	12	14	16	18	20	22	24
Key tasks:												
1. Baseline survey												
Development of survey instrument	■											
Baseline survey data collection		■										
Baseline survey data analysis		■										
2. Analysis of routine activity data and resource used data												
Activity and resource use data collection (after 1 year and after 2 years)				■						■		
Data analysis					■	■				■		
3. Case studies												
Pilot case study				■								
Case study data collection					■	■	■	■	■			
Case study analysis												
4. Focus groups												
Focus groups with project co-ordinators at pre-arranged workshops × 2				■								
Transcription and analysis of focus groups					■	■						
Dissemination												
Interim report to Regional Advisory Group						■						
Feedback to project sites, dissemination and writing of final report for Regional Advisory Group										■	■	■

identify milestones, stating the date by which each stage of the research will be completed, though this is obviously subject to change as the inevitable obstacles and delays come into play. It is customary to include a breakdown of resources required and a justification of why they are needed.

Clearly, the research proposal cannot be written until the researcher has thought through all the stages of the research process in some detail. However, the proposal is of necessity one of the early stages in the process, as it is impossible to proceed without one.

GAINING ACCESS TO THE DATA

Because of the sensitivity of much of the research that takes place in healthcare, and the vulnerability of many of its subjects, a complex system of governance has been developed in the UK to ensure all research is approved for its ethical soundness, scientific quality and legal propriety. NHS trusts are also concerned to ensure that all research that takes place within the trust is properly funded and insured against liability. A system of ethical regulation via the National Research Ethics Service (www.nres.npsa.nhs.uk/) is in place, and all applicants carrying out research in healthcare must follow this system. In addition, since 2001 a system of research governance has been developed to guard against research that has not been properly scrutinised and approved, after various high-profile scandals concerning NHS research (Department of Health 2005).

Chapter 10 deals with this topic in depth. Suffice to say at this stage that the system is necessary, but rather bureaucratic and time-consuming. Depending on arrangements at each local trust, it is likely to take anything from 4 to 20 weeks from completing a research proposal to having all the required permissions in place to begin data collection (Gerrish & Guillaume 2006).

In addition to formal permission, however, access to the data may require negotiation of a more informal nature with local personnel who act as 'gate-keepers'. If access to patients or their records is needed, for example, it may be necessary to gain the co-operation of the appropriate consultant, practice manager or audit department in addition to ethical and research governance committees. Access to a nursing home or school will require the permission of the appropriate senior manager. Chapter 10 also deals in more depth with this informal process of negotiating access.

SAMPLING

Once the research begins, the first stage is likely to be selecting the sample. Unless it is a complete census, researchers collect data from a selected group, rather than an entire population. In our earlier examples, samples might be taken from antenatal class attenders, nursing homes in a particular region of the country, consultants in paediatric medicine or relatives of patients requiring palliative care. How are the samples to be selected, and how many is enough? These questions are dealt with in detail in Chapter 12, but the answers are rarely simple, particularly about sample size.

A quantitative study involving a comparison between two groups is likely to require a *power calculation*, a statistical technique to estimate minimum sample size. This is comforting to the researcher as it gives a scientific answer to the question, but is also based on various assumptions and decisions that any statistician making the calculation will ask the researcher to make. In qualitative research samples tend to be smaller, but again there is no hard and fast rule as to how big they must be. Data saturation, or achieving the stage where no new information is being revealed by additional data collection, may be the stated goal, but it is impossible to predict beforehand when that stage may be reached.

As to the method of selection of the sample, there is a range of well-developed methods to choose from (see Chapter 12). The type of sampling will depend on the research design. Random sampling, and its variants, is the method of choice in traditional survey research, whereas theoretical sampling may be more appropriate for grounded theory. Whatever approach is adopted, it is essential for the validity of the research that the sample is chosen in a rigorous way, and sampling techniques adopted are adhered to closely.

The size and selection of the sample will have an effect on the timescale and cost of the research. Usually, the cost increases with sample size, although this is less significant for, say, a postal survey than for a randomised controlled trial. Similarly, in-depth interviewing and subsequent transcription of tape recordings is resource-intensive, and each increase in sample size will require significant extra resources. A realistic assessment of how quickly a particular sample size can be obtained is necessary before embarking on a piece of research – all too often patients with the relevant condition seem to disappear as soon as a research study starts recruiting.

PILOT STUDY

It is always advisable to conduct a pilot study before embarking on the research. This may take the form of a 'dummy run' to see if the whole recruitment process works, or may simply involve testing out a data collection instrument. Questionnaires are usually piloted on a small sample of people with similar characteristics to those in the full study, to pick up questions that are misinterpreted or items that are frequently missed out. Modifications can then be made to the questionnaire before large numbers are printed and money wasted. If interviews are to be used, a wise researcher will conduct one or two pilot interviews to test out the interview schedule, ensure technical equipment (such as a tape recorder) works satisfactorily and assess how long the interview is likely to take. Data collected in a pilot study is not usually included with the main results, but may be reported separately and even published if the pilot study is a substantial one.

DATA COLLECTION

A wide range of data collection techniques and methods is available, and Chapters 28 to 33 describe the commonest of these. Nursing research relies heavily on interviews, focus groups and question-naires as methods of choice, but observation, clinical measurement and the use of documents as data are also appropriate methods to be considered. In our earlier Research Examples data collection methods would include clinical observations and documents (length of second stage of labour), questionnaires (prescribing practice of doctors) and focus groups (experience of palliative care link nurses). The stage of data collection is, in many ways, the most straight-forward and rewarding stage of research. It frequently involves interaction with patients, the public or other research participants after a long stage of filling in forms and writing research proposals. At last, the researcher gets to ask the questions they started out with.

Data collection tools will usually have been selected at the research proposal stage. Ethical and research governance committees like to see the intended instruments, or at least to have a draft of an interview schedule or questionnaire. The instruments will need to be refined and developed ready for use, however, and practicalities of how the data will be collected, by whom and when are often done as data collection begins.

It is at this stage that the researcher needs to keep tight control over the data collection process. Failure to keep index numbers on documents, or to record the time of a clinical observation, can render data collected useless. It is also important to consider who should be involved in data collection. Using our earlier example, in Question 1 it might be unwise to use the physiotherapist who taught the pelvic floor exercises to collect the data, as they might feel some conscious or unconscious interest in showing that their teaching was effective.

All data collected needs secure storage, whether this is in hard copy (paper records or audiovisual material) or electronic form. Paper copies and tapes need to be locked in a cabinet or drawer to preserve confidentiality, and electronic records need to be stored on a secure computer and backed up on a sepa-rate disk or server. Many researchers will preserve both paper and electronic records, as either can be destroyed or corrupted by unexpected events such as fire, theft or computer breakdown.

DATA ANALYSIS

This is perhaps the most crucial phase of any research project. Once data are collected, they need to be assembled and organised in such a way that conclu-sions can be drawn from them. A huge spreadsheet of numbers or multiple pages of narrative cannot be disseminated to others or used in practice until some analysis has taken place. It is also the phase that is most demanding from an intellectual point of view. Whether using qualitative or quantitative methods, data analysis is hard work. Contrary to many people's expectations, computer software analysis packages such as NVivo (for qualitative analysis) and SPSS (for quantitative analysis) do not do the analysis, they simply provide practical tools to manage the data more easily. The researcher still has to manage and guide the process, and do some serious thinking about the meaning of the data.

If the data collected are qualitative, data analysis techniques such as those described in Chapter 34 can be used. The exact methods used will vary according to the qualitative methodology adopted. In practice, there are few universally accepted methods of analys-ing qualitative data, but the researcher must make the process 'transparent' by describing in detail how the results were derived.

Quantitative data are usually analysed statistically, and Chapters 35 and 36 provide guidance on the standard techniques available. With anything other than a small project, a quantitative piece of research should include a statistician in the research team, or at least be able to access professional statistical advice.

Some research projects use 'mixed methods' that include both qualitative and quantitative approaches. Here, the analysis may attempt to combine the two sets of results, perhaps using the qualitative data to provide interpretation of the quantitative results. See Chapter 27 for more on this issue.

DISSEMINATION OF THE RESULTS

Of course there is little point in conducting any research if the results are never made known to anybody except the researcher. Dissemination can take many forms. At the local level, research can be presented to colleagues at team or unit meetings, or as a more formal seminar to local professionals who may be interested. The study in Research Example 2.1 about pelvic floor exercises might be of interest to pregnant mothers, consultant obstetricians, general practitioners and physiotherapists, as well as to midwives themselves. Many nurses have access to a specialist group of health professionals in their discipline at local or national level, and this is also a suitable forum in which to disseminate the results of small- or large-scale research.

The increasing use of the internet has provided opportunities for researchers to post details of their research on a website, perhaps hosted by an NHS trust or university. This ensures that research results are widely and freely available, but, like most online resources, provides no guarantee of quality. Increasingly, however, information is being disseminated via the web, and online discussion groups are also enabling informal exchange of ideas.

Publication in written form, in academic and professional journals, remains the most widely accepted method of dissemination of research, but presentation of results at conferences, by oral presentation or by poster, is also common. All of these media enable fellow researchers and practitioners to discuss the results and provide some feedback about the useful-

ness of the research, and possible avenues for further studies. Chapter 37 discusses methods of dissemination more thoroughly.

IMPLEMENTATION OF THE RESULTS

This topic is dealt with in depth in Chapters 38 and 39. Needless to say, the purpose of nursing research is to improve practice in some way, whether by direct application of the results of a trial, by better informing practitioners of the culture in which they are working, or by evaluating the effects of an innovation. While it is not the direct responsibility of the research community to ensure implementation of the findings of research, it is incumbent on researchers to ensure that their findings are being shared with those who implement nursing policy and engage in clinical practice. This implies that research findings should be published in places where practitioners, managers and policy makers will read them, and taken to professional as well as academic conferences. The findings from the study in Research Example 2.3, for example, will not be implemented unless they reach the managers and owners of nursing homes, who may not attend the research conferences or read the academic journals where the results are first presented.

ENSURING RIGOUR

Rigour refers to the strength of the research design in terms of ensuring that all procedures have been followed scrupulously, that all possible confounding factors have been eliminated and that the user can be confident that the conclusions are dependable. Of course, this is always a relative concept; social research can very rarely be said to have eliminated all possible sources of error, but the quality of the research will be judged by the extent to which this has been done.

There are two key concepts that concern the quality of research: validity and reliability. *Validity* concerns the extent to which the research measures what it purports to measure without bias or distortion. A study to assess the health effects of air pollution in a community would not be valid if it simply collected people's views about the air quality, without measuring actual levels of disease or even mortality rates. In the study in Research Example 2.1, validity would be reduced if the pelvic floor exercises were taught poorly or if some women were given additional written materials while others were not. Validity would also be affected by the representativeness of the sample chosen – if this included only well-educated, middle-class women from the UK, for example, it would not be valid to apply the results to a mixed community living in Brazil.

Reliability refers to the consistency of measurement within a study. A set of weighing scales that gave a person's weight as 52kg at 10am and 55kg at 10.05am could not be said to be reliable. Repeated measurement is the usual test of reliability, and can be done by second administration of a questionnaire under similar conditions, or by two researchers making the same set of observations and comparing results. Data collection tools such as quality-of-life scales are extensively tested for reliability before being used as a standard measure in research studies. Unreliable measurement tools will always mean that the validity of a research study is compromised, as confidence in the quality of data collection is reduced. A study might use perfectly reliable instruments, however, and still not be valid. Meticulous collection of body mass index of patients in primary care, for example, will not generate a valid measure of the prevalence of diabetes in the practice, though the two may be related. In the study in Research Example 2.2, a poorly designed questionnaire which gave ambiguous answers or low completion rates would have made the results unreliable.

Some qualitative researchers reject the terms validity and reliability because of their association with the quantitative research tradition, and the assumption implicit in their definition that research can be entirely objective and free from bias (Holloway & Wheeler 2002). Such researchers may prefer to use concepts such as credibility, trustworthiness and transparency to describe the quality of the research, but the underlying concept of rigour and the use of a systematic approach remains the same. Chapters 11, 13, 14 and 15 will discuss these issues further.

CONCLUSIONS

The research process outlined in this chapter will be adapted according to the research design, the scale of the undertaking, resources available and the context in which the research is conducted. However, all research needs to be systematic and rigorous in its approach. This chapter began by discussing the relative complexity of conducting research in a social, rather than laboratory, context. Robson (2002) sums up the situation with characteristic frankness.

> 'One of the challenges inherent in carrying out investigations in the "real world" lies in seeking to say something sensible about a complex, relatively poorly controlled and generally "messy" situation' (Robson 2002: 4)

One of the particular complexities is the need to conduct research that involves people according to ethical principles, and this requirement frequently impinges on the design and conduct of the research process. This question is addressed in the next chapter.

References

Chevalier I, Benoit G, Gauthier M, Phan V, Bonnin A, Lebel M (2008) Antibiotic prophylaxis for childhood urinary tract infection: a national survey. *Journal of Paediatrics and Child Health* **44**: 572–578.

Department of Health (2005) *Research Governance Framework for Health and Social Care*. London, Department of Health.

Frasure J (2008) Analysis of instruments measuring nurses' attitudes towards research utilization: a systematic review. *Journal of Advanced Nursing* **61**: 5–8.

Gerrish K, Guillaume L (2006) Whither survey research: the challenges of undertaking postal surveys within the UK research governance framework. *Journal of Nursing Research* **11**(6): 485–49.

Graziano AM, Raulin ML (2004) *Research Methods: a process of inquiry*, 5th edition. Boston, Pearson.

Hasson F, Kernohan W, Waldron M, Whittaker E, McLaughlin D (2008) The palliative care link nurse role in nursing homes: barriers and facilitators. *Journal of Advanced Nursing* **64**(3): 233–242.

Hek G, Judd, M, Moule P (2006) *Making Sense of Research: an introduction for health and social care practitioners*, 3rd edition. London, Sage.

Holloway I, Wheeler S (2002) *Qualitative Research in Nursing*, 2nd edition. Oxford, Blackwell.

Moule P, Goodman M (2009) *Nursing Research: an introduction*. London, Sage.

Parahoo K (2006) *Nursing Research: principles, process and methods*, 2nd edition. Basingstoke, Macmillan.

Robson C (2002) *Real World Research: a resource for social scientists and practitioner-researchers*, 2nd edition. Oxford, Blackwell.

Salvesen KA, Morkved S (2004) Randomised controlled trial of pelvic floor muscle training during pregnancy. *British Medical Journal* **329**: 378–380.

Websites

www.dh.gov.uk/en/Researchanddevelopment/index.htm – Department of Health section on research and development, where you can find information about research funding, ethical approval and research governance.

www.nres.npsa.nhs.uk – National Research Ethics Service gives full information about the system of ethical regulation for the NHS and social care research.

www.rdinfo.org.uk – R&D info 'Support and Help' section gives information about the research process, writing research proposals and getting approval.

3 Research Ethics

Martin Johnson and Tony Long

Key points

- The main ethical issues that require attention when planning and conducting research include the importance of respecting participants, responding to the needs of vulnerable individuals and groups, gaining consent and maintaining confidentiality.

- Strategies for conducting ethical research include balancing the potential disadvantages of participation in the research with the likely benefit to participants, minimising the risk of harm to participants and the formal ethical scrutiny of research proposals.

- When evaluating a research report consideration needs to given to the ethical conduct of the study.

THE IMPORTANCE OF ETHICS IN RESEARCH

Early nurse researchers paid scant attention to ethics as such. Nurses were assumed to be professionals with integrity and a vocation in which putting patients' interests before their own could be assumed. Even from these times, however, researchers were confronting moral dilemmas and sometimes used methods which, when made public, were seen to have infringed human rights and possibly caused harm.

More recently, because of increasing public concern that not all health professionals have behaved with complete integrity, procedures to assure ethical probity of research programmes have become increasingly rigorous, some might even say tiresome (Howarth & Kneafsey 2003, 2005). Chapter 10 examines these procedures in some detail. Arguments

regarding the adequacy and appropriateness of some approaches are provided by Long and Fallon (2007), while examples of studies where the ethical issues are controversial are considered elsewhere (Johnson 2004).

In this chapter we aim to introduce basic issues that researchers need to think about when designing their studies. We will suggest that while it is essential to keep the core principle of respect for individuals firmly in mind, it will also be necessary in most cases to focus carefully on balancing potential disadvantages of participating in the research study with the likely benefits for participants. The chapter has two main parts: issues that require the researcher's attention, and strategies that may be employed to deal adequately and ethically with these issues. This chapter can present only a brief introduction to the key ideas and a wide range of resources are available, some of which we refer to here. We have dealt with most of the issues and some of their solutions at much greater length and with more concrete examples elsewhere (Long & Johnson 2007).

ISSUES FOR RESEARCHERS TO ADDRESS

Respect for participants

This key principle is based on the belief that every individual matters and has the right to be treated with respect. Most adults are autonomous: that is, they have the mental ability to deliberate about issues that affect them and to make decisions (however wise, foolish or capricious) for themselves. Respecting the individual implies respecting their decisions. Many factors may conspire to limit the autonomy of an individual.

Adequate information on which to base choices

Many decisions in life would be flawed if vital pieces of relevant information were not available – or even deliberately withheld. A constant concern for researchers in healthcare is how much information to give people (particularly about unlikely risks) without worrying them unduly. However, the key aspects of participation should be made clear to potential recruits for them to make an informed choice, together with at least the most important risks in terms of likelihood of occurrence or extent of potential impact.

Understanding and evaluating the issues involved

While most adults (and, indeed, many children) are able to understand a sufficient depth of information or detail to allow for rational decision making, this is not the case for all. It is possible for this ability to be temporarily or permanently lost through illness, trauma, or degenerative processes of ageing or disease. Under normal circumstances, potential participants need to know what harm, if any, might result. However, in circumstances where this is simply not possible, and when the research results might be important, different approaches may need to be adopted (see Research Example 3.1).

Perceived or actual coercion

Health professionals generally accept a role in persuading their patients to do what they consider to be good for them. Nurses regularly encourage and cajole people to mobilise after surgery, to take medication and to abstain from harmful behaviours. Coercion, however, involves using 'undue' pressure or leverage to engage compliance. In practice, the distinction is often blurred, particularly in circumstances of increased vulnerability of the patient, when the consequences of a poor choice are potentially disastrous or at times when staff are under strain. These pressures are easily transferred to the research arena, too.

Freedom from undue social restriction

While the individual's ability to make decisions may be compromised by severe intellectual disability resulting, for example, from dementia or head injury, it may also be limited by the social diminution of status which is inherent in the stereotyping and stigmatisation of some forms of illness or disability (Johnson 1997). Health researchers therefore need to be aware that personal autonomy can become limited for both pathological and social reasons, rendering the individual more vulnerable and less autonomous.

Vulnerable individuals and groups

Every recipient of healthcare is in some way vulnerable, but those with more limited ability to act autonomously can also be more vulnerable to the impact of research activity. For example, those whose first language is not English, notably some members of minority ethnic communities, can find it difficult to make their preferences known or to understand the issues (RCN 2007). Similar difficulties may attach to other individuals, such as some deaf people who use only sign language (whether using English or some other language in the written form).

Most young children are self-evidently vulnerable. In light of several scandals in which the poor standard of care of children has led to their deaths, great prominence has been given to safeguarding children, and responsibility has been passed to OFSTED *'to ensure*

RESEARCH EXAMPLE

3.1 Practical Ethics

Lawton J (2000) *The Dying Process: patients' experiences of palliative care*. London, Routledge.

Julia Lawton used open participant observation to avoid long and possibly exhausting interviews with dying people in a hospice. In this edited extract from her excellent book she illustrates how, while attempting to get consent, wherever possible, she had to be practical.

'Formal interviews not only seemed to be too obtrusive to many patients and their families; in a substantial number of cases they were simply not viable. Some patients, for example, were heavily sedated during their stay in the hospice, whilst others experienced changes in their mental state, such as becoming very paranoid or confused. It was, of course, impossible to interview a patient in a coma.

I worked as an "in-house" volunteer within the hospice because this particular role enabled me to have substantial and regular contact with patients and their visitors in the wards, side rooms and other communal areas within the building ...

I often found that performing a practical task, such as making a bed, gave me an ideal excuse to enter a ward and make observations in situations when it might have been too awkward and obtrusive to have a researcher present; for instance, when one of the patients had just died ...

Whenever possible, patients were informed by staff about my research and given the option of "opting out" of any observations I made. In cases where a patient was admitted in a coma, or was suffering from confusion, the consent of his or her relatives was obtained instead.'

(Lawton, 2000: 30–31)

---

that services for children, young people and their families whose circumstances make them vulnerable ... are as good as possible' (OFSTED 2008). However, continued failures mean that concern for the safety and wellbeing of children and young people must remain high on the agenda of all professionals, including researchers. The ability to act and decide autonomously develops with maturity, but even very young children of primary school age can be capable of holding reasoned, well-informed views on issues that affect them. When children are unable to determine what is in their best interests, parents are normally the best alternative decision makers.

In situations where the planned research participants are children under the care of the Social Services, special care needs to be taken to ensure that decisions are made by the appropriate legal guardian. Despite the difficulties inherent in researching with children and young people, such research is essential if advances in treatment and better understanding of their needs are to be achieved (Long 2004). Without such efforts to find ways to make inclusion in a study

compatible with the best interests of children and young people, we risk double jeopardy by adding denial of the chance of improvement to the misfortune of suffering from a health or social problem.

It is equally tempting to assume that older people are automatically vulnerable to inappropriate clinical or research interventions. On the other hand, the majority of healthcare recipients *are* older people, and this trend will continue. Although it may sometimes be more convenient, excluding people from research on the grounds of age alone is not equitable and constitutes ageism.

The same applies to other groups that might require extra efforts and resources to reach, but that should not be excluded inappropriately from studies. Minority ethnic populations are sometimes difficult to involve in research, especially where there are language and cultural differences. For this reason, sensitive efforts should be made to include people with such backgrounds where possible, since everyone should have the opportunity to take part in and potentially benefit from research (Gunaratnam 2003).

This applies to both individuals and whole groups defined by ethnicity, age or gender.

In some cases nurses care for, and may need to be involved in, research with individuals who are considered to be no longer cognitively competent to give consent. For example, some patients may have progressive dementia or brain damage to a degree that leaves them in a persistent vegetative state. Leslie Gelling (2004) discusses approaches that he and colleagues took when carrying out research with patients in a vegetative state and their families. Gelling discusses the different degrees of loss of competence and autonomy that can occur as a result of brain damage. He shows that research with this group and their families can help to clarify diagnosis and prognosis, and help in arriving at more appropriate plans of care and treatment. He argues that despite the complexity involved, it would be quite wrong to avoid doing research with this group of individuals who have been largely ignored by the research community. In England and Wales, the provisions of the Mental Capacity Act have clarified the position that already pertained in Scotland, that an appropriate advocate, such as a relative, can make decisions on behalf of those who lack the capacity do so, for example about treatment or participation in research (HM Government 2005).

Nurse researchers commonly wish to study their own clients, students or staff. In this context it is important to ask why these particular participants are more appropriate, given the possibility for an existing power relationship (e.g. teacher/student) that might affect the individual's decision to participate or the outcomes of the study. Even those who are not affected by illness may become vulnerable in circumstances of power differential.

To summarise, research samples should be inclusive and should represent the diversity of society across all relevant groupings. In particular, vulnerable people should not be excluded from participation in research except for well-justified reasons, which do not include mere convenience to the researcher. A mature approach to such cases is needed in which extra efforts are made to ensure protection of vulnerable individuals without denying them the chance to participate and potentially benefit from the research.

Gaining consent

People who are able to consider what participation will involve should be able to decide whether or not to take part in a study. Researchers should provide full information that is easy to understand, and software is now available to evaluate the readability of such information. For example, Microsoft Word for Windows features such a facility within the spelling and grammar-checking tool, while standard tests of readability based on sentence length and other criteria are also available. Useful resources in this area are listed at the end of the chapter. The participant should give their consent freely and there should be opportunities for consent to be withdrawn at a later stage. In some studies it may be necessary to ensure continuing consent on several occasions over a long period. However, it should be noted that an excess of concern in this respect could make respondents feel that research is more harmful than it really is. It is important to establish a sense of balance here. For example, participating in a trial of a new anti-cancer drug carries far greater dangers than being part of a focus group to evaluate a new service. The potential harms and possible benefits are of a different order of magnitude.

Consent freely given to participate in research that might hold dangers does not absolve the researcher of accountability for these dangers. It has long been established that responsibility for the welfare of research participants rests with the researcher, who must prioritise the best interests of participants. Perhaps less serious, but no less challenging, is what to do when the researcher discovers a clear and present need, for example for pain relief. In such cases, where the demands of the research design and the more immediate needs of participants conflict, the researcher needs to be clear in advance what they will do. It is debatable whether or not registered nurses retain an overriding professional duty to pursue the best interest of patients and clients when acting solely as a researcher. Such issues cannot be left until the point at which a decision is needed, but must be resolved clearly by the individual before embarking on the study.

In practice, obtaining consent should involve giving clear, unambiguous information to potential respondents so that they (or their advocate) can make an autonomous decision. Information on participant information sheets and consent forms is given in Chapter 10. Further guidance is available for nurses from the Royal College of Nursing (RCN 2007).

Maintaining confidentiality

The collection of data, usually about people, is the principal strategy of nursing research. Often these data include personal, biographical and demographic information, which, while essential to the analysis, should normally be used for this purpose only. In some cases, such as focus groups, research participants and others may need to be asked to keep matters discussed confidential to the group. This is illustrative of the need to be responsive to the nature of the data and address issues of confidentiality accordingly. The possibilities for collecting and holding data of a novel or non-standard nature have expanded to a large degree to include:

- still photography
- video images and voices
- computerised patient records
- paintings, sculpture, drama and other forms of expression
- human tissues.

Each of these forms of data poses different problems for the researcher, and sometimes creative means are required for both analysis and safe storage (Haigh & Jones 2005). However, there is nothing inherently unethical about their use and we feel that the potential of some of these tools is insufficiently exploited in nursing research where the semi-structured interview seems to predominate (Long & Johnson 2002).

Collected data must be stored securely, and in many cases arrangements are made to dispose of data safely once they have been used for their main purpose, on the grounds that data used for one purpose should not, without permission, be used for any other. Certainly, there is a convention that data should not normally be put to a use that has not previously been made clear to research participants. However, it seems to us that the value of data, suitably ano-

nymised and carefully stored, should never be underestimated. There is no way to know what great benefit it may offer in the future. What is important is that people know that data may be kept, and that it might be used to support research in due course. It is wise to make clear that such data may be used on more than one occasion for research and publication purposes. Before data are destroyed we must ask what undertakings were made regarding storage or destruction of data, and what harm such data could do now.

It has become traditional in much nursing and health research to assure research participants and organisations of the confidentiality of the data collected. However, researchers need to be aware that in a research context (as in a clinical one) they may become privileged with information of great importance, for example in a criminal matter. We take the view that in the overriding interest of personal safety or the protection of vulnerable people, confidentiality cannot be considered an absolute duty. This should be made clear to participants. Declarations by participants that suggest the potential for harm to themselves or third parties should prompt the serious consideration of the researcher divulging the essential information to an appropriate authority or professional.

The place of anonymity

A common way of assuring confidentiality of responses is to anonymise both individuals and organisations. In large surveys this may be relatively straightforward. In smaller, qualitative studies, anonymising data can be much more difficult. Certainly, erring on the side of safety, it has become common to remove identifying characteristics and to assign pseudonyms to respondents and organisations in much health and social care research. However, we need to remember that in some research traditions, such as nursing history, the preservation of anonymity is inappropriate and may even be contrary to respondents' interests. A historian of British nursing research would inevitably collect data from, and name, key individuals and reserve the right to evaluate their contribution critically.

The unlinked anonymous prevalence monitoring programme (UAPMP) began in the UK in 1990 and has tested nearly 10 million samples of human tissue (mostly blood) from adults since then (Health Protection Agency 2008). Much of the activity is related to genitourinary medicine clinic attendees, injecting drug users and pregnant women – all potentially vulnerable groups. Consent is not sought, but the samples are acquired through a process that irreversibly removes any link to the identity of the donor. The purpose of the programme is to measure the distribution of undiagnosed infection, particularly human immunodeficiency virus (HIV), in parts of the adult population. This programme – essentially a public health data collection activity – meets with the ethical requirements laid down by the National Research Ethics Service, the Department of Health, the Medical Research Council and English law, and it is a prime example of large-scale data collection in which consent is not sought but otherwise the research subjects are protected by the maintenance of their anonymity.

STRATEGIES FOR ETHICAL RESEARCH

Balancing risks and benefits

We would argue that, in general, decisions about healthcare interventions, and about research, are ones in which we weigh the possible risks and benefits in the interests of individuals and wider society. A problem with this notion of balancing risks and benefits, however, is that it implies a degree of certainty about what these may be. It suggests a calculation that cannot actually be performed. Instead, a human judgement needs to be made which accepts the disadvantages of an approach and takes account of the benefits research may bring, either now or in the future.

In some forms of experimental research, the evidence for and against the planned intervention may already be substantial and can be summarised for both approval bodies and research participants. Certainly, obvious risks (such as allergic reaction) and discomfort or pain should be made very clear to all concerned in the context of a rationale that includes the likely benefits of the research. In exploratory research, which is often qualitative, these outcomes may be less clear. Nevertheless, compared to the quite profound iatrogenic risks of much healthcare, serious physical or emotional harms are rare in nursing research.

Potential benefits from participation in research

Before any research project is undertaken, the possible benefits should be clear to all concerned. First among these might be a direct improvement in the health or care of individuals participating in the study. Second are longer-term benefits for others. Third, as a report by Doyal (2004) has argued, is the development of research skills, which is itself a legitimate aim of research. Each of these possible benefits must be carefully balanced with any likely disadvantages.

Predicting the benefits of a particular study can be difficult even with the most rigorous of experiments. In qualitative research with less foreseeable outcomes, this estimation can be even harder to make. For this reason, approval committees and other gatekeepers sometimes find it difficult to approve such studies. However, the more such studies are undertaken, the greater the likelihood that some may be very beneficial, and few would doubt the influence and importance of works of this kind by Glaser and Strauss (1965), which drew attention to the way the dying were treated; by Stockwell (1984), who explored the inappropriate labelling of patients; and more recently by Lawton (2000), who shows clearly how grim the process of dying can be, even in a hospice.

Minimising harm

Most patient care and treatment contains an element of risk of harm or, at the very least, discomfort. Nurses give injections, dress painful wounds and detain patients with a clear sense of proportion between the discomfort or denial of liberty and the likely future benefit. Research is little different, but the level of risk depends on the nature of the research.

The trial of new products may cause harm, such as allergic reaction or worsening of the condition, to particular individuals. Other risks are less obvious, such as the possibility of upsetting people during research about sensitive subjects or inadvertently stimulating or revealing cause for conflict between participants. It is therefore important to be clear about harms and discomforts and to discuss these openly with research participants. In many cases, nursing research will involve minor inconvenience at most. This should be kept to a minimum, but complete avoidance may be impossible.

Watson (1996) argues that 'the concept of a test or trial immediately raises ethical issues' (Watson 1996:7). Above and beyond the risk of actual harm, he argues that it is almost impossible to conduct a clinical trial without a measure of deceit. For example, even though respondents know they are in a trial, they may be blinded to which, if any, intervention they are receiving. Once again, the risk of harm must be minimised, and in such cases truly informed involvement means that the subject accepts this element of potential deception.

It may be that this situation of conflict – between ensuring high-quality research that can result in positive outcomes and protecting participants – is compounded by being a health professional. It could be argued that non-professionals would feel less responsibility to rescue research subjects from minor discomforts and dangers. With the aim of minimising harm, health professional researchers appreciate that they should intervene to prevent or reduce harms in certain circumstances. Occasionally, the issue is potentially too serious for a nurse to ignore. Researchers learn, however, that many dilemmas are much less clear-cut, and some tolerance of standards and procedures different to one's own is part and parcel of doing research in practice settings. Such issues are best discussed with experienced research colleagues or supervisors.

Personal integrity and professional responsibility

Although there are many safeguards such as research ethics committees, NHS research governance proce-dures and university approval arrangements, the protection of participants' interests in matters of research still often relies on the professionalism and personal integrity of the members of the research team.

Promises to keep data safely should be kept, and research processes should be carried out rigorously. Research approval processes increasingly have a brief reporting procedure, but sadly this can hardly be relied on to assure quality and proper adherence to high standards of research conduct. Perhaps more reliable, although far from foolproof, is effective training of researchers and accountability to departmental or unit-based supervisors. Being overseen by a steering committee that contains suitably briefed representatives of the population being studied and a genuine peer-review process are also usually of great help, if time-consuming. Additional guidance on personal responsibility for nurses in research is provided by the Royal College of Nursing (2007).

The ethical evaluation of research studies

The methodological literature in nursing research is expanding, but it is clear that despite the current fashion in the UK for procedural control of research in an attempt to prevent problems, little exists by way of ethical evaluation of the nursing research literature. An edited collection of essays (de Raeve 1996) examines some dilemmas and legal problems that researchers have faced themselves, but there is a general reluctance to debate the issues and problems faced by others. Matthews and Venables (1998) offer areas or criteria that might be used to such a purpose, such as the degree to which participation was voluntary, whether informed consent was achieved and the risk–benefit ratio. Unfortunately, they shrink from identifying genuine studies to illustrate their use of this approach. Instead they offer four brief hypothetical examples. Their general intention is sound, however.

It is important that as part of the reader's and especially the advanced student's evaluation of any research report they give thought to its ethical conduct. Achieving this may sometimes require the reader to dig a little deeper than the published article, since not all authors are equally robust in reporting

Box 3.1 Questions to ask about research conduct

For each question the reviewer ought to consider: did this exert any impact on the worth of the findings?

- What were the aims of the study? How important were they and why?
- Who undertook the study and how did their background prepare them?
- Who supervised or monitored the study?
- What sort of ethics approval was given, if any?
- What information were participants given and how readable and accurate was this?
- What checks were made to ensure that consent was given and remained in force?
- What opportunities were given for participants to withdraw?
- How were issues of power between researcher and respondents dealt with?
- Were any social groups excluded and, if so, how powerful was the justification?
- Were participants deprived of a known helpful intervention? If so, on what grounds?
- What risks/harms were associated with the study? Were these acceptable in the context of the potential benefits?
- What benefits were likely from the study and for whom?
- Did the effort made to disseminate the study outcomes to all concerned match the promises made?

the mistakes made and problems encountered while undertaking research. In Box 3.1, we offer a list of questions that might be asked about studies being reviewed or developed. It would be useful if more attention were given to these issues in the review of literature than has been customary in the past. It is possible to bring moral theory such as consequentialism, duty and 'ethics of care' to bear on these discussions (Long & Johnson 2007), but much can be achieved generally by critical debate of the issues raised by these questions.

CONCLUSIONS

Despite the developing bureaucracy that is meant, at least in part, to assure ethical conduct of research, much will continue to rely on the integrity and training of the researchers themselves and their supervisors. They should try not to be intimidated from undertaking an important study by myths that the proposed study may be unethical. Such myths include the involvement of children or the very ill as participants, and the use of technology to record data. The

ethics approval mechanisms should review what, if any, real harm might result, and, in balance with this, what benefits might accrue. Provided these are addressed clearly in the proposal, and the approach defended with rigour and obvious integrity, it should be possible to negotiate the bureaucracy.

Of course, for those who are less experienced, it is wise to work with a supervisor to design a study that is realistic and avoids putting the approval mechanisms, and the researcher, under too much strain. Reading widely and considering some of the more difficult issues that we can refer to only briefly here can also help. Certainly, novice researchers should try to develop the skill of identifying the ethical issues in every study they read or hear about, but they should also maintain a realistic sense of proportion.

References

de Raeve L (ed) (1996) *Nursing Research: an ethical and legal appraisal*. London, Baillière Tindall.

Doyal L (2004) *The Ethical Governance and Regulation of Student Projects: a draft proposal*. Working group on ethical review of student research in the NHS, Chair: Professor Len Doyal.

Gelling L (2004) Researching patients in the vegetative state: difficulties of studying this patient group. *NT Research* **9**(1): 7–17.

Glaser BG, Strauss AL (1965) *Awareness of Dying*. Chicago, Aldine.

Gunaratnam Y (2003) *Researching 'race' and ethnicity*. London, Sage.

Haigh C, Jones N (2005) An overview of the ethics of cyber-space research and the implications for nurse educators. *Nurse Education Today* **25**: 3–8.

Health Protection Agency (2008) *The Unlinked Anonymous Prevalence Monitoring Programme*. London, HPA. Available at *www.hpa.org.uk/web/HPAweb&Page& HPAwebAutoListName/Page/1201094588821*

HM Government (2005) *The Mental Capacity Act*. London, The Stationery Office.

Howarth ML, Kneafsey R (2005) The impact of research governance in healthcare and higher education organisations. *Journal of Advanced Nursing* **49**: 1–9.

Howarth ML, Kneafsey R (2003) Research governance: what future for nursing research? *Nurse Education Today* **23**: 81–82.

Johnson M (2004) Real world ethics and nursing research. *NT Research* **9**: 251–261.

Johnson M (1997) *Nursing Power and Social Judgement*. Aldershot, Ashgate.

Lawton J (2000) *The Dying Process: patients' experiences of palliative care*. London, Routledge.

Long T (2004) *Excessive Crying in Infancy*. London, Whurr Publishers.

Long T, Fallon D (2007) Ethics approval, guarantees of quality, and the meddlesome editor. *Journal of Clinical Nursing* **16**(8): 1398–1404.

Long T, Johnson, M (2007) *Research Ethics in the Real World: issues and solutions for health and social care*. Edinburgh, Churchill Livingstone-Elsevier.

Long T, Johnson M (2002) Research in *Nurse Education Today*: do we meet our aims and scope? *Nurse Education Today* **22**(1): 85–93.

Matthews L, Venables A (1998) Critiquing ethical issues in published research. In: Crookes P, Davies S (eds) *Research Into Practice*. Edinburgh, Baillière Tindall.

OFSTED (2008) *The Annual Report of Her Majesty's Chief Inspector of Education, Children's Services and Skills 2007/08*. London, OFSTED, available at www.ofsted. gov.uk/Ofsted-home/Publications-and-research/Browse-all-by/Annual-Report/2007-08/The-Annual-Report-of-Her-Majesty-s-Chief-Inspector-2007-08

Royal College of Nursing (2007) *Research Ethics: RCN guidance for nurses*. London, RCN, available at www. rcn.org.uk/__data/assets/pdf_file/0010/78742/003138. pdf

Stockwell F (1972, 1984) *The Unpopular Patient*. London, Croom Helm.

Watson R (1996) Product testing on trial. In: de Raeve L (1996) *Nursing Research: an ethical and legal appraisal*. London, Baillière Tindall, pp 3–17.

Websites

www.hpa.org.uk/web/HPAweb&Page&HPAwebAuto ListName/Page/1201094588821 – details of the un-linked anonymous prevalence monitoring programme (UAPMP), an example of a major survey undertaken without consent from participants.

www.invo.org.uk – INVOLVE is a national advisory group, funded by the Department of Health, which aims to promote and support active public involvement in NHS, public health and social care research.

www.nres.npsa.nhs.uk – the UK National Research Ethics Service offers comprehensive guidance to researchers.

The websites of the relevant government departments in the four countries of the UK contain relevant information for researchers:

England – *www.dh.gov.uk/policyandguidance/researchan-ddevelopment/fs/en*

Northern Ireland – *www.dhsspsni.gov.uk*

Scotland – *www.show.scot.nhs.uk/cso*

Wales – *www.wales.gov.uk*

Sources of standard tests for readability:
www.literacytrust.org.uk/campaign/SMOG.html;
www.usingenglish.com/glossary/readability-test.html

4 User Involvement in Research

Gordon Grant and Paul Ramcharan

Key points

- User involvement has emerged in the context of new research approaches, in the political move towards consumerism, the public service orientation and localisation of services, and within a policy and practice context that recognises that those best placed to inform service development are those on the receiving end of such services.

- User involvement in research ranges on a continuum between consultation with users through partnerships in a collaborative model to complete user control. Each of these may apply to different parts of the research process.

- User control in a politicised, emancipatory model led by users differs from a participatory model in which, via collaboration, there is joint ownership, accountability to host research organisations or funding agencies, an emergent methodological process and dissemination to a multiplicity of audiences.

- More work is required in the development of user involvement in research and in making judgements about different approaches. Involvement itself should be seen as being fit for purpose and not an end in itself. Attention should be paid to the inclusion of groups that have been marginalised, hard to reach or lacking in capacity.

INTRODUCTION

Recent government endorsement of the importance of the user voice has served to strengthen a growing commitment to user involvement in nursing research from many quarters: charitable trusts that fund research, user organisations and activists, as well as advocacy organisations and the wider research community. Evidence has been accumulating about the engagement of service users in different parts of the research process (INVOLVE 2004, 2006a,b,c; Lowes & Hulatt 2005; Nolan et al. 2007; Staniszewska et al. 2007; Smith et al. 2008). Though many first-hand accounts by users themselves are anecdotal, there is a growing body of more robust evidence garnered by users about their experiences of engagement in planning and carrying out health and social care research (Department of Health 2006). The rhetoric of user involvement in research has, however, encountered methodological and other challenges in its practical implementation.

In this chapter, we therefore consider:

- why user involvement in health and social care research has become popular
- how user involvement in research has been depicted
- some experiences of user involvement in research
- ethical and methodological questions associated with a commitment to user involvement in research
- shifting the focus from process to outcome questions.

A BRIEF HISTORY OF USER INVOLVEMENT IN RESEARCH

User involvement in research has a rich and long history and extends at least as far back as the genesis of action research (see, for example, Lees & Smith 1975) and the early forays into community development research commonly associated with developing countries (see for example, Freire, 1968; Richards, 1985). Within social science circles the 1980s saw major questions raised about Grand Theory (i.e. those social theories designed to understand the whole of society and human action) and a similar rejection of such meta-narratives by post-structuralism. Policy during this period also saw the emergence of localisation and user involvement in health and social care (Hadley & Hatch 1981) and the emergence of participatory politics (Richardson, 1983). The problem was, and remains, how ordinary citizens are best involved in decisions about how public services affect their lives.

The political response in the UK in the 1970s and 1980s under Margaret Thatcher and then later under John Major was the marketisation of health and social welfare and consumerism such as that represented by the Citizen's Charter (1991). This 'public service orientation' (Clarke & Stewart 1987) involved promoting:

- closeness to the customer and citizen
- listening to the public
- access for the public
- service from the public's point of view
- the views, suggestions and complaints of users

- the public's right to know
- an emphasis on service quality
- public opinion as a test of quality.

Recognition of the importance of the user voice quickly found its way into national policy. More than 20 years ago it featured in the innovative All Wales Strategy for the Development of Services for Mentally Handicapped People (sic) (Welsh Office 1983), which emphasised the right of service users and their families to be involved in the planning, management, delivery and review of services. The primacy of public and user involvement has been firmly embedded for some time within the NHS Plan (Department of Health, 2000a), reinforced more recently by Lord Darzi's next steps review of the NHS (Department of Health 2008). It is profiled in the National Service Frameworks, and in the White Paper *Valuing People* (Department of Health 2001a), in which people with learning disabilities helped to shape policy itself under the banner of 'nothing about us without us' (People First London *et al.* 2000). Though user inclusion has been a feature of declared government research strategy for some time too (Department of Health 2000b), the new National Institute for Health Research (NIHR), formed in 2006 to co-ordinate a more strategic approach to clinical, policy and applied health research in England, has placed user involvement in research high on its new strategic agenda by making a more principled commitment to the active involvement of patients a requirement in its core programmes.

It is easy for researchers to claim that users are involved in research, but in conventional forms of research this typically means that users are passive or compliant subjects with no hand in prioritising, commissioning, planning, undertaking, disseminating or utilising research. More recently, users have been challenging this position, the disability movement being particularly vocal and effective in this respect (see Moore *et al.* 1998). For some years now leading research funding bodies such as the Joseph Rowntree Foundation and the National Lottery Charities Board (now the Big Lottery Fund) have been exceptions in adopting a more open and inclusive approach to research that includes service users, especially those who are vulnerable. As mentioned above, the NIHR has recognised the growing importance of user involvement in research. One of its new programmes, the Research for Patient Benefit Programme, is dedicated to applied research with user involvement in mind. Now operating under the aegis of the NIHR, INVOLVE (formerly the Consumers in NHS Research) was established by the government to promote good practice in research committed to user involvement, but with a remit extending to social care as well as healthcare research. INVOLVE (2004) suggests user involvement in research may be valuable because people who use services:

- will offer different perspectives
- can help to make sure that research priorities are important to them
- can help to ensure that money and resources are not wasted on research that has little or no relevance
- can ensure that research does not just measure outcomes that others (academics and professionals) consider important
- can recruit their peers for research projects
- are better placed to access people who are often marginalised (i.e. 'hard-to-reach' groups in research terms)
- can help with the dissemination and implementation of research findings
- can be empowered through taking part
- are involved in the increasing political priority of involving consumers around the services they receive.

So what does this growing experience add up to? Are assumptions about the value of user involvement in research, such as those identified by INVOLVE, mirrored in practice? To address such questions we need to be rather more discriminating in how we account for user involvement in research.

MAPPING USER INVOLVEMENT IN NURSING RESEARCH

A cursory glance at the nursing and nursing-related research literature now shows growing evidence of user involvement in different fields of enquiry, for example learning disabilities (Richardson 2002; Ham *et al.* 2004; Department of Health 2006; Grant & Ramcharan 2007), mental health (Trivedi & Wykes 2002; Simpson *et al.* 2004; Telford & Faulkner 2004), forensic mental health (Faulkner & Morris 2003; Sainsbury Centre for Mental Health 2008), elder care and dementia care (Tetley & Hanson 2000; Tetley *et al.* 2003; Cowdell 2006), cancer and palliative care (Seymour & Skilbeck 2002; Maslin-Prothero 2003; Wright *et al.* 2007), primary care (Thornton *et al.* 2003) and back pain care (Ong 2003), among many others. The practicalities, lessons and emergent models of user involvement in nursing, midwifery and health visiting research have recently been reviewed by Smith *et al.* (2008).

Research Example 4.1 provides an example of user involvement. The Faulkner and Morris report is

---

RESEARCH EXAMPLE

4.1   User Involvement in Mental Health Research

Faulkner A, Morris B (2003) *User Involvement in Forensic Mental Health Research and Development*. NHS National Programme on Mental Health Research and Development, Liverpool.

In this expert paper the authors report that user involvement in forensic mental health research is currently limited to small-scale consultations and audits. Issues associated with the need to maintain security, confidentiality and the protection of individuals appear to be challenging user involvement in research as well as in services. At the present time there is thought to be no magic formula, implying therefore that it is necessary to continue testing and evaluating different ways of involving users in research. Based on evidence assembled, the report suggests principles, encompassing procedures and ethics that may be helpful in guiding good practice.

applied to the field of forensic mental health. Consider your own practice field. How far has user involvement in research gone?

In describing the range of activity conducted under the banner of user involvement in research there has been a tendency to adopt one or both of two extremes, i.e. user control versus researcher control. Similarly the Consumers in NHS Research group (2001) suggests that involvement may entail:

- *consultation* – where consumers are consulted with no sharing of power in the decision making
- *collaboration* – that involves an active ongoing partnership with consumers in the research process
- *user control* – where consumers design, undertake and disseminate the results of a research project.

There are advantages and disadvantages associated with each of these levels of involvement. We briefly examine these in relation to a case study (Research Example 4.2) provided by Rodgers (1999).

The main advantage of a *consultation* approach is that it is simple. It enables people to express their views without a commitment to act on them, and it can feel safe when people have not been involved before. The disadvantages are that involvement without action can lead to frustration; consultation fatigue can set in; and ideas may be constrained by

the agenda of those in power, so some people may not see it as worthwhile unless they are full partners.

The case study shows that there was consultation involved in establishing the research interest and in various parts of the research process. It also indicates that the development of the research idea was not purely an unencumbered product of the users' interests. However, the gatekeeping role of ethics committees and services tended not to confer as high a value on the user voice independent of those of 'professionals'.

In a *collaborative* approach there are more likely to be outcome measures, assessment criteria and forms of evaluation relevant to consumers. As collaborators, consumers can help to recruit research participants and deal with consent issues, and they can feel a greater sense of ownership. The disadvantages appear to be related to the heightened user commitment and associated issues of time and cost; the supports that may be needed to sustain commitment; and the problematical nature of power sharing. In the case study article, Rodgers reports that although people with learning difficulties were supposed to be interviewers they seldom took a lead role.

Finally, in the *user control* approach, the main advantages are tied to the greater likelihood of being able to address questions not thought of by academic researchers; the prospect of revealing evidence

---

○ RESEARCH EXAMPLE

4.2 Involving People with Learning Disabilities in Research

Rodgers J (1999) Trying to get it right: undertaking research involving people with learning difficulties. *Disability and Society* **14**(4): 421–433.

Rodgers aimed to examine the health of 30 people with learning difficulties from their own point of view. The research interest was partly prompted by a consultation with a group of women with learning difficulties who raised issues about health and medical care. However, it also reflected the interests of both the researcher and the local health services. Rodgers had to gain permission for the research from several quarters (ethics committees, GPs, parents and services) as well as from the research participants. People with learning disabilities were employed as consultants to the study and developed research questions that gave new insights into health from their point of view. They also helped in developing plain language findings summaries and took part in the interviewing with the main researcher. However, Rodgers found it hard to include them in the analysis of data.

missed by other researchers; and an even higher sense of ownership and therefore a fuller commitment to research dissemination. There are also raised prospects for the empowerment of service users. Disadvantages relate to the relative lack of experience and expertise of users in the conduct of the research; higher research costs; the lack of evidence about what constitutes good research facilitation and support for user researchers; and, therefore, some fears that user-controlled research may not be as independent as it seems.

Rodgers reports in the case study article that analysis continued as the research took place so that subsequent interviews could reflect emergent issues, but she adds that:

> 'I found it hard to contemplate how methodological considerations that I found challenging could be made more accessible to people with learning difficulties' (Rodgers 1999: 431).

Rodgers does claim that there was success in turning complex ideas into plain language in report-ing the findings, and that this could not have been done without the co-researchers. However, despite her best efforts, the research was commissioned neither by people with learning difficulties nor their allies; it was not wholly controlled by people with learning difficulties; and it was greatly affected in its orientation by other stakeholders from service, professional and governance sectors. In short, user control of research is not an easy ideal to accomplish.

We can see in the case study an implicit reliance on understanding levels of involvement alongside different parts of the research process, a position formalised by Faulkner and Morris (2003) and summarised in Figure 4.1. However, while it provides a framework for understanding, Figure 4.1 does not directly address what value should be placed on each combination of activities, and whether any are meaningful and relevant to service users. One way of approaching this last issue is to ask about the values and principles that should be attached to user involvement in research.

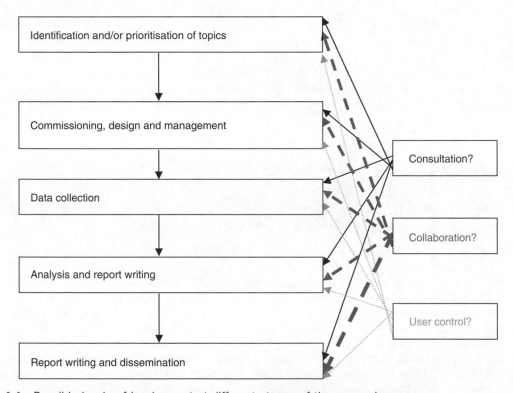

Figure 4.1 Possible levels of involvement at different stages of the research process

In a consensus study, Telford *et al.* (2004) developed a series of principles and indicators about the successful involvement of consumers in research. Consensus was reached on eight principles among a wide range of research participants. The principles are worth listing.

- Research roles of consumers and researchers are agreed.
- Budgets should include all costs of consumer involvement in research (useful guidance about payments to users participating in research has been provided by INVOLVE 2006c).
- Researchers respect the differing skills, knowledge and experience of consumers.
- Consumers are offered training and personal support to aid their research involvement.
- Researchers ensure that they have the necessary skills to involve consumers in the research process.
- Consumers are involved in decisions about how participants are both recruited and kept informed about the progress of the research.
- Consumer involvement is described in research reports.
- Research findings are made available to consumers in formats and in language they can easily understand.

(Adapted from Telford *et al.* 2004)

Consensus-based principles have an instant appeal, but as the authors themselves suggest, the value and utility of these principles have yet to be established with reference to different research methodologies and models of consumer involvement.

The application of general principles like these may well have rather limited utility when considered against forms of participatory or participatory-action and emancipatory research. This may become clearer when we consider how these forms of research differ in their stated purposes, philosophy and methods, and therefore in terms of the roles and allegiances required of users. These are summarised in Table 4.1.

It is important to say that Table 4.1 is very much a simplification of broad categories of research.

Traditional research as used here refers to those forms of scholarly endeavour that are based on careful hypothesis testing, coupled with testing of the generalisability of findings. Experimental designs, randomised controlled design studies, population sample surveys and many kinds of service evaluation studies fall within this broad category and generally require high technical expertise.

Participatory research is another very broad category. For Cocks and Cockram (1995), participatory research involves a research question being brought to the attention of (disabled) people; (disabled) people and researchers working together to achieve a collective analysis; and alliances being formed between (disabled) people and others to make changes following research. The potential methods of research have been suggested as discussion groups, public meetings, the establishment of investigative research teams, community seminars, fact-finding tours, the collective production of educational material, the use of popular theatre and educational camps or retreats (Cocks & Cockram 1995: 32).

Emancipatory research, on the other hand, represents the overt politicisation of research in which the researcher struggles for 'transformative change' (Barnes 2003) as a direct product of the research experience. Chappell (2000), reviewing the contributions of Zarb, Morris and Oliver, points to key features of emancipatory research as:

- being a tool for improving people's lives
- providing opportunities for (disabled) people to be researchers themselves
- involving a more reflexive stance
- being commissioned by democratic organisations of (disabled) people
- having an accountability to democratic organisations of (disabled) people.

Yet Chappell argues that very little emancipatory research has been funded by or accountable to organisations of (disabled) people. Of course, a possible reason for this is that few such organisations are in the financial position to fund programmes of research. The difficulties of accomplishing such an approach are also clear in our consideration of the earlier case study.

Taking *traditional*, *participatory* and *emancipatory* research as points of reference allows us to pose rather more discriminating questions about the status of user involvement, as well as emergent good practice.

Table 4.1 Parameters of traditional, participatory and emancipatory research

Parameter	Traditional	Participatory	Emancipatory
Ownership of research	Held by academic researchers	Joint/shared	Held by service users
Values	Value-neutral	Shared/negotiated	Political, partisan, reflecting user interests
Accountability	To academic peers, host organisation, funding agency	To research group, host organisation, funding agency	To co-researchers (service users), host organisation, funding agency
Focus of enterprise	Science and accumulation of generalisable knowledge; an emphasis on limited forms of research dissemination	Articulation of user voice; an emphasis on research dissemination and utilisation	Orientation towards changing or improving people's lives and opportunities; an emphasis on research utilisation to bring about change in people's everyday lives
Locus of control for change	External	Internal and external	Internal, generated by service user research group
Concepts, methodology	Imposed	Product of process, evolutionary	Product of process, evolutionary
Research dissemination	Written for academic audiences, therefore likely to be published in academic journals	Could be written for a multiplicity of audiences, therefore found in academic and popular outlets, and grey literature	Likely to be written mostly for user audiences, often located in grey literature and on user organisation websites
Costliness	Can be costly	Can be costly	Expensive
Sources of funding	Widespread	Growing	Very limited; still constrained by lack of official backing for putting evidence into practice

In the case of *traditional* research it would be wrong to assume that user involvement does not have an important place. Research governance and ethics arrangements (Department of Health 2005, 2001b) should at least ensure that inclusion/exclusion criteria and consent and capacity issues affecting users are accorded their proper status, much as with any kind of research. Hence the right to participate in research, but also the accompanying rights to protection and wellbeing, are to be afforded to everyone. However, some categories of service users are frequently excluded from traditional research, possibly on spurious grounds. For example, in the earlier case study, Rodgers was instructed to 'seek permission' from both the GP and family carer of each interviewee in the research and this affected who was finally recruited. People with serious mental health problems or severe learning disabilities, and others whose capacity to consent may be an issue, are often subject to exclusion. Policy guidance on this matter is unfortunately rather confused at this time. It asserts the presumption of capacity, while stating that:

> 'It is not appropriate to carry out research on adults who cannot give consent for themselves, if the research can instead be carried out on adults who are able to give or withhold consent. The only exception to this rule would be where clinicians believe that it is in the person's best interests to be involved in research' (Department of Health 2001c: 15).

RESEARCH EXAMPLE

4.3 Involving Users in Low Back Pain Research

Ong BO (2003) Involving users in low back pain research. *Health Expectations* **6**: 332–341.

The aim of this study was to determine how patient and professional perceptions of low back pain and its treatment relate to the use of healthcare and to subsequent outcomes. Focus groups were held with GPs, other healthcare practitioners and low back pain sufferers. Tensions arose between involving patients (users) as co-researchers both in designing research tools and in sharing their experiences of low back pain. However, sharing experiences became a problem over emotive issues, with some contributors seeking to place an emphasis on areas relating to their own experiences over those of others. It was therefore considered that agreeing a certain distance from personal experiences may be a prerequisite for formulating a research agenda, especially when discussing emotive issues and that this kind of dilemma might be the product of the focus group process.

Given the contradictions and ambiguities, it is easy for researchers to 'play safe' by excluding people in these categories. The wider research ethics issues involved are discussed more fully in Chapter 3.

Most published evidence about user involvement concerns *participatory* research. By its very nature, participatory research is predicated on strong alliances and partnerships between those involved. In principle, potentially all the stages of the research process are shared. In practice, this is much less the case. As the example from Ong's study (see Research Example 4.3) indicates, there is no guarantee of a strong alliance between people who share particular symptoms. There are also potential variations between what constitutes such alliances dependent on the user groups themselves. People with learning disabilities, for example, are likely to experience their alliances over a lifetime. In contrast, pregnant women or those with treatable critical illnesses may only be users over a short period. The concept and meaning of alliances may therefore differ substantially between different user groups.

Moreover, it is not uncommon for academic researchers to go looking for user organisations as partners, pre-armed with research questions where the research interest is a product of several competing interests such as in the case of Rodgers (see Research Example 4.2). Participatory research can also be a messy business:

- power relations between those involved have to be tested and re-tested
- accommodations are required between the various partner organisations that fund the research, employ workers or support users
- research methods have to be worked out as things proceed.

The rhetoric of participation sounds very rosy; the reality, on the other hand, can be quite different (see Walmsley & Johnson 2003).

Emancipatory research, much of it tied to social model thinking within the disability field (Barnes 2003), seeks to address and deal with social, political and environmental factors that perpetuate forms of exclusion or oppression in people's lives and, given a paucity of research using its principles, remains largely aspirational. It takes a particular kind of person to commit themselves to this kind of research, and resilience to see things through to the end, particularly in the later action stages. As the example in Research Example 4.3 also demonstrates, there are often 'structural impediments' such as lack of funding through user organisations, lack of support from services and professionals, differences in the language of research and the language of those seeking to be involved, and with ethical and governance issues that make such research difficult to accomplish in practice (see Staniszewska *et al.* 2007).

CHALLENGES FOR USER INVOLVEMENT IN NURSING RESEARCH

The practicalities of user involvement in research leave some important unanswered questions that are illustrated below.

Fitness for purpose

As has been illustrated, different kinds of research require different commitment from users, their supporters, researchers and others – a point further developed recently by Smith *et al.* (2008). It is useful to think of user involvement strategies being informed and led by the purposes and goals of individual research projects, that is they need to be *fit for purpose*. To involve people as an 'end in itself' can lead to tokenism, where there is no role to be played by users and no clear gain for either side. There are as yet no published criteria against which to measure fitness for purpose in relation to traditional, participatory and emancipatory research, although a range of guidance for involvement in parts of the research process have recently been published by INVOLVE (for example, INVOLVE 2006a,b,c).

Questions remain about why user involvement has been more likely in some parts of the research process than others. INVOLVE's website revealed a database of 181 projects in 2004 and 228 in November 2008. These confirm that users are involved to varying extents in key stages of the projects listed, and that over time the contributions in different areas remain relatively stable (see Table 4.2). Early stages of the process, especially prioritising research topic areas and planning research, appear to have quite high proportions of users involved. Writing publications and implementing action appear to involve users least of all. Why users appear to be less involved in writing publications is less clear at this time, although collaborative writing, especially when directed towards academic publishing, can generate tensions between users and academic researchers. More accounts are required about how these issues are best addressed.

User involvement and excluded groups

As suggested in relation to traditional forms of research, it is easy to exclude categories of people on grounds of mental capacity. Unfortunately, people can be excluded for other reasons too. People may be 'invisible', meaning that they can be 'lost' in service systems through poor case records; they may be lost 'outside the service system' because they have lost contact with services (for example many people with mild learning disabilities); or they may 'lack voice' or articulacy (for example following stroke, head injury or the onset of dementia). Those who are marginalised may pose researcher–user translation problems, both at a cultural and language level, especially where there are no assistive technologies for communication. Indeed, in Research Example 4.2 above, Rodgers notes that:

Table 4.2 Summary of user involvement in research projects listed on the INVOLVE website*

Stage of involvement	Percentage of projects 2004 (n = 181)	Percentage of projects 2008 (n = 228)
Prioritising research topic areas	66 (n = 120)	61 (n = 140)
Planning research	77 (n = 139)	73 (n = 167)
Managing research	50 (n = 91)	48 (n = 109)
Designing research instruments	72 (n = 131)	68 (n = 155)
Undertaking research	52 (n = 94)	48 (n = 109)
Analysing research	47 (n = 85)	44 (n = 101)
Writing publications	34 (n = 61)	32 (n = 72)
Disseminating	56 (n = 101)	54 (n = 124)
Implementing action	35 (n = 63)	33 (n = 75)

*As at December 2004 and November 2008

'the inclusion of people with more severe impairments meant that there were times when I was not able to talk directly with the person concerned'' (Rodgers 1999: 427)

This forced her to rely instead on carers or advocates who knew the person well. The roles that advocates, proxies and guardians play here as spokespersons or enablers for such users in research are matters warranting closer study.

The indications are that articulate service users or those closely connected to user organisations are most likely to be involved in participatory and emancipatory research. If this is indeed the case, it raises further issues about whose voices are being represented in such research, and whether this matters.

WEIGHING USER EXPERIENCES – LEARNING DISABILITY AS A CASE EXAMPLE

In this light, user views and experiences also prove complex. Such experiences are seldom unitary. For example, in a review of the views and experiences of people with learning disabilities, Ramcharan and Grant (2001) point to a range of research products:

- 'testaments of life' (e.g. life histories, narrative accounts)
- 'user movement media' incorporating materials published by self-advocacy groups and those available on the web
- 'research-based studies' in which a range of experiences are collected from people with learning disabilities.

Moreover, as Telford and Faulkner (2004: 549) assert, the 'alternative literature (including what is commonly called the grey literature) offers a rich source to learn from'. In these varied accounts there are issues relating to how best to judge:

- the extent to which non-disabled researchers have set the agenda of experiences from which to draw
- the difficulties of translation that are often required to bring the voices to a wider audience

- the representativeness of the voices heard relating their experiences
- the power of users in the research process.

As part of our own work as academic co-ordinators of the Department of Health Learning Disability Research Initiative (LDRI) linked to the implementation of Valuing People (Department of Health 2001a), we have involved people with learning disabilities in commissioning a nationally funded research initiative as well as advising on dissemination strategies. Service users were paid accepted consultancy rates and involved as:

- members of the research commissioning group
- reviewers whose expert knowledge was used in assessing proposals against criteria relating to the involvement of people with learning disabilities in the funded research projects and whether the research was likely to change the lives of people for the better.

Research applicants were asked to provide easy-to-read as well as technical research proposals so that judgements could be made about the capacity of researchers to produce information in accessible formats. Dissemination at three annual research seminars has brought together service users with academics, managers and civil servants. Newsletters about the LDRI have incorporated plain language summaries to reach user as well as academic and policy audiences. The final project to be commissioned under the initiative was a user-led study supported by INVOLVE and Values into Action (VIA), which evaluated the arrangements for user involvement in the remaining 12 projects.

Comments from participants have suggested that involvement was welcomed, though the practice related to implementation was not seen by users as unproblematic. Among the issues they raised were:

- more time for their personal assistants to 'talk them through' their allocated proposals
- prior training
- feedback to know where the funding was allocated
- quicker financial reimbursement.

Users on the research commissioning group felt that people listened to them and that their views made a real difference to decision making, although they would have liked more service users to be members of the group.

In cancer care research it has similarly been shown that there are creative avenues for involving consumers in regional and local forums where research priority setting and commissioning takes place, for example in the North Trent Cancer Research Network (NTCRN) (Stevens *et al.* 2003). In the NTCRN consumers have an equal say in deciding what research ideas should be developed and funded, identifying topics of particular interest to themselves, and being part of a recruitment panel that appoints researchers. In addition, sponsored conferences for consumers have added to this voice. Dimensions of this experience are being independently evaluated.

SHIFTING THE FOCUS FROM PROCESSES TO OUTCOMES

With much of the focus having been placed on the experiences or *processes* of user involvement in research, attention now needs to be turned to *outcomes*. At the moment evidence about outcomes is embryonic. Until this changes, the credibility of this form of research will continue to be questioned. With this in mind, and drawing from theorising about individual and social capital (McKenzie & Harpham 2005), we suggest below some criteria for considering outcomes of user research at three levels: individual, social and project.

Individual

- *Technical/analytic* – what understanding do users have of research opportunities? What research skills can users acquire?
- *Psychological* – improvements in self-confidence, assertiveness, self-esteem.
- *Project management* – capacity for decision making, advice giving, exercise of control.

Social/partnerships

- *Security* – feeling safe in relationships (ethics).
- *Belonging* – feeling part of things (valued as a contributor).

- *Continuity* – experiencing links and consistency over time; possibilities of research career development.
- *Purpose* – meaningfulness of shared activity.
- *Achievement* – using knowledge to change services.
- *Significance* – feeling that you matter (external or institutional recognition).

Project

- *Rigour of data analysis* – attention to reliability/validity or authenticity criteria.
- *Transparency* – of data analysis and interpretation.
- *Complementarity of knowledge contributions* – from service user and academic researchers.
- *Mutual appraisal of knowledge claims* – service user appraisal of academic knowledge; academic appraisal of service user knowledge.
- *Transformational potential* – in terms of theory testing; practice and policy impacts; research capacity building.

An attempt to apply some of these criteria can be found in McClimens *et al.* (2007).

CONCLUSIONS

In this chapter we have considered how and why user involvement has become popular. We have shown how it might be categorised in terms of the level of involvement, i.e. via consultation, collaboration or control. Categorisations emerging from theoretical research perspectives have been outlined, i.e. the consumer involvement, participatory and emancipatory models. We have sought to examine how each of these categorisations might be used in understanding the place of users within the research process and, most importantly, we have pointed out using a case study that there remain a substantial number of issues still to be addressed in the field of user involvement in research. There is much potential to the involvement of users in research but this potential remains to be more fully demonstrated and substantiated, especially with respect to generating better evidence about outcomes. The survival of the approach is therefore at a critical point in its history.

References

Barnes C (2003) What a difference a decade makes: reflections on doing 'emancipatory' disability research. *Disability and Society* **18**: 3–17.

Chappell AL (2000) Emergence of participatory methodology in learning disability research: understanding the context. *British Journal of Learning Disabilities* **28**: 38–43.

Clarke M, Stewart J (1987) The public service orientation: issues and dilemmas. *Public Administration* **65**: 161–177.

Citizen's Charter (1991) Cm. 1599. London, HMSO.

Cocks E, Cockram J (1995) The participatory research paradigm and intellectual disability. *Mental Handicap Research* **8**(1): 25–37.

Consumers in NHS Research (2001) *Getting Involved in Research: a guide for consumers*. Eastleigh, Consumers in NHS Research.

Cowdell F (2006) Preserving personhood in dementia research: a literature review. *International Journal of Older People Nursing* **1**: 85–94.

Department of Health (2008) *High Quality Care for All: NHS next stage review final report*. Cm. 7432. London, The Stationery Office.

Department of Health (2006) *Best Research for Best Health: a new national health research strategy*. London, Department of Health.

Department of Health (2005) *Research Governance Framework for Health and Social Care*, 2nd edition. London, Department of Health.

Department of Health (2001a) *Valuing People: a new strategy for learning disability for the 21st century*. Cm. 5085. London, Stationery Office.

Department of Health (2001b) *Research Governance Framework for Health and Social Care*. London, Department of Health.

Department of Health (2001c) *Seeking Consent: working with people with learning disabilities*. London, Stationary Office.

Department of Health (2000a) *The NHS Plan: a plan for investment, a plan for reform*. Cm. 4818. London, Stationery Office.

Department of Health (2000b) *Research and Development for a First Class Service: R&D funding in the new NHS*. London, Department of Health.

Faulkner A, Morris B (2003) *User Involvement in Forensic Mental Health Research*. Liverpool, NHS National Programme on Forensic Mental Health Research and Development.

Freire P (1968) *Pedagogy of the Oppressed*. New York, Seabury Press.

Grant G and Ramcharan P (2007) *Valuing People and Research: the Learning Disability Research Initiative – overview report*. London, Department of Health.

Hadley R, Hatch S (1981) *Social Welfare and the Failure of the State: centralized social services and participatory alternatives*. London, Allen and Unwin.

Ham M, Jones N, Mansell I, Northway R, Price L, Walker G (2004) 'I'm a researcher!' Working together to gain ethical approval for a participatory research study. *Journal of Learning Disabilities* **8**(4): 397–407.

INVOLVE (2006a) *Getting Involved in Research Grant Applications*. London: Department of Health. Available from www.invo.org.uk/key_publications.asp

INVOLVE (2006b) *Being a Member of a Commissioning Board: guidelines for members of the public*. Available from www.invo.org.uk/key_publications.asp

INVOLVE (2006c) *Guide to Reimbursing and Paying Members of the Public Actively Involved in Research*. London: Department of Health. Available from www.invo.org.uk/key_publications.asp

INVOLVE (2004) *Involving the Public in NHS, Public Health, and Social Care Research: briefing notes for researchers*. Eastleigh, INVOLVE.

Lees R, Smith G (1975) *Action-Research in Community Development*. London, Routledge and Kegan Paul.

Lowes L, Hulatt I (2005) *Involving Service Users in Health and Social Care Research*. Abingdon, Routledge.

Maslin-Prothero S (2003) Developing user involvement in research. *Journal of Clinical Nursing* **12**: 412–421.

McClimens A, Grant G, Ramcharan P (2007) Looking in a fairground mirror, reflections on partnerships in learning disabilities research. In: Nolan M, Hanson E, Grant G, Keady J (eds) *User Participation in Health and Social Care Research: voices, values and evaluation*. Maidenhead, Open University Press and McGraw Hill Education, pp 104–119.

McKenzie K, Harpham T (2005) *Social Capital and Mental Health*. London, Jessica Kingsley Publishers.

Moore M, Beazley S, Maelzer J (1998) *Researching Disability Issues*. Buckingham, Open University Press.

Nolan M, Hanson E, Grant G, Keady J (eds) (2007) *User Participation in Health and Social Care Research: voices, values and evaluation*. Maidenhead, Open University Press and McGraw Hill Education.

Ong BN (2003) Involving users in low back pain research. *Health Expectations* **6**: 332–341.

People First London, Change, Speaking Up in Cambridge, Royal Mencap (2000) *Nothing About Us Without Us – The Learning Disability Strategy: the user group report.* London: Department of Health.

Ramcharan P, Grant G (2001) Views and experiences of people with intellectual disabilities and their families. (1) The user perspective. *Journal of Applied Research in Intellectual Disabilities* **14**: 348–363.

Richards H (1985) *The Evaluation of Cultural Action: an evaluation study of the parents and childrens' program.* London, Macmillan.

Richardson A (1983) *Participation*. London, Routledge.

Richardson M (2002) Involving people in the analysis: listening, reflecting, discounting nothing. *Journal of Learning Disabilities* **6**(1): 47–60.

Rodgers J (1999) Trying to get it right: undertaking research involving people with learning difficulties. *Disability and Society* **14**(4): 421–433.

Sainsbury Centre for Mental Health (2008) *A Review of Service User Involvement in Prison Mental Health Research.* London, Sainsbury Centre for Mental Health.

Seymour J, Skilbeck J (2002) Ethical considerations in researching user views. *European Journal of Cancer Care* **11**(3): 215–219.

Simpson EL, Barkham M, Gilbody S, House A (2004) Involving service users as researchers for the evaluation of adult statutory mental health services. *Cochrane Database of Systematic Reviews* **4**.

Smith E, Ross F, Donovan S, Manthorpe J, Brearley S, Sitzia J, Beresford P (2008) Service user involvement in nursing, midwifery and health visiting research: a review of evidence and practice. *International Journal of Nursing Studies* **45**(2): 298–315.

Staniszewska S, Jones N, Newburn M, Marshall S (2007) User involvement in the development of a research bid: barriers, enablers and impacts. *Health Expectations* **10**(2): 173–183.

Stevens T, Wilde D, Hunt J, Ahmedzai SH (2003) Overcoming the challenges of consumer involvement in cancer research. *Health Expectations* **6**: 81–88.

Telford R, Boote JD, Cooper CL (2004) What does it mean to involve consumers successfully in research? A consensus study. *Health Expectations* **7**: 209–220.

Telford R, Faulkner A (2004) Learning about service user involvement in mental health research. *Journal of Mental Health* **13**(6): 549–559.

Tetley J, Hanson E (2000) Participatory research. *Nurse Researcher* **8**(1): 69–88.

Tetley J, Haynes L, Hawthorne M, Odeyemi J, Skinner J, Smith D, Wilson V (2003) Older people and research partnerships. *Quality in Ageing* **4**(4): 18–23.

Thornton H, Edwards A, Elwyn G (2003) Evolving the multiple roles of 'patients' in health-care research: reflections after involvement in a trial of shared decision-making. *Health Expectations* **6**: 189–197.

Trivedi P, Wykes T (2002) From passive subjects to equal partners: qualitative review of user involvement in research. *British Journal of Psychiatry* **181**: 468–472.

Walmsley J, Johnson K (2003) *Inclusive Research with People with Learning Disabilities: past, present and futures.* London, Jessica Kingsley Publishers.

Welsh Office (1983) *All Wales Strategy for the Development of Services for Mentally Handicapped People.* Cardiff, Welsh Office.

Wright, DNM, Corner, JL, Hopkinson JB, Foster CL (2007) The case for user involvement in research: the research priorities of cancer patients. *Breast Cancer Research* **9** (Suppl 2: S3): 1–4.

Further reading

Oliver M (1997) Emancipatory research: realistic goal or impossible dream? In: Barnes C, Mercer G (eds) *Doing Disability Research*. Leeds, Disability Press, pp 15–31.

Ramcharan P, Grant G, Flynn M (2004) Emancipatory and participatory research: how far have we come? In: Emerson E, Hatton C, Thompson T, Parmenter TR (eds) *The International Handbook of Applied Research in Intellectual Disabilities*. Chichester, John Wiley, pp 83–113.

Royal College of Nursing (2007) *User Involvement in Research by Nurses*. RCN Guidance. London. The guidance contains links to useful websites about planning, design, ethics, costing and payment issues.

Smith E, Manthorpe J, Brearley S, Ross F, Donovan S, Sitzia J, Beresford P (2006) *User Involvement in the Design and Undertaking of Nursing, Midwifery and Health Visiting Research*, Report to the National Co-ordinating Centre for NHS Service Delivery and Organisation R&D, London. Available from *www.sdo.lshtm.ac.uk/sdo692003.html*

Websites

www.alzheimers.org.uk/site/scripts/documents.php?categoryID=200296 – Alzheimer's Association.

The Quality Research in Dementia Programme (QRD) website has information for member and prospective members of the QRD consumer network and researchers.

www.biglotteryfund.org.uk/ – the website for the Big Lottery Fund provides details of funding programmes to support research involving users.

www.ceres.org.uk – Consumers for Ethics in Research (CERES) is an independent charity set up to promote informed debate about research and help users of health services to develop and publicise their views on health research.

www.invo.org.uk – INVOLVE is a national advisory group, funded by the Department of Health, which aims to promote and support active public involvement in NHS, public health and social care research.

www.scmh.org.uk – the Sainsbury Centre for Mental Health is a charity that works to improve the quality of life for people with severe mental health problems. It carries out research, development and training work to influence policy and practice in health and social care.

5 Research for a Multi-ethnic Society

Sarah Salway and George Ellison

Key points

- Conducting research that appropriately and sensitively pays attention to ethnicity presents an important challenge to researchers and requires particular competencies.

- Researchers must recognise the multifaceted nature of ethnicity and the varied ways in which health-related experiences and outcomes may be associated with ethnicity.

- Ethnic identities are complex and fluid, therefore using fixed ethnic categories in research requires careful consideration.

- Describing and explaining differences between ethnic 'groups' demands careful attention to sampling, data generation and analysis so that partial or misleading interpretations are avoided.

- Researchers should be alert to the potential for research on minority ethnic groups to do more harm than good and should seek to ensure that their research focus and approach are informed by the experiences and priorities of these groups.

INTRODUCTION

The UK is now widely regarded as a multi-ethnic society. In the 2001 Census, 8% of the UK population self-identified as non-White, with 13% of the population of England identifying as belonging to an ethnic group other than White British. The terms 'ethnic group' and 'ethnicity' are commonly heard in public policy, the media and even everyday conversation (Eriksen 2002). Likewise, health and social research pays increasing attention to 'ethnic diversity' and 'ethnic inequalities' in experiences and outcomes. As Anthias (2001) and others have argued, ethnicity is one of the major social divisions in modern societies and ethnic identities have important implications for people's lives. However, the meaning of such terms remains ambiguous and research that engages with these issues is inherently politicised and often controversial in nature. Conducting research that appropriately and sensitively pays attention to ethnicity presents an important challenge to researchers and requires particular competencies (see Box 5.1).

There is substantial evidence that health and healthcare provision vary along ethnic lines and that minority ethnic groups are at risk of significant disadvantage across a range of indicators (Nazroo 1997; Gill *et al.* 2007; Henry 2007). UK health policy and

Box 5.1 Cultural competence in research

Papadopoulos and Lees (2002) suggest the following model of cultural competence in research:

Cultural awareness: examining and challenging your own personal value base and behaviours and reflecting on how these may affect the research process.

Cultural knowledge: understanding the similarities, differences and inequalities between and across ethnic 'groups' and the multiplicity of factors that might account for these patterns. Such knowledge should help to avoid stereotyping, prejudice and discrimination in research.

Cultural sensitivity: challenging power relationships and oppressive practices to offer true partnership to the participants of research studies founded on trust, respect and empathy.

Cultural competence: synthesis and application of awareness, knowledge and sensitivity, enabling racism, discrimination and ethnocentricity to be recognized and challenged.

Both culture-generic and culture-specific competence are considered necessary, the former being the acquisition of knowledge and skills that are applicable across ethnic groups, the latter being the knowledge and skills that relate to a particular ethnic group which enable an understanding of that group's particular values and behaviours.

practice directives over the past four decades have repeatedly acknowledged the need to understand and tackle ethnic health disparities (DoH 2003), identifying nursing as a key profession to contribute to this endeavour (Culley & Dyson 2001). Further, the Race Relations (Amendment) Act (RR(A)A) 2000 places legal obligations on all public organisations to consider the need to eliminate unlawful discrimination and to promote equality of opportunity and good relations between people from different ethnic groups.

Given that it is now commonly accepted that healthcare policy and practice should be evidence based, these policy directives and legal duties clearly imply the need for researchers to generate an evidence base that reflects the needs of our ethnically diverse population. This requirement has been formally acknowledged by the Department of Health in its Research Governance Framework for Health and Social Care in which it sets out a number of general principles that should apply to all research:

'Research, and those pursuing it, should respect the diversity of human society and conditions and the multi-cultural nature of society. Whenever relevant, it should take account of age, disability, gender, sexual orientation, race, culture and religion in its design, undertaking and reporting. The body of research evidence available to policy makers should reflect the diversity of the population' (DoH 2005: Para 2.2.7)

However, much health research does not include participants from minority ethnic groups and/or fails to give considered attention to ethnicity as an element of analysis (Hussain-Gambles 2003). Furthermore, despite government directives and some recent improvements, routine data collection systems such as the Hospital Episodes Statistics still achieve low coverage and poor-quality information on ethnicity (Aspinall & Anionwu 2002).

A number of factors appear to have contributed to the inadequate attention to ethnicity in health (and nursing) research, including:

- a lack of awareness of the potential significance of ethnicity
- a tendency to consider ethnicity as a specialist area of investigation

- conscious exclusion of minority ethnic individuals on the grounds of added cost and complexity
- a lack of researcher confidence and skills to engage with individuals from ethnic groups that are perceived to be 'hard to reach'.

At the same time, growing awareness of past abuses and negative experiences of research may also make individuals from minority ethnic groups reluctant to participate in research.

However, research interest in ethnicity and health is growing in the UK and elsewhere (Drevdahl *et al.* 2006). Yet, as the volume of research addressing ethnicity and health expands, so too do concerns regarding the *quality* of this research, its potential to inform changes in policy and practice that benefit minority ethnic populations, and its potential role in stereotyping and stigmatising ethnic minority populations (Gunaratnam 2007). Indeed, much of the previous research in this field has been of dubious ethical and scientific quality and a number of persistent pitfalls are identified, including:

- the use of outdated, inappropriate models of ethnicity that present ethnic groups as stable, discrete entities
- a failure to research issues that are of concern to minority ethnic people
- a lack of cultural competence in research practice
- a failure to incorporate a broader social, historical and political analysis of ethnicity (Stubbs 1993).

Against this rather unpromising history, it is salient to stress that poorly designed and poorly conducted research will, at best, fail to contribute to a better understanding of the links between ethnicity and health and how ethnic inequalities in health might be addressed and, at worst, serve to perpetuate the stereotyping and disadvantage experienced by minority ethnic groups. Conducting research into ethnicity and health appropriately and sensitively raises a range of complex theoretical, methodological and practical issues, and researchers require support and guidance if their work is to make a positive contribution to the health and healthcare received by minority ethnic groups.

This chapter introduces the reader to some of the most important issues for consideration. We encourage researchers to recognise that there are often no simple, 'cook book' solutions to the complex issues that arise in researching ethnicity and health, and to aim instead for heightened critical reflexivity in the research they conduct.

THE CONCEPT OF ETHNICITY

So far our discussion has employed the term 'ethnicity' without further elaboration. However, frequent, everyday reference to 'ethnicity' and 'ethnic groups' belies the complex and contentious nature of these terms. As Mulholland and Dyson (2001) argue, researchers must look beyond the popular everyday use of these terms and the implicit meanings such use reflects, and seek a more informed appreciation of their complex and dynamic nature.

In health research (as well as wider societal and policy discourse), the term 'ethnicity' is used in diverse and contradictory ways. In its most generic form, ethnicity represents a form of social or group identity, which draws on notions of shared origins or ancestry. However, different conceptualisations of ethnicity tend to emphasise different aspects of such group identity and to view the processes of identification through which ethnic affiliations arise very differently. Some conceptualisations emphasise the cultural commonality within ethnic groups, identifying shared beliefs and behaviours, sameness and belonging; essentially an *internal* identification. In contrast, other ideas about ethnicity place emphasis on geographical origins and shared biological features among the members of ethnic groups. Still others focus on sociopolitical dimensions, viewing ethnicity as the *process* through which boundaries between hierarchically organised 'groups' are constructed and symbolised, with the emphasis on the imposition of categories and labels by external forces. Indeed, some conceptualisations appear to invoke a combination of all three of these dimensions. This is why some have called ethnicity a 'biosocial' or 'biocultural' concept. Similar variability exists in the ways in which the term 'race' is employed (see Box 5.2).

Box 5.2   Ethnicity or race?

Though the term 'ethnicity' is currently more commonly employed in UK health research than the term 'race', the two concepts are closely related and both are used somewhat interchangeably. It is commonly suggested that while 'race' refers to biological features (such as skin colour) to distinguish different groups of people, 'ethnicity' focuses primarily on differences in cultural practices and beliefs. In practice, however, this neat distinction is not consistently applied in either research practice or social discourse. As Gunaratnam (2003) and others have noted, 'race' may often emphasise differences in physical characteristics (such as skin colour) but 'race' has always been a far broader concept that *also* sought to reflect differences in a range of social and cultural characteristics. Likewise, though ethnicity tends to emphasise cultural and religious attributes, these characteristics are frequently represented as relatively fixed and inherent, being passed down from one generation to the next through endogamous marriage as well as processes of socialisation. Given the complex inter-relationships between the two terms it is not surprising that there is little standardisation of research practice, and there are disparate opinions as to which of these two terms should be employed by health researchers. While some advocate avoiding the use of the term race because of its association with discredited 19th-century work labelled 'scientific racism', other researchers retain its use as a biological, social and/or biosocial construct. Some researchers go one step further and place the term race in scare quotes – 'race' – both to signal its contested meaning and to acknowledge that as long as racism exists within society, then 'race', however problematic, will be needed in research. Few comparable concerns have been raised over the use of the term 'ethnicity' in health research, and this partly explains why it is more commonly used in the UK. However, some researchers have argued that 'race' is preferable to 'ethnicity' since the latter tends to obscure the importance of external forces, power and exploitation in the lives of people from minority ethnic groups, and instead ascribes disadvantage to the internal attributes of the groups themselves. Other researchers have suggested a compromise of sorts, in which the two terms are conflated in a joint formulation – 'race/ethnicity' – to encapsulate and signal the diverse biosocial character of both terms while retaining a focus on the role each have played in stereotyping, discrimination and disadvantage.

There is also variation across research contexts in the extent to which the boundaries and characteristics of ethnic groups are seen as fixed and stable. Recent years have witnessed increasing criticism of health-focused research that portrays ethnic identities as immutable and ethnic groups as distinct, homogenous and unchanging. On the one hand, researchers who have taken the discredited view that ethnic groups display wholesale genetic differences (claimed to be the result of their different geographical and socio-cultural ancestries) have tended to interpret ethnic disparities in health as resulting primarily from biological differences, ignoring the importance of culture, socioeconomic status and discrimination. On the other, there are researchers who portray the culture of ethnic groups (together with related beliefs and behaviours) as homogeneous, distinct, immutable and, in some respects, 'innate'. Such 'cultural determinism' ignores the diverse, fluid and context-dependent nature of cultural characteristics, overlooks the potential role of socioeconomic status and discrimination, and contributes to the stereotyping and stigmatisation of minority ethnic populations as culturally deviant or inferior (Gerrish 2000).

Researchers must therefore recognise the multifaceted nature of ethnicity and the varied ways in which health-related experiences and outcomes may be associated with ethnicity. It is useful to think of two broad modes of impact: first, the ways in which an individual's experience of their own ethnic identity informs their health-related attitudes, beliefs and behaviours (and thus their risks and responses to ill health); and second, the role of ethnic identification in processes of inclusion and exclusion that can importantly determine access to a wide range of resources relevant to health (including appropriate health services). Researchers must take care to 'unpack' the concept of ethnicity so that it is clear which of its various biosocial dimensions are being explored in their work. Furthermore, researchers need to recognise the dangers of conceptualising ethnicity in ways that inadequately capture its multi-faceted, dynamic and context-dependent nature.

Adopting this inherently reflexive approach to research on ethnicity and health will frequently require researchers to explore not only the implications of ethnic identities for health experiences and outcomes, but also the mechanisms through which ethnic identification occurs (at both the inter-personal level and between groups within society at large). As Gunaratnam (2003) argues, researchers need to ask questions about why and how ethnic categories, such as 'Chinese', come to stand for diverse groups of people, and what implications this labelling and homogenisation has for people's lives.

IDENTIFYING A RESEARCH FOCUS

Before embarking on the details of study design, we suggest that researchers should give careful consideration to whether or not attention to ethnicity is warranted within a particular study. Clearly, there are some research issues in which ethnic identity is unlikely to play a role, such as studies exploring the functioning of a new medical device or the effects of new technologies on healthcare policies. There may also be reasons for excluding attention to ethnicity in some studies on the grounds of cost and/or complexity. However, since ethnicity is such an important axis of identity and inequality in contemporary societies there are unlikely to be convincing arguments for overlooking ethnicity in most areas of nursing research.

Where the broad topic of inquiry makes a compelling case for paying attention to ethnicity, the researcher then needs to carefully consider how to focus the research. As Johnson notes:

> 'from the perspective of minority populations there may be both "too much" research – insofar as their particular ('peculiar') specific characteristics may attract research attention that is unwelcome or serves to stigmatise their community – or "too little", insofar as they may be excluded from research that has measureable benefits or informs policy and practice shaping the provision of services they want or need' (Johnson 2006: 49)

Framing research questions in such a way that the knowledge generated contributes positively to understanding and tackling ethnic inequalities in health requires careful thought. Key issues to consider include the following.

- Does the study aim to explore processes of ethnic identification (how and why individuals identify themselves and others as belonging to particular ethnic groups in particular contexts)?
- Does the framing of the research avoid presenting ethnic categories as taken for granted, natural or neutral?
- Does the research aim to describe differences between ethnic groups?
- Does the study hope to go further and seek to explore the possible reasons behind differences between ethnic groups?
- Does the study seek to identify similarities as well as differences across ethnic groups?
- Does the research focus too narrowly on any particular dimension(s) of ethnicity thereby closing off potentially important avenues of investigation?
- Does the research over-emphasise ethnicity to the exclusion of other aspects of identity and difference, such as gender, age, social class and so on?

More fundamentally, researchers must ask themselves whether their focus is important and meaningful to those who are the subject of the research. Engagement with people from minority ethnic backgrounds can help ensure that research is adequately informed by the experiences and perspectives of these groups. However, this requires careful planning to achieve adequate representation of diverse views and experiences, cultural sensitivity and meaningful involvement (Johnson 2006).

ETHNIC CATEGORIES AND LABELS

In studies that gather new data, the researcher must decide how to operationalise, or measure, ethnicity within their research. Studies that explore ethnic identification as a process will need to examine the multiple and diverse constructions of ethnicity and will most often employ qualitative, inductive approaches (though some quantitative studies have offered important insights; see, for example, Karlsen 2004). In such studies the researcher will generally avoid the use of predetermined, fixed ethnic categories and will instead operationalise ethnicity as a fluid property of individuals and groups. Nevertheless, there is clearly a need to start somewhere and, in most studies, to identify potential respondents who might be included as sources of data. For this reason, researchers will often be guided by what Mason (2002) calls 'real-life' categories – using, for instance, self-reported religion or ethnicity, physical appearance or perhaps membership of an ethnically affiliated organisation, to identify a selection of respondents who seem likely to have a range of relevant social positions and experiences.

Studies that seek to understand ethnicity as a potentially important determinant of health experiences and outcomes tend to be framed differently. Here the focus is usually on the characteristics, outcomes or experiences of a set of individuals categorised as belonging to an ethnic 'group'. Frequently, comparisons are made between two or more such 'groups', and these can be useful in identifying areas of inequality or minority ethnic disadvantage. These studies usually need to operationalise ethnicity as a discrete categorical variable, and this can be challenging for those researchers who regard ethnicity as a fluid and context-specific concept. Furthermore, attempts at categorisation and the labels employed vary over time and place, calling into question their meaningfulness, and making comparison and synthesis of findings from different studies difficult. However, while accepting that ethnic classifications will *always* be crude, researchers can nonetheless seek to identify the best available categorisation for the study in hand (Ellison 2005).

It is important to consider the extent to which the categories chosen can serve as adequate proxies for the components of interest in the current study (whether cultural, sociopolitical and/or genealogical factors). As such, it should be recognised that particular categorisations will have utility in some research studies but be less helpful in others. For instance, Bhopal *et al.* (1991) argue that the collective ethnic category 'Asian' or 'South Asian' is inappropriate for understanding coronary heart disease risk and treatment in the UK and can lead to false interpretations, advocating instead the use of the more refined categories: Indian, Pakistani and Bangladeshi. In contrast, Ali *et al.* (2006) in their study of patient–general practitioner interactions employed the grouping 'South Asian' and found that the 'finer distinctions' of Indian, Pakistani and Bangladeshi were neither relevant nor necessary within the context of their study.

Notwithstanding the observation that some categorisations will be more or less useful depending on the research topic, any attempt at categorising ethnicity will not get over the fundamental tension that exists in 'fixing' socially mediated categories that are inherently complex and variable.

In many instances, researchers interested in exploring ethnic variation in health and healthcare will be forced to rely on secondary data collected using standardised and statutory classifications, categories and labels (such as those developed for use in the 2001 UK Census, see Box 5.3). When undertaking new data collection more options are available, but there will be pros and cons to adopting bespoke, rather than standard, classifications.

The disadvantages of standardised schemes include the fact that they may not be precise measures of the key dimension(s) of ethnicity that the study aims to examine, or they may not be sufficiently refined to differentiate between important ethnic subgroupings (such as those with different religious, socioeconomic or ancestral characteristics). For instance, the category 'Black African' frequently employed in UK

Box 5.3   Measurement of ethnic group in the UK Census

The most recent census in the UK, carried out in 2001, asked people the following questions.

What is your ethnic group?
Choose ONE section from A to E then tick the appropriate box to indicate your cultural background.

A White

☐ British   ☐ Irish
☐ Any other White background (please write in).

B Mixed

☐ White and Black Caribbean,   ☐ White and Black African,   ☐ White and Asian
☐ Any other Mixed background (please write in).

C Asian or Asian British

☐ Indian   ☐ Pakistani   ☐ Bangladeshi
☐ Any other Asian background (please write in).

D Black or Black British

☐ Caribbean   ☐ African
☐ Any other Black background (please write in).

E Chinese or other ethnic group

☐ Chinese
☐ Any other (please write in).

Questions were also asked on religion and country of birth.
Adapted from information provided by the Office for National Statistics, www.statistics.gov.uk/

national surveys has doubtful utility in many contexts because of the substantial heterogeneity with respect to national origins, religion and language concealed within (Aspinall & Chinouya 2008). However, statutory categories have often gone through substantial testing and development to ensure that they are both acceptable and meaningful to respondents, a factor that may be worth bearing in mind in terms of how research findings are received and acted on. Moreover, statutory classifications and categories are often used by a large number of studies and agencies, and there-

fore facilitate comparisons. However, when studies (only) use these types of classifications, they are generally constrained in the analyses and explanations they can offer.

A final issue for consideration is how ethnic category should be assigned. An individual's self-reported ethnicity will best reflect their own perceptions of who they are, and some would argue is the only ethical way to measure ethnicity. Nonetheless, assignment of ethnicity by a third party may be appropriate, particularly when the focus of study is how one person's view of other people's ethnicity (e.g. a health-care practitioner's view of a patient's ethnicity) affects the way they treat those people.

Regardless of the exact approach to categorisation and labelling adopted, it is important to be explicit about the methods employed and their rationale, so that any inherent problems and potential limitations are clearly articulated.

SAMPLING

Researchers interested in exploring the ways in which health experiences and outcomes are influenced by ethnicity will commonly engage with individual people – be they patients, providers or members of the public – to elicit data that are relevant to their focus of inquiry. Though the logic behind sampling in qualitative and quantitative research is very different, the approaches share important elements. First, the sample's purpose is to provide access to data that will allow the research questions identified to be answered. Second, a sample must have an explicit and meaningful link with a 'wider universe' – a larger population to which the results of the research can then be applied. Third, as Mason (2002) notes, the drawing of a sample implies that other selections would have been possible and therefore demands a clear rationale for why that particular sample was chosen. Sampling must therefore link clearly to both the study's research questions and any planned analyses.

As suggested above, studies that seek to understand *processes* of ethnic identification will usually adopt sampling strategies that access a diverse range of individuals capable of capturing the full scope of ethnic identity as understood and experienced by the populations of interest. Such sampling schemes tend not to be fixed but rather are flexible and involve the selection of participants in a purposive, non-random manner. Often data analysis and theory building take place alongside data collection, so that new participants are chosen intentionally to fill gaps in understanding or to test out emerging hypotheses from the data gathered so far.

Studies that are framed more in terms of describing the experiences and circumstances of delineated ethnic groups and those that aim to explain any differences (or similarities) found between these groups, can essentially adopt one of three different sampling strategies: exclusive, comparative or representative.

Exclusive sampling strategies aim to recruit participants from just one ethnic group and can be justified on two grounds: first, for studies that aim to generate evidence on an issue that only, or disproportionately, affects the population concerned; and second, for studies that aim to generate evidence for an ethnic group that has not previously been adequately studied with regard to the topic concerned. In quantitative work, such exclusive samples should be representative of the wider population that could be categorised as belonging to the specific ethnic group concerned. In qualitative work, the exclusive sample drawn will relate to the wider ethnic group in a more theoretical or interpretive way. Bearing in mind the tendency for research to stereotype and homogenise the experiences of minority ethnic groups, exclusive qualitative samples will often usefully aim to capture a diverse set of respondents.

Comparative sampling strategies aim to recruit participants from two or more ethnic groups to assess any similarities and differences in the outcome of interest (e.g. health or healthcare) among different ethnic groups. An important consideration in such quantitative designs is the need to ensure that the ethnic categories used are equally diverse, capture an equivalent focus on ethnic identity (and on the cultural, sociopolitical and/or genealogical dimensions of ethnicity) and that the samples of each are of a comparable size. These are complicated technical issues that need not undermine simple *descriptive* comparisons, but are worthy of consideration by a qualified statistician when designing studies that aim to explore causal relations between health/healthcare and ethnicity. Similar concerns arise in qualitative work when comparisons are drawn between predefined ethnic groups that do not necessarily include individuals with uniform or meaningful experiences, and thereby lead to misleading or partial interpretations. However, the qualitative researcher has greater flexibility to investigate ethnic group identification and, if appropriate, to modify the sampling strategy as analysis proceeds. For instance, a study initially designed as a comparison between two ethnic groups might, as analyses proceed, be reconfigured as a three-way comparison if the findings reveal important unforeseen diversity within one of the groups as originally delineated. Such a development in theory might lead to subsequent sampling of respondents to allow further investigation of these intra-group differences.

Comparative sampling strategies, whether qualitative or quantitative, also need to generate an equivalent volume of data relating to each of the ethnic groups of interest to ensure that any comparisons are not compromised by spurious or inaccurate findings that more often arise with smaller samples. Quantitative surveys often include so-called 'boosted' samples to generate adequate data for minority ethnic 'groups'. Researchers using comparative sampling also need to consider how many different ethnic groups to include. Qualitative studies should generally not try to include too wide a range of ethnic groups because they are likely to provide greater clarity and depth of understanding when fewer categories are considered (Atkin & Chattoo 2006). Practical considerations may also limit the number of groups that a quantitative study can sample, particularly since costs can be considerable when seeking to generate 'boosted' samples from small and geographically dispersed populations.

Finally, representative sampling strategies aim to ensure that the ethnic diversity found within the study's sample is the same as that found in the wider target population to which the study's results are intended to apply. This notion is fundamental to quantitative research and researchers should strive to ensure that their sampling strategies generate samples that are representative of their target population. However, the fluid and context-specific nature of ethnicity means that careful consideration should also be given to specifying the target population to which findings can be most safely extrapolated (for instance in terms of geographical location). A final word of caution is also offered. Representative samples from ethnically diverse populations will ordinarily include participants from a range of different ethnic groups and it is important to recognise that samples of this sort are often inappropriate to use for comparative analyses. This is because, except in the case of extremely large study samples, representative sampling strategies inevitably generate samples of different ethnic groups that are of very different size with very different statistical power (see Chapter 36).

The principle that a sample should be empirically representative of the wider (target) population is rarely adopted by qualitative researchers on both theoretical and practical grounds. Nevertheless, qualitative researchers should consider whether their samples adequately offer the potential to generate data that are generalisable. Indeed, even when there is no intention to perform systematic comparative analyses across ethnic groups, it will often be desirable for qualitative work to generate findings that have a wider resonance with the diverse experiences of multi-ethnic communities.

DATA COLLECTION

Researchers have a wide range of methods to choose from when deciding how to generate the data needed to address the research questions at hand. Here we highlight some general issues relating to data generation that are worth considering when researching the field of ethnicity and health.

First, ethnicity is a multifaceted concept that can be a marker or proxy for a wide range of factors. Studies that seek to do more than simply document differences between ethnic groups will therefore need to adopt data generation methods that yield information on a variety of potentially important dimensions of ethnicity. In particular, there are concerns that health-related research has been poor at addressing the sociopolitical dimensions of ethnicity (including the effects of racism) (Gill *et al.* 2007), and that innovative tools are needed to effectively capture these dimensions (Gunaratnam 2007). Studies that exclude attention to particular dimensions of ethnicity run the risk of producing partial and superficial findings.

Second, ethnicity research will frequently imply the need for researchers to work across languages and cultural contexts. In quantitative work, careful attention is needed to ensure the equivalence of standardised measurement tools, and caution should be exercised when employing measures and tools for which cross-cultural/cross-language validity and reliability have not been established. Standard guidelines exist for translating between languages (Behling & Law 2000), and in general the focus should be on ensuring conceptual equivalence (Atkin & Chattoo 2006). We would strongly recommend the inclusion of multilingual researchers within the research team rather than reliance on interpreters and translators who are unfamiliar with the context and purpose of the research.

More generally, researchers must be alert to the possibility that their data-generation methods may operate differently among different sets of participants. For instance, methods that depend heavily on respondents' narratives may lead to erroneous interpretations if there is significant diversity in forms of expression among groups of study participants. Further, the identity of the researcher/data gatherer and their interactions with research participants deserve attention. Notions of 'insider' and 'outsider' status are complex and there are no simple rules regarding ethnic matching (Gunaratnam 2003). Indeed, the personal characteristics and skills of the data gatherer are likely to be just as important as any marker of social identity in gaining the trust of participants and generating credible findings.

DATA ANALYSIS AND INTERPRETATION

As we have seen, much health-related research that pays attention to ethnic diversity takes a comparative approach, often comparing outcomes and experiences of minority ethnic groups to the majority (usually the White or White British group). While this approach may be a useful way of flagging up inequalities, caution is needed in both the analytical procedures employed and the interpretations drawn.

First and foremost, researchers should recognise, and counter, any tendency for *associations* to be interpreted as *explanations*. It is important that analyses seek to identify underlying causal factors rather than simply inferring their existence. Where data on potential causal attributes are unavailable, analysis and interpretation must be cautious and speculative. It is also important that researchers are aware of factors that may be significant in shaping minority or

majority experiences but may be beyond the scope of their analysis (such as geographical concentration of particular ethnic groups, historical factors or wider social structures). As described earlier, researchers should recognise that analyses taking an ethnicity-focused approach may fail to capture the diversity of experiences *within* groups. In both qualitative and quantitative work it is useful to explore the ways in which other factors, such as age, gender, class and so on, inter-relate with ethnicity to create divergent experiences and circumstances within delineated groups.

Finally, it is important that analyses explore absolute levels of particular outcomes and experiences, in addition to relative differences between 'groups', and that comparisons are drawn with a range of 'groups' rather than with the majority/'White' category alone. This approach helps to avoid the tendency to overlook important issues facing minority ethnic 'groups' just because they are similar to those experienced by the majority 'White' group.

ETHICAL ISSUES

Many general issues of research ethics apply to research that gives attention to ethnicity. However, a further point worth emphasising is the potential for group harm that can ensue from research that includes minority ethnic individuals. Attention to this issue is warranted at all stages in the research cycle, but particular care is needed in the presentation and dissemination of findings. Researchers must be alert to, and should manage from the outset, the ways in which the findings of their work might be interpreted, distorted and (mis)used by the media and others – particularly in establishing or contributing to the stereotyping and stigmatisation of ethnic groups, and the threat of breaching the confidentiality of data collected from very small ethnic groups. Indeed, it has been argued that researchers should even consider withholding findings from dissemination where there is the potential for more harm than good to the individuals and communities represented.

In general, researchers should consider carefully the best way to represent and disseminate the findings of their research. As with all good research, it is important to ensure effective communication to all stakeholders, but particularly to ensure that the minority ethnic individuals and communities who are the subject of the research have ready access to the findings in a format that is accessible and relevant.

CONCLUSIONS

Many of the issues raised above are fundamental to sound research practice. Clear conceptualisation, careful measurement, strategic sampling, rigorous analyses and accurate representation are clearly generic elements of good research. However, the dangers of poor research are much greater when the focus of the research is ethnicity. Indeed, there are concerns that such research, if poorly executed, may do more harm than good. While there are no simple answers to some of the issues raised in this chapter, critical reflexivity and a cautious approach to interpretation can go a long way to improving the quality of research and the usefulness of findings.

We urge nursing researchers not to shy away from these complex and contentious issues, but rather to accept their responsibility to generate an evidence base that informs positive change in nursing policy and practice for all members of contemporary multiethnic societies.

References

Ali N, Atkin K, Neal RD (2006) The role of culture in the general practice consultation process. *Ethnicity and Health* **11**(4): 389–408.

Anthias F (2001) The concept of 'social division' and theorising social stratification: looking at ethnicity and class. *Sociology* **35**: 835–854.

Aspinall P, Anionwu E (2002) The role of ethnic monitoring in mainstreaming race equality and the modernization of the NHS: a neglected agenda? *Critical Public Health* **12**:1. Online document accessed on 23 January 2009 at *pdfserve.informaworld.com/185559_751317704_713658297.pdf*

Aspinall P, Chinouya M (2008) Is the standardised term 'Black African' useful in demographic and health research in the United Kingdom?' *Ethnicity & Health* **13**: 3183–3202.

Atkin K, Chattoo S (2006) Approaches to conducting qualitative research in ethnically diverse populations. In: Nazroo J (ed) *Health and Social Research in Multiethnic Populations*. Routledge, London, pp 95–115.

Behling O, Law KS (2000) *Translating Questionnaires and Other Research Instruments: Problems and Solutions*. London, Sage.

Bhopal RS, Unwin N, White M, Yallop J, Walker L, Alberti KGMM *et al.* (1991) Heterogeneity of coronary heart disease risk factors in Indian, Pakistani, Bangladeshi, and European origin populations: cross sectional study. *British Medical Journal* **319**: 215–220.

Culley L, Dyson S (2001) Introduction: sociology, ethnicity and nursing practice. In: Culley L, Dyson S (eds) *Ethnicity and Nursing Practice*. Basingstoke, Palgrave, pp 1–14.

Department of Health (2005) *Research Governance Framework for Health and Social Care*, 2nd edition. Online document accessed 10 June 2009 at www.dh.gov.uk/en/Publicationsandstatistics/Publications/PublicationsPolicyAndGuidance/DH_4108962

Department of Health (2003) *Tackling Health Inequalities*. London, HMSO.

Drevdahl DJ, Philips DA, Taylor JY (2006) Uncontested categories: the use of race and ethnicity variables in nursing research. *Nursing Inquiry* **13**(1): 52–63.

Ellison GTH (2005) 'Population profiling' and public health risk: when and how should we use race/ethnicity? *Critical Public Health* **15**: 65–74.

Eriksen TH (2002) *Ethnicity and Nationalism: anthropological perspectives*, 2nd edition. London, Pluto.

Gerrish K (2000) Researching ethnic diversity in the British NHS: methodological and practical concerns. *Journal of Advanced Nursing* **31**(4): 918–925.

Gill PS, Kai J, Bhopal RS, Wild S (2007) Black and minority ethnic groups. In: Stevens A, Raftery J, Mant J *et al.* (eds) *Health Care Needs Assessment: the epidemiologically based needs assessment reviews*. Abingdon, Radcliffe Publishing, pp 227–239.

Gunaratnam Y (2007) Complexity and complicity in researching ethnicity and health. In: Douglas J, Earle S, Handsley S, Lloyd C, Spurr S (eds) *A Reader in Promoting Public Health: challenge and controversy*. Basingstoke, Palgrave, pp 147–156.

Gunaratnam Y (2003) *Researching Race and Ethnicity: methods, knowledge and power*. London, Sage.

Henry L (2007) Institutionalized disadvantage: older Ghanaian nurses' and midwives' reflections on career progression and stagnation in the NHS. *Journal of Clinical Nursing* **16**: 2196–2203.

Hussain-Gambles M (2003) Ethnic minority under-representation in clinical trials: whose responsibility is it any way? *Journal of Health Organisation and Management* **17**(2): 138–143.

Johnson M (2006) Engaging communities and users: health and social care research with ethnic minority communities. In: Nazroo J (ed) *Health and Social Research in Multiethnic Populations*. Routledge, London, pp 48–64.

Karlsen S (2004) 'Black like Beckham'? Moving beyond definitions of ethnicity based on skin colour and ancestry. *Ethnicity & Health* **9**(2): 107–137.

Mason J (2002) *Qualitative Researching*. London, Sage.

Mulholland J, Dyson S (2001) Sociological theories of 'race' and ethnicity. In: Culley L, Dyson S (eds) *Ethnicity and Nursing Practice*. Basingstoke, Palgrave, pp 17–37.

Nazroo J (1997) *The Health of Britain's Ethnic Minorities*. London, PSI.

Papadopoulos I, Lees S (2002) Developing culturally competent researchers. *Journal of Advanced Nursing* **37**(3): 258–264.

Stubbs P (1993) 'Ethnically sensitive' or 'anti-racist'? Models for health research and service delivery. In: Ahmad WIU (ed) *'Race' and Health in Contemporary Britain*. Buckingham, Open University Press, pp 34–47.

Further reading

Nazroo J (2007) (ed) *Health and Social Research in Multiethnic Populations*. London, Routledge.

Websites

mighealth.net/index.php/Main_Page – information network on good practice in minority and migrant healthcare. The website aims to give professionals, policy makers, researchers, educators and representatives of migrant and minority groups easy access to an evolving body of knowledge and a virtual network of expertise on migrant health.

www.jiscmail.ac.uk/cgi-bin/webadmin?A0=MINORITY-ETHNIC-HEALTH – discussion list on minority ethnic health. This listserve is aimed at professionals working in the academic, NHS and local government sectors who seek to improve the health of minority ethnic communities in the UK via a multidisciplinary approach.

www.library.nhs.uk/ethnicity – NHS Evidence – ethnicity and health (formerly a Specialist Library of the National Library for Health). This site provides information on the best available evidence about management of healthcare services and specific needs in healthcare for migrant and minority ethnic groups.

www2.warwick.ac.uk/fac/med/research/csri/ethnicity-health/ – Centre for Evidence in Ethnicity, Health and Diversity (CEEHD) supports interdisciplinary, collaborative research in the field of ethnicity and health, working with NHS Trusts, community groups and other academic centres. The website contains various resources on the topic.

Preparing the Ground

At the beginning of any research enterprise, a considerable amount of work needs to be undertaken before the active stages of data collection and analysis can begin. This section deals with five major issues that require attention in the early stages of a research project, leading on to research design that will be the subject of Section 3.

Chapters 6 and 7 are linked, and draw on the discipline of information science. Chapter 6 takes the reader through the essential preparatory stage of reviewing existing evidence in the field of interest for research. Chapter 7 builds on this base using the now well-established science of critical appraisal and equipping the reader with tools with which to test the validity and applicability of published research to their own situation. It is impossible to overstate the importance of these preparatory stages in research; unless new knowledge is developed from a sound base of previous well-validated evidence, the credibility of nursing research will be called into question. More than this, those who implement research findings must also develop the skills of finding and appraising the evidence that is available.

Chapters 8, 9 and 10 are concerned with practical issues of preparing to undertake a specific project. Chapter 8 has been written by a new author for this edition, but as before, guides the reader through the formal process of writing a research proposal. The proposal might be for an academic dissertation or for a national funding body, but the process is the same in principle. Getting the proposal right is likely to make the difference between obtaining approval and funding or not, but writing the proposal also helps to clarify the researcher's thinking. Chapter 9 is newly written for this edition of the book, and deals with planning and managing a research project. The chapter focuses particularly on the needs of students pursuing higher degrees and their relationship with supervisors and other sources of support. Many of the users of this book will be engaged in research in the course of academic study and will find this chapter a valuable source of advice. Chapter 10 completes the section by discussing in detail the complex process of obtaining formal permissions for research and the regulatory frameworks that exist in the UK for research in health and social care. No research project that takes place in a healthcare context in the UK can proceed without going through the ethical and governance approval procedures, and successful negotiation of the regulations depends on careful and informed preparation and planning.

6 Finding the Evidence

Claire Beecroft, Andrew Booth and Angie Rees

Key points

- Effective literature searching is an essential skill for research, audit and evidence-based practice in nursing.

- The research literature consists of journals, reports, theses, conference proceedings, government publications and web-based resources.

- Much literature searching now uses electronic databases and the internet.

- A focused question is important in developing a good literature search.

- High-quality sources of evidence include systematic reviews and evidence syntheses.

- Reference management skills are important when writing a literature review.

INTRODUCTION

As the nursing and healthcare literature grows, so does the need for individuals to acquire and maintain the skills to search it effectively. Increasingly, nursing education programmes are including teaching on literature searching and its application to evidence-based practice – demonstrating the increasing importance being placed on these skills (Mohide & Matthew-Maich 2007). While databases such as CINAHL (the Cumulative Index to Nursing and Allied Health) continue to be key for those seeking to access the nursing and healthcare literature, resources such as the Cochrane Library (www.thecochranelibrary.com) now complement traditional information sources.

The nursing literature is expanding rapidly as more nurses are encouraged to become involved in research (Purkis *et al.* 2008). Searching the literature is also essential when developing policy, evaluating practice or attempting to implement change. When auditing a service, up-to-date, high-quality evidence is required on which to base the proposed standards. So, consider the ability to search the literature as a skill to support you throughout your career and to enhance your life-long learning.

ELECTRONIC INFORMATION RESOURCES AND THE INTERNET

Recent years have seen dramatic increases in access to the internet by healthcare staff. It is now recognised that all staff need to be able to access the necessary resources if they are to obtain timely, high-quality information to support clinical effectiveness and evidence-based practice. UK National Health Service staff have access via the internet to a host of specialist resources developed to meet their needs via the national NHS Evidence – Health Information Resources (www.library.nhs.uk). Such resources underpin the use of high-quality research. Before carrying out any research you should undertake a systematic search of the literature to identify previous studies that are similar or identical to the proposed study.

In this chapter, the 'internet' is not considered as an information source in itself; strictly speaking, it is primarily a means of delivering access to information. The internet, while undoubtedly useful, is unsystematic and provides materials of variable quality. However, once a useful report or journal article has been identified it is worth checking to see whether the internet provides access to this specific item.

THE RESEARCH LITERATURE

We have already referred to the 'research literature', but it is important to be aware of the full range of literature available to support research and practice. The word 'evidence' is now widely used to describe the information on which clinical decisions should be based, and this evidence comes from a variety of sources (Ehrlich-Jones *et al.* 2008). Below we consider some key forms of 'evidence'.

Journals and journal articles

Journals and journal articles perhaps come to mind first when thinking about the 'research literature'. Journals not only contain research (such as clinical trials), but also opinion, editorials, letters, case studies and reports. All contribute evidence to support practice and research. However, background questions such as general information on a disease or condition may best be answered from a current textbook. Knowledge in journal articles tends to be specialised rather than general.

Most of the key health and social care databases now offer increasing numbers of articles electronically as full text. With a few clicks of a mouse you can move from the database results to the full version of an article. This potentially saves a visit to the library and the effort of photocopying articles that have been identified.

Books

While books are not always sufficiently up to date to support research they can provide useful background information to assist in developing a research question. Many library users enjoy browsing the shelves to find books of interest, but electronic library catalogues now feature in most health libraries. These enable relevant books to be identified much more efficiently.

Reports

In addition to research published in journals, some research findings are published as reports. Research reports may yield useful facts and figures such as statistics and cost data and thus complement information from books and journals. Bear in mind that some research that has not been successful in getting published in the journal literature may be issued as a report as a 'last resort', so quality may be variable. However, reports are not included in many of the major databases such as MEDLINE. It is possible to identify reports using specialist databases such as the Health Management Information Consortium (HMIC) database or by searching appropriate internet sites.

Theses

Theses are usually the end product of research degrees either at master's or doctoral level. They provide an extensive record of a student's research project and are therefore considerably longer than most journal articles. To identify relevant theses, major databases and specialised sources such as *Dissertation Abstracts* (an electronic database of abstracts for theses) and *Index to Theses* need to be searched. Most university libraries hold an extensive collection of theses by their own students so are a good place to look.

Conference proceedings

Papers presented by speakers at a conference are often collected together and published either in print or electronic form as 'Conference Proceedings'. This allows those not at the conference to read through the papers that were presented. Conferences are frequently used as a forum for presenting the results of ongoing or recently completed research. They can therefore provide up-to-date information if proceedings are published soon after the conference has ended. Not all papers presented at a conference are necessarily included in the proceedings – sometimes a peer-review process will approve those papers to be included. Bear in mind too that less than half of all conference abstracts result in published papers (Scherer *et al.* 2007) and, even when they do, there may be inconsistencies between interim results and what is ultimately printed (Toma *et al.* 2006). Conference proceedings are often referenced in the main databases (such as MEDLINE and CINAHL). If you are trying to locate the proceedings of a particular conference, it might be worth searching the internet to see if the conference has a website, as proceedings are sometimes published in this way.

Government circulars

Circulars are published by governmental departments, groups and committees. Such documents are usually available via the relevant government department's website, such as the UK Department of Health's publications site (www.dh.gov.uk/publications), though a health library may maintain a small print collection.

Grey literature

'Grey literature' describes literature, ranging from pamphlets and leaflets to governmental or health service documents, which is often not collected by libraries and is frequently not referenced in electronic databases (Conn *et al.* 2003). The key characteristic of this literature is that it is elusive and fugitive. Again, the internet has made such literature easier to identify and obtain. Specialist databases, such as HMIC (available via NHS Evidence Health Information Resources) and OpenSIGLE (http://opensigle.inist.fr/), offer access to selected grey literature. Local health library staff are able to identify available resources to locate grey literature.

ACCESSING THE LITERATURE

The existence of the internet has resulted in major changes in not only how the literature is accessed, but also where it can be accessed from, be that in the workplace or at home. Many resources discussed earlier can now be accessed in electronic format. Clearly, information technology skills are an important factor in how an individual searches the available literature, so both traditional and modern methods will be examined.

Finding the nearest/best library

Most health organisations maintain their own libraries and additionally many negotiate 'access agreements' with local libraries to complement their own resources. However, certain services, such as printing, borrowing materials or photocopying, may be unavailable or only available on a fee-paying basis. If you are unsure of what services are available, enquire at the nearest hospital-based library. Training in the use of electronic resources is usually provided, either as hands-on practical sessions, e-learning modules, lectures or on a one-to-one basis.

Going further afield

Some of the above resources may not be available via a local library. In going further afield, there are three main things to consider

- Are the cost of services such as photocopying and printing affordable if they are not provided free?
- How feasible is it to travel to use the library?
- How can the best use be made of libraries that are not nearby?

Making sure that resources you are seeking further afield are not available locally prevents wasting valuable time.

National/international electronic resources

Many public healthcare systems fund access to major electronic databases, journals and books. For example the NHS Evidence Health Information Resources (www.library.nhs.uk) offers access to a variety of databases that match the needs of staff in the NHS. You should also bear in mind that some nursing organisations provide access to databases and/or electronic journals. For instance, the Royal College of Nursing provides its members with electronic access to a core collection of nursing and health-related journals. Key international databases available online via the NHS Evidence Health Information Resources include the following.

- AMED: an allied and complementary medicine database compiled by the British Library, with references from nearly 600 journals.
- CINAHL: the Cumulative Index to Nursing and Allied Health has references to almost all English-language journals in the nursing and allied health literature, plus conference proceedings and reports. It is the most comprehensive nursing database.
- MEDLINE: a major medical database of more than 16 million records, with references from more than 3,900 journals, covering a broad and expanding range of medical specialities. It also includes some references to conference proceedings
- EMBASE: similar to MEDLINE but with an emphasis on drugs and pharmacology, and superior coverage of European publications. It has references from more than 3,500 journals and also includes some references to books and conference proceedings.
- PsycINFO: this specialised database covers psychology and allied fields. It contains references from more than 1,900 journals plus

books, reports, etc. Ninety-eight percent of journals indexed are peer reviewed.
- HMIC: a database produced jointly by the King's Fund and the UK Department of Health. It contains references to health and social care management literature, including journal articles, conference proceedings, grey literature and policy documents.

In addition to the databases provided by the NHS Evidence Health Information Resources, nurses may also find the following databases useful. All of these databases are web-based, free to access and do not require a login or password.

- Social Care Online (www.scie-socialcareonline. org.uk/): this database abstracts social work and social care literature. It contains more than 75,000 references to books, journal articles, government reports, etc. The database covers English language publications from the UK, North America and beyond.
- PubMed (www.pubmed.com): is produced in the US by the National Library of Medicine and is a search interface to a collection of databases, the key database being MEDLINE. Although PubMed has powerful searching facilities, you will generally find it more useful to use locally available commercial versions of MEDLINE, particularly if you require links to full-text journal subscriptions held by your local library.
- Cochrane Library (www.thecochranelibrary. com): more details about the Cochrane Library are provided later in this chapter. It is not a single database but a collection of databases that can be searched simultaneously. It is an essential source for information on the effectiveness and cost-effectiveness of healthcare interventions.
- OpenSIGLE (http://opensigle.inist.fr/): is the System for Information on Grey Literature in Europe. It contains references to research reports, dissertations and policy documents from European countries.

Information about access to other databases, e-journals and e-books can be obtained from a local health library.

Access to PCs

PCs are normally available in wards and hospital libraries, or via local research and development offices or postgraduate education centres. Booking in advance is wise as it may save a wasted trip.

PLANNING A LITERATURE SEARCH

Planning a literature search is vital and yet this stage is often neglected. Remember, much time and effort can be saved by planning a search strategy before you begin searching. Furthermore, such planning will dramatically improve the quality of the search.

The importance of a focused search question

A focused search question is critical when searching the literature (Cleary-Holdforth & Leufer 2008). If the question is not sufficiently focused you will find yourself wrestling with large sets of mostly irrelevant search results. A focused question helps to ensure that the search is precise and accurate and that you are able to manage the volume of literature rather than drowning in it (McKibbon & Marks 2001).

The anatomy of a question

It is helpful to develop a focused question using one of the available models (see PICO or SPICE below). These will assist you in planning the search strategy.

PICO

The PICO model is an acronym made up as follows (Stone 2002).

- **P**atient/Problem (e.g. common cold)
- **I**ntervention/Exposure (e.g. vitamin C supplements)
- **C**omparison (e.g. no vitamin C supplements)
- **O**utcome (e.g. reduced incidence of common cold)

PICO works well for questions about healthcare interventions. Once the four elements to the question are identified, the next step is to make a list of all the words and phrases needed to search for each PICO element. Remember to think of synonyms, alternative spellings and plurals. Box 6.1 provides an illustration of the PICO model. Within the specific context of systematic reviews, where you also need to identify the types of study required to answer the review question, you will frequently see PICO become PICOS where the additional **S** is used to designate **S**tudy design (see Chapter 24).

Box 6.1 Illustration of the PICO model

Patient/Problem	Intervention/Exposure	Comparison	Outcome
Cold/s Common cold/s	Vitamin C Ascorbic acid	Placebo	Prevention Prevents Preventative Incidence

There will be many additional terms, so Box 6.1 is a simplified version. Under the 'comparison' heading the term 'placebo' (i.e. vitamin C is being compared with no treatment) is provided as a suggestion. The 'comparison' element of PICO is sometimes implicit and it may be possible to obtain a good set of results by simply identifying the other elements and then combining them.

SPICE

The SPICE model is a useful alternative to the PICO model for questions that relate to qualitative methodologies or the social sciences. Using a similar format to PICO, the SPICE model breaks a search question down into the following.

- **S**etting (e.g. general practice)
- **P**erspective (e.g. smokers)
- **I**ntervention (e.g. smoking cessation advice)
- **C**omparison (e.g. variation from patient to patient)
- **E**valuation (e.g. reasons for giving/not giving advice)

As Box 6.2 illustrates, it is not necessary to identify terms for all aspects of the SPICE model to produce a useful list of terms and a search strategy. In this example combining the terms from the 'S' 'P' and 'I' sections may be sufficient to find relevant articles. Adding additional terms from the 'E' section might help to identify papers that investigate how GPs decide to provide or not provide smoking cessation advice to smokers. A search using just the S' 'P' and 'I' sections of this strategy retrieves the article from MEDLINE shown in Research Example 6.1.

Clearly, analysing the information using these models helps to produce a more relevant set of results. Once the PICO or SPICE model has been developed, each element is searched *separately* and then each search statement is combined to produce a smaller set of results using Boolean operators.

Boolean operators

Boolean operators are simply the words 'AND', 'OR' and 'NOT' that are used to combine search concepts. Box 6.3 shows how they work for the example given earlier.

When using the 'OR' operator you are asking the database to identify papers that feature either of the terms you have searched. In the example above, the 'Patient' element retrieves papers that contain the word 'cold' or the phrase 'common cold', as both could be relevant. Similarly for the Intervention, 'ascorbic acid' is a synonym for 'vitamin C', so 'OR' is used to find papers that feature either term. When combining across PICO elements the 'AND' operator is used. When combining the Patient and Intervention columns we are instructing the database to find papers featuring the terms 'cold' OR 'common cold' AND also the terms 'vitamin c' OR 'ascorbic acid' within the same paper.

Box 6.2   Illustration of the SPICE model

Setting	Perspective	Intervention	Comparison	Evaluation
General Practice	Smokers	Advice	No terms required	Motivation?
Primary care	Smoking	Support		Selection?
Family Practice		Counselling		Reason?
				Choice?

RESEARCH EXAMPLE

6.1   A Medline Abstract

Authors

Murray, Rachael L; Coleman, Timothy; Antoniak, Marilyn; Stocks, Joanne; Fergus, Alexia; Britton, John; Lewis, Sarah A

Institution

Division of Epidemiology and Public Health, University of Nottingham, Nottingham, UK; rachael.murray@nottingham.ac.uk

Title

The effect of proactively identifying smokers and offering smoking cessation support in primary care populations: a cluster-randomised trial

Source

Addiction **103**(6): 998–1006; discussion 1007–8 (Jun 2008)

Abstract

Aims: To establish whether proactively identifying all smokers in primary care populations and offering smoking cessation support is effective in increasing long-term abstinence from smoking. **Design:** Cluster randomised controlled trial. **Setting:** Twenty-four general practices in Nottinghamshire, randomised by practice to active or control intervention. **Participants:** All adult patients registered with the practices who returned a questionnaire confirming that they were current smokers (n = 6856). **Intervention:** Participants were offered smoking cessation support by letter and those interested in receiving it were contacted and referred into National Health Service (NHS) stop smoking services if required. **Measurements:** Validated abstinence from smoking, use of smoking cessation services and number of quit attempts in continuing smokers at 6 months. **Findings:** Smokers in the intervention group were more likely than controls to report that they had used local cessation services during the study period [16.6% and 8.9%, respectively, adjusted odds ratio (OR) 2.09, 95% confidence interval (CI) 1.57–2.78], and continuing smokers (in the intervention group) were more likely to have made a quit attempt in the last 6 months (37.4% and 33.3%, respectively, adjusted OR 1.23, 95% CI 1.01–1.51). Validated point prevalence abstinence from smoking at 6 months was higher in the intervention than the control groups (3.5% and 2.5%, respectively), but the difference was not statistically significant (adjusted OR controlling for covariates: 1.64, 95% CI 0.92–2.89). **Conclusions:** Proactively identifying smokers who want to quit in primary care populations, and referring them to a cessation service, increased contacts with cessation services and the number of quit attempts. We were unable to detect a significant effect on long-term cessation rates, but the study was not powered to detect the kind of difference that might be expected.

Box 6.3 Example of Boolean operators

Patient/Problem		Intervention/Exposure		Comparison		Outcome
cold/s		Vitamin C		placebo		prevention
or		or				or
common cold/s		Ascorbic acid				prevents
	and		**and**		**and**	or
						preventative
						or
						incidence

SEARCHING THE LITERATURE

Electronic searching

Despite differences between databases in terms of interfaces and search terminologies, many key techniques are common to many different databases. Once you have mastered these techniques on one database it becomes correspondingly easier to approach the next one (Poynton 2003).

Free-text searching

Most databases allow you to type in words and phrases and search for references that feature those terms in the title, abstract, authors, journal name, etc. This is how most people instinctively search databases, but it has its drawbacks. As mentioned above, you need to be able to think of all the synonyms and alternative spellings for each term to be sure not to miss anything important. 'Truncation' is a technique that saves time when typing in variations of a word. Most databases allow you to enter a truncation mark (often a $ or a *) after a word stem. For instance, if you want to search for:

- prevent
- prevents
- prevention
- preventative

you can simply enter Prevent$ (or Prevent* depending on the database) to find all the above words.

It is important to note that such a search will generate numerous results that make a fleeting reference to the search term but are not fundamentally about that subject. The abstract in Research Example 6.2, found by searching MEDLINE for the free-text terms 'vitamin C' and 'cold', illustrates this. Although vitamin C and cold are mentioned in the abstract, this paper is not about these subjects but is using an analogy about how regulation of telemedicine is as annoying as a common cold.

Subject headings

Due to the limitations of free-text searching, it may be necessary to search for subject headings that relate to the topic. Subject headings are standardised terms used to describe the content of an article. They enable searchers to avoid typing multiple terms for the same subject, as a single subject heading is assigned to replace them all. For instance, for a free text search for papers about 'vitamin C', you would need to enter all of the following terms (and possibly others):

- vitamin C
- ascorbic acid
- hybrin
- l-ascorbic acid.

6.2 A Retrieval Error from MEDLINE

Bilimoria NM (2003) Telemedicine: laws still need a dose of efficiency. *Journal of Medical Practice Management* **18**(6): 289–294.

RESEARCH EXAMPLE

Ever have a **cold** that just won't go away? You try lozenges, **vitamin C**, and a humidifier. Nothing seems to work. Telemedicine still has the same **cold** today in the form of laws and regulations that make the practice of telemedicine onerous. The best a health practitioner can do today is weather the **cold** that plagues telemedicine and make the best of it until legislators and regulators work on solutions to remove the barriers to effective telemedicine practice. This article provides a view of the landscape of telemedicine law today, outlines the barriers to the effective practice of telemedicine and offers strategic concerns for health care providers to consider before entering into telemedicine arrangements.

However, indexers may assign a single subject heading 'ascorbic acid' to describe all papers about this subject, regardless of the terminology used by the authors. Once a paper has been assigned a list of subject headings, the terms that describe the main concepts of the paper are emphasised as 'major subject headings'. Several subject heading systems are used by health-related databases. The most well known is MeSH (Medical Subject Headings), used by the US National Library of Medicine for the MEDLINE database.

Limiting searches

Once you have completed initial free-text and subject heading searches you may wish to limit your results set further. Typical limits include the following.

- Age: to restrict the search to patients within certain age groups.
- Language: to confine the search to publications in a specified language.
- Date range: to identify papers that have been published in the past few years, or if historical articles are required.
- Full text: to limit the search to papers available in full to print or download.

Limits are a useful way of making the results set more focused and smaller. They should be used with caution to ensure that relevant material is not missed.

Grey literature

A good starting point for health-related grey literature is the homepage of a national governmental health department, such as the Department of Health (www.dh.gov.uk) in England or the US Department of Health and Human Services (www.hhs.gov). In terms of electronic databases, in addition to HMIC (mentioned earlier), there is the OpenSIGLE (System for Information on Grey Literature in Europe) database. Ask at your local health library about access to these databases or to others that they can recommend.

Manual searching

Some techniques used for manually searching the literature are mentioned earlier in this chapter. These are particularly useful when searching for grey literature which often 'slips through the net' of the major electronic databases.

Journal indexes

Many journals produce an annual printed index to help users find the articles they need. This is published either as a separate volume or in the back of the last issue of a volume or year. The index usually enables a reader to look up articles by a particular author or that contain a specific keyword. These indexes are useful if you wish to browse a key journal in a subject area but do not want to go through each table of contents individually.

Reference lists

It is useful to search through the lists of references of any relevant articles that you have found. When a useful reference has been identified this way, it is worth trying to retrieve the reference from databases you have already searched to identify why it was not found by your search strategies. It will also allow you to read the abstract for the paper and helps you to decide whether the paper is worth obtaining.

Tables of contents

For journals that do not produce an annual index, the best alternative is to browse tables of contents. This can be a lengthy process so you will need to target key journals in your subject area and simply read through the titles in the table of contents of each issue to find relevant articles.

Further help with literature searching

Literature searching is an important skill for nurses to develop. This chapter has attempted to introduce the key concepts and methods, but you will need to seek further assistance. Always ask for help from your local health library or the research support facilities in your area. In the UK, NHS regional Research Design Services (RDSs) for the National Institute for Health Research (NIHR) (www.nihr.ac.uk/) provide a range of services to NHS staff involved in research, including support for literature searching. Your NHS trust Research and Development Office should be able to provide information about available support.

SPECIALIST INFORMATION SOURCES

'Digested' forms of evidence: reviews and syntheses

While there is a wealth of literature available to help nurses answer clinical questions, it is often difficult and time-consuming to wade through the enormous quantities of studies published. One approach is to limit a search to a particular type of study design (Littleton *et al.* 2004; Flemming & Briggs 2007).

However, even within one study design studies will vary considerably in quality, due to such factors as poor resourcing, inappropriate methodology, etc. The need to provide healthcare professionals with reliable evidence on which to base decisions has led to the increasing importance of published reviews (Docherty 2003). Reviews aim to bring together and 'digest' a body of research on a subject and find common themes in the results, enabling the reviewer to draw conclusions for their proposed research question. Broadly speaking there are two different types of review, 'traditional' and 'systematic'.

Traditional reviews take many forms, but they are usually highly selective in the literature that is reviewed. For instance, in a literature review, a reviewer may include only papers published in the past year or in certain key journals. Reviews such as this are useful for keeping up to date and managing the volume of literature in a subject area, as they provide a brief summing-up of several papers in a single article.

Systematic reviews are the focus of Chapter 24. They are the 'gold standard' research method for reviewing the literature on effectiveness in healthcare. They aim to bring the same rigour and discipline that characterises primary research to the review process, leaving a reproducible audit trail of methods. Systematic reviews are often, though not always, characterised by the presence of 'meta analysis': a combination of statistical techniques enabling the reviewer to produce an overall estimate of the results of the individual studies. They are mentioned here as an invaluable starting point for your own research.

Cochrane Library

The Cochrane Library is produced by the Cochrane Collaboration, an international organisation comprising numerous subject-specific groups conducting systematic reviews in their topic areas. The Cochrane Library comprises seven different databases. The most prominent of these is the Cochrane Database of Systematic Reviews (CDSR), which contains reviews undertaken by the Cochrane Collaboration. Other databases include the Cochrane Central Register of Controlled Trials containing randomised controlled trials used in Cochrane systematic reviews. This database is now considered the single best source of information on controlled trials of quality. The Cochrane Library also includes a database of appraised reviews *not* produced by the Cochrane Collaboration, the Database of Abstracts of Reviews of Effects (DARE).

Evidence-based journals

The number of journals devoted to summarising key research findings has grown significantly in recent years. The BMJ Publishing Group alone numbers three such titles, *Evidence-Based Medicine, Evidence-Based Mental Health* and *Evidence-Based Nursing*. Digests of systematic reviews, reviews and meta-analysis such as *Bandolier* (www.medicine.ox.ac.uk/bandolier/) make the findings from research even more accessible. Another journal that will be of interest to nurses is *World Views on Evidence-Based Nursing*.

Web 2.0 technologies

Increasingly, web 2.0 technologies are used to disseminate research and popularise evidence-based practice. An excellent example is the 'Nursing Research: Show me the evidence!' blog from St Joseph's Hospital, California, used by nursing staff to communicate their research activity (evidencebasednursing.blogspot.com/).

Evidence summaries

Clinical Knowledge Summaries (www.cks.nhs.uk/home) is a service delivered via the NHS Evidence Health Information Resources (www.library.nhs.uk/). It enables practitioners to put research into practice by summarising evidence on the effectiveness of healthcare interventions, providing guidance on diagnosis and management and offering printable leaflets that practitioners can pass on to their patients. Arranged alphabetically by clinical specialty (e.g. 'child health'), it enables the healthcare practitioner to make decisions about patient care based on up-to-date evidence about treatments. Similar resources are available via the internet and are easily accessible.

WRITING A LITERATURE REVIEW

Once the literature search is completed and papers are identified to answer the search question, the next stage is to write a review. There are three key stages.

- *Sorting the 'wheat from the chaff'* – this involves examining retrieved papers critically to decide whether they meet the criteria for the review and whether they really help to answer the question. Chapter 8 considers this in more detail.
- *Identifying key points, results and themes* – this involves interpreting research findings and applying them to your own questions (see Greenhalgh 2001).
- *Writing up your findings* – this involves using a clearly structured approach. It may be helpful to look at examples of reviews or digests to get a feel for different ways of presenting the results.

MANAGING REFERENCES

Why you need to record and manage your search results

When the electronic and manual searches are completed it is important to document the search strategies. First, providing examples of search strategies demonstrates the quality and efficacy of the search effort; second, it may later be necessary to update the searches or to re-run them. Searches can be recorded manually (by printing out the search strategies) or electronically. Many bibliographic databases now permit users to store their search strategies online for later recall. This is particularly useful if you need to conduct the searches again or modify them, saving you the time-consuming task of retyping the search terms. The databases that have been used should also be documented, with the dates on which they were searched.

Consideration should also be given to using a system to manage all the references as they are obtained (Nicoll 2003). Using an organised system to manage your references will help you when you are obtaining copies of papers and appraising them. It will also prove valuable when you come to write up your work and need to produce bibliographies, footnotes, etc.

Electronic reference management software

There are several software packages available to help researchers manage their references. Popular commercial examples include Procite, Reference Manager and Endnote. Other products are available to download free of charge from the internet. A principal advantage of using an electronic method is that most reference management software allows you to produce bibliographies in various formats very efficiently. Many also interact with word-processing software to enable references to be inserted directly into the text. References can be individually annotated and keywords identified as they are imported into the software. This allows subgroups of different records to be kept within the database.

Figure 6.1 shows a screen-shot for the popular reference management software package Reference Manager. Individual references are displayed at the top of the screen and a full list of references appears below. This makes browsing and checking references simple and speedy.

Manual methods

Manual methods of organising your references still have their advantages. They are cheaper and easier to manage, and do not require special training. However, they will typically be more time-consuming. One method is to maintain a simple card index. A manual, hand-written index card might look like Box 6.4.

Whichever method you choose, it is important to get into the habit of recording references as they are obtained. This will help to prevent references 'slipping through the net' and becoming lost. Managing

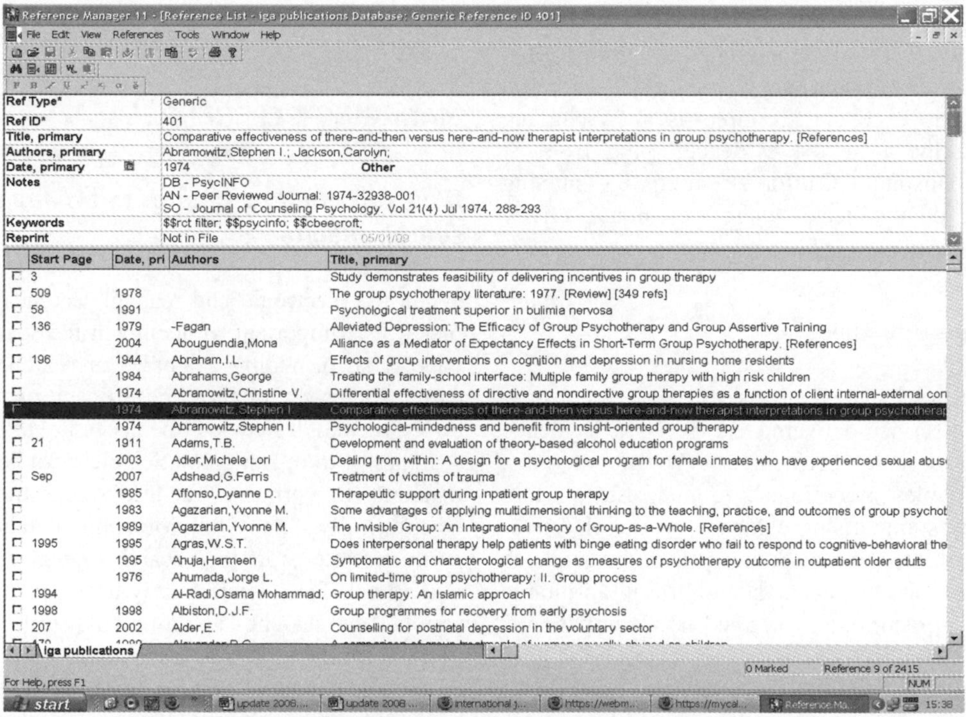

Figure 6.1 Screen shot of Reference Manager software

Box 6.4 A manual index card

Author/s:	Smith A, Jones B
Title:	Manual reference cards versus reference management software: a review of the literature
Source:	International Journal of Reference Management
Year:	2008
Volume:	52
Part:	3
Pages:	79–93
Notes:	mentioned in footnote 2

references effectively as the search progresses will save much hard work at the conclusion of your project.

CONCLUSIONS

This chapter has examined the importance of focusing a search question and planning the search to save both time and frustration. It has outlined the various methods of searching and using the literature. Here are a few key points to remember.

■ First, focus your question and plan your search strategy. Make notes on paper and do not be tempted to go straight to the computer to start searching.
■ Get to know your local health library and the librarians who work there. They are a valuable resource for your research and can save you time and effort.
■ Familiarise yourself with the resources that are most relevant to you by using them regularly.
■ Try to practise your searching as frequently as you can. Repeated searching is the best way to hone your search skills.

Finally, remember that the skills of searching and using the literature are not just useful for research, they will support you throughout your professional career. Taking the time to gain these skills now will pay great dividends both immediately and for many years to come.

References

Cleary-Holdforth C, Leufer T (2008) Essential elements in developing evidence-based practice. *Nursing Standard* **23**(2): 42–46.

Conn VS, Isaramalai S, Rath S, Jantarakupt P, Wadhawan R, Dash Y (2003) Beyond MEDLINE for literature searches. *Journal of Nursing Scholarship* **35**: 177–182.

Docherty B (2003) How to access online research reviews to inform nursing practice. *Professional Nurse* **19**(1): 53–55.

Ehrlich-Jones L, O'Dwyer L, Stevens K (2008) Searching the literature for evidence. *Rehabilitation Nursing* **33**(4): 163–169.

Flemming K, Briggs M (2007) Electronic searching to locate qualitative research: evaluation of three strategies. *Journal of Advanced Nursing* **57**(1): 95–100.

Greenhalgh T (2001) *How to Read a Paper: the basics of evidence-based medicine*. London, BMJ Publishing.

Littleton D, Marsalis S, Bliss DZ (2004) Searching the literature by design. *Western Journal of Nursing Research* **26**: 891–908.

McKibbon KA, Marks S (2001) Posing clinical questions: framing the question for scientific inquiry. AACN Clinical Issues: *Advanced Practice in Acute and Critical Care* **12**: 477–481.

Mohide EA, Matthew-Maich N (2007) Engaging nursing preceptor-student dyads in an evidence-based approach to professional practice. *Evidence-Based Nursing* **10**: 36–40.

Nicoll LH (2003) A practical way to create a library in a bibliography database manager: using electronic sources to make it easy. *CIN: Computers, Informatics, Nursing* **21**(1): 48–54.

Poynton MR (2003) Information technology and the clinical nurse specialist. Recall to precision: retrieving clinical information with MEDLINE. *Clinical Nurse Specialist* **17**(4): 182–184.

Purkis J, Jackson J, Hundt F (2008) Increasing nursing research capacity in the workplace. *Nursing Times* **104**(37): 28–31.

Scherer RW, Langenberg P, von Elm E (2007) Full publication of results initially presented in abstracts. *Cochrane Database of Systematic Reviews* April **18**(2): MR000005.

Stone PW (2002) Popping the (PICO) question in research and evidence-based practice. *Applied Nursing Research* **15**(3): 197–198.

Toma M, McAlister FA, Bialy L, Adams D, Vandermeer B, Armstrong PW (2006) Transition from meeting abstract to full-length journal article for randomized controlled trials. *Journal of the American Medical Association* **295**(11): 1281–1287.

Further reading

Aveyard H (2007) *Doing a Literature Review in Health and Social Care*. Maidenhead, Open University Press.

De Brún C, Pearce-Smith N, Heneghan C (ed), Perera R (ed), Badenoch D (ed) (2009) *Searching Skills Toolkit: finding the evidence*. Chichester, Wiley-Blackwell.

Guyatt G, Drummond R (eds) (2001) *Users' Guides to the Medical Literature: essentials of evidence-based clinical practice*. Chicago, AMA Press.

Hart C (2001) *Doing a Literature Search: a comprehensive guide for the social sciences*. London, Sage.

Katcher BS (2006) *Medline: a guide to effective searching in PubMed and other interfaces*. San Francisco, Ashbury.

Websites

www.evidence.nhs.uk/AboutUs.aspx – NHS Evidence has a wide range of electronic health resources intended to act as a source of evidence and best practice to support healthcare and research.

www.nihr.ac.uk/ – Information on NHS funding opportunities and support for research design can be accessed via the NIHR website.

7 Critical Appraisal of the Evidence

Angie Rees, Claire Beecroft and Andrew Booth

Key points

- Critical appraisal is needed by researchers and practitioners to assess the validity of a research study or group of studies, and whether their results can be applied to a particular situation.

- Three concepts are of key importance to critical appraisal: validity, reliability and applicability.

- Checklists are available to assist with critical appraisal of both quantitative and qualitative research, and for systematic reviews.

- Ready-made critically appraised products are becoming more available and frequently appear in evidence-based healthcare journals.

INTRODUCTION

Critical appraisal focuses on the practical application of research, whether it be in applying the findings of research to clinical or managerial practice or in establishing an evidence base to which our own research will add a distinctive contribution.

Critical appraisal skills enable us to assess whether an individual study has particular value for us. Equally, they help us to reconcile dissonant, even conflicting, messages from different research studies. For example, one study conducted in a very selective population may show that a treatment works. A similar study in a general population may show less favourable results. Critical appraisal helps us to understand reasons for such differences and to decide which study, if any, we will use to inform our practice. Critical appraisal is equally valuable whether we have to start from scratch ourselves in assessing a research study for a new treatment or whether we seek to interpret the appraisals of others in the form of systematic literature reviews, guidelines or critically appraised topics (CATS) (Guyatt *et al.* 2000).

For a profession with a justifiable reputation for challenging 'nursing ritual', critical appraisal is a key skill. Critical appraisal of relevant research helps us to cease ineffective procedures and put a brake on unquestioning acceptance of novel or fashionable technologies. For example, after critically appraising evidence supporting vitamin C in the healing of pressure sores, a dietitian and information specialist were able to challenge textbook recommendations based on a 20-year-old flawed study. They were thus able to 'encourage disinvestment from an ineffective, though non-harmful, treatment in favour of spending resources on treatments for which there is at least sufficient proof of benefit' (North & Booth 1999: 243).

WHAT IS CRITICAL APPRAISAL?

Critical appraisal is 'the process of assessing and interpreting evidence by systematically considering its validity, results and relevance' (Parkes *et al.* 2001: 10). This definition not only values the technical skills of 'assessing evidence', understanding study design and research quality, but also the contextual knowledge of 'interpreting evidence', based on clinical experience. This combination of skills and knowledge, while recognising the values and preferences of the individual patient, constitutes evidence-based practice.

A key principle of critical appraisal is that a good study usually provides enough information to help a researcher to judge that it *is* a good study. Unfortunately, the reverse is not necessarily true – the IMRAD (Introduction, Methods, Results And Discussion) structure used to present published research may make research appear superficially plausible. To help 'scratch beneath the surface' you typically use a published checklist. Many such checklists exist for different audiences or different types of study. However, checklists should focus on the actual quality of the methods and not merely on how well the study is reported. Avoid checklists that focus on factors external to the study itself, such as 'Have you heard of the author? What qualifications do the authors have? Is the journal peer-reviewed?' The study should speak for itself. A useful critical appraisal checklist focuses on the validity, reliability and applicability of a study. These three associated concepts are central to all critical appraisal, regardless of whether the research being appraised is quantitative or qualitative, or whether it is a primary study (e.g. a randomised controlled trial) or a secondary study (e.g. a guideline or systematic review). Each concept will be considered in turn.

Validity (are the results of the study valid?)

Suppose you were to stand in your work area with a clipboard. What effect might this have on patients or colleagues? Given that even the smallest observational study can, like a pebble in a lake, disturb the 'real world', what might we expect if we design a large and complex experimental study? Clearly we want limitations arising from our chosen research method to be outweighed by the 'trueness' of the findings. If we suspect that the picture obtained by the research no longer relates to the 'world' that we are investigating, then the study is invalid. The researchers may have based their study on flawed assumptions, there may be some inherent weakness in the study design they have chosen (bias) or they may have failed to take into account an important complicating factor (confounding).

Reliability (what are the results?)

All research results are subject to the possible effects of chance. When we measure outcomes we want to be sure that the results are reliable. If we were to measure the same outcomes repeatedly, would we still obtain the same results? Statistical measures allow us to interpret whether the results fall within the bounds of reasonable expectation. Finally, when the variability of results from repeated measurements is taken into account, we want to be able to judge whether we would make the same decision based on the best possible result as we would when faced with the worst possible result.

Once we have established that the results are reliable we want to ascertain whether an effect is meaningful – is it large enough to be clinically significant? For example, a study may demonstrate a change of five points on a pain scale. However, you may know from experience that a change of less than 10 points makes no difference at all to how a patient is feeling. A change of five points may be *statistically significant*, but as a clinician you may decide that only a change of 10 points or more is *clinically significant*.

Applicability (will the results help locally?)

If the study is well designed and shows a reliable enough result, we need to consider its implications for both current clinical practice and future research. It is helpful to separate the strength of the evidence (in terms of validity and reliability) from the strength of recommendations or action (in terms of applicability). Most practitioners will broadly agree whether a study has been designed well or a result is meaningful. However, when they come to determine whether the results can be applied locally they will take into account available resources, the skills of involved staff, and local policies and politics.

THE NEED FOR CRITICAL APPRAISAL

Critical appraisal has become increasingly important for several reasons. First, the sheer volume of information available, in printed form or via the web, has meant that any aspiring researcher needs to filter out unreliable lower-quality studies. Second, even the best journals can publish poor or misleading information. Even where information is of good quality, delays of up to 10 years may occur before research findings become standard practice in textbooks (Antman *et al.* 1992).

Researchers need to judge whether the study design used to conduct research makes the findings either potentially useful or unusable. If an inferior study design has been used, you may be able to examine the same research question with a more robust design. If a robust design has been used and the findings are still open to doubt you may wish to repeat the study with a larger sample size. Finally, if the research has been conducted well and has conclusive results you are free to concentrate on other aspects that need to be researched. Critical appraisal skills are required throughout a research career and are thus skills for lifelong learning.

Any research study is prone to two potential flaws: bias and confounding.

'Bias is a systematic tendency to underestimate or overestimate the parameter of interest because of a deficiency in the design or execution of a study' (Coggon *et al.* 2003: 21)

For example, when patients self-report whether they have given up smoking, some may convey a more positive image than is truthful. Whereas self-report is open to bias, biochemical confirmation of nicotine in their blood or saliva would be a more objective (less biased) way of establishing the facts. Confounding is where you cannot ascertain whether an effect is caused by the variable you are interested in or by another variable. So, for example, a study may demonstrate a link between alcohol consumption and lung cancer. However, alcohol consumption is commonly associated with smoking. Smoking is therefore a potential confounder for your study. Ideally, a researcher identifies potential confounders before they begin and then adjusts their results accordingly in the analysis. Common confounding variables are age, sex, ethnicity and co-morbidity.

VALIDITY OF RESEARCH DESIGNS

An optimal research design minimises bias and anticipates confounding. The researcher therefore has the responsibility to choose the best research design to answer the question that they are asking. This choice is limited by ethical or practical considerations (Ploeg 1999; Roberts & DiCenso 1999). For example, if a researcher believes that keeping pigeons causes bird-fanciers' lung it is not ethical to randomise subjects to keep pigeons or not within a randomised controlled trial. The strongest available design would be an observational study that simply observes what the population chooses to do. A researcher selects the most appropriate research design from within a so-called 'hierarchy of evidence' (Sackett 1986) (see Box 7.1).

This hierarchical approach has several limitations. By emphasising the study design over the features of an individual study it gives the false impression that a poor randomised trial is better than a good observational study. Nor can it handle conflict between the findings of several observational studies and a single randomised controlled trial or a situation where

---

Box 7.1 The hierarchy of evidence

1 Systematic reviews and meta-analyses
2 Well-designed randomised trials
3 Well-designed trials without randomisation (e.g. single-group pre-post, cohort, time-series or matched case-controlled studies)
4 Well-designed non-experimental studies from more than one centre
5 Opinions of respected authorities based on clinical evidence, descriptive studies or reports of expert committees

---

randomised controlled trials are split in favour of and against the same intervention. It is more important to trade off the strength of a paper's findings against the weaknesses of its methodology than slavishly follow a hierarchy of evidence (Edwards *et al.* 1998). Alternatives to Sackett's hierarchy are being developed to take some of these limitations into account (Evans 2003).

HOW TO APPRAISE QUANTITATIVE RESEARCH STUDIES

As a researcher you will encounter many checklists that claim to be useful when appraising different types of quantitative study. A useful checklist will only include criteria that are relevant for a given paper. For example, a clinical trial should demonstrate that it has avoided selection and observer bias and that the large majority of subjects (80% or more) are accounted for by the results. We also want to ensure that the outcomes chosen measure the right thing over the right time period. Finally, quantitative studies need large enough numbers of patients to avoid being wrong because of the random play of chance. In summary, then, for a quantitative paper to provide strong evidence, it must be high quality, valid and well powered.

For an individual researcher, checklists provide a framework for analysing a published article. Similarly, for the reviewer producing a systematic review or a clinical guideline, a checklist provides a standardised, explicit tool for consistently examining all articles being considered. Two main sources for checklists are the Critical Appraisal Skills Programme and the influential Users' Guides to the Medical Literature (Box 7.2).

Getting started

While every quantitative article is different LoBiondo-Wood and colleagues (2002) suggest that critical reading falls into four stages:

- *preliminary understanding* – skimming or quickly reading to gain familiarity with the content and layout of the paper
- *comprehensive understanding* – increasing understanding of concepts and research terms
- *analysis understanding* – breaking the study into parts and seeking to understand each part
- *synthesis understanding* – pulling the above steps together to make a (new) whole, making sense of it and explaining relationships.

Experience confirms that several practical strategies prove useful when appraising a research article. First, quickly read the abstract. Increasingly, articles use a structured abstract to make it easier to identify the study design, the participants and the intervention being studied. Pay particular attention to the main outcome measures – most studies contain multiple measurements, but you should isolate the outcome measures of importance. If the study is a randomised controlled trial you should look for a table describing the baseline characteristics. This enables you to assess whether the experimental and controlled

Box 7.2 Sources of critical appraisal checklists

Critical Appraisal Skills Programme: www.phru.nhs.uk/Pages/PHD/CASP.htm
Evidence Based Medicine Tool Kit: www.med.ualberta.ca/ebm/ebm.htm
Guyatt G, Rennie D *et al.* (eds) (2008) *Users' Guides to the Medical Literature: a manual for evidence-based clinical practice*. Ontario, McGraw-Hill Professional.
Guyatt G, Rennie D *et al.* (eds) (2008) *Users' Guides to the Medical Literature: essentials of evidence-based clinical practice*. Ontario, McGraw-Hill Professional.
Users' Guides to Evidence Based Practice: www.cche.net/usersguides/main.asp

groups are similar at the beginning of the study. Having established a 'level playing field', you can look for a detailed description of the study design. While the Introduction, Discussion and Conclusions may inform an understanding of the issue, it is the Methods section that enables you to decide whether or not it is a good study. The Methods and Results sections should command most attention. Increasingly, randomised controlled trials present a flowchart that shows how withdrawals and dropouts are handled within the study – a requirement of the CONSORT agreement among journal editors (Begg *et al.* 1996), which dictates clearer standards of trial reporting. You should also focus on results that are considered significant (i.e. that have a p value of 0.05 or less), as these are where the research team has demonstrated a measurable (and possibly important) difference. However, you should make sure that these relate to primary outcomes of the study, because a significant difference is not always an important one.

Examples of published checklists include those for randomised controlled trials (Box 7.3), those for surveys (Box 7.4), and those for observational and epidemiological studies. Research Example 7.1 gives a sample critical appraisal of a survey.

HOW TO APPRAISE QUALITATIVE RESEARCH STUDIES

While critical appraisal of quantitative research studies is relatively well established and uncontrover-sial, appraisal of qualitative studies is less widely accepted. Appraisal of qualitative studies seems more intuitive and less deductive; less of a science and more of an art (Booth & O'Rourke 2001). In addition, tools used for data collection (such as interviews and focus groups) seem more prone to the influence and bias of the observer. Indeed, some argue that such research does not seek a result that is replicable, and hence generalisable, but rather to provide a valid observation of an individual phenomenon.

Research into the use of checklists in appraising qualitative research suggests that it is neither desirable nor practical to select a single instrument or tool (Barbour 2001). With so many different approaches to qualitative research, one checklist might privilege, for example, grounded theory, while another might be more appropriate for ethnographic studies. Nevertheless qualitative research should still demonstrate:

- a clear aim for the project
- an appropriate methodology
- justification for the sampling strategy, i.e. who was and who was not included.

In addition, qualitative research should be reflexive on the possible effect that the relationship between investigators and subjects might have had on interpretation of the phenomenon. Ironically, given general mistrust of subjectivity in qualitative research, approaches to handling bias in quantitative research appear crude and formulaic by comparison.

While much is made of differences between quantitative and qualitative research, both should

Box 7.3 Questions for critical appraisal of a randomised controlled trial

A Are the results valid?
  1 Did the study address a clearly focused issue? Are you able to describe the study participants, the intervention under study, the outcomes being measured and the comparison(s) being made?
  2 Was the assignment of subjects to treatments randomised?
  3 Were all the subjects who entered the trial properly accounted for at its conclusion?
  4 Blinding: were the subjects, workers, study personnel 'blind to the treatment'?
  5 Were the groups similar at the start of the trial?
  6 Aside from the experimental intervention, were the groups treated equally?
B What are the results?
  7 How large was the difference between the two groups? (consider what outcomes were recorded, and how the differences between the groups were expressed)
  8 How precise was the estimate of the treatment effects? (hint: look for confidence intervals)
C Will the results help locally?
  9 Can the results be applied to your work? (or, how different are the subjects in the study to the population you are interested in?)
  10 Were all the important outcomes considered? (would you make a different decision if other important outcomes had been included?)
  11 Are the benefits worth the harms and costs?

essentially pose and answer the same three questions:

- what is the message?
- can I believe it?
- can I generalise?

The recent growth in so-called mixed-methods research has made it more necessary to establish a common approach between the two types of research (Gilbert 2006).

While it is clear that qualitative research has an important and expanding role within nursing research, the researcher should be aware that there remains much opposition to criteria-based approaches to appraisal. In an attempt to sidestep such objections, Dixon-Woods and colleagues (2004) have proposed a minimal set of prompts designed to stimulate appraisal of different dimensions of qualitative

research while remaining explicitly methodology-neutral. They argue that any approaches to critical appraisal of qualitative studies should recognise the importance of distinctive study designs and theoretical perspectives within qualitative research. They conclude that any such approach should distinguish fatal flaws from minor errors. They further assert that:

'the more important and interesting aspects of qualitative research may remain very difficult to measure except through the subjective judgement of experienced qualitative researchers' (Dixon-Woods *et al.* 2004: 225)

Box 7.5 and Research Example 7.2 show examples of how a qualitative research article might be appraised.

Box 7.4   Questions for critical appraisal of a survey

A   Are the results valid?
1   Objectives and hypotheses
   ● Are the objectives of the study clearly stated?
2   Design
   ● Is the study design suitable for the objectives?
   ● Who/what was studied?
   ● Was this the right sample to answer the objectives?
   ● Did the subject represent the full spectrum of the population of interest?
   ● Is the study large enough to achieve its objectives? Have sample size estimates been performed?
   ● Were all subjects accounted for?
   ● Were all appropriate outcomes considered?
   ● Has ethical approval been obtained if appropriate?
   ● What measures were made to contact non-responders?
   ● What was the response rate?
3   Measurement and observation
   ● Is it clear what was measured, how it was measured and what the outcomes were?
   ● Are the measurements valid?
   ● Are the measurements reliable?
   ● Are the measurements reproducible?
B   What are the results?
4   Presentation of results
   ● Are the basic data adequately described?
   ● Are the results presented clearly, objectively and in sufficient detail to enable readers to make their own judgement?
   ● Are the results internally consistent, i.e. do the numbers add up properly?
5   Analysis
   ● Are the data suitable for analysis? Are the methods appropriate to the data? Are any statistics correctly performed and interpreted?
C   Will the results help locally?
6   Discussion
   ● Are the results discussed in relation to existing knowledge on the subject and study objectives?
   ● Is the discussion biased?
   ● Can the results be generalised?
7   Interpretation
   ● Are the authors' conclusions justified by the data? Does this paper help me answer my problem?
8   Implementation
   ● Can any necessary change be implemented in practice? What are the enablers/ barriers to implementation?

7.1   Sample Critical Appraisal of a Survey

Question: How do older people's expectations regarding ageing affect their physical and mental health status and how do health-promoting behaviours mediate the relationship between expectations and health status?

Kim SH (2009) Older people's expectations regarding ageing, health-promoting behaviour and health status. *Journal of Advanced Nursing* **65**(1): 84–91.

Aim

The objective of the research reported here was to investigate how older people's expectations of ageing influence their physical and mental health, and also to assess how health-promoting behaviours might mediate the relationship between expectations of ageing and physical and mental health.

Design and setting

A survey of older Korean people residing in the community. *There is reason to suppose that* **community-dwelling residents may not be representative of the more general older population in Korea**, *and that* **Korean culture may differ from other cultures** *in ways that* **could influence the results of this study and affect its applicability to older people in another population**.

Methods

Three standardised measures were used – a short version of the Expectations Regarding Aging questionnaire, the Health Promoting Lifestyle Profile II and the Medical Outcomes Study 12-item short form. ***Measures used are well established and have been previously validated.***

Results

Ninety-nine community-dwelling older Korean people responded. The participants were a **convenience sample** – meaning they were **chosen for reasons of ease of data collection** by the researchers – this affects the validity of the study as the researchers may have been biased in their choices, for instance choosing (consciously or unconsciously) participants who would be most likely to provide data that supports the study hypothesis.

The study found a **statistically significant relationship between higher expectations of ageing and better physical and mental health**. *The study also* **proved statistically** *that* **health-promoting behaviours partially mediated both expectations of ageing and physical and mental health**.

Conclusions

The results confirm that older people who plan to maintain high levels of health when they are older have better physical and mental health. Nursing care of older people should therefore focus on improving older people's expectations about ageing. Additionally, the study found that those older people who plan to maintain high levels of health as they age are more likely to participate in health-promoting behaviours, which in turn improve their physical and mental health status. This suggests that older people should be encouraged and supported to promote and manage their own health.

Box 7.5   Critical appraisal checklist for a qualitative research article

A   *Are the results of the study valid?*
  1 Was there a clear statement of the aims of the research? Why is it important?
  2 Is a qualitative method appropriate?
  3 Sampling strategy
     [Includes selection and purpose of sample, who was selected and why, how they were selected and why, whether the sample size is justified and why some participants may have chosen not to take part]
     Was the sampling strategy appropriate to address the aims?
  4 Data collection
     [Includes whether it is clear why the setting was chosen, how the data were collected and why (e.g. focus group, structured interview, etc.), how the data were recorded and why (e.g. tape recording, note taking, etc.) and if the methods were modified during the process and why]
     Were the data collected in a way that addresses the research issue?
  5 Data analysis
     [Includes a description of the analysis, how categories and themes were derived from the data, whether the findings have been evaluated for credibility and whether we can be confident that data have not been overlooked]
     Was the data analysis sufficiently rigorous?
  6 Research partnership relations
     [Includes whether the researchers examined their own role, the setting in which data were collected and how the research was explained to participants]
     Has the relationship between researchers and participants been adequately considered?

B   *What are the results?*
  7 Findings
     Is there a clear statement of the findings?
  8 Justification of data interpretation
     [Includes whether sufficient data are presented to sustain the findings and how the data used in the paper were selected from the original sample]
     Do the researchers indicate the links between the data presented and their own findings on what the data contain?

C   *Will the results help locally?*
  9 Transferability
     Are the findings of this study transferable to a wider population?
  10 Relevance and usefulness
     [Includes whether the research is important and relevant in addressing the research aim, in contributing new insights and in suggesting implications for research, policy and practice]
     Are the findings of this relevant and important to your patients or problems?
  11 Eliciting your patient's preferences and values
     Do you and your patient have a clear assessment of their values and preferences?
  12 Meeting your patient's preferences and values
     Are they met by this regimen and its consequences?

7.2   Sample Critical Appraisal of a Qualitative Research Study

Question: What are the self-management behaviours of patients with chronic obstructive pulmonary disease?

Chenk H, Chenm L, Lee S, Choh Y, Wengl C (2008) Self-management behaviours for patients with chronic obstructive pulmonary disease: a qualitative study. *Journal of Advanced Nursing* **64**(6): 595–604.

Design and setting

The **aims of the research** *are clearly indicated in the paper.* A qualitative design using semi structured, face-to-face interviews is **appropriate** *because the researchers are investigating* **patients' perceptions or attitudes** *to their self-management. If researchers wished to ensure that this self-reported behaviour is what is happening in practice then they might follow this up with a quantitative observational study.*

Patients

18 male COPD patients aged 55–81 years again chosen from a convenience sample **for ease of data collection** by the researchers. The study took place in Taiwan, all patients were Taiwanese or Mandarin speakers. *As with the example of the survey above (Box 7.5) there may be issues about the extent to which results in a Taiwan-based, non-English speaking population may be* **transferable** *to a different cultural setting.*

Methods

Face-to-face, semi–structured interviews were conducted with all patients. Interviews were transcribed by a research assistant and verified by the first author of the study. The taped interviews and transcripts were analysed by two researchers for consistency. *Use of a second researcher helps to add* **rigour and ensure that the analysis is based on the data** *and that each researcher has not imposed their own interpretation without it being verifiable from the data.* Data collection from the transcripts continued until 'theme saturation' was achieved. Analysis of data was completed using a three-step process: **data reduction, data display and conclusion drawing**. *The researchers have described* **how they derived the categories from the data**. *We are not able to tell if* **the researchers took their own role (reflexivity) into account** *when collecting and interpreting the data.*

Main findings

Self-management techniques mapped to five main themes:

1 *symptom management*
2 *activity and exercise implementation*
3 *environmental control*
4 *emotional adaptation*
5 *maintaining a healthy lifestyle*

> Thirteen subthemes were also identified. *The reader can examine these themes and the supporting data extracts to establish the extent to which they believe them to apply to COPD patients in their own culture or setting.*
>
> ### Conclusions
>
> Patients chose self-management techniques to help prevent or reduce episodes of exacerbated lung disease. Patient's choice of technique depended on lifestyle, personal preference and ability to maintain stable health. *A reader seeking to meet **the preferences and values of their own patient** and to apply these findings in their own practice will consider lifestyle and personal preferences as important alongside disease-related factors.*

HOW TO APPRAISE SYSTEMATIC REVIEWS, PRACTICE GUIDELINES AND ECONOMIC ANALYSIS

Up to this point we have focused on single research studies, either quantitative or qualitative. However, basing research plans on the results of a single research study in isolation may prove misleading. As a researcher you need to examine the entire body of evidence as captured by a systematic review (overview); typically this provides a rigorous summary of all the research evidence that relates to a specific question (Engberg 2008).

Systematic reviews make strenuous attempts to overcome possible biases (see Chapter 24). They follow a rigorous methodology of search, retrieval, appraisal, data extraction, data synthesis and interpretation. To protect against possible bias, explicit, pre-set inclusion criteria are used in selecting studies for inclusion. Similar protections are used when producing clinical guidelines. Much time and resources are expended in assuring the quality of the process by using more than one reviewer to independently select studies and by recording explicit details of methods used at every stage.

Systematic reviews focus on high-quality primary research reports in attempting to summarise research-based knowledge on a topic. Nevertheless, not every systematic review is of high quality and critical appraisal remains essential. Box 7.6 gives guidelines on appraising a review article.

Systematic reviews are one type of research synthesis, other examples include practice guidelines and economic evaluations. These integrative studies frequently draw on the results of systematic reviews and so share common principles for critical appraisal. Economic evaluations compare costs and consequences of different strategies, with consequences and the values attached to them frequently being generated from systematic reviews.

APPLYING THE RESULTS OF CRITICAL APPRAISAL

Reading, appraising and applying the results from research articles is a time-consuming concern. While the evidence-based healthcare movement originally aspired for all practitioners to locate and appraise their own evidence, recent years have seen the lowering of this bar (Guyatt *et al.* 2000). Now proponents suggest all practitioners should learn the skills of critical appraisal primarily to enable them to use other people's products of critical appraisal with confidence. Such products fall into one of two categories: article-based and topic-based. Article-based critical appraisal is represented by a plethora of evidence-based journals such as *Evidence-Based Nursing*, *Evidence-Based Medicine*, etc. These summarise the cream of current journal articles in single-page summaries that present the main methodological features of each study and appraise them for quality. Each

Box 7.6 How to critically appraise review articles

A *Are the results of this systematic review valid?*
  1 Is this a systematic review of randomised trials?
  2 Does the systematic review include a description of the strategies used to find all relevant trials?
  3 Does the systematic review include a description of how the validity of individual studies was assessed?
  4 Were the results consistent from study to study?
  5 Were individual patient data or aggregate data used in the analysis?
B *What are the results?*
  6 How large was the treatment effect?
  7 How precise is the estimate of treatment effect?
C *Will the results help locally?*
  8 Are my patients so different from those in the study that the results do not apply?
  9 Is the treatment feasible in our setting?
  10 Were all clinically important outcomes (harms as well as benefits) considered?
  11 What are my patient's values and preferences for both the outcome we are trying to prevent and the side effects that may arise?

summary is arranged under an indicative title that captures the study's principal result in a clinically relevant 'bottom line'. Similarly, databases such as those from the NHS Centre for Reviews and Dissemination at the University of York provide free internet access to article-based summaries of particular types of research synthesis, notably systematic reviews (the Database of Abstracts of Reviews of Effects, DARE) and economic evaluations (the NHS Economic Evaluations Database, NEED).

Topic-based critical appraisal is question driven, rather than literature driven. Important questions from clinical practice are identified and specialist staff or volunteer clinicians search for answers from the research literature. Results identified from the literature are summarised and presented in a concise and meaningful summary, for example as a Critically Appraised Topic (CAT). Alternatively, this process may contribute to some wider publishing enterprise such as the clinical handbook, *Clinical Evidence* published by BMJ Publishing Group, or results posted on a website, as with the Manchester-based *BestBETS* initiative. Concern has been expressed over the quality of CATS – not with regard to appraisal, which is largely found to be satisfactory, but because search

procedures have frequently failed to identify the most relevant items to address the clinical question (Coomarasamy *et al.* 2001). Clearly the value of appraisal depends on first finding the most appropriate research study.

Successful application of appraisal results also assumes that the study population is similar enough to the local population. Questions such as those given below are key when deciding whether we need to replicate research carried out elsewhere or simply to extrapolate findings from existing research.

- Can I apply results from a study that only includes patients between 70 and 80 years old to those in the 65 to 70 age group?
- What about relatively fit and 'biologically young' 81-year-olds?
- Can the results of studies conducted in Edmonton, Alberta, be extrapolated to Edmonton, north London?
- Are rural practices in Finland different to those in Wales?

For the researcher the value of pre-appraised products is twofold. First, they provide a quality-fortified environment for assessing key research studies that contribute to knowledge within a particular topic area (for example, hospital infection or hand-washing). Second, and more importantly, studies critically appraised by experienced researchers provide a useful benchmark against which you, as a less-experienced researcher, can chart your progress as you become more aware of methodological issues.

CONCLUSIONS

This chapter demonstrates that critical appraisal has become increasingly important. It can be used by the researcher as a quality control tool to assess individual studies. Alternatively, if the researcher is reviewing multiple studies, it provides a standardised approach for producing systematic reviews and clinical guidelines. The key concepts of validity, reliability and applicability have been emphasised together with the usefulness of a checklist-led approach. Notwithstanding essential differences between quantitative and qualitative research, this chapter demonstrates the value of a common approach. Above all, the take-home message is that critical appraisal is not simply a pure academic skill – it is an ongoing strategy to help you in your continuing clinical and research career.

References

Antman EM, Lau J, Kupelnick B, Mosteller F, Chalmers TC (1992) A comparison of results of meta-analysis of randomised controlled trials and the recommendations of experts. *Journal of the American Medical Association* **268**: 240–248.

Barbour RS (2001) Checklists for improving rigour in qualitative research: a case of the tail wagging the dog? *British Medical Journal* **322**: 1115–1117.

Begg C, Cho M, Eastwood S, Horton R, Moher D, Olkin I *et al.* (1996) Improving the quality of reporting of randomized controlled trials. The CONSORT statement. *Journal of the American Medical Association* **276**: 637–639.

Booth A, O'Rourke AJ (2001) Critical appraisal and using the literature (www.shef.ac.uk/scharr/ir/units/critapp/appqual.htm).

Coggon D, Rose G, Barker DJP (2003) *Epidemiology for the Uninitiated*, 5th edition. London, BMJ Publishing Group.

Coomarasamy A, Latthe P, Papaioannou S, Publicover M, Gee H, Khan KS (2001) Critical appraisal in clinical practice: sometimes irrelevant, occasionally invalid. *Journal of the Royal Society of Medicine* **94**: 573–577.

Dixon-Woods M, Shaw RL, Agarwal S, Smith JA (2004) The problem of appraising qualitative research. *Quality and Safety in Health Care* **13**: 223–225.

Edwards AG, Russell IT, Stott NC (1998) Signal versus noise in the evidence base for medicine: an alternative to hierarchies of evidence? *Family Practice* **15**: 319–322.

Engberg S (2008) Systematic reviews and meta-analysis: studies of studies. *Journal of Wound, Ostomy & Continence Nursing* **35**(3): 258–265.

Evans D (2003) Hierarchy of evidence: a framework for ranking evidence evaluating healthcare interventions. *Journal of Clinical Nursing* **12**(1): 77–84.

Gilbert T (2006) Mixed methods and mixed methodologies: the practical, the technical and the political. *Journal of Research in Nursing* **11**(3): 205–217.

Guyatt G, Meade MO, Jaeschke RZ, Cook DJ, Haynes RB (2000) Practitioners of evidence based care. Not all clinicians need to appraise evidence from scratch but all need some skills. *British Medical Journal* **320**: 954–955.

Guyatt G *et al.* (eds) (2008a) *Users' Guides to the Medical Literature: a manual for evidence-based clinical practice*. Ontario, McGraw-Hill Professional.

Guyatt G *et al.* (eds) (2008b) *Users' Guides to the Medical Literature: essentials of evidence-based clinical practice*, Ontario, McGraw-Hill Professional.

LoBiondo-Wood G, Haber J, Krainovich-Miller B (2002) Critical reading strategies: overview of the research process. In: LoBiondo-Wood G, Haber J (eds) *Nursing Research: methods, critical appraisal, and utilization*, 5th edition. St Louis, Mosby, pp 33–49.

North G, Booth A (1999) Why appraise the evidence? A case study of vitamin C and the healing of pressure sores. *Journal of Human Nutrition and Dietetics* **12**: 237–244.

Parkes J, Hyde C, Deeks J, Milne R (2001) *Teaching Critical Appraisal Skills in Health Care Settings* (Cochrane Review). The Cochrane Library **4**. Oxford, Update Software.

Ploeg J (1999) Identifying the best research design to fit the question. Part 2: qualitative designs. *Evidence-Based Nursing* **2**: 36–37.

Roberts J, DiCenso A (1999) Identifying the best research design to fit the question. Part I: quantitative designs [editorial]. *Evidence-Based Nursing* **2**: 4–6.

Sackett DL (1986) Rules of evidence and clinical recommendations on the use of antithrombotic agents. *Archives of Internal Medicine* **146**: 464–465.

Further reading

Ajetunmobi O (2002) *Making Sense of Critical Appraisal.* London, Arnold.

Critical Appraisal Skills Programme, www.phru.nhs.uk/Pages/PHD/CASP.htm

Cullum N (2001) Evaluation of studies of treatment or prevention interventions. Part 2: Applying the results of studies to your patients. *Evidence-Based Nursing* **4**: 7–8.

Cullum N (2000) Evaluation of studies of treatment or prevention interventions [editorial]. *Evidence-Based Nursing* **3**: 100–102.

Cutcliffe J, Ward M (2007) *Critiquing Nursing Research*, 2nd edition. London, Quay Books.

Dixon-Woods M, Booth A, Sutton AJ (2007) Synthesising qualitative research: a review. *Qualitative Research* **7**: 375–422.

Greenhalgh T (2006) *How to Read a Paper: the basics of evidence-based medicine*, 3rd edition. Oxford, Wiley-Blackwell.

Satherley P, Allen D, Lyne P (2007) Supporting evidence-based service delivery and organisation: a comparison of an emergent realistic appraisal technique with a standard qualitative critical appraisal tool. *International Journal of Evidence-Based Healthcare* **5**(4): 477–486.

Scottish Intercollegiate Guidelines Network (SIGN) (2008) *Critical Appraisal: Notes and Checklists*. www.sign.ac.uk/methodology/checklists.html

Young JM, Solomon MJ (2009) How to critically appraise an article. *Nature Clinical Practice Gastroenterology & Hepatology* **6**(2): 82–91. www.nature.com/ncpgasthep/journal/v6/n2/full/ncpgasthep1331.html

8 Preparing a Research Proposal

Julie Taylor

Key points

- A research proposal helps researchers to clarify their intentions and communicate these to funding bodies and committees granting ethical or research governance approval.

- A research proposal should present a reasoned argument about the need for the study; provide explicit details on how it will be carried out; and clearly state the deliverables.

- A proposal should include a clear statement of the rationale for the study, the research questions, details of the methods to be used, the resources required and the methods of dissemination.

- Research methods should be appropriate to the research question(s), costed appropriately and undertaken by people who demonstrate the potential to deliver.

- The format of a research proposal will vary depending on the target audience, but all share common features.

INTRODUCTION

One of the most rewarding tasks in a researcher's life is writing a successful research proposal. It is also a task that can be the most frustrating, because writing a proposal is always time-consuming and, if written to seek funding to support the proposed study, it may not always be successful. However, there are a number of key principles that can be applied to preparing a research proposal and a few tactics that can increase the success rate. This chapter provides an overview of how to construct a robust research proposal, whether this is for an education programme or as an application for funding. It will address the main points that are needed in the proposal, and also how to meet the requirements of the intended audience.

Research proposals are written for a number of reasons. These include:

- for a dissertation towards the end of a period of study (e.g. for a master's degree)
- to undertake doctoral studies
- to respond to a specific research or development tender
- to answer a competitive grant application call
- to seek funding for your own research idea
- to obtain research governance and research ethics approval.

Although the reasons for writing a research proposal may vary, the components of a successful proposal are the same whatever the purpose. All research proposals need to be able to meet a few essential criteria, it is just a matter of scale or emphasis.

Once a proposal has been written it will generally be subject to some form of review, for example by supervisors or examiners, members of an independent scientific review committee or ethics committee, or reviewers acting on behalf of a funding agency. Reviewers will make decisions about the quality of the proposal, and in cases where funding is being sought, make recommendations about whether or not the proposal should be funded.

So why may a research proposal be rejected? The main reasons are:

- poorly phrased research question
- flawed research design
- no articulation with the aims of the funder/ programme/university/supervisor
- the research has been done before
- no evidence that the applicant(s) have the skills or potential to be able to deliver the work
- over-ambitious in terms of timescale, expected outcomes or funds
- under-ambitious for the amount of money or 'reward' being asked for
- did not respond to feedback given at an earlier stage.

Even when a proposal is judged to be of a high quality it may still be rejected because there is limited funding available and it did not score as highly as others.

Paying careful consideration to the above points when developing a proposal will enhance the likelihood of success.

IDENTIFYING A RESEARCH IDEA

One might think that identifying a research idea is easy. However, the feasibility, practicality and usefulness of ideas is another matter. There are several key questions to consider.

- Is my idea something that can be researched?
- Is it something that could be made into a proposal?
- Is it something I could do in the time that is available?
- If I need to apply for external funding, is it an idea that would appeal to the funding body?
- If I am undertaking an education programme, is my idea likely to appeal to a potential supervisor. This is especially important with PhD proposals.

Some universities produce a list of topics or research questions that supervisors are interested in and students may select to develop into their own project. This can be especially useful when students have to complete a research project in a relatively short period of time and can provide a close match between the student's and the supervisor's interests. Alternatively, hospitals and primary care organisations may identify research areas that merit investigation. Selecting a topic that is of interest to the organisation in which you work and to the managers, may help in securing support for the study and in disseminating the findings.

As discussed in Chapter 2, there are many sources of research questions; however, in a practice-based profession such as nursing, clinical practice is an important source of ideas. We talk a lot about evidence-based practice, but it is equally as important that nursing research is driven from and informed by practice. So what do nurses and midwives need to know that would make the patient experience better? Are there perceived gaps in knowledge that practitioners want to know about, or problems they think they have to deal with unnecessarily? What do patients and carers require to be done?

IDENTIFYING SOURCES OF FUNDING

If your research proposal is for an education programme, for example a master's course, funding may not be an issue, although you might want to seek funding to support some parts, for example transcribing interview tapes. However, for most people engaged in research, identifying a source of funding is essential. With increasing financial pressures on healthcare organisations and universities, the luxuries of researching a project as part of the job just for personal satisfaction are largely gone. Researchers need to ensure that the full costs of their proposed project are covered, including in many instances overheads specified by their employing organisation.

Securing funding can be difficult; the requirements of funding bodies are stringent and they will only fund high-quality applications. If this is the first time a researcher has sought funding, it is advisable to start with a relatively small and less competitive funding body, but it will still have to be a high-quality application to stand a chance of success. It is good practice to identify potential funding bodies from the outset and tailor the proposal to meet their requirements. Funding bodies are usually very clear about what they will and will not fund. There is no point submitting a proposal on educational methods for student nurses, however good it is, to a funder who is only concerned with funding clinical trials for interventions on neuromuscular disease.

It is therefore important to seek out information on possible funding bodies to ascertain whether your interests match those of the funder. Most organisations that fund research display details of the topic areas they are interested in funding, and details of past projects they have funded, on their websites. There is usually a contact name and it is often worth discussing your research interests with this person. Do you know anyone who has had success with this funder before? If so, talk to them. Do you know someone who sits on the scientific panel that will review proposals? If so, get in touch.

In the UK, there are small charities, local health service grants, professional awards, etc., that do not receive enough applications of sufficient quality each year. Even if an organisation does not offer a large amount of funding, it may be possible to approach them to support a particular part of a project (e.g. a systematic review of the literature) and to apply to another organisation to support a different component (e.g. data collection and analysis). Additionally, two or three small-scale projects on related aspects of the same topic can be very convincing when it comes to putting in a PhD proposal or a larger grant application

to pursue the topic further, especially if the findings have been published. So targeting a particular funder from the outset is a good strategy.

THE RESEARCH PROPOSAL

Whatever the purpose of the proposal, the main topics that need to be covered will probably be dictated by the university or funding body, and they generally fall under the same main headings.

Title and summary

Research projects become known by their title so it is important to provide a brief but accurate summary of the project. An acronym may be helpful as long as it is not too contrived. The title should give a clear indication of the purpose of the study and it can be helpful to indicate the methodology used, for example 'survey', 'randomised controlled trail', 'evaluation'.

For example, the titles for three recently funded proposals from the Chief Scientist Office (Scotland) (CSO 2008) are given below.

- Perceptions of future fertility among people of reproductive age with cancer, and their professional carers
- Cross-sectional survey of the individual, social and environmental determinants of physical activity participation in older people
- Response to oral agents in diabetes (ROAD) – pilot study

These titles all give enough information to describe the study and provide an indication of how they will be approached. And importantly, they are short and readable.

The summary that follows the title often has a specified word limit or number of characters (for example 150 words), so it is important to be succinct to ensure that all key areas relating to the proposal are covered. The summary should normally be written for a lay audience and provide an accessible overview of the focus of the study, how it will be undertaken and what the intended outcomes will be. Although the title and summary are usually written last of all, they are the first things that the reviewers will read and therefore give a strong indication of the quality of the proposal.

Background and justification of the study

Explaining why the proposed research study is important is absolutely pivotal. From my experience of reviewing proposals, it is often the flimsiest part of a proposal. There is often a misconception that the background literature can be reviewed as part of the actual study, either during the first few months of the PhD study or by a research assistant employed on a funded project.

Although an in-depth consideration of the known evidence base on the topic is usually included as part of an actual study, a research proposal needs to provide a strong case for the intended research, which draws on relevant literature. It is therefore paramount to undertake a review of key literature on the topic to demonstrate that the proposed study is needed because there is a gap in knowledge.

Proposals are usually sent out to reviewers who are experts in the topic area. So if I am making an argument that child neglect is under-researched on a particular aspect, I can be sure that the proposal will be sent to someone in the field of safeguarding children. I need to convince the reviewer that I have a good understanding of the main literature on the topic. In preparing the proposal it is essential that, as a nurse, I do not restrict my initial review solely to nursing journals. The two articles on child neglect (for example) that appeared in *Journal of Advanced Nursing* or *Journal of Clinical Nursing* this year may have been excellent, but these are not the key journals for child neglect research. So assume that the proposal will be sent to the key researchers on this topic (who may not be nurses) and write the proposal to persuade them of the need for the research. Knowing who the lead researchers are in a field is crucial, and including their work is obvious (but oft-forgotten). Venture beyond nursing journals to really contribute to nursing research.

As well as being thoroughly steeped in the literature and contemporary debates on a topic, it is also worthwhile considering the likely impact of the research on healthcare policy and/or practice.

Moreover, simple statistics can be used to provide a convincing argument for the research, for example the percentage of the population who experience a particular health problem, the incidence of hospital-acquired infection among a patient population or the ratio of the number of qualified to unqualified staff in a particular healthcare setting.

So, for example, we may want to undertake a small-scale, local study of student nurses' understanding of drug calculations. To provide a convincing case for the proposed research we can explain how many drug errors occur each year at a local and national level; we could project the costs of these errors to the health service, to the legal system, to the trade unions, as well as the emotional impact on the nurse or the patient if errors occur. We can locate the argument in the topical Patient Safety agenda and expose numerous benefits on a range of levels for undertaking this research. A small-scale study cannot possibly solve all the problems, but we could make links between our small local topic and the much wider political agenda. We could demonstrate that the proposed study could lead to a better understanding of the risks and lead to identifying potential interventions, to be tested in subsequent work, which may ultimately save the NHS money.

Box 8.1 identifies 10 key points that should be considered when preparing the background and rationale sections of a research proposal.

Research question and aims

The research question is arguably the most important part of a research proposal and requires careful consideration. Chapter 6 provides more detail of how to develop a research question. It is important to keep the question(s) simple and concise. Ideally, the background discussion will have led directly to the question, demonstrating a lack in current knowledge and why this is a worthwhile area of study. It is also acceptable to have more than one research question, although the design will need to demonstrate that they can all be answered.

Rather than research questions, or indeed in addition to these, you may prefer to describe the aims and objectives. This is a matter of style, but it may also be a requirement of the target audience for the pro-

Box 8.1   Background and rationale

- Cite key literature in the field (and if you or one of the team has written this, so much the better)
- Make clear linkages between different theories and models
- Summarise the main methods and findings in the field
- Leave an impression of thoroughness and mastery on the topic
- Succinctly describe what is already known
- Expose the gaps in the evidence
- Make a strong argument as to the benefits to practice, to policy, to the funding body
- Highlight the value to the health service, to users and carers, to practitioners
- Point out the consequences of not doing this research
- Locate the arguments in current and forthcoming priorities and concerns

posal. The same principles apply: research aims and objectives need to be clear and precise. Clearly articulating a research question/aim that comes directly from what has been found missing in the literature review and can be investigated is crucial.

The design (or plan of investigation)

At this point in the proposal the study area should be clear; a good case will have been made for it; and there should be a well-constructed question that clearly states the focus of the proposed study. The design of the study (sometimes referred to as a plan of investigation) should then follow. Chapter 2 provides an overview of the main issues to consider in designing a research study, which include selecting a suitable research methodology (quantitative or qualitative), the methods of data collection and analysis, and identifying an appropriate sample. It is essential that the research methodology is selected to address the research question rather than the other way round. A researcher may have a personal preference for undertaking qualitative research, but it is wholly inappropriate to use a qualitative approach to investigate a research topic that requires a quantitative design, for example investigating the effectiveness of a particular intervention. Use quantitative methods to answer quantitative questions, and qualitative methods to answer qualitative questions. Mixed

methods may be helpful if the research question has elements of both approaches (see Chapter 27 for more detail on this approach).

The research design should:

- demonstrate clearly how the research questions will be answered
- describe and justify the proposed sample
- explain how the research participants will be identified, approached and recruited to the study
- provide a robust account of how data will be collected and analysed.

Chapter 12 provides an overview of factors that should be considered in identifying the sample for both quantitative and qualitative studies. In quantitative studies, for example a clinical trial, power calculations may be undertaken to ascertain the correct sample size, but even if power calculations are inappropriate, it is still important to justify the proposed sample size in some other way. The advice of a statistician can be usefully sought at this stage.

Although it can be against the ethos of qualitative research to specify a precise sample size in advance, some indication of the number of research participants will need to be provided to demonstrate that sufficient data will be collected to answer the research questions and that the proposed data collection and

---

Box 8.2 The plan of investigation

- Will the methods answer the questions?
- Is the sample size defined?
- Is access to the population clear (and even agreed)?
- How will the data collection be undertaken, and by whom?
- What tools will be used for data collection?
- Are there examples of these tools (e.g. questionnaire, interview schedule)?
- Is the timeline clear and feasible?
- How will the data be analysed? By whom? When?
- What feedback will be given to participants and funders and at what stages?
- What are the likely outputs of the research?

---

ensuing analysis is feasible within the timescale of the study and funding available.

An account should also be provided of the proposed methods of data collection, justifying their inclusion and explaining how they will be carried out. For example, in undertaking a survey it will be important to state whether an existing validated questionnaire will be used and if so, to justify its appropriateness for the proposed study. Alternatively, if a new questionnaire is to be developed for the project, an explanation needs to be provided as to how it will be developed, piloted and validated. Likewise in an interview-based qualitative study, the choice of methods needs to be justified and an explanation provided as to how the interviews will be conducted, including venue, means of recording, etc.

This section of the proposal also needs to take account of how data will be analysed, by whom, using which methods and at what point in the timeline. It is important to provide as much clarity as possible. It is not sufficient to say that data will be analysed using SPSS v18. What tests will be undertaken using SPSS? Is the appropriateness of such tests demonstrated? Chapters 35 and 36 introduce the reader to statistical analysis; however, it can be useful to involve a statistician to help write this section of the proposal. Clarity regarding the analytic methods used for qualitative research is also required. It is not enough to suggest that themes will be derived from the transcripts. How will this happen? Using what tools and techniques? The analytic methods need to

be clearly described and reference made to appropriate frameworks for analysis. Chapter 34 provides an overview of different approaches to qualitative data analysis.

The plan of investigation should clearly demonstrate that every part of the research process has been carefully thought through. Box 8.2 provides 10 areas that should be considered.

The research team and project management

If writing a proposal for an education programme (e.g. a master's degree or PhD) the research 'team' will comprise primarily the student. However, when applying for research governance and ethical approval, the proposal will need to include details of the student's supervisor, as approval bodies consider the supervisor (as the more experienced researcher) to have overall responsibility for the research project. Chapter 9 provides guidance on identifying an appropriate supervisor.

If funding is being sought for the proposal, the composition of the research team will be crucial. The lead applicant (known as the principal investigator or PI) should have the experience, reputation and previous research success to give the proposal stature. Of course, everyone has to be principal investigator for a first time, but the PI should still have a reasonable publication record in the field, and if they do not have a track record of successful grant capture, there should be more senior people on the team who can offer support. Crucially, the composition of the research team needs to convince the funder that there is the necessary experience and expertise to deliver the grant successfully. Usually this means that one or two people have had previous successes, preferably with the same funder or at least a similar one. The best way to get this experience is to be co-applicant on some proposals first. Funders are cautious, and will be more inclined to fund studies undertaken by people who they consider are most likely to deliver.

The members of the team should provide complementary expertise. The curriculum vitae of each team member (which usually have to be provided as part of the submission) should demonstrate the range of experience in both the topic area and the proposed methods. There should be no glaring gaps in the team's expertise. If the team (or some combinations within the team) have worked together before, so much the better.

Approaching senior people who you want to be part of the research team can be daunting. However, if it is a good research idea and a well-formed proposal, they may well be willing to participate. With a large team it is important to gain agreement before submission on exactly what and how much everyone will be doing. The PI will have overall responsibility for the management of the project, but individual duties, tasks and areas of responsibility should all be articulated. Contracts of employment should be agreed with relevant human resource departments before commencement, as should agreement about office space and equipment. If there are likely to be issues relating to intellectual property rights (IPR) these should be discussed with the research contracts team at the researcher's place of employment.

Ethical considerations

A research proposal needs to include an account of the main ethical issues associated with undertaking the project and explain how these will be addressed. In the UK, it is almost certain that ethical approval will be required from either the National Research Ethics Service (NRES) or from another appropriate body (e.g. the university research ethics committee). Chapter 4 introduces the reader to the main ethical issues that need to be considered in developing a proposal, and Chapter 10 outlines the mechanisms required to gain ethical approval for health research in the UK. The application form for seeking approval from an NHS research ethics committee is extensive and there are potential benefits in starting to complete the application at the same time as you are developing the research proposal. The questions asked on the ethics application form may help the researcher select scientifically sound as well as ethically appropriate methods. The ethical application can then be held on file and submitted once funding has been secured.

Value for money

Reviewers of funded research proposals are always asked to consider whether a study represents good value for money, and will weigh up the costs of the study against the likely outputs. Contrary to popular opinion, this is not only whether people have asked for too much, but also if they have asked for too little.

All costs need to be justified, and fortunately universities and NHS R&D departments provide help with this aspect. Indeed, proposals normally have to be signed off by an appropriate finance officer prior to submission to a funding body.

Salaried time is usually the largest expense incurred. Is the research assistant employed at the appropriate rate? Costs may have been kept low, but the study may require someone on a higher salary scale because of the nature of the work. Employing someone full time for two years to undertake 10 interviews and a focus group is unlikely to be seen as good value. Conversely, is the proposal realistic in how much time is likely to be needed? Are the associated travel, consumables and equipment fully costed? Table 8.1 identifies the main points that need to be considered when costing a research proposal.

Dissemination

The dissemination plan requires careful consideration to demonstrate to the reviewers how the research team plan to share their findings with research

Table 8.1 Preparing the budget

Description	Explanation	Justification
Human resource	Salary costs of those employed; the time of those who are applicants if this is allowable; on-costs (national insurance, superannuation). The finance office will help, but it is the applicant's job to estimate as accurately as possible how much time everyone is going to spend on the study. This section should also include administrative or secretarial support	What exactly will people be doing with that time? Does the study really need an administrator as well as two research nurses?
Data collection	The costs that will be incurred by the study, such as travel expenses, meeting venues, catering costs for steering group members, participant incentive vouchers, equipment, postage, photocopying, etc.	Check what is allowed. Do not ask for equipment that is provided as standard in your place of work
Data processing	There may be costs associated with entering data into SPSS, or transcribing costs	Do not double-count: these costs may be covered under human resource
Dissemination	Include the costs of stakeholder events, booklet production, conference attendance, etc.	Check what is allowed. Many funders will not support conference attendance
Miscellaneous	Will there be a cost for inter-library loans or books? What about printing, consumables and product development?	Think through every stage of the research and if is going to cost something, put it in
Overheads	There is always a cost for lighting, heating, office space, insurances, etc. Do you have permission to waive this if the funder does not pay?	In UK universities, the introduction of 'full economic costing' (FEC) means that 'overheads' is no longer in common usage. Some funders have agreed to pay up to 80% of the costs of a study to cover the 'actual' costs of research. It is complicated, but the finance office will help. You need to check what the funder will cover

participants and potential users of the research. Funders are increasingly looking for innovative and targeted means of dissemination that take account of practitioners, academics, patients and carers, policy makers and the public. As outlined in Chapter 37, although journal articles and conference presentations are common forms of dissemination, researchers would do well to consider other avenues. For example, research websites, 'good practice' leaflets or stakeholder events are worth considering. Increasingly, funders are giving high weightings to dissemination plans as they seek assurance that the studies they fund have the potential for wide impact.

User involvement

The time has gone (thankfully) when research was undertaken on patients or other service users and they were then possibly told about what was found at the very end. As Chapter 5 has demonstrated, patients/service users and carers should be involved in every part of a study. A well-constructed proposal will demonstrate how public engagement has informed the development of the proposal and how they will be involved in the study itself. There is a fine line between tokenism and active participation and reviewers will be seeking evidence that where claims are made for user involvement it is meaningful and has been articulated clearly.

SUBMISSION REQUIREMENTS

Before spending hours writing a proposal it is important to check the requirements of the funding body. When does the proposal have to be submitted, by which date, electronically or in hard copy or both, how many copies and whose signatures need to be secured? These small bureaucratic details can be enormously time-consuming and can unravel everything right at the end. It is worth trying to get everything into place as early as possible. The rules for each submission will be slightly different, but one thing is certain: if the deadline is 12 noon on Tuesday, then the proposal must not be submitted at 4 pm Wednesday! If the proposal can be a maximum of eight pages in font size 12, then 10 pages in font size 6 will be discarded. Whereas it may be possible to adjust the margin width, most reviewers do not want to read a tightly condensed proposal with a magnifying glass. If not specified in the submission requirement, use a plain font (e.g. Arial or Verdana) and a font size of at least 10.

Even with excellent organisational skills, collating signatures can be a challenging undertaking. For larger grants it is not unusual to require all the applicants' signatures and those of their respective line managers. This should not too problematic, but you may also need the signature of the research sponsor (usually the head of the research services department in your organisation), who will not sign until they have read and understood the full proposal; the financial manager, who will not sign until all costings have been approved; the head of the NHS research and development office, who may not sign until the others have signed; and possibly various other people as well. It is worth alerting such individuals to the timescales and proposal development as early as possible, finding out what they require to be in place before they sign; and checking when and where they will be available. This all needs to be completed before final copies of the proposal are made and posted.

Most successful researchers will have had problems at this stage; mine include having to drive the submission to another city at 4am to deliver by hand, and racing around in a taxi to gather disparate signatures from across the region because I had overlooked the fact that every applicant had to complete an individual equal opportunities form. So the key message is to check the rules of submission and not wait until the last minute. If you have not followed the rules exactly, you will be giving the supervisor/committee/ funder the message that you are not reliable or careful, and that you cannot follow instructions. This is not a message likely to help you on your way to success. Box 8.3 suggests 10 points to consider before submission for a grant application for funding.

MAXIMISING SUCCESS

Even experienced researchers are not always successful in seeking funding for their proposals. Having a proposal turned down after all the hard work that has gone into its development is very disappointing and frustrating. It can be difficult to pick yourself up when this happens and the temptation is to discard the proposal. But while there are lots of reasons why proposals are not accepted, very few proposals are worth discarding altogether. It is always worth taking some time to reflect on the reasons why it was turned down and then trying again in a modified way, possibly with an application to a different funding body. It is a fact of life that more proposals will be rejected than are ever accepted. The acceptance rates of the larger research councils run at about 25%, and this is probably average for many other funders. This means that for every four proposals written by an experienced researcher, three are likely to be rejected. For novice researchers this rate is likely to be higher, so the effort:reward ratio in proposal writing is fairly imbalanced. However, the satisfaction that comes from having a grant accepted is perhaps worth the disappointments.

Proposals may not be rejected outright and the reviewer may provide guidance on how the proposal might be further developed. Because of the personal investment that has gone into developing the research

Box 8.3 Checklist for final submission

- Date and time of submission
- Number of copies required and in which format – paper or electronic?
- All signatures have been obtained
- Costings have been signed off by the relevant department(s)
- All applicant CVs are complete and in the required format
- All additional forms required from the applicants have been completed and signed
- Word limits have been checked for each section (if applicable)
- Font sizes and types and line spacing have been adhered to, and the proposal is easy to read
- Accompanying letter written by the principal investigator (either introducing the study, or responding to earlier feedback)
- Arrangements for posting/courier/hand delivery are in place

proposal it may be tempting to ignore the advice and stick to the original ideas. This kind of behaviour rarely pays off and on the whole it is worth responding to feedback from reviewers – even if you submit to a different funder. A proposal submitted after a response to feedback will almost certainly be enhanced. Of course, there may be some areas of disagreement, or it may appear that the reviewer had not fully understood some aspects of the proposal. Clarifying these points in a revised proposal and sending an accompanying letter in which you indicate that you have given careful consideration to the reviewer's comments and explain why you may not have addressed some of the concerns will often satisfy the funding body.

CONCLUSIONS

This chapter has charted the journey through writing a research proposal. The overall message is that the proposal needs to be written clearly, fit for purpose, robust and explicit. While there is no easy way of preparing a proposal, there are various strategies that can be used to increase the quality of the proposal. Working with more experienced researchers is an extremely useful way to begin. Although some of the bureaucratic detail required can be off-putting, there

should be people available to help with this side and engaging them from the beginning will maximise success. Resilience is key, as is the ability to learn through the process, even when a proposal is turned down for funding.

Well-constructed proposals using appropriate methods for the research question are generally successful. We owe it to our professional identity and reputation to make sure nurses submit high-quality, appropriately argued, well-constructed research proposals. If nursing is to truly make a difference to clinical practice, then rigorous research proposals that extend our knowledge and evidence base are essential.

Reference

CSO (2008): Recently funded projects [online]. Available at www.sehd.scot.nhs.uk/cso/index.htm (accessed 12 December 2008).

Further reading

Day Peters A (2003) *Winning Research Funding*. Farnham, Gower.

Fricker L (2004) *How to Write a REALLY Bad Grant Application (and Other Helpful Advice for Scientists)*. Milton Keynes, Authorhouse.

Krathwohl DR, Smith NL (2005) *How to Prepare a Dissertation Proposal: suggestions for students in education and the social and behavioral sciences*. New York, Syracuse University Press.

Mores J (2004) Preparing and evaluating qualitative research proposals. In: Seale C, Gobo G, Gubrium J, Silverman D (eds) *Qualitative Research Practice*. London, Sage, pp 493–503.

Phillips EM, Pugh DS (2000) *How to Get a PhD*. Buckingham, Open University Press.

Punch K (2006) *Developing Effective Research Proposals*. London, Sage.

Reif-Lehrer L (2005) *Grant Application Writer's Handbook*. Sudbury MA, Jones and Bartlett.

Thody A (2006) *Writing and Presenting Research*. London, Sage.

Websites

www.esrcsocietytoday.ac.uk – Economic and Social Research Council (ESRC). Click the 'academic' button and follow the links to writing a good proposal.

www.mrc.ac.uk/Fundingopportunities/Applicanthandbook/index.htm – Medical Research Council (MRC). The applicant handbook provides detailed advice on how to apply for an MRC grant, information that is useful more broadly.

www.rdinfo.org.uk/flowchart/Flowchart.html – R&D funding provides an overview of all stages of the research process, with useful sections on writing a successful proposal.

9 Planning and Managing a Research Project

Carol Haigh

Key points

- Various resources are available to enable the research student to identify and find funding for their study.

- Academic support is crucial to the success of the research study. Students need to be aware of:

  ○ how to choose a supervisor

  ○ what to expect from a supervisor

  ○ what a supervisor will expect from a research student.

- Sources of emotional and peer support need to be identified and used appropriately.

INTRODUCTION

For many research students, finding funding for their studies is the first hurdle they have to overcome in their educational advancement. Students need to be aware of how to identify and secure various sources of funding. However, funding is only one aspect of the support necessary to undertake a research study. The supervisor/student role is crucial to the successful completion of a research dissertation or thesis and cannot be taken for granted. Both supervisor and student need to understand how to get the most out of the supervisor–student relationship by being clear from the outset about expectations, roles and responsibilities. This chapter offers practical advice on how to identify and secure the necessary funding resources

and ensure appropriate supervisory, peer and emotional support to ensure success.

IDENTIFYING AND FINDING FUNDING

One of the first challenges facing the potential student is how to fund their study. Some employers are open to the idea of supporting students to undergraduate level; however, support for higher levels of study can be harder to obtain. There are a number of funding bodies that will provide financial support for individuals undertaking advanced study. Some of these may be disease-specific, such as the Parkinson's Disease Society, which will provide scholarships for nurse undertaking higher-level studies in Parkinson's disease, and there are other similar schemes run by healthcare organisations such as BUPA, professional organisations such as the Royal College of Nursing and the pharmaceutical industry.

One way of finding funding opportunities is to sign up for email alerts from funding databases such as RD Info (www.rdinfo.org.uk/), an organisation that is part of the National Institute for Health Research (NIHR) in the UK and which offers scholarship information for those researchers in the field of health and social care. Other professional groups or disciplines, such as the Joseph Rowntree Foundation (www.jrf.org.uk/) for social policy research, offer similar schemes. Many universities subscribe to the ResearchResearch website (www.researchresearch.com), which allows you to search by discipline, country and programme/level when seeking funding, as does the Postgraduate Studentships website (www.postgraduatestudentships.co.uk/). There are a number of other such sites and inserting the search term 'research student funding' into any internet search engine will bring them up. In addition, research scholarships for masters and doctoral studies are offered by the seven UK Research Councils, all of whom offer doctoral and postdoctoral fellowships in their associated disciplines (Haigh 2008).

For UK students wishing to study overseas, or for international students wishing to study in the UK, there are a number of fellowships run by organisations such as The British Council (www.britishcouncil.org) and The Fulbright Commission (www.fulbright.co.uk). UK universities occasionally offer scholarships for overseas students and these are advertised in the press and on websites such as the previously mentioned RDInfo.

Be aware that if you are planning to go for any kind of scholarship or funding for training from a specific funding body, time lines are usually quite tight. If you have already selected the institution in which you plan to study, and especially if you already have a contact in that institution, it might be a good idea to involve the programme leader or your potential doctoral supervisor in any scholarly funding bid. Not only will this give you the advantage of having an experienced mentor to help with the bid, it will indicate to funding bodies that you have identified a research mentor and a host organisation in which to carry out your research activity. Indeed, some funders expect the application to come from the supervisor rather than the student, so you need to be clear about who can actually apply before you start. Competition for studentships and fellowships is fierce, so you need a well-crafted project that makes a clear contribution to your discipline.

ACADEMIC AND PRACTICAL SUPPORT

Most students, at any academic level, find the thought of completing their dissertation or thesis a challenging one. A suitable supervisor and a clear understanding of the roles and expectations of both parties in the supervisory relationship can go some way to making the preparation and production of a dissertation or thesis achievable and fulfilling.

How to choose a supervisor

The relationship between a research student and their supervisor is one that can be argued to develop longitudinally as the student moves through the different strata of academia. The roles of both student and supervisor change over time; as the student acquires more knowledge they will require different things from their supervisor and the supervisor, in turn, has different expectations of the student (Thompson *et al.* 2005). It is appropriate at this point to explore what these needs and expectations are before exploring the student–supervisor relationship in greater detail.

Undergraduate supervision

Generally, at undergraduate level the relationship is very much that of a student and teacher. The student is starting out on the research path and can be seen to be a novice seeking support and direction from a more experienced colleague. At this stage the student often finds that they are allocated a supervisor and expected to make contact with them.

The main advantage of this approach is that the student, who may have little or no insight into the practicalities of the research process, is spared the stress of selecting someone to support them by an educationalist who has a good overview of the research skills and interests of the university staff and can try to match students with supervisors who will be best placed to help them through the process. The two main disadvantages are, first, that students may be allocated a supervisor based on their research topic rather than their approach. This may result in the student being supervised by a subject specialist who may have little expertise in the research methodology chosen. It is unfortunate when this scenario occurs because undergraduate research is often designed to introduce the student to research methods and processes that can be used in a wider context than in a confined, specific disciplinary field. It can also present a challenge if the student is choosing to explore a methodology that is not widely used in their specific field. For example, person-centred disciplines such as counselling tend to used person-centred research methods, so the undergraduate student who wishes to undertake a randomised controlled trial in that area may struggle to find a supervisor with the relevant experience.

In addition, students are usually allocated only one person to supervise their study at this level and this can present difficulties if the relationship is not an amiable one. Undergraduate students are generally unaware that they have any sort of influence in the selection of supervisors; it is not inappropriate for a student to approach academic staff with supervision requests, although it is sensible to select such staff on their suitability rather than their personality. If a student wants to change supervisors they should negotiate this with the undergraduate research tutor who may be able to help. It is never in the student's interest to simply disregard their supervisor, no matter how difficult the relationship or the synchronisation of diaries for tutorial time.

Postgraduate supervision

As with undergraduate research, there is some element of pedagogy in the student–supervisor relationship at postgraduate level. In the UK, the impact that the research governance system had on times-cales for research approval led to universities making changes to undergraduate dissertations such that master's level may be the first time the student has attempted a research project. So there needs to be a strong element of educational input from the supervisor. However, at the postgraduate level, particularly in the healthcare professions, a degree of professional expertise can be assumed and it is therefore, potentially, more useful to the student to have a supervisor with research rather than clinical expertise.

The relationship between doctoral student and supervisor is, it must be said, different from any other supervision relationship to which the student may have been exposed. The pedagogy of undergraduate and master's level supervision is subsumed by a partnership approach to project management in which it is as acceptable to challenge as be challenged by your supervisor.

TYPES OF SUPERVISOR

Work carried out by Trocchia and Berkowitz (1999) suggests that there are four main categories of supervisor and supervision.

- Nurturing – in this relationship the student obtains a great deal of help and support from their supervisor and other members of the faculty. Supervision tends to be formal and directive.
- Top down – similar to the formal nurturing role with the exception that the student is expected to show more signs of independent self-management.
- Near peers – this model is best suited to those students who value a high degree of independence in the direction of their study but who appreciate having access to their supervisor within a relationship of collegial equality.
- Platonistic – can be summed up in the phrase 'go away, do something, come back when it's good'. Students who benefit most from a platonistic supervisor are those who are extremely self-motivated and individualistic.

It can be seen that different supervision styles are appropriate at different academic levels and for different study styles. A supervisor's supervision style is something a student may wish to consider when selecting an academic mentor to support them through their research process. Standards for postgraduate student supervision are articulated in the UK by the Quality Assurance Agency for Higher Education (2004), and most universities base their own guidelines and regulations on them across all of the academic levels.

SUPERVISION SELECTION CRITERIA

At postgraduate and doctoral level, students will find that they have a degree of input into the make up of the supervisory team. Ellis (2006) and Lee (2008) have suggested that the following criteria should be considered when selecting a supervisor.

- Find a supervisor who is knowledgeable in their field.
- Whether methodologically focused or subject-specific, it is not inappropriate to expect potential supervisors to be fully conversant with the topic or methods to be used.
- Expect to have or find a supervisor who understands the nature of master's or PhD work.
- Any supervisor involved should be familiar with the standards expected of students studying at these specific academic levels.
- The potential supervisor should have enough time for meetings.
- Sometimes this can only be assessed once the student–supervisor relationship has been established, but a simple rule of thumb is that students should expect to have at least an undisturbed hour of their supervisor's time.
- Find someone with whom you can get on.

For doctoral students, the relationship with their supervisor will be one that lasts at least three years or even longer for part-time students, so it is important that the association is one that is founded on mutual regard. Life can be very difficult for both student and supervisor if that regard is absent.

THE RESPONSIBILITIES OF THE SUPERVISOR

As has already been emphasised, the relationship between supervisor and PhD student is very different from other supervisory relationships. For the relationship to be a success, the expectations of both parties should be made clear at the start.

At the earliest point of the relationship negotiation is of key importance. A wise supervisor will use initial meetings to ensure that supervision arrangements and the role of progress meetings are clear and agreed. At undergraduate and master's level, when students are working to an extremely strict time schedule, the supervisor may expect such meetings to be regularly scheduled. However, doctoral students have the luxury of more time for the completion of their study so some supervisors may well be more flexible and less prescriptive about contact (Malfroy 2005).

In the early stages of research, particularly at undergraduate but often at higher levels as well, the student can feel as if they are drifting because they may have an idea of what they wish to study but no concrete plans as to how to collect information. In these cases, the supervisor may be able to assist in the planning and operation of a realistic plan of research and provide guidance about literature.

Although at undergraduate and at master's level the dissertation is the end point of a programme of study – the task that draws all previous work into a coherent whole – one of the defining characteristics of doctoral study is the expectation that the student will develop and enhance research skills throughout the process. To this end, a good supervisor will provide an example of good research and academic conduct, arrange instruction in research techniques and supplementary classes as required, and support access to any doctoral training programmes on offer. They can also encourage integration with the wider academic community via conferences and seminars.

One of the biggest challenges for students who are undertaking healthcare research is the obligation to obtain ethical approval from an ethics review committee and, in the UK, this is further complicated by the need to obtain research governance approval as well. This is the point when supervisors and students should discuss the personal safety of the student throughout the research process and delineate lone-worker policies or strategies if appropriate. It is not inappropriate for students to expect help with ethical approval, risk assessment and governance forms and attend local research ethics committee meetings when appropriate. Ethics committees appreciate it when supervisors attend to support their students, as do most students. Chapter 10 provides more detail of the processes involved in securing ethical approval.

On the more practical side of the supervision process, all supervisors have a significant role to play in monitoring the standard of the work produced and the student's progress. This includes ensuring that the appropriate documents and milestones are met in order for the student to progress.

At doctoral level the supervisor has a responsibility to make sure that the student understands the nature and process of thesis examination; for many students this can include setting up practice viva voce events. The thought of the viva is one that many doctoral students dread. The challenges of the examination can to some extent be obviated by careful selection of examiners and the supervisor has a key role in this respect. The recruitment of and liaison with examiners is the sole responsibility of the supervisor, as is approving submission of the finished thesis. Students should be aware that, even though the supervisor approves the thesis for submission, final approval of the thesis is a matter for the examiners not the supervisor.

What supervisors should do to keep students happy

While the practical element of the supervisory role clearly helps to facilitate the student's progress, there are a number of simple things that a supervisor can do to promote peace of mind in their supervisees.

Set clear goals. The first meeting of any supervisory relationship is the most crucial since it is the one at which the tone and direction of all future meetings will be set. Clear outlines of the roles, requirements and expectations can be discussed and agreed by all

parties. It is crucial that the student is clear on what is expected of them and what they can expect of the supervisor if the relationship is to flourish.

Be prepared for supervisory meetings. It is important that the supervisor and student view supervision sessions with the same degree of importance. For the supervisor this means ensuring that work the student has submitted for the session has been thoroughly read and critiqued and, if necessary, feedback prepared. It is also a good idea to review the notes made at the previous meeting to ensure that there are no outstanding tasks for the supervisor to complete before the next encounter.

Answer emails. One of the biggest criticisms levelled at supervisors by their students is the dilatory nature of email response. Even a simple response acknowledging receipt of the student work and providing a broad timetable for a more detailed response will help to make the student happy.

Be available to attend seminars, local research ethics committees, etc., to support the student. One of the crucial sources of support that a supervisor can offer is to be present at some of the presentations or professional encounters the student will undertake at various stages of their programme of study. It can be very comforting to a student to have their supervisor present when they are making their first conference presentation for example, if only to field some of the challenging questions that are often posed to novices on the conference circuit (Haigh 2007).

It is also very important that the supervisor makes every effort to attend the local research ethics committee with their student. Although ethics committees are generally sympathetic to student research, especially at the undergraduate and postgraduate levels, doctoral students are regarded as researchers first and students second. Having their supervisor with them can provide much-needed confidence and support and also, incidentally, shows the ethics committee that the student is adequately supervised.

Be there at all the important milestone events – especially the viva. As a student progresses through their postgraduate and doctoral studies there are various points of assessment that require the reassuring presence of the supervisor. Different education institutions mange these in different ways, but the one event that the supervisor must not miss is the PhD viva. Although, often the supervisor is not permitted to participate in the viva process, merely having them in the room taking notes on the proceedings is a source of tremendous support for the student.

In summary, whether at undergraduate, postgraduate or doctoral level, the supervisor is there to help to support and guide the student to a greater or lesser degree. The relationship develops and changes across the academic levels, but students should remember that a fundamental part of the supervisor's role is to facilitate them through the process.

THE RESPONSIBILITIES OF THE STUDENT

The section above clearly delineates the responsibilities of the supervisor. However, it must be acknowledged that the supervisor–supervisee relationship is a two-way street, with the student having a significant part to play. It may seem evident to suggest that the student should undertake to study conscientiously and at a level appropriate to the research degree. However, this is a fundamental student responsibility. It is not appropriate for the student to interpret the supervisory relationship as one in which they only do what the supervisor suggests or, an even worse scenario, they expect the supervisor to do the majority of the work.

It is incumbent on the supervisee to seek the advice and constructive criticism of the supervisor. In many cases, with the exception of doctoral study, the supervisor is involved in the marking of the finished work and it is therefore sensible to listen to the suggestions they make. Having said that, it is also important to remember that it is *your* study, so do not allow your supervisor to sidetrack your project if you do not feel it is an appropriate or fruitful direction in which to go. However, it is in the student's best interest to attend regular supervisory meetings. This can be difficult if study is being undertaken on a part-time basis, especially as many healthcare students are fitting their studies around the demands of the clinical environment. If it has been difficult to make contact with or keep appointments with supervisors and some period of time has elapsed since the last meeting, students sometimes feel reluctant to make contact.

However, most supervisors will be pleased to hear from their student no matter how much time has gone by and will understand the pressures inherent in balancing study with clinical practice. It is important that students do not lose contact with supervisors or allow themselves to 'drift' simply because they are too embarrassed to get in touch. At all levels of study there is an obligation on the student to undertake to submit the finished dissertation or thesis within the scheduled registration period, and doctoral students will be expected to attend such research training as is offered or provided by the supervisor or the research institute – regular contact with supervisor(s) will facilitate this.

Every university has a number of milestones inherent within the dissertation/thesis route that are designed to assess progress. These milestones tend to be more formalised at the doctoral level. The doctoral student will be expected to work with the supervisor to meet all important milestones, producing any written work expected to deadline and to a suitable standard. Participation in these progression meetings are another useful source of support, since they often constitute an opportunity for a student's work to be scrutinised by people who are external to the supervisory team. This brings the advantage of a new perspective to the work.

The opportunity to integrate with the wider academic community is one that is more likely to be offered to postgraduate and doctoral students rather than undergraduates. However, most undergraduate students can expect to be called on to undertake presentations to their peers at some point in their programme of study. Although this can seem daunting, and even experienced presenters often find it easier to present to strangers rather than peers, it is an essential skill to possess. Research that is not promulgated is pointless and so the early development of confidence in presenting your own work is essential.

Many master's-level students are encouraged by their supervisors to turn their dissertations into conference presentations or published papers. This is an excellent thing to do. Such presentations, developed and produced by the student, are sometimes reviewed and edited by the supervisor. If that is the case then it is not inappropriate for the supervisor to be credited as an author. Authorship, order of authors and potential publications should be discussed early on in the writing process.

At doctoral level there is an absolute expectation that the student will publish, if not during, then very soon after the completion of their work. In this instance the supervisor will expect to be credited as an author. Students are strongly encouraged to publish their work only with the prior knowledge of their supervisor, since more than their own reputation may be at stake. Conference presentations, particularly at the national and international level, are also key to the doctoral student's development and the supervisor can be helpful in signposting which ones will be most useful to the student. The doctoral student, particularly in the latter stages of their study, will be on the look out for suitable examiners and such events are often a good way of getting a feel for those people who may be potential assessors.

What students should do to keep supervisors happy

So far, this chapter has focused on the practical support inherent within the supervisory relationship. However, the key to a successful supervisor–supervisee relationship, as with any other, is understanding the small things that can be done to ensure the co-operation and regard of the other party. So, to ensure that supervisors come to supervision sessions in a tranquil and positive frame of mind, the following strategies are recommended.

Do not expect them to comment on written work that they have not seen in advance. Nothing can annoy a supervisor more than if the student arrives for a supervision session equipped with their latest draft chapter (or even the entire first draft of their thesis) expecting the supervisor to read it and comment on the content intelligently while the student sits expectantly at their side. Likewise, if the focus of the supervision session is to be your latest 20,000-word literature review, sending it to your supervisor at 3.30 on a Friday afternoon does not mean you can expect them to have reviewed it by 10.30 on Monday morning.

Make proper appointments. One of the difficulties inherent for most supervisors when supervising

work colleagues or full-time students who work on campus is the informal 'pop-in'. Slipping into your supervisor's office to say 'hello' and leaving 2 hours later having discussed your latest data collection problems is likely to become irksome to your supervisor sooner rather than later. It is always advisable to make a follow-up appointment at the end of each scheduled supervision session. If you do not need it you can cancel it at a later date, whereas trying to make an appointment at short notice can be troublesome.

Bring an agenda. One of the expectations of undertaking a dissertation or thesis is that the student will develop or enhance their organisational skills. Whether working at undergraduate level, when you want your supervision to be direct and to the point, or at master's or doctoral level, where supervision may be more discursive, bringing an agenda to meetings will ensure that you cover all the points on which you want an opinion and thus derive the maximum benefit from the encounter.

Be prepared for constructive criticism. It can be quite difficult, as you nurture your thesis to its conclusion, to expose it to scrutiny and criticism. However, your supervisor will comment on both the strengths and the weakness of the work you produce and you should expect such criticism to be constructive. Your supervisor will probably expect you to take their criticism into account. It is not compulsory, but if the criticism is constructive and you choose not to address it, you should have a strong rationale for your decision.

Keep in touch. It has already been shown how easy it is to lose contact with your supervisor and how difficult it is to re-establish that contact as time goes by. Most supervisors see maintenance of contact as a student responsibility and so would be unlikely to chase up communication defaulters. However, they will value the occasional email to reassure them that your work is continuing.

Do not demand or agree to unrealistic deadlines. Many students, especially at the earlier stages of their academic career, find the setting of goals or deadlines to be met before the next supervision meeting gives a structure and focus to their work. However, if having demanded such deadlines of their supervisor, the student is regularly unable to meet them, the supervisor may become annoyed or begin to question the student's commitment to the study.

Keep comprehensive records. Some supervisors are very efficient in the record they keep of supervision sessions, others less so. It is always in the student's best interest to keep records of the discussion and goal setting that occurs in the supervisory session, but sharing and agreeing these records with the supervisor will help to facilitate the relationship.

In summary, the student must be aware that the supervision process is a collaborative one. The amount of power and autonomy the individual has within the relationship varies across the academic levels, but students should remember that a fundamental part of the success of supervisory support is their participation in the process (Thompson *et al.* 2005).

SOURCES OF EMOTIONAL AND PEER SUPPORT

Your supervisor is there to offer academic advice and support. Boucher and Smyth (2004) have suggested that it is possible for a satisfactory supervisory relationship to be maintained between two people who are also friends. However, Sullivan and Ogloff (1998) have warned that the supervisor's objectivity may be jeopardised if a more personal relationship is in existence, and Lee (2008) cautions that boundaries may become blurred to the detriment of both the supervisory and the personal relationship. For the supervisory relationship to serve the student's best interests it is wise to ensure that boundaries are clear and to seek emotional support from other sources.

Personal tutors

Many universities insist on students having a personal tutor. This person is generally external to any academic supervision team, exists to act in a pastoral role and is usually concerned with the students welfare. Very often the personal tutor role is a loose and casual one and students only seek out their tutor when in the throes of a personal crisis. Malik (2000) noted that uptake of and satisfaction with the personal

tutor role was enhanced when regular meetings were formally scheduled and the student and tutor worked to develop a relationship early on in the education process.

Family, friends and other students

There is no doubt that undertaking a dissertation or thesis can impact significantly on family life. Family and friends will have to become accustomed to your long periods of absence as you write up your research. However, they can also be a good source of emotional support and may be counted on to act as passive listeners when things go wrong. They can also help to counteract 'writing-up syndrome' by encouraging you to take a break from the computer.

Thomas (2002) noted that the 'family' played a significant role in undergraduate student retention, citing the support offered as a major factor contributing to completion of a programme of study. She also acknowledged that the identity of the family changed to include other students on the programme who provided support and understanding. This can be an issue for part-time students who may lose out on this camaraderie, and/or doctoral students who very often work in isolation, and these groups should be encouraged to make extra effort to connect with their peers.

Thus, it can be seen that other students are a good source of emotional support throughout the process. It is ironic that, at doctoral level, where input from peers could be seen to be crucial to mental wellbeing, students tend to work alone with little engagement with the academic community. However, peers understand the challenges and pressures inherent in the course of study and can often provide both practical and emotional support.

External support mechanisms

Although friends, family and other students can provide good levels of emotional care, it is also a good idea to seek such support from people who are external to the institution of study. This is especially true at the doctoral level, when conversation with other PhD students allows for comparison of supervisory styles, institutional expectations and a sharing of concerns and worries. There are a number of doctoral student support networks around the UK; some are organised by universities while others, such as the Doctoral Student Network (www.rcn.org.uk/development/researchanddevelopment/rs/networking/phd_student_network), are hosted by professional organisations, in this case the Royal College of Nursing. These networks are similar in that they attempt to provide an arena for doctoral students across the UK to meet and exchange experiences. In addition, a number of clinical and research-focused conferences have fringe events that are explicitly aimed at students of all levels who are undertaking the research element of a programme of study or a PhD, and it is often worthwhile making an effort to attend them.

Online communities and social network sites

One of the difficulties that face practitioners is finding enough time to attend support events in the 'real' or offline world. That is why online communities and social networking sites can be an attractive source of support. An asynchronous discussion board, that is a site where messages are posted but interaction does not take place in real time, can allow students to post their concerns at any time of the day or night. An added advantage of using international rather than national or university-specific discussion groups is that, as the internet transcends geographical boundaries, there is always likely to be someone online to talk with.

A number of research students finding blogging a cathartic and useful way of seeking emotional support from others. Blog is a portmanteau word that is a contraction of the term 'web log'. A blog is a website that has regular entries of commentary that can be read and commented on by others. There are a number of student blogs of all academic levels on the internet and at the very least they can reassure students that they are not alone in their experiences.

Finally, social networking sites such as Facebook or Bebo can also be attractive to students. Social networking sites are places where users can join networks organised by city, workplace, school and region to connect and interact with others. People can also add contacts and send them messages, and update their personal profile to notify contacts about themselves. It must be noted that some social networking sites are banned in certain overseas countries and so this option may not be so useful to some international students.

CONCLUSIONS

This chapter has signposted some of the sources that are available to research students for the funding of their studies. Nurses and other health-related professionals have not had a tradition of seeking funding from external bodies that is other than their employing institution or from their personal finances. However, as more healthcare professionals enter academe an awareness of alternate sources of funding is important.

The main focus of this chapter, however, has been the roles and responsibilities inherent in the supervisor–supervisee relationship: the nature and style of supervision, and strategies for emotional and peer support. Students of all academic levels need to be aware that they have varying degrees of autonomy in the supervisory relationship and that they should exercise this autonomy if they are to get maximum benefit from the experience.

References

Boucher C, Smyth A (2004) Up close and personal: reflections on our experience of supervising research candidates who are using personal reflective techniques. *Reflective Practice* **5**(3): 345–356.

Ellis L (2006) The professional doctorate for nurses in Australia: findings of a scoping exercise. *Nurse Education Today* **26**(6): 484–493.

Haigh C (2008) Life after your professional doctorate: what happens next? In: Lee NJ *Achieving your Professional Doctorate. A handbook.* Buckingham, McGraw Hill, pp 187–204.

Haigh C (2007) Peacocks and jellyfish; steps and strategies for successful conference chairing. *Nurse Education Today* **27**: 91–94.

Lee NJ (2008) *Achieving your Professional Doctorate. A handbook*. Buckingham, McGraw Hill.

Malfroy J (2005) Doctoral supervision, workplace research and changing pedagogic practices. *Higher Education Research & Development* **24**(2): 165–178.

Malik S (2000) Students, tutors and relationships: the ingredients of a successful student support scheme. *Medical Education* **34**: 635–641.

Quality Assurance Agency for Higher Education (2004) *The Code of Practice for the Assurance of Academic Quality and Standards in Higher Education*. Available at www.qaa.ac.uk

Sullivan L, Ogloff J (1998) Appropriate supervisor graduate student relationships. *Ethics and Behavior* **8**(3): 229–248.

Thomas L (2002) Student retention in higher education: the role of institutional habitus. *Journal of Education Policy* **17**(4): 423–442.

Thompson D, Kirkman S, Watson R, Stewart S (2005) Improving research supervision in nursing. *Nurse Education Today* **25**: 283–290.

Trocchia PJ, Berkowitz D (1999) Getting doctored: a proposed model of marketing doctoral student socialization. *European Journal of Marketing* **33**(7/8): 746–759.

Websites

www.fulbright.co.uk – the Fulbright Commission offers awards and advice for study, research, lecturing or professional development in any academic field.

www.jrf.org.uk/ – the Joseph Rowntree Foundation issues calls for research proposals in two main areas: (a) examining the root causes of poverty, inequality and disadvantage and identifying solutions; (b) contributing to the building and development of strong, sustainable and inclusive communities.

www.rcn.org.uk/development/researchanddevelopment – the Royal College of Nursing Research and Development Co-ordinating Centre provides information on a doctoral student network and scholarly awards.

www.rdinfo.org.uk – RD Info provides information on research funding and training events for health researchers.

www.researchresearch.com – ResearchResearch offers a research funding alert service and regular news bulletins of research opportunities.

10 Gaining Access to the Research Site

Leslie Gelling

Key points

- All research involving human participants requires ethical review by an appropriate research ethics committee (REC). Research involving NHS patients, staff or property requires the opinion of an NHS REC.

- In addition to obtaining a favourable ethical opinion from an appropriate REC, all researchers wishing to undertake research in the NHS must obtain approval from an NHS R&D department in accordance with research governance requirements before the study can begin.

- Researchers should pay particular attention to issues around confidentiality and informed consent.

- Researchers should consider recent changes to the law and the legal context in which research is undertaken.

- Seeking the required approvals to access the research site can be complex and time-consuming, so adequate time should be allowed to plan the research and prepare necessary applications and paperwork.

- Researchers should treat seeking the required approvals as an integral and useful stage in the planning of their research project.

INTRODUCTION

Of all the chapters undergoing revision for this sixth edition of *The Research Process in Nursing*, none can be more in need of update than this one. Since publication of Amanda Hunn's chapter in the 2006 edition, the multiple processes for seeking permissions and approvals to access research sites have

moved on considerably. In addition, significant changes and additions to the law in European Union (EU) and the UK have transformed the legal context within which research is now undertaken. This chapter will offer a practical overview of the approvals required to access research sites, drawing on the author's experience as a researcher, as chair to an NHS research ethics committee (REC) and as chair to a university faculty research ethics panel.

THE NEED FOR REGULATION OF RESEARCH

In recent years researchers have been expected to adhere to a wealth of regulations, guidance and codes of practice when undertaking their research endeavours. Most professional bodies and research organisations have published their own guidance, including the Royal College of Nursing (RCN 2005; 2007) and the Medical Research Council (MRC 2005). The problem with these and other multiple guidelines is that they are not mandatory and can offer conflicting advice. Researchers have also been expected to comply with the principles of the World Medical Association's Declaration of Helsinki since its publication in 1964. There have been multiple revisions, most recently in 2008, but again the Declaration is not compulsory and there has been much discussion about how the Declaration should be used in different forms of research and in a climate very different to that in which the Declaration was first published (Goodyear *et al*. 2008). Despite the differences of opinion, the Declaration of Helsinki remains the foundation upon which ethical practice in all biomedical research, including nursing research, involving human participants is performed.

What is clear is that these various guidelines and codes of practice have repeatedly failed to halt unethical research in the past (Beecher 1966; Pappworth 1967) or more recently (Smith 2006; Saunders & Savulescu 2008; Wells & Farthing 2008). Repeated high-profile incidences of unethical and potentially harmful research, including the retention of children's organs without informed consent at Alder Hey Children's Hospital in Liverpool, resulted in the Department of Health publishing its *Research Governance Framework for Health and Social Care* in 2001, which was revised and updated in 2005 (DoH 2001a; 2005). This framework clarified the roles of all those involved in health and social care research and added the requirement that researchers seek local NHS approval in addition to seeking an ethical opinion. Researchers are now required to undertake this dual review process before they are able to access research sites or to begin their research.

The UK has had a system for ethical review in place since the 1970s, but it is only more recently that ethical review has been regulated by the law. The EU Clinical Trials Directive 2001/20/EC (European Parliament and Council of the European Union 2001) and the Directive's implementation into UK law through the Medicines for Human Use (Clinical Trials) Regulations (2004) have placed particular legal requirements on RECs, not least the obligation that they make their final opinion available within 60 days of a valid application being submitted. In addition to dealing with practical matters related to the management and organisation of RECs, the Directive also outlined the important points to be considered during the process of ethical review. The Directive was written primarily to harmonise the management of clinical trials across the EU and its implementation by member states, including the UK, has undoubtedly improved the processes of ethical review for both RECs and researchers. Although the Directive strictly relates to clinical trials only, there have also been advantages for researchers undertaking all other forms of research in health and social care. For examples, the 60-day rule has been applied to *all* research reviewed by NHS RECs in the UK, not just to clinical trials.

Past failures by researchers to comply with ethical guidelines and codes of practice have resulted in an increasing reliance on the law to provide a structure to the context within which research is undertaken. In addition to the *EU Clinical Trials Directive*, researchers are also now required to comply with a number of legal requirements when seeking approvals to access research sites (see Box 10.1).

Box 10.1 Research ethics and the law

The Children Act 1989
The Data Protection Act 1998
EU Clinical Trials Directive
   2001/20/EC
The Human Tissue Act 2004
The Medicines for Human Use
   (Clinical Trials) Regulations 2004
The Mental Capacity Act 2005

During the process of ethical review, a REC will need to be convinced that all data and personal information will be handled in compliance with the Data Protection Act 1998, that the collection and storage of human tissue samples complies with the requirements of the Human Tissue Act 2004, and that the acquisition of informed consent always complies with the requirements of the Mental Capacity Act 2005. This is further complicated because the law can be different in different parts of the UK. For example, in Scotland the Children (Scotland) Act 1995 and the Adults with Incapacity (Scotland) Act 2000 take precedence over the above Acts of Parliament.

Recent changes to the law have placed greater emphasis on the need for researchers to always act in a manner deemed acceptable by society and the wider scientific community. RECs and R&D departments play important roles in ensuring that researchers comply with the law, act in an ethical manner and do not put research participants or themselves in positions of unacceptable risk while undertaking scientifically rigorous research that will contribute to existing knowledge. Ultimately, the aim is to generate high-quality evidence to inform clinical practice, an aim shared by researchers, RECs and R&D departments. Evidence would suggest that researchers have repeatedly failed to always act in an ethical manner, so it is through a meticulous and rigorous dual review process that society can have confidence in the safety and value of health and social care research.

RESEARCH ETHICS

All research involving human participants requires ethical review by an appropriate REC. Research involving NHS patients, staff or property requires the opinion of an NHS REC. Although NHS RECs will give an opinion on any health and social care research placed before them, there are RECs outside the NHS, including university research ethics committees (URECs), RECs in social care organisations and independent RECs. These non-NHS RECs undertake important work and make a significant contribution to supporting health and social care research in the UK. The remainder of this chapter will focus on

ethical review by NHS RECs, but it is usually possible to find information about URECs on individual university websites. Although the organisation, management and membership of different RECs may vary, the principles underpinning ethical review are constant. This is demonstrated by the membership and work of the Association of Research Ethics Committees (AREC). Members are drawn from all of the above RECs with the shared aim of protecting research participants from unduly risky or unethical research, while also encouraging research of high quality.

The remit of research ethics committees

NHS RECs (from here on known as RECs) will consider all research involving the NHS or research requiring review by an NHS REC as a result of recent changes to the law. This includes research that needs to meet the requirements of the Medicines for Human Use (Clinical Trials) Regulations 2004, the Mental Capacity Act 2005 and the Human Tissue Act 2004. In addition, RECs will review any human research submitted from any source related to health and social care.

RECs have evolved over time but it remains their principal objective to protect potential and actual research participants from harm associated with research (Gelling 1999). RECs do not attempt to eliminate all risk but they do try to balance risks against possible benefits. Almost all research involves risk, either physical or psychological. In particular, much research, including clinical trials of medicinal products, has a high degree of uncertainty about possible side effects. RECs will want to be reassured that the risks are not excessive and do not exceed the possible benefits. As importantly, the REC will want to be confident that research participants are made aware of the risks to which they might be exposing themselves before and during the research.

In addition to protecting research participants, RECs will also be keen to protect others, including the researchers, from possible risks associated with a research project. For example, if researchers plan to visit participants in their own homes, the REC will want to be reassured that all possible steps are being taken to protect the researchers from harm. Many research groups now have lone-worker policies that address such matters, and details should be provided to the REC reviewing the research.

RECs will also want to know that appropriate indemnity arrangements are in place should anything go wrong. For student projects, indemnity is usually arranged through their university. For all other research, indemnity is usually arranged through the chief investigator's employer. In all instances where the application for ethical approval is being made to an NHS REC, the sponsor will sign to confirm that the appropriate indemnity arrangements are in place. Other RECs, including university RECs, will also want to be sure that arrangements are in place.

The system for ethical review

While there has been a formal research ethics system operating in the UK for many years, such systems only acquired legal status in 2004 as a result of *the EU Clinical Trials Directive 2001/20/EC* and the Directive's implementation into UK law through *the Medicines for Human Use (Clinical Trials) Regulations*. As a result of this legislation it became a requirement to obtain a favourable ethical opinion for all clinical trials of medicinal products. In addition to the 60-day rule highlighted above, it also became a requirement that researchers need only to seek the opinion of a single REC regardless of the number of sites involved in the research.

The ethical review of research came under the control of a single authority known as the UK Ethics Committee Authority (UKECA), headed by the Secretary of State for Health. The day-to-day management and governance of all NHS RECs came under the control of the Central Office for Research Ethics Committees (COREC), established by the Department of Health in 2000. In 2007, COREC was replaced by the National Research Ethics Service (NRES), part of the National Patient Safety Agency (NPSA). All REC members are now recruited through a transparent process and receive letters of appointment from the NHS.

Since its establishment, one of the main objectives for NRES has been to standardise the process for seeking the opinion of RECs in the UK. In the past each REC had its own application processes, its own ways of working and its own application forms. This made the process of seeking an ethical opinion hugely time-consuming, especially with multi-site studies. The processes have now been standardised and all RECs adhere to *The Governance Arrangements for Research Ethics Committees* (DoH 2001b) and work within a single set of standard operating procedures. This process of standardisation means that all applications submitted in the UK, to whichever REC, should be treated and reviewed in a similar manner.

The most important change to the process for ethical review has been the introduction of the single standard application process and application form called the Integrated Research Application System (IRAS). Launched in 2008, IRAS is an online application system that enables researchers to input data once for the majority of possible approvals required to access research sites. Much of the criticism of the past online application form concerned the length of the form and the repeated appearance of irrelevant questions. The new, 'intelligent' form begins with a number of filter questions that then determine which questions the researcher needs to answer, and unnecessary questions do not appear. The new IRAS form makes seeking the necessary approvals easier for researchers and for those reviewing the applications.

Applying for an ethical opinion

The first point to consider is whether it is necessary to seek an ethical opinion at all. RECs will offer an opinion on all research submitted to them but their opinion is not required if the project is audit or service evaluation. NRES offers a useful document that differentiates between these three forms of investigation (NRES 2008). It is important that researchers do not describe their research as anything other than research in an attempt to avoid the need to seek the opinion of an REC. Deliberately avoiding the opinion of an REC in this way would be considered a form of research misconduct and could result in serious repercussions for the researcher.

An important early consideration is to determine which REC an application should be submitted to. There are still more than 100 RECs in the UK and

Box 10.2 Types of
research requiring review
by specialised RECs

Clinical trials of medicinal products
Medical devices
Research involving prisoners
Adults with incapacity
Children and young people
Human tissue and samples
Prison research

many specialise in the review of different types of research, so it is important that applications are submitted to a REC able to undertake the review. Box 10.2 highlights some of the types of research requiring review by specialist RECs. These types of research will need the applicant to contact the NRES Central Allocation System (CAS) to be allocated to an appropriate REC. If an application is submitted to a REC that cannot undertake its review, it is possible that there will be a considerable delay for the researcher and unnecessary work for the REC. For many types of research the application will be submitted to the most convenient local REC.

Applicants are required to submit three sets of paperwork: the protocol; the application form; and additional papers, including participation information sheets and consent forms. It is the author's experience that fewer than 10% of projects receive an unfavourable opinion because of ethical issues and only 14% have an uninterrupted passage through the process (NRES 2007). Of the remaining applications, a small number will have minor ethical problems, but nearly all will display flaws in the paperwork. It is important, therefore, that great care is taken in the preparation of the application form and accompanying papers. If there are inconsistencies between the application form and the protocol or if the application is full of spelling and grammatical errors, the REC will seek clarification and amendment before an application can proceed to a favourable opinion. It is also important that all required documents are submitted with the necessary signatures.

Despite many improvements in the application form, completion can remain a burdensome task, not least because few researchers ever have to use the form sufficiently frequently to become comfortable with it. The time required to complete the form should not be underestimated. The perceived burden can be somewhat eased if researchers make themselves aware of the ethical requirements and expectations of RECs from the outset. This allows for 'built-in' rather than 'bolt-on' ethics and increases the likelihood of smooth passage through the review process. In addition to reading the guidance made available on the NRES website, researchers might consider attending a REC meeting as an observer, enabling them to gain an insight into how the REC works, how it deals with applications and the key points the REC is likely to consider when reviewing an application.

The application form should be completed in lay language, making it accessible to all members of the REC. Challenging technical text copied verbatim from the protocol may leave REC members unable to understand the research and unable to reach an informed opinion. This is particularly important for the free-text responses that describe the research questions and objectives, scientific justification and methods. To further ensure clarity, it is recommended that every effort is made to attend the REC meeting to discuss the project with the committee. By attending the meeting, the applicant is able to clarify misunderstandings and to answer the REC's questions. This can help ease the progress of the application through the review process.

The Patient Information Sheet (PIS) is the document most rigorously scrutinised by the REC and also the one most frequently requiring modification following review. There should be no conflicting information between the PIS and the application form. Such inconsistency is surprisingly frequent and makes it hard for the REC to reach an informed opinion, especially if the researcher is not available to provide clarity. Researchers should note that many REC members start their review by reading the PIS as this is the document most likely to provide a lay introduction to the proposed research.

When appropriate, the PIS template on the NRES website can be used. NRES suggests a two-part PIS; part 1 provides general information about the research and part 2 provides more detailed information about specific points. They also provide a list of the questions that might be included in both parts of the PIS (see Box 10.3). This can be amended according to the nature of the research; it may not be appropriate to use all the headings in the template and it may be helpful to add additional headings. It is also permissible to reorder the questions so that information is presented in a logical order. Many applicants stick rigidly to the NRES template with the result that the PIS is often difficult to read.

Research participants are often members of the general public, so paperwork should be written in appropriate language (Franck & Winter 2004), remembering that the average reading age in the UK is that of a 9-year-old. This can be tailored if the research targets a particular group, including illiterate or more educated participants. It should be

---

Box 10.3   Design of participant information sheets

Part 1

Study title
Invitation paragraph
What is the purpose of the study?
Why have I been chosen?
Do I have to take part?
What will happen to me if I take part?
Expenses and payments
What will I have to do?
What is the drug, device or procedure that is being tested?
What are the alternatives for diagnosis or treatment?
What are the possible disadvantages and risks of taking part?
What are the side effects of any treatment received when taking part?
Harm to the unborn child: therapeutic studies
What are the possible benefits of taking part?
What happens when the research study stops?
What if there is a problem?
Will my taking part in the study be kept confidential?

Part 2

What will happen if I don't want to carry on with the study?
What if there is a problem?
Will my taking part in the study be kept confidential?
Involvement of the general practitioner/family doctor
What will happen to any samples I give?
Will any genetic tests be done?
What will happen to the results of the research study?
Who is organising and funding the research?
Who has reviewed the study?
Further information and contact details

remembered that participants with long-term conditions will become familiar with some of the medical terminology but it should still be explained. This tailoring is sensible and is encouraged. Patients and representative groups are often happy to review copies of the PIS and other documents before submission. It is usually quite apparent to the REC where this knowledgeable input has been provided.

The ethical review process

REC members are volunteers who take pride in their work and the service they offer to researchers. RECs have both lay and expert members covering many disciplines, including pharmacists, statisticians, nurses and medical practitioners. Professional members are expected to consider matters pertinent to their expertise. For example, the pharmacist will scrutinise more closely the responses to questions about any investigational medicinal products and the statistician will focus most closely on the responses to questions about the planned sample size and data analysis. Despite their particular expertise, professionals are not polymaths so you should assume that every REC member possesses only lay understanding for the majority of the areas covered on the form.

After submitting your application, the REC coordinator will check that all the necessary information, papers and signatures have been provided and, if they have been, the application will be deemed valid and added to the agenda for the review at the next meeting (see Figure 10.1). All members of the REC will review all the applications, receiving them about 10 days before the meeting. Two members of the committee are usually nominated to act as lead reviewers for each new application. It is the lead reviewer's role to undertake a thorough review and to lead the discussion of the application during the meeting.

The researchers will have been invited to attend the meeting at which their application will be reviewed and, as noted above, it is essential that they make every effort to attend if they can. It is not uncommon for a REC to misunderstand an element of a research project, so it is helpful if the researcher is present to clarify any uncertainties and answer any other questions. Researchers should remember that REC members are faced with up to eight new applications and protocols at each meeting so it can be difficult for them to have a comprehensive understanding of each one.

Following discussion, the committee will form an opinion of the research. The options available to them are:

- *favourable opinion* – in this instance the REC is completely satisfied with all parts of the research. The researcher will be informed and their research can begin
- *conditional opinion* – the committee will use this opinion if the researcher is able make a simple change or clarify a minor point. Once the condition of the opinion has been met, the favourable opinion will be confirmed
- *provisional opinion* – this opinion is offered if the committee needs revisions to documentation or needs matters clarifying. The researcher usually responds by dealing with each of the matters raised by the committee. If all the matters raised are dealt with to the REC's satisfaction, then a favourable opinion will be confirmed and the research can begin. If the committee is not satisfied then an unfavourable opinion will be issued. The researcher's response is usually dealt with by the chair or by a subcommittee as soon as it is received
- *unfavourable opinion* – although uncommon, a small number of unfavourable opinions are given and they usually involve a significant flaw with the application requiring a major revision
- *no opinion* – the committee uses this opinion when it believes it has not been provided with sufficient information with which to form a decision.

Once an application has been validated, the REC is required to inform the researcher of its final opinion within 60 days. A written summary of the REC's opinion is sent to applicants within 10 working days of the review meeting. If a provisional opinion is granted, all required points of clarification and suggested amendments will be listed in the REC's post-review letter. The 60-day clock stops after the REC

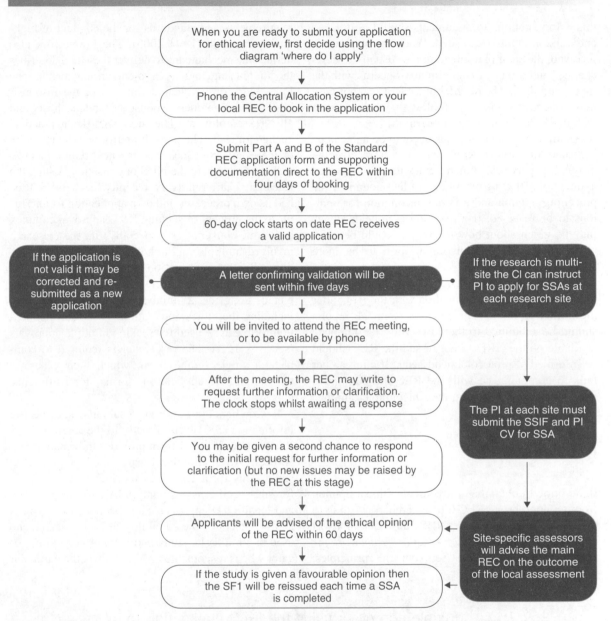

Figure 10.1 How to apply for approval from an NHS research ethics committee
CI – chief investigator; PI – principal investigator; SSA – site-specific assessment; SSIF – site-specific information form; SF1 – site approval form
Reproduced with permissions from National Research Ethics Service (2007) *Guidance for Applicants to the National Research Ethics Service.* London, National Patient Safety Agency.

has informed the researchers of its opinion if a response is required from the researcher. This ensures that a researcher who is slow to respond to the REC's post-review letter does not cause the clock to tick over the 60 days. Once the REC receives the researcher's response, the clock starts ticking again. Although the REC has 60 days to inform the researcher of its decision, it usually takes considerably less time than this. Modifications to documents should be tracked and version numbers updated. When the response is received, the chair or a subcommittee usually reviews changes and offers a final opinion. Concerns with the modifications can be raised, but the REC cannot raise new concerns at this time (unless they arise from a lack of clarity in the new information).

An unfavourable opinion is uncommon and can be appealed to another REC, which will receive the original paperwork. When reviewing an appealed application, REC members do not feel bound by the preceding opinion and it is not uncommon for opinions to be reversed. If a rejection is upheld, advice may be given about how the project could be redesigned to enable a future application to be more successful.

It is important that researchers remember the need to continue their communication with the REC after the initial opinion. For example, annual reports should be submitted to the REC using the template available on the NRES website and the REC should be informed of protocol amendments. If a researcher fails to communicate with the REC the committee may consider withdrawing their favourable opinion.

R&D APPROVAL

In addition to obtaining a favourable ethical opinion from an appropriate REC, all researchers wishing to undertake research in the NHS must obtain R&D approval. The *Research Governance Framework for Health and Social Care* sets out the principles, requirements and standards for the conduct of high-quality research (DoH 2005). The Framework also defines the mechanisms to deliver these and describes the monitoring and assessment arrangements. The Framework offers clear definitions of the responsibilities of researchers, sponsors, funders, hosts and all NHS employees. The most significant practical change for researchers resulting from implementation of the Framework has been the new requirement to seek approval from the NHS organisation hosting the research. Until relatively recently, each NHS trust had its own processes and own application form. This made the process of seeking R&D approval complex and time-consuming, especially if the research involved multiple research sites and NHS organisations. With the introduction of the IRAS form this has changed and now the R&D application form is completed alongside a number of other applications, including the ethics application. The IRAS application form can be used for seeking multiple approvals (see Box 10.4). The researcher is required to complete a single online form, which then generates the necessary application forms for difference approvals.

Researchers are required to submit a site-specific information (SSI) form directly to the relevant NHS R&D office. The SSI form provides information that is specific to a particular research site in a multi-sited study. This form combines the information needed for site-specific assessment (SSA), where required, and local R&D approval. Site-specific assessment is an assessment of the suitability of each research site used in a multi-site study and local principal investigator who is responsible for the study at the particular

---

Box 10.4 Multiple approvals using the IRAS application form

Administration of Radioactive Substances Advisory Committee (ARSAC)
Gene Therapy Advisory Committee (GTAC)
Medicines and Healthcare Products Regulatory Agency (MHRA)
Ministry of Justice (including research involving prisoners)
NHS research offices
NRES research ethics committees
Patient Information Advisory Group (PIAG)

site. The R&D office will also wish to review the study-wide form, generated through the IRAS application, and other documents, including PIS, consent forms and any letters or questionnaires to be used.

In November 2008, the National Institute for Health Research (NIHR) Co-ordinated System for gaining NHS Permissions (NIHR CSP) was introduced for NIHR Clinical Research Network Portfolio studies. Portfolio studies are those that meet eligibility criteria set by the NIHR Clinical Research Network Coordinating Centre (CRNCC). For example, studies funded by the NIHR, research councils and national charities where grants are awarded through open competition and subject to rigorous independent scientific review. This system should streamline the process by which NHS trusts provide R&D approval for new research and should reduce duplication in NHS review processes. NIHR CSP has a single entry point, via IRAS, so that researchers are able to apply for permission from all NHS sites in England through a single gateway. It is important to remember that this process can only be used by those whose research fits within the NIHR Clinical Research Network Portfolio. Research outside this portfolio will still need to apply to individual NHS trusts.

Another new initiative is the use of research passports with the aim of simplifying the administrative procedures associated with issuing honorary research contracts to those not employed directly by the NHS trust hosting the research. Research passports should be available to NHS, university and other researchers working in partnership with the NIHR, but other researchers will need to seek advice about honorary contracts from local NHS trusts.

INFORMAL ACCESS TO RESEARCH SITES

While there are formal approvals processes to be negotiated before research can commence, it is also advisable for researchers to ensure that they have informal approval to access research sites. Once a favourable ethical opinion and R&D approval have been gained, researchers will still encounter numerous 'gatekeepers' who can control access to participants or data. In the vast majority of cases these gatekeepers are willing to facilitate research, but it helps this process if researchers approach appropriate individuals during the early stages of the project so that they can build up a rapport. Gatekeepers might include the following.

- *Ward sisters or managers.* Ward sisters and managers, or their deputies, are responsible for the day-to-day management of many clinical settings. It can be extremely difficult to undertake research in these settings without the support of these gatekeepers. If the research involves interviewing nursing staff, the scheduling of interviews could be much easier with the ward manager's support.
- *Caldicott Guardians.* Since 2001, and in response to the Caldicott Committee's report (DoH 1997), each NHS trust has appointed a Caldicott Guardian, usually a senior manager, who is responsible for the safekeeping of patient records to ensure their rights are protected and to oversee how staff use personal information. Research requiring access to patient information may also need the approval of the Caldicott Guardian.
- *Patient support groups.* Research frequently focuses on patients in particular groups, so it can help if the appropriate patient group supports a research project. They can facilitate recruitment and even encourage patients to participate. One of the biggest ways that patient groups can help researchers is in the preparation of the PIS. As noted earlier, RECs will spend considerable time reviewing this paperwork and the PIS can be much improved if it is developed with the support of those representing the target patient group.

It is important that negotiations with gatekeepers happen as early in the research planning as possible. It is also not uncommon for these individuals and groups to suggest useful changes to the planned research. If these negotiations are left until after the formal approvals are gained it is more difficult and time-consuming to make any amendments that might be necessary, because they will need to be approved by both the REC and R&D departments before they can be implemented.

BUILDING THE APPROVAL PROCESS INTO RESEARCH PLANNING

Criticising the approvals processes has become a popular pastime for many researchers in recent years (Robinson *et al.* 2007). As a result, researchers have treated seeking the required approvals as hurdles to be jumped or barriers to be knocked down before their research can begin. This attitude fails to appreciate the great value that can result from using these necessary processes as an integral part of the research process. Navigating one's way through the appropriate approvals processes is also an important part of the learning experience for research students.

The remit of RECs is to maximise benefit and minimise risk while protecting the rights of participants (Gelling 1999). These objectives are best achieved through mutual respect between researchers, RECs and others involved in the approvals processes. Within this relationship an application receives constructive criticism and advice, in a timely manner, before the research is able to proceed. It is also important that the work of researchers is treated with due respect. The view that RECs are intent on obstructing research is misguided, compromises such relationships and achieves nothing. It is similarly misguided for those involved in the approvals processes to treat every researcher as if they were planning to cause harm to research participants in order to advance their research careers. Seeking approvals is an important part of the research process and has much to contribute to the development of new knowledge if there is mutual respect between all those involved.

Many researchers refine their research project as a direct result of planning applications for a research ethics opinion and approval from an R&D department. This process helps to ensure that research combines ethical standards with the most rigorous science in a way that is most likely to result in meaningful evidence to guide practice.

Consideration of science and ethics

There has been much discussion, sometimes heated, relating to the review of science by RECs. Some have argued that RECs should only consider matters relat-

ing to ethics and should leave the scientific review to others (Dawson & Yentis 2007). RECs, however, will argue that ethical review without consideration of the science would be incomplete and inadequate. This is based on the notion that bad science is bad ethics. In many instances, a REC is able to feel confident in the science because the research had undergone adequate scientific peer review prior to submission to the REC. Scientific reviews are frequently undertaken before seeking an ethical opinion as part of the process of applying for research funding or they are required by universities, NHS trusts or other organisations. When scientific review has been undertaken the REC will need to focus very little of its attention on the science and can focus on matters related directly to ethics. If a review has not been undertaken, or if the REC deems the review to be inadequate, then the REC will feel obliged to consider the science. In many instances this will result in the researcher being asked to have a scientific review undertaken before the REC can form an opinion. It is worth noting that RECs are keen to see an independent external review of the science rather than a review undertaken in the same organisation or the same department. This contributes to ensuring transparency for all those involved in the research process.

Planning the application

There is considerable advice available to anyone planning an application for an ethical opinion or R&D approval. In addition to the wealth of guidance available on the NRES and IRAS websites, advice can be sought from the NRES helpline and from REC chairs and co-ordinators. R&D departments also offer advice during the preparation phase of a research project. Both RECs and R&D departments are keen to promote high-quality research and it can save much wasted time, for both researchers and the reviewing bodies, if advice is sought as early as possible. As noted in the introduction to this chapter, the approvals processes for health and social care research have undergone considerable change in recent years. It is likely that changes will continue to be implemented, so it is advisable to seek advice when preparing an application.

CONCLUSIONS

The key to navigating successfully through the approvals processes and gaining access to the research site is planning and allowing sufficient time to prepare the application forms and accompanying paperwork. In most cases, it is not major ethical concerns that delay approvals, but poorly prepared and inadequately thought through application forms and supporting paperwork. Researchers would be advised to treat seeking the required approvals as an integral and useful part of the research process and to use this process to help refine their research project.

References

Beecher H (1966) Ethics and clinical research. *New England Journal of Medicine* **274**: 1354–1360.

Dawson AJ, Yentis SM (2007) Contesting the science/ethics distinction in the review of clinical research. *Journal of Medical Ethics* **33**(3): 165–167.

Department of Health (2005) *Research Governance Framework for Health and Social Care*. London, Department of Health.

Department of Health (2001a) *Research Governance Framework for Health and Social Care*. London, Department of Health.

Department of Health (2001b) *Governance Arrangements for NHS Research Ethics Committees*. London, Department of Health.

Department of Health (1997) *The Caldicott Committee: report of the review of patient-identifiable information*. London, Department of Health.

European Parliament and Council of the European Union (2001) Directive 2001/20/EC of the European Parliament and of the Council (EU Clinical Trails Directive). *Official Journal of the European Committee* **L121**: 34–344.

Franck L, Winter I (2004) Research participant information sheets are difficult to read. *Bulletin of Medical Ethics* **195**: 13–16.

Gelling L (1999) Role of the research ethics committee. *Nurse Education Today* **19**: 564 569.

Goodyear MDE, Eckenwiler LA, Ells C (2008) Fresh thinking about the Declaration of Helsinki. *British Medical Journal* **337**: 1067–1068.

Medical Research Council (2005) *Good Research Practice*. London, MRC.

Medicines for Human Use (Clinical Trials) Regulations (2004) Statutory Instrument 2004 No. 103. London, The Stationery Office.

National Research Ethics Service (2008) *Defining Research*. London, National Patient Safety Agency.

National Research Ethics Service (2007) *Cambridgeshire 4 Research Ethics Committee Annual Report*. Cambridge, NRES.

Pappworth MH (1967) *Human Guinea Pigs*. Boston, Beacon Press.

Robinson L, Murdoch-Eaton D, Carter Y (2007) NHS research ethics committees. *British Medical Journal* **335**(7609): 6.

Royal College of Nursing (2007) *Research Ethics: RCN guidance for nurses*. London, RCN.

Royal College of Nursing (2005) *Informed Consent in Health and Social Care Research: RCN guidance for nurses*. London, RCN.

Saunders R, Savulescu J (2008) Research ethics and lessons from Hwanggate: what can we learn from the Korean cloning fraud? *Journal of Medic Ethics* **34**(3): 214–221.

Smith R (2006) Research misconduct: the poisoning of the well. *Journal of the Royal Society of Medicine* **99**(5): 232–237.

Wells F, Farthing M (2008) *Fraud and Misconduct in Biomedical Research*. London, Royal Society of Medicine Press.

Further reading

Beauchamp TL, Childress JF (2009) *Principles of Biomedical Ethics*. Oxford, Oxford University Press.

Long A, Johnson M (2006) *Research Ethics in the Real World: issues and solutions for health and social care*. London, Churchill Livingstone.

Manson NC, O'Neill O (2007) *Rethinking Informed Consent in Bioethics*. Cambridge, Cambridge University Press.

Websites

http://ohsr.od.nih.gov/guidelines/nuremberg.html – the Nuremberg Code provides a full version of the Nuremberg Code.

www.arec.org.uk – Association of Research Ethics Committees (AREC) is an independent organisation for members and administrators from research ethics committees, including NHS, university and other committees. Its website includes information about courses and conferences for those interested in research ethics and those involved in ethical review.

www.mrc.ac.uk – the Medical Research Council (MRC) provides information about the many activities of the MRC, including guidance on matters relating to research ethics.

www.myresearchproject.org.uk/Signin.aspx – Integrated Research Application System (IRAS) allows access to registration and use of the IRAS form.

www.nres.npsa.nhs.uk – the National Research Ethics Service (NRES) provides a wealth of information and guidance on matters relating to research ethics and seeking ethical opinion.

www.rcn.org.uk/__data/assets/pdf_file/0004/56695/ researchethicsmay07.pdf – Royal College of Nursing (RCN) guidance on research ethics intended for nurses and others involved in research.

www.rcn.org.uk/__data/assets/pdf_file/0003/56703/ informedconsentdec05.pdf – Royal College of Nursing (RCN) guidance on informed consent.

www.rdforum.nhs.uk – the NHS R&D Forum is a network for those involved in planning and managing research in health and social care.

www.wma.net/e/policy/b3.htm – the Declaration of Helsinki includes a full version of the Seoul 2008 revision of the Declaration of Helsinki.

Choosing the Right Approach

This section forms the heart of this book, as research approaches in nursing are many and diverse, and it is important to understand the range of approaches available before choosing a specific one to answer a particular question.

The section begins with a theoretical chapter tackling the two broad approaches available to the nurse researcher. Chapter 11 considers the philosophical underpinning of the qualitative and quantitative paradigms in research, and emphasises the necessity to engage in the complex debates raised in the extensive literature on this subject. Both approaches, however, are valid for nursing research, and the perspective adopted should be guided by the nature of the question to be answered.

Chapter 12 stands alone as an essential pre-requisite to any research design, be it qualitative or quantitative. Sampling procedures are well established for many methodologies, and this chapter discusses a variety of the most common sampling strategies used in nursing research, with appropriate examples from the literature. Sampling cannot be considered separately from issues of research design, as it will determine the resources required and therefore the feasibility of the project.

The following three chapters introduce the major approaches used in qualitative research: grounded theory, ethnography and phenomenology.

Chapter 16 is newly written for this edition, and introduces a relatively new approach known as narrative research. This has much in common with other qualitative methods, but does not fall readily into the major categories. Narrative research has particular relevance to nursing research because of its use to uncover the experience of patients through 'illness biographies'.

The focus then moves on to the major quantitative approaches with a series of chapters that deal with mixed methods. Chapter 17 introduces experimental design and Chapter 18 surveys. Both these approaches have a long and well-established history in medical and social sciences, and both are also widely used in nursing research. These chapters discuss the strengths and weaknesses of the methodologies and highlight examples from the nursing and medical literature where they have been used to good effect. Chapter 17 includes a critical discussion of the randomised controlled trial and its place as the 'gold standard' of medical research evidence. Chapter 18 includes a short section on epidemiology, a well-established research tradition that has perhaps been overlooked in nursing research.

There follow nine chapters that each take a very specific approach used in nursing research. Five of the nine chapters have been newly written for this 6th edition of the book, reflecting the dynamic state of nursing research methodology. The Delphi approach (Chapter 19) and historical research (Chapter 26) have both been used for some years in nursing research, but were not included in the 5th edition of the book. This omission, it was felt, needed to be rectified. Action research (Chapter 20), evaluation research (Chapter 21), case study research (Chapter 22) and systematic reviews (Chapter 24) are all still deservedly well-used methodologies, and the chapters on these have been updated accordingly. The increasing need for guidance on research undertaken by, and for, practitioners has been addressed in Chapter 23, where those who are engaged in healthcare practice are encouraged to engage in systematic and rigorous research that arises directly from their everyday experience. Chapter 25, on the emerging methodology of realist synthesis, complements the previous chapter on the more established discipline of systematic reviews. Realist synthesis is particularly appropriate for assessing the impact of complex interventions in their context and for developing theory. Finally in this section, Chapter 27 discusses mixed methods, combining qualitative and quantitative approaches in the same research project.

11 The Quantitative–Qualitative Continuum

Annie Topping

Key points

- Qualitative and quantitative research have different characteristics and derive from different scientific traditions and forms of knowledge.

- Quantitative research methods assume that the world is stable and predictable, and phenomena can be measured empirically. The positivist tradition of quantitative research derives from the biomedical sciences.

- Qualitative research methods take an interpretivist perspective, emphasising meaning and the understanding of human actions and behaviour. The tradition of qualitative research derives from the social sciences.

- Both are appropriate approaches for nursing research; the choice of methodology depends on the nature of the research question. In some cases the two approaches can be blended in the same study.

INTRODUCTION

Not that long ago the unique characteristics and differences between qualitative and quantitative research would have been described in a way more akin to an intellectual battleground, with researchers aligned to a particular camp. That position has undergone considerable revision across many disciplines and is particularly marked in nursing. Today, there is a growing recognition that the use of a range of approaches strengthens, rather than divides, nursing enquiry. Researchers, irrespective of their preferred way of approaching problems or questions, are involved in

an endeavour with a shared purpose. Quality in research is about using the most appropriate approach for investigating research problems and about researchers adopting a systematic, rigorous and transparent approach for exploring, discovering, confirming and understanding. Underlying the practice of research and its findings are fundamental questions about the nature of knowledge, termed as epistemology, and what we understand as reality. In recognition of the fact that nursing, as a research active profession, does not function in isolation, the assumptions and contribution of the natural sciences, western medicine and the social sciences will be examined.

THE CHARACTERISTICS OF QUANTITATIVE AND QUALITATIVE RESEARCH

First, let us turn our attention to the defining characteristics of the two approaches. Philosophically, quantitative research is underpinned by a tradition that proposes that scientific truths or laws exist; this is called *positivism*. These truths emerge from what can be observed and measured, and can be studied as objects. Methods that minimise, or are free from, bias are used to do this so that greater confidence can be given to any findings. This approach is often referred to as the *scientific* or *empirical method*. Qualitative research, in contrast, fits more neatly within an *interpretivist* tradition which is based on assumptions that in order to make sense of the world, human behaviour should be interpreted by taking account of interactions between people. So research that seeks to understand human behaviour and the social processes we engage in must employ approaches and techniques that allow interpretation in natural settings. This interpretative stance goes further, as qualitative methodologies also strive to emphasise that there is no single interpretation, truth or meaning, but recognise that just as human beings are different, so are the societies and cultures in which they live their lives. Box 11.1 sets out the different qualities and characteristics that have been used to describe the two approaches. Although of some value, the information is presented in stark contrast to emphasise the differences, and you may not always be able to recognise all these characteristics in any single report of a quantitative or qualitative study.

INFLUENCES AND CONTRIBUTIONS TO THE DEVELOPMENT OF NURSING RESEARCH

It might seem a little odd to discuss the influence of other disciplines in a textbook targeted to a nursing readership, but it would be naive not to recognise the shared history and mutual dependency. Biomedicine, like contemporary nursing, has it roots in the nineteenth century. This period of accelerated social upheaval and industrialisation brought many scientific breakthroughs and technological innovations.

Box 11.1 Characteristics of quantitative and qualitative research

Quantitative research	Qualitative research
Hard science	Soft science
Objective	Subjective
Political	Value-free
Reductionist	Holistic
Logico-deductive	Dialectic, inductive, speculative
Cause and effect relationships	Meaning
Tests theory	Develops, advances and reinterprets theory
Control	Shared interpretation
Instruments as data collection tools	Listening and talking, observation as ways of gathering data
Basic unit of analysis: numbers	Basic unit of analysis: words
Statistical analysis	Interpretation
Generalisation	Uniqueness/transferability

Sources: Burns & Grove (2008), Silverman (2005, 2007)

These changes inevitably challenged previously held notions of illness. The premise that illness was caused by an imbalance, a loss of harmony between individual and the environment, was questioned, and more rational, objectively based approaches were adopted. During the same time period modern nursing began to emerge under the leadership of such figures as Florence Nightingale and Mrs Bedford Fenwick in response to the plight of soldiers injured in the Crimean War and the growing demand for a different type of workforce to support the organisation and delivery of what has become hospital medicine.

What is now described as *reductionism* emerged as a way of studying the causes and treatment of disease(s). This approach allows disease to be objectified, and the experience of ill health to be reduced to the signs and symptoms that allow it to be better classified and diagnosed, and the response, if any, to treatment to be monitored. This view of illness as an object inevitably distances the doctor or nurse, encouraging detachment from the influencing effects of subjectivity. You can still see this approach in medical practice where routine assessment involving taking a patient's history to establish diagnosis might more correctly be described as an illness history.

Objectification and distancing is ingrained in the scientific tradition through separation of the subject of research from the investigator. The belief that removing the doctor or researcher from the context in which healthcare is delivered, or research undertaken, provides a sense of security that neither doctor nor researcher impacts on illness or makes judgements about it. That picture of medicine and research performed by an objective yet fundamentally altruistic scientist fails to recognise that 'medical knowledge is never disinterested' (Annandale 1998: 5). Indeed, scientific neutrality has itself received considerable attention from a number of social scientists (Foucault 1973; Hammersley 1989; Shipman 1997) and nurse researchers (Johnson & Webb 1995; Porter 1995).

The study of societies, the people within them and the ways in which they organise themselves is the focus of sociology, which at its most basic is an acceptance that people are different from objects. Objects do not have thought or consciousness, they do not reason, think or reflect, and therefore are qualitatively different from people. Importantly, objects, unlike people, do not have free will or choice. For that reason the ways in which a researcher might study and understand objects will, by necessity, be different from the approaches used to understand human society or indeed nursing. However, this argument becomes quite complex when applied to healthcare, where people become patients. In so doing they can be viewed objectively as a dysfunctioning machine, and subjectively as an individual interacting with people and systems designed to support their illness. This complexity of the subjective person and objective body, aligned philosophically as interpretivisim and positivism respectively, reinforces why both quantitative and qualitative approaches can and do make important contributions to our understanding.

The positivist approach to investigating the social and natural world draws on empiricism and the scientific method. It is based on the assumption that social life, like natural sciences, can be studied as facts. That is not to say that the ways in which individual, groups and societies organise themselves or their beliefs and practices are objects, but more that they can be examined as such. Interpretivism, on the other hand, asserts that the purpose of research is to examine meaning, and therefore interpretation must remain central. Groundbreaking research undertaken nearly 50 years ago introduced the interpretative approach and continues today to inform thinking about medicine (Becker *et al.* 1961), mental illness and stigma (Goffman 1964), and the dying (Glaser & Strauss 1965).

EMPIRICISM AND THE SCIENTIFIC METHOD

Science, Western modern medicine and quantitative approaches have their origins in the philosophical movements of the 16th and 17th centuries. A logical approach for developing knowledge emerged, built on the three principles of scepticism, determinism and empiricism. First, anything, irrespective of its origin or authority, is open to analysis and doubt and thus is susceptible to *scepticism*. Second, regular laws and rules of causation determine all things – *determinism*. Third, *empiricism* asserts that enquiry or problem solving such as research should be undertaken through observation and verification. The application of the scientific method was a major developmental shift in thinking from previously held explanations and it encouraged a way of looking at the natural world, one freed from mystery and superstition clouded by religious explanations (Shipman 1997). The scientific method became a formula for the production of knowledge and, as Figure 11.1 illustrates, is based on the processes of *induction* and *deduction*.

It might be useful to consider how the scientific method has become part of how we understand events around us and, moreover, how information is presented to us through the media. Try to remember your first encounter with science at school. Probably early in your school career you learnt how to undertake and report a simple experiment. This no doubt involved learning how to make accurate descriptions, reliable measurements and diligent recordings of your observations about what occurred to help you understand whatever you were investigating. From that first exposure to the scientific method, schoolchildren are taught to describe the equipment used, how to undertake a test and record any deviations from the approved recipe, what they used to measure any reaction or outcome, and to document the results. These skills form the basis of *observation*, *description* and *measurement* that underlie much of the conduct of science. By using this approach findings can be translated into explanations. These explanations are often expressed as *hypotheses* or *theories* that are themselves amenable to testing. This progression from observation to statement of a relationship between different observations (*hypotheses*) to *theory* and ultimately generalisation is termed *induction*. So theories derived through the process of induction move from the particular to the general and can be seen as an organising system for what are essentially conjectures or tentative proposals based on observation (Polgar & Thomas 2008).

An essential feature of any scientific theory is the account of how the theory works and its potential to predict. These predictions enable the researcher to *deduce* causal relationships, expressed through theory but testable through controlled observation. The results of testing (*experimentation*) will produce data that can be translated into findings that may be consistent with the predictions expressed in the original hypothesis. This verifies or provides support for the theory. Alternatively, the results may fail to support the hypothesis and contradict the theory. Ultimately, the volume of conflicting evidence may swell to such proportions that the original theory is discarded.

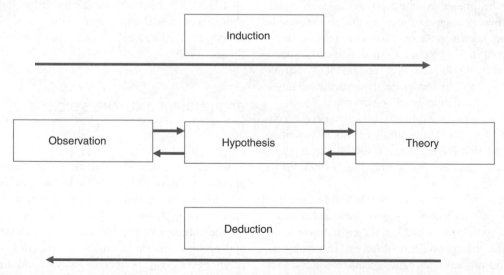

Figure 11.1   The scientific method

Hence any scientific theory is not an absolute truth, but only provisional, and therefore can be modified, refined, disputed or invalidated (Popper 1972, 2002).

It might be helpful to illustrate the scientific method with an example. Imagine you are working on a surgical ward where patients are admitted for elective surgery. You observe that those patients who have not received preoperative preparation about the proposed procedure experience greater distress postoperatively than those who have received preparation. You also observe that the unprepared patients require more analgesia and appear to mobilise more slowly. You develop a theory that suggests a relationship between information and postoperative outcomes. In fact, two seminal studies undertaken by Hayward and Boore in the 1970s did just that (Hayward & Boore 1994). These studies demonstrated a relationship between information and the level of pain experienced by patients recovering from surgery. You could ask whether the relationship between information and pain was an existing theory that Boore and Hayward sought to test using hypothetico-deductive reasoning, or whether the theory emerged from them observing patients who received pre-operative information. Probably the initial idea came from the latter, but the former approach was used to demonstrate the relationship. As discussed in Chapter 2, initial ideas for research often come from observation, and are checked by literature searching and analysis prior to undertaking an investigation. In this way, existing understanding can be examined to avoid embarking prematurely on ill thought through research, and also to refine and hone original research ideas.

To extend this discussion, Wilson-Barnett (1988), drawing on many of the same theoretical ideas associated with the positive benefits of information, deduced that anxiety associated with radiological investigations could be reduced by information giving. Her results supported in part the value of information in reducing anxiety, but also found that in some cases information could make people more anxious. Although a deductive approach was used to undertake the work, the interpretation of the findings led to an inductively driven revision and modification of the original theoretical assumptions. This reinforces the assertion that any knowledge is only provisional.

Today we have far greater insight about the beneficial effects of information giving and best ways to provide that information to patients, their relatives and carers (Davies *et al.* 2008). Technological advances such as the worldwide web and mobile technology continue to increase the volume of information available to patients (Murray *et al.* 2005; Antiila *et al.* 2008; Atack *et al.* 2008). Even so, some users of health services still have cause to complain about the poor quality of information received, despite the wealth of evidence confirming that the experience of healthcare is enhanced by effective education and information (Kinnersley *et al.* 2007). This problem of translating what is known – the evidence base – into practice will be developed in much more detail in Chapters 38 and 39. Yet, even for something as fundamental as information giving, there are still many unanswered questions that deserve further investigation.

- How do we ensure that information giving is appropriately targeted?
- Is information provided at the appropriate level?
- Do healthcare professionals have the skills or wherewithal to provide information effectively?
- What is it about healthcare organisations and the way(s) in which health professionals interact with users that prevents them from communicating effectively?

These questions as research problems may require a number of different research approaches, as it is unlikely that one approach will provide all the answers.

In research that is largely deductive, the theory normally directs and drives the design and interpretation. In inductively driven work theory serves to provide a commitment to a particular way of looking at the world, such as feminism, or to justify a methodological approach (Sandelowski 1993). This is why you may be able to identify the theoretical framework that informed a research design in research reports. This explicit reference to the theoretical basis of the work can help the reader to navigate the interpretation offered, but it can also provoke criticism when the theoretical framework itself appears to create a tension within the work, particularly if it appears incongruent with the research approach. For example, Patricia Benner's (1984) influential work *Novice to Expert*, which explored how nurses developed competence, became the focus of some critical censure on these grounds (Cash 1995), albeit firmly countered by the author (Benner 1996). A further consideration concerns the role of theory in research. If data are collected in the absence of an organising framework or theory it could attract the criticism that the researcher is merely confirming their own biases (Grbich 1999). At this juncture it might be helpful to look at the two approaches in more detail.

QUANTITATIVE RESEARCH

Quantitative research is a broad, umbrella term for research that uses methods that collect evidence that can be transformed into numerical data and are based on a *positivist* position. Often the numerical data produced in quantitative research can be statistically manipulated to confirm (or sometimes fail to confirm) the original hypothesis or research question. The findings can then be used to make predictions or indicate trends. Formal, objective and systematic processes are used to explain causal relationships between events or things (variables). Underpinning quantitative research is the principle that the world is stable and predictable and the quantitative researcher, by controlling external influences, can seek to minimise bias that might otherwise explain the findings. The ultimate aim is for the researcher and the consumer of the research to be assured that any results are *valid* and *reliable* (see Chapter 2). Classical experimental design is one such method. but surveys, analysis of official statistics and structured or non-participant observation are all quantitative methods (Silverman 2005).

The use of quantitative research methods is illustrated in the study undertaken by Todd *et al.* (2008), where the research team set out to establish when was the best time for women undergoing surgery for breast cancer to commence full shoulder movements as part of an exercise regime (see Research Example 11.1). They defined, for the purposes of the study, the clinical outcomes most amenable to measurement and presentation as numerical data. Outcomes included incidence of lymphoedema, reduced shoulder mobility and health-related quality of life. Using these outcomes, statistical analysis suggested women should not commence above shoulder exercise until at least seven days after surgery.

From this example you can see how in quantitative research the focus of study has to be broken down into those component parts that can be readily defined and are measurable. This provides greater assurance to the researcher and reader that the results are the product of consistent, reproducible measurement that describes what the researcher sought to understand. The accuracy of any instruments developed to measure whatever is under investigation and their ability to consistently reproduce results is fundamental to undertaking quantitative research. This also allows other researchers to replicate the study and therefore compare, confirm and question existing findings. The problem for the researcher is that dependency on measurement of what can be complex theoretical ideas or models is reliant on the clarity of the conceptualisation of the underlying concept, the technology available and the reliability of the researcher to use the instrument consistently. No matter how diligent a researcher is, or how well designed a study, the instrument used to test the findings could be reliable yet will not necessarily give valid results. In other words, the research may measure something, but not necessarily the thing that was under investigation. That is why it is often more of a challenge in research to establish with any confidence that findings represent facts or truths about something than it is to construct an approach to measure the phenomenon under investigation or some part of it.

Another feature of quantitative research is that it aspires to objectivity, and therefore different approaches are used to keep the researched (participants) at a distance from the researcher. Detachment is used as a strategy for reducing bias and minimising any involvement that might contaminate the results or influence outcomes. There are numerous ways to increase detachment, including randomisation of participants. This ensures the researcher remains unaware (blind) of which subjects receive an intervention and

RESEARCH EXAMPLE

11.1 A Quantitative Research Study

Todd J, Scally A, Dodwell D, Horgan K, Topping A (2008) A randomised controlled trial of two programmes of shoulder exercise following axillary node dissection for invasive breast cancer. *Physiotherapy* **94**: 265–273.

This British study compared the incidence of treatment-related complications including lymphoedema and shoulder mobility from use of a shoulder exercise programme. Traditionally, women undergoing breast cancer surgery involving the axilla have been taught shoulder exercises and encouraged to persist with exercise regimes long term. The literature was inconclusive regarding timing (when exercises should commence postoperatively) and extent (above-shoulder mobilisation). This study compared early (within 48 hours postoperatively) versus delayed (day 7) introduction of full shoulder exercise. At three months following initial treatment 116 women patients were randomised to either full or restricted shoulder mobilisation programmes. Exercises were taught by nurses and women received additional written and diagrammatic material. Patient outcome measures were incidence of lymphoedema (arm volume increase >200 ml), wound drainage volumes, range of shoulder movement, grip strength and health-related quality of life (shoulder disability questionnaire, Functional Assessment of Cancer Therapy – Breast). Results showed that women who underwent early full shoulder mobilisation had a higher incidence of lymphoedema one year postoperatively. Other outcomes, including grip strength, shoulder movement and quality of life, indicated patient acceptability was also similar. The researchers concluded that women undergoing axillary surgery should undertake exercise regimes that delay full shoulder mobilisation.

which do not by referring to all subjects by a coded descriptor, thus promoting anonymity and separating those delivering an intervention from those responsible for collecting data. In the study by Todd *et al.* (2008), an independent researcher recruited the women, allocated them to either the control or intervention group and collected the outcome data, thus removing any danger of bias. Nurses who were directly involved in advising the women on their allocated exercise programme were not involved in these activities.

QUALITATIVE RESEARCH

Defining qualitative research is often made more difficult by the absence of a common, unified set of techniques, philosophies or underpinning perspectives (Mason 2002). Qualitative research methods are used across a range of disciplines, such as the social sciences, management and nursing, and are beginning to be used more widely in the biomedical sciences.

Qualitative researchers use an array of terms, concepts and assumptions that may appear less familiar on initial encounter than scientific terms. This can be particularly confusing to the novice researcher, who not only has to contend with the challenge to previously held notions of what is robust research, but also has to acquire what at times appears to be a new language. An analogy might be trying to cook from a recipe where all the ingredients and terms for techniques such as sieving, mixing, beating and combining were different and possibly unfamiliar. This would inevitably make you feel uncertain about what you had to use, how to use it and what the final product might be like. Moreover, the uncertainty if you persevere would require you to interpret to make sense of the recipe. This is not dissimilar from the processes involved in doing qualitative research. Ethnography, phenomenology, grounded theory and case study are just some of the *methodologies* that are part of the cluster of approaches that can be considered qualitative. Various attempts have been made to categorise what seems an incomprehensible array (see Creswell 2007; Denzin & Lincoln 2005). Some of these different methodological approaches will be examined in more detail in subsequent chapters, particularly Chapters 13–15. Research Example 11.2 presents a summary of a qualitative study by Reid-Searl *et al.* (2008) using a particular methodological approach – grounded theory.

The subjectivity of using an approach where the researcher and the research are closely intertwined has its problems, and reflexivity (critical self-reflection on the research process and interpretation of data) is an important part of the qualitative researcher's toolkit (Schwandt 1997). Reflexivity has some similarities to the strategies used in reflective practice. In qualitative research the acknowledgement of the influence, and hence the critical scrutiny, of the researcher is often subject to the same level of examination as the research itself (Carolan 2003). For this reason, emphasis is placed on recording in field notes a description of what was seen, said and done in the act of doing the research, as well as interpretation of meaning in memos.

This emphasis on involvement and analytical detachment can seem paradoxical to the reader. The research approach encourages involvement, as the researcher frequently designs the study and collects, interprets and reports the data themselves. They can therefore influence and exert a bias on all stages of the research process. Yet the researcher(s), even though the report may be written in an engaging style, more often than not using first person pronouns, employs a number of different devices to assure the reader that the study is trustworthy. For example, Koch *et al.* (2004) in a study examining how people with long-standing asthma manage the condition use the pronoun 'we' to signal to the reader the subjectivity of the approach, yet provide a transparent description of how the research was conducted, which of the research team undertook specific activities, and how the findings were created and corroborated by the participants. They also suggest that readers can judge the authenticity of the findings by the inclusion of selected snippets of interview data in the report.

Data collection or generation is reliant on using approaches that are sensitive to the social context in which the data are produced. So qualitative studies often lack standardisation, as too rigid or unsympathetic an approach might reduce the authenticity of the data. Semi- or unstructured interviewing and participant observation are commonly used methods in data collection and are often used in combination. Raw data may be recorded on to audiotapes or video-

---

RESEARCH EXAMPLE

11.2 A Qualitative Research Study

Reid-Searl K, Moxham L, Walker S, Happell B (2008) Shifting supervision: implications for safe administration of medication by nursing students. *Journal of Clinical Nursing* **17**: 2750–2757.

This study adopted a grounded theory approach to explore undergraduate nursing students' experience of medication administration in practice settings. Data were collected from in-depth interviews with volunteer final year students (n = 28) recruited from a university in Queensland, Australia. Data were analysed using a constant comparative method that involved open, axial and selective coding. A central category emerged, *supervision*, which was refined to *shifting levels of supervision*. This is offered as a framework to illustrate how the level of supervision given by registered nurses to students when engaged in medication administration changed. The levels were described as *being with*, *being over*, *being near* and *being absent*. The researchers concluded that the potential for errors associated with medication administration is widely recognised as a major safety issue in healthcare. Registered nurses need to *be with* students if they are to acquire the requisite skills and embed knowledge required for safe practice. From this study the level of supervision was reported to be inconsistent and this has serious implications for safety including error minimisation.

tapes or in field notes and then transcribed and transformed into words for analysis. Qualitative analysis inevitably involves breaking the data up and coding the different segments. Increasingly, researchers use software packages to assist in managing data. Irrespective of whether the researcher uses paper-based or electronic software for handling the data, the process involves a fracturing process that includes breaking down, coding, re-ordering and reconstituting in order to describe, explain or generate theory.

CRITICAL ACCOUNTS OF RESEARCH EPISTEMOLOGY

Numerous commentators have offered critical accounts of the epistemology, methodologies and methods used in the name of research, irrespective of perspective. Criticism should not necessarily be seen as negative, and debate could be considered an indicator of the health of a discipline and its practitioners. Much of the criticism centres on the rigour of the approaches used to manufacture results and the questionable disinterest of research and researchers. Two of the arguments that cast doubt on the validity of many assumptions inherent in scientific enquiry are those offered by Popper (1972, 2002) and Kuhn (1972). Popper's argument is philosophical, examines the provisional nature of any knowledge or truth, and maintains that researchers should seek to challenge hypotheses rather than set out to prove them. Kuhn offers a critical account of the culture of research communities and how they are self-maintaining and constraining. He terms this a paradigm that arguably limits the development of new ways for looking at problems. An example from history is how understanding of infection transmission was overturned by germ theory. This change took considerable time before finally it was adopted, despite the considerable efforts of the Austrian obstetrician Semmelweiss (1818–1865). He encountered bitter resistance and incarceration in a mental hospital when he tried to disseminate his evidence relating to the positive benefits of hand washing. This shift in understanding ultimately led to the introduction of routine hand washing in healthcare – still a pressing issue today.

It might be useful to apply these two critiques to nursing. To do this, think of nursing as a culture. One of the enduring narratives in the nursing literature is that associated with the concept of caring. Considerable effort has been exerted to define caring, understand it better through research and to theorise about the significance of caring to the experience of nursing and, importantly, being nursed. Indeed, recently Juliet Corbin (2008) pondered the question: is caring a lost art? This has become the focus of a debate (see Brearley 2008; Ehlers 2008; Griffiths 2008; Maben 2008; Pajnkihar 2008; Rolfe 2009). For the purposes of this discussion, accept as given that caring is a paradigmatic framework for nursing, an explanation for the nature of nursing and, by extension, presents a way of interpreting what is done as nursing. In effect, the way caring is theorised prescribes the way(s) in which research will be undertaken to better understand it. It is not difficult, using a Kuhnian analysis, to distinguish a link between the volume of effort invested in understanding caring, its elevation as the primary contribution of nursing to care delivery and an explanation for the rapid assimilation of qualitative approaches into nursing research (Ramprogus 2002).

A different but associated criticism of research about nursing is that the work fails to make visible the caring aspect of nurses' work (Maben 2008). This is said to make nurses' efforts and the unique contribution of nursing invisible, with the consequence that the impact of nurses' caring skills on health and patient outcomes has gone unrecognised (Oakley 1984; Weinberg 2003; Enns & Gregory 2007). Applying a Popperian analysis, the research activity seeking to uncover caring should focus on critical appraisal of caring as the essential concept of nursing. In effect, this would challenge the hypothesis or at least encourage critical analysis of any understandings that emerge. Numerous arguments have been put forward to explain why particular methods used to demonstrate the concept of 'caring' are not sensitive enough or are inappropriate to capture the nature of caring, or that the assumptions underlying the concept have not been considered critically (Barker *et al.* 1995; Johnson 1999; Nelson & McGillon 2004). Kuhn would contend that it is only when there is enough substance to cast doubt, or a competing set of assumptions emerge, that a paradigm shift ultimately occurs. This is when a discipline changes its way of understanding problems. A recent reorientation can be seen in the policy and research attention given to nurses' work across the globe. The research focus has shifted towards the organisational constraints that impact on care delivery (Weinberg 2003) and identification of the outcomes of nursing that can be measured (Rafferty *et al.* 2007). This has transformed understanding of nurses' contribution to patient safety and quality care. Interestingly, the shift to a focus on outcomes has by necessity used quantitative methods.

BLENDING QUANTITATIVE AND QUALITATIVE APPROACHES

A solution offered as an alternative to using one or other research approach is to blend qualitative and quantitative approaches through the use of mixed or combined methods (Becker 1996; Brannen 2005; Burke Johnson & Onwuegbuzie 2004; O'Cathain 2009). Chapter 27 deals with this issue in more depth, but we will consider it briefly here. The advantage of blending approaches is the added value that using different yet complementary approaches can provide, particularly if the relative weaknesses of one are offset by another. The approach is not without its critics, however (Brannen 2005). The use of a number of methods within a research design is termed *triangulation*. The term has more traditionally been coined to refer to procedures used in surveying to pinpoint a particular geographic position by taking reference measurements from three or more points. In research, it is used to describe a way to increase the types of information obtained from participants to produce a more holistic picture (Begley 1996).

There is, however, a difference between using a number of methods to provide convergent views yet still provide a coherent account and an approach where a range of data collection strategies are used to provide a more complete but layered analysis. According to Denzin (1989), triangulation in research can take a number of forms – data, investigator, theory and method. Data triangulation involves using a number of different data sources that can shed light

on a particular phenomenon. That said, Hammersley and Atkinson (2007) warn that using multiple data sources may not always confirm inferences but it may make differences more blatant and act as a further check to credibility. Theoretical triangulation encourages the use of competing theory to compare and contrast interpretations of data. By this means theory can be advanced and revised. Methodological triangulation can be within methods where compatible data collection methods such as participant observation, qualitative interviewing and field notes can be used. Alternatively, dissimilar data collection strategies from different research traditions may be used to illuminate the same phenomenon, such as using a structured questionnaire with focus group interviews.

Criticisms of triangulation include concerns about philosophical incongruity between the position of positivism, with its emphasis on objective truth, and the interpretative traditions that make no claims to any single reality (Silverman 1985; Johnson *et al.* 2001). Another criticism is that it can merely compound sources of error (Armitage & Hodgson 2004) inherent in the methods employed. There is also the issue of how the reader should judge quality, particularly if competing research traditions are used in the same study (Creswell & Tashakkori 2007).

JUDGING THE QUALITY OF QUANTITATIVE AND QUALITATIVE RESEARCH

Judgement inevitably introduces a comparison. In order to contrast one thing with another, the individual making the comparison uses criteria to judge the two things. In quantitative research these are normally the concepts of reliability and validity. Various commentators have questioned the appropriateness of using these concepts that fit with a positivist world view with research methodologies that do not sit comfortably with that way of thinking (Koch 1994; Koch & Harrington 1998; Mays & Pope 2000). Those voicing this position maintain that distinctive criteria are required to assess qualitative research. Lincoln and Guba (1985, 1989) offered one such set of

Table 11.1 Comparison of the criteria used to judge the trustworthiness of a study

Quantitative research	Qualitative research Trustworthiness Criteria (Lincoln & Guba 1985)
Internal validity: extent to which what is observed truly represents the variable under investigation	Credibility – fit between participant's views and researcher's representation of them
External validity: extent that the results of a study can be generalised to other contexts and populations	Transferability – relates to the adequacy of the description to judge similarity to other situations so findings might be transferred
Reliability: refers to the consistency and accuracy of the data collection approach or instrument	Dependability – relates to transparency of the research process and decision trail
Objectivity	Confirmability – establishing that data, findings and interpretation are clearly linked

criteria based on the concept of trustworthiness, later refined as authenticity criteria (see Table 11.1). An alternative position proposed is that researchers should adopt a more tentative position referred to as subtle realism (Mays & Pope 2000). This is a more conciliatory position and recognises that research is more concerned with representing what is perceived as reality rather than trying to present truth accurately.

CONCLUSIONS

This chapter has examined the key assumptions underpinning the research process. In doing so it has attempted to move attention away from quantitative and qualitative research as two approaches divided by irreconcilable differences and instead to consider them as different approaches with strengths and weaknesses, whether used separately or in combination. Subsequent chapters will emphasise that the purpose of research is to adopt the right tools for the task in hand. Just as a driver faced with a punctured tyre would select the appropriate equipment and most effective way to approach the task, arguably the same principles apply to research problems. It would be naive not to recognise that a researcher experienced in the use of a particular methodology or method, or holding a particular set of beliefs about the world, would be more inclined to explore research problems amenable to their preferred approach(es), just as a

chef will return to a tried-and-tested recipe. Research includes a broad constituency of competing perspectives, assumptions, methodologies and methods. All approaches can be criticised or found insufficient, and rightly so. Healthy constructive disrespect should be encouraged. Nevertheless, this chapter has sought to emphasise that research problems or the pursuit of answers, however incomplete, should drive approaches, not vice versa.

References

Annandale E (1998) *The Sociology of Health & Medicine*. Cambridge, Polity Press.

Antiila M, Koivunen M, Välimäki M (2008) Information technology-based standardized patient education in psychiatric inpatient care. *Journal of Advanced Nursing* **64**(2): 147–156.

Armitage G, Hodgson I (2004) Using ethnography (or qualitative methods) to investigate drug errors: a critique of a published study. *NT Research* **9**: 379–387.

Atack L, Luke R, Chien E (2008) Evaluation of patient satisfaction with tailored online patient education information. *CIN – Computers Informatics Nursing* **26**(5): 258–264.

Barker PJ, Reynolds W, Ward T (1995) The proper focus of nursing: a critique of the 'caring' ideology. *International Journal of Nursing Studies* **32**: 386–397.

Becker HS, Geer B, Hughes EC, Strauss AL (1961) *Boys in White: student culture in medical school*. Chicago, University of Chicago Press.

Becker H (1996) The epistemology of qualitative research. In: Jessor R, Colby A and Scheweder R (eds) *Essays on Ethnography and Human Development: context and meaning in social inquiry.* Chicago, University of Chicago Press, pp 53–71.

Begley CM (1996) Using triangulation in nursing research. *Journal of Advanced Nursing* **24**: 122–128.

Benner P (1984) *Novice to Expert.* Menlo-Park, Addison-Wesley.

Benner P (1996) A response by P Benner to K Cash Benner and expertise in nursing: a critique. *International Journal of Nursing Studies* **33**: 669–674.

Brannen J (2005) *Mixed Methods Research: a discussion paper.* ESCR National Centre for Research Methods NCRM Methods Review Papers (available at www.ncrm.ac.uk/research/outputs/publications/documents/MethodsReviewPaperNCRM-005.pdf, accessed 17 December 2008).

Brearley S (2008) The cost if caring: commentary on Corbin (2008). *International Journal of Nursing Studies* **45**(6): 805–806.

Burke Johnson R, Onwuegbuzie AJ (2004) Mixed methods research: a research paradigm whose time has come. *Educational Researcher* **33**(7): 14–26.

Burns N, Groves SK (2008) *The Practice of Nursing Research: appraisal, synthesis and generation of evidence*, 6th edition. Philadelphia, WB Saunders.

Carolan M (2003) Reflexivity: a personal journey during data collection. *Nurse Researcher* **10**(3): 7–14.

Cash K (1995) Benner and expertise in nursing: a critique. *International Journal of Nursing Studies* **32**: 527–534.

Corbin J (2008) Guest editorial: Is caring a lost art in nursing? *International Journal of Nursing Studies* **45**: 163–165.

Creswell JW (2007) *Qualitative Inquiry and Research Design*, 2nd edition. Thousand Oaks, Sage.

Creswell JW, Tashakkori A (2007) Editorial: Developing publishable mixed methods manuscripts. *Journal of Mixed Methods Research* **1**(2): 107–110.

Davies MJ, Heller S, Skinner TC, Campbell J, Carey ME, Cradock S *et al.* (2008) Effectiveness of the diabetes education and self management for ongoing and newly diagnosed (DESMOND) programme for people with newly diagnosed type 2 diabetes: cluster randomised controlled trial. *British Medical Journal* **336**(7642): 491–495.

Denzin N (1989) *The Research Act: a theoretical introduction to sociological methods*, 3rd edition. New Jersey, Prentice Hall.

Denzin NK, Lincoln Y (eds) (2005) *The Sage Handbook of Qualitative Research*, 3rd edition. Thousand Oaks, Sage.

Ehlers VJ (2008) Editorial debate: Is caring a lost art in nursing or is it a changing reality? Commentary on the editorial written by Juliet Corbin. *International Journal of Nursing Studies* **45**: 802–804.

Enns C, Gregory D (2007) Lamentation and loss: expressions of caring by contemporary surgical nurses. *Journal of Advanced Nursing* **58**(4): 339–347.

Foucault M (1973) *The Birth of the Clinic.* London, Tavistock.

Glaser BG, Strauss AL (1965) *Awareness of Dying.* New York, Aldine.

Goffman A (1964) *Stigma: notes on the management of a spoiled identity.* Harmondsworth, Penguin.

Grbich C (1999) *Qualitative Research in Health.* London, Sage.

Griffiths P (2008) The art of losing … ? A response to the question 'is caring a lost art?' *International Journal of Nursing Studies* **45**: 329–332.

Hammersley M (1989) *The Dilemma of Qualitative Method.* London, Routledge.

Hammersley M, Atkinson P (2007) *Ethnography Principles in Practice*, 3rd edition. London, Taylor & Francis.

Hayward J, Boore JRP (1994) *Research Classics from the Royal College of Nursing. Volume 1. Information: a prescription against pain and prescription for recovery.* Harrow, Scutari.

Johnson M (1999) Observations on positivism and pseudo-science in qualitative nursing research. *Journal of Advanced Nursing* **39**: 67–73.

Johnson M, Long AJ, White A (2001) Arguments for pluralism in qualitative health research. *Nurse Education Today* **22**(1): 85–93.

Johnson M, Webb C (1995) Rediscovering unpopular patients: the concepts of social judgement. *Journal of Advanced Nursing* **21**: 466–475.

Kinnersley P, Edwards A, Hood K, Cadbury N, Ryan R, Prout H *et al.* (2007) *Interventions Before Consultations for Helping Patients Address Their Information Needs.* Cochrane Database for Systematic Reviews Issue 3. Art No: CD004565. COI: 10.1002/14651858. CD004565.pub2.

Koch T (1994) Establishing rigour in qualitative research: the decision trail. *Journal of Advanced Nursing* **19**: 976–986.

Koch T, Harrington (1998) Reconceptualizing rigour: the case for reflexivity. *Journal of Advanced Nursing* **28**: 882–890.

Koch T, Jenkin P, Kralik D (2004) Chronic illness self management: locating the 'self'. *Journal of Advanced Nursing* **48**: 484–492.

Kuhn TS (1972) *The Structure of Scientific Revolutions*, 2nd edition. Chicago, University of Chicago Press.

Lincoln Y, Guba E (1985) *Naturalistic Inquiry*. Thousand Oaks, Sage.

Lincoln Y, Guba E (1989) *Fourth Generation Evaluation*. Thousand Oaks, Sage.

Maben J (2008) Editorial debate: The art of caring: invisible and subordinated? A response to Juliet Corbin: 'Is caring a lost art in nursing?' *International Journal of Nursing Studies* **45**: 335–338.

Mason J (2002) *Qualitative Researching*, 2nd edition. London, Sage.

Mays N, Pope C (2000) Assessing quality in qualitative research. *British Medical Journal* **320**: 50–52.

Murray E, Burns J, See Tai S, Lai R, Nazereth I (2005) *Interactive Health Communication Applications for People with Chronic Disease*. Cochrane Database of Systematic Reviews 2005 Issue 4 Art No: CD004274. DOI: 10.1002/14651858.CD004274.pub4.

Nelson S, McGillon M (2004) Expertise or performance? Questioning the rhetoric of contemporary use of narrative use in nursing. *Journal of Advanced Nursing* **47**: 631–638.

Oakley A (1984) The importance of being a nurse. *Nursing Times* **80**(59): 24–27.

O'Cathain (2009) Editorial: Mixed methods research in the health sciences: a quiet revolution. *Journal of Mixed Methods Research* **3**(1): 3–5.

Pajnkihar M (2008) Editorial debate: Is caring a lost art in nursing? *International Journal of Nursing Studies* **45**: 807–808.

Polgar S, Thomas SA (2008) *Introduction to Research in the Health Sciences*, 5th edition. Edinburgh, Churchill Livingstone.

Popper K (1972) *Conjectures and Refutations*, 4th edition. London, Routledge & Kegan Paul.

Popper K (2002) *The Logic of Scientific Discovery*. London, Routledge.

Porter S (1995) *Nursing's Relationship with Medicine*. Aldershot, Ashgate.

Rafferty A-M, Clarke SP, Coles J, Ball J, James P, McKee M, Aiken LH (2007) Outcomes of variation in hospital nurse staffing in English hospitals: cross-sectional analysis of survey data and discharge records. *International Journal of Nursing Studies* **44**(2): 175–182.

Ramprogus V (2002) Eliciting nursing knowledge from practice: the dualism of nursing. *Nurse Researcher* **10**(1): 52–64.

Reid-Searl K, Moxham L, Walker S, Happell B (2008) Shifting supervision: implications for safe administration of medication by nursing students. *Journal of Clinical Nursing* **17**: 2750–2757.

Rolfe G (2009) Commentary: Some further questions on the nature of caring. *International Journal of Nursing Studies* **46**: 142–145.

Sandelowski M (1993) Rigor or rigor mortis: the problem of rigor in qualitative research. *Advances Nursing Science* **16**(2): 1–8.

Schwandt TA (1997) *Qualitative Inquiry: a dictionary of terms*. Thousand Oaks, Sage.

Shipman M (1997) *The Limitations of Social Research*, 4th edition. London, Longman.

Silverman D (1985) *Qualitative Methodology and Sociology: describing the social world*. Aldershot, Gower.

Silverman D (2005) *Doing Qualitative Research: a practical handbook*, 2nd edition. London, Sage.

Silverman D (2007) *Very Short, Fairly Interesting Book about Qualitative Research*. London, Sage.

Todd J, Scally A, Dodwell D, Horgan K, Topping A (2008) A randomised controlled trial of two programmes of shoulder exercise following axillary node dissection for invasive breast cancer. *Physiotherapy* **94**: 265–273.

Weinberg DB (2003) *Code Green*. New York, Cornell University Press.

Wilson-Barnett J (1988) Patient teaching or patient counselling? *Journal of Advanced Nursing* **13**: 215–222.

Websites

http://onlineqda.hud.ac.uk/index.php – Online QDA is a set of training support materials that address common problems (both early and advanced) of using qualitative data analysis (QDA) methods and selected computer-assisted qualitative data analysis (CAQDAS) packages.

www.data-archive.ac.uk/ – ESDS Qualidata is a specialist service of the ESDS led by the UK Data Archive (UKDA) at the University of Essex. The service provides access and support for a range of social science qualitative data sets, promoting and facilitating increased and more effective use of data in research, learning and teaching.

www.nova.edu/ssss/QR/web.html – the Qualitative Report is an online journal dedicated to qualitative research.

www.ncrm.ac.uk/ – ESRC National Centre for Research Methods (NCRM) is a network of research groups, each conducting research and training in an area of social science research methods.

www.qualitative-research.net/fqs/fqs-eng.htm – Qualitative Social Research is an online, peer-reviewed, multilingual journal for qualitative research.

12 Sampling

Susan Procter, Teresa Allan and Anne Lacey

Key points

- Sampling techniques aim to produce the best science within the constraints of resources available.

- A variety of sampling strategies are used in both qualitative and quantitative research, depending on the context and the research design.

- Sample selection and sample size affect the validity of the research and so should be done with maximum rigour.

INTRODUCTION

Sampling is a necessary aspect of all social research, as by definition it is not possible, except in exceptional and limited circumstances, to carry out a census that collects data from the total population. Sampling reduces the costs of research projects and also reduces the time required to gather the data. As this chapter will demonstrate, research is a pragmatic activity and researchers are constantly trying to produce the best science within the constraints of time, resources and feasibility.

There is considerable overlap between the sampling techniques used in both qualitative and quantitative research, but also some important differences. This chapter will guide the reader through the sampling procedures that need to be considered when undertaking both quantitative and qualitative research.

POPULATIONS AND SAMPLES

In all research it is important to distinguish between the target population, study population and the sampling frame used in the study. These are described below.

Target population

The target population is the total population that forms the focus for the study. In quantitative research it is the population to whom the study results will be generalised or applied. For instance, in the example given in Research Example 12.1, the target population was all adults over 18 living in the Isle of Man.

Qualitative research increases knowledge and understanding about the features of the target population under study. In Research Example 12.2, the target population was recently employed dietitians

12.1   Systematic Random Sampling

Plant ML, Miller MA, Plant MA, Ozenturk T (2007) Drinking patterns and alcohol-related experiences amongst adults on the Isle of Man: a comparison with the United Kingdom. *Journal of Substance Use* **12**(4): 243–252.

This cross-sectional survey compared alcohol consumption among adults in the Isle of Man with data from a previous survey conducted in UK. A simple systematic random sample of 2350 adults over the age of 18 was selected from the Isle of Man Electoral Register, and names selected were approached to take part in the study. One thousand adults eventually took part in the survey, which was conducted using face-to-face interviews with trained interviewers. Results suggested that there were more abstainers in the Isle of Man than in the comparable UK sample, but among those who drank, frequency and amount consumed was comparable. Nine percent of women and 22% of men were drinking above safe levels, and there were many reported alcohol-related problems. This survey did not find, however, any upsurge in drinking among young women in the Isle of Man, whereas this was found in the UK survey.

12.2   Purposive Sampling

Lordly D, Taper J (2008) Assumptions lead to the devaluation of dietician roles in long-term care practice environments. *Journal of Allied Health* **37**(2): 78–81.

This mixed methods study used a purposive sample of eight recently qualified dietitians and six supervisors working in two contrasting settings. Half of the sample was working in acute care, and half in long-term care settings. All the recently qualified dietitians came from a single degree programme. A questionnaire completed by all participants yielded both quantitative and qualitative data, and interviews were also conducted. Results suggested that, although basic competencies were gained in both environments, the role of the dietitian was devalued in long-term care settings, and newly qualified dietitians working in these settings were seen as gaining inferior experience and skills compared with those working in acute settings. Long-term care was seen as a second-choice career.

and their supervisors in two different care settings in Canada.

Study population

The study population is a subset of the target population from whom the sample is taken. It is not always practical to recruit respondents from across an entire country or even one geographical area. Instead, researchers may recruit respondents who fit the inclusion criteria for the study and are accessible locally. In

Research Example 12.2, for example, the study population was restricted to newly qualified dietitians from one graduate programme in Canada only. In Research Example 12.1, the target population was all adults living in the Isle of Man, but the study population consisted only of those on the electoral register.

Sampling frame

A sampling frame is a comprehensive, itemised list of all people, patients, practices, hospitals or events, which comprise the study population, from which a sample will be taken. It includes the settings or individuals of interest to the researcher, and provides a transparent framework from which to derive a sample. When devising a sampling frame it is important to distinguish between the target population and the study population. The sampling frame is normally taken from the study population, which is assumed to broadly reflect the characteristics of the target population. If there are important differences between the two populations, these will limit the generalisability or transferability of the study findings and this should be noted as a study limitation. Once the sampling frame has been compiled it is possible to use it to derive a sample. In the example in Research Example 12.1, the sampling frame was all names on the electoral register of the Isle of Man, which the researchers estimated to be 91% of the population.

TYPES OF SAMPLING

There are two basic sampling schemes in research – probability, and non-probability sampling schemes. Quantitative research studies tend to use probability schemes, as the errors or biases are more easily calculated and thus accounted for in the sampling procedures and analysis. This allows for generalisation to the study and target population more readily than non-probability schemes. Qualitative researchers predominantly use non-probability schemes as this allows for theoretical sampling, and the aim is not so much to generalise but to uncover truths about a phenomenon.

Probability sampling

Probability sampling means that each unit in the target population has a known chance of selection. Usually it is an equal chance (as in the National Lottery), but sometimes it may be unequal, but known. Probability sampling can only be used when an accurate and up-to-date sampling frame is available. Where the study population is known in advance (e.g. all names on the electoral register as in Research

Example 12.1) this provides a useful sampling frame for research. The strength of probability sampling arises from the fact that it generates a representative sample, which should ensure that the sample has the same characteristics as the study population, and where the study population is similar to the target population.

Non-probability sampling

Non-probability sampling is used when it is necessary to derive a sample from an unknown (hidden) population. It is frequently the case that the study population cannot be identified in advance or, more usually, that no up-to-date and complete list is available from which a sample can be derived. When it is not possible to obtain a comprehensive list of the study population, researchers must use non-probability sampling schemes. In quantitative research, these are considered less rigorous because bias may inadvertently be introduced, making the sample not representative of the total population.

Nevertheless, the alternative of not undertaking the research because a sampling frame is not available may impoverish our knowledge about important groups of people such as the homeless, family carers, single parents and other groups where a register does not exist. In-depth qualitative studies and descriptive surveys that identify the key characteristics and features of the sample population can be used to increase our knowledge and explanatory theories of the population, and can be generalised to other populations that match the sample in ways identified as important by the researchers.

Non-probability sampling schemes are widely used in nursing research. In quantitative research, they may be used in preliminary or exploratory studies, where random sampling is too costly, where an appropriate sampling frame is not available or when it is the only way of getting the information required. In qualitative studies they are used to study the population of interest and to ensure that the research samples rich sources of data that generate in-depth conceptual and theoretical understanding.

SAMPLING SCHEMES IN QUANTITATIVE RESEARCH

Simple random sampling

In simple random sampling, each member of the sampling frame has a known and equal chance of being selected for the sample. To derive a sample of 390 from a list of 2,600, the list should be numbered systematically and a random number table or a statistical software package used to randomly generate the required number of 390. Simple random sampling can produce 'rogue' samples, especially if the sample size is small. To overcome this, either systematic or stratified random sampling can be used.

Systematic random sampling

Again a numbered list is used, but this time a sampling fraction is calculated. The sampling fraction depends on the sample size and how long the list is. If there are 400 on the list and 40 are required, this gives a sample fraction of 10% and selects 1 in 10. So the starting point on the list for selection (the start value) must be a number between 1 and 10, chosen randomly. Every tenth item on the list is chosen thereafter, e.g. 6, 16, 26, etc. Research Example 12.1 gives an example of a systematic random sample drawn from an electoral register list. Systematic random sampling leads to a more evenly spaced distribution of the sample from the list than simple random sampling (Bowling & Ebrahim 2005). But even this can introduce bias if there is a cyclical pattern in the underlying list, e.g. operations in hospitals that follow a weekly pattern would give the same type on the same day. Blocking schemes (Pocock 1983) can be used to overcome cyclical patterns. For instance, over seven weeks a different day each week is chosen at random before sampling takes place (using systematic random or random sampling) within each block.

Stratified random sampling

This is where the population is divided into well-defined subgroups or strata, e.g. males/females, age groups, operation types, illness type, nurse grades. This means that people within a stratum are more similar to each other than across the different strata. There are two forms of stratified random sampling: *proportionate* and *disproportionate* sampling.

In *proportionate* sampling the same sampling fraction (e.g. 15%) is used to draw a sample from each group/stratum. This means that the different groups in the population (strata) are correctly represented in the sample, with larger groups contributing proportionately more people to the sample, as demonstrated in the example in Table 12.1. This increases the precision of the estimates of error compared with simple random sampling and gives more confidence in the results. In Research Example 12.3, stratified random sampling ensured an accurate representation of healthcare workers in three different language regions of Wales, and in different care settings.

In *disproportionate* sampling, a variable sampling fraction is used to increase representation of particular groups that may have small numbers in the study or total population. For instance, if an area had a very mixed ethnic population, the sample fraction might be increased to include people from a wider range of different ethnic backgrounds in the study. Similarly, some strata may be very small, giving rise to only a few members being selected if the standard sampling fraction is used. A 15% sampling fraction of band 5 staff nurses in a hospital, for example (see Table 12.1), yields a much higher number than a 15% sample of band 8 senior clinical nurses. However, because in disproportionate sampling the sample is no longer representative of the study or total

Table 12.1 Proportionate sampling from nurse grades

Population stratum nurse banding/ grades	Number of people in the stratum	Number sampled from the stratum (15%)
5	1,500	225
6	800	120
7	200	30
8	100	15
Total	2,600	390

12.3   Stratified Random Sampling

Roberts GW, Irvine FE, Jones PR, Spencer LH, Baker CR, Williams C (2007) Language aware-ness in the bilingual healthcare setting: a national survey. *International Journal of Nursing Studies* **44**: 1177–1186.

This Welsh national survey investigated the language awareness of healthcare professionals working in different types of healthcare setting, and in three different language regions of Wales. The sample of 3,358 health professionals was drawn from a range of public, private and voluntary organisations across Wales, and was stratified by three regions according to the proportion of Welsh language speakers in each. Data were collected by means of a postal questionnaire, which achieved a 57% response rate. The survey found that positive attitudes towards cross-cultural communication was strongly correlated with use of the Welsh language, but that there were positive language attitudes even among those who spoke little Welsh or worked in areas with low Welsh-speaking populations. Language awareness training was rec-ommended as a way of enhancing care delivery for minority language speakers.

12.4   Cluster Sampling

Greenough PG, Lappi MD, Hsu EB, Fink S, Hsieh Y, Vu A, Heaton C, Kirsch TD (2008) Burden of disease and health status among hurricane Katrina-displaced persons in shelters: a popula-tion based cluster sample. *Disaster Medicine* **51**(4): 426–432.

Two weeks after Hurricane Katrina hit Louisiana in 2005, this research study investigated the health status of victims of the hurricane who were staying in temporary shelters. A cluster sample of 499 evacuees was selected from 20 Red Cross shelters, a random sample of 30 heads of households being selected from each of the selected shelters. Results indicated that the respondents were predominantly female and black, and of low socioeconomic status. Over half arrived at the shelter with a chronic disease such as hypertension, diabetes or psychiatric illness. Of those with chronic disease, nearly half lacked access to their usual medication. One-third arrived with symptoms requiring immediate intervention, such as dehydration, dysp-noea, chest pain and injury.

population, some variables will be over-represented. The analysis has to be adjusted to account for this over representation.

Cluster sampling

Here, the entire population is divided into groups or clusters based on closeness of some kind (e.g. geographical) or similarity (e.g. type of hospital) or speciality (e.g. orthopaedic or cardiac) or particular wards (medical or surgical). First, a sample of the clusters is taken using simple, systematic or stratified random sampling. Then all members of each cluster selected are recruited, or members of each cluster are sampled using simple, systematic or stratified random sampling. Cluster sampling reduces the costs of research as it ensures that the population sampled is clustered together, so making access and communica-tion easier. It also enables probability sampling to be used when a sampling frame of the population is not available. The clusters may be schools, hospitals, villages, wards or departments for which a sampling frame is available. In the example in Research Example 12.4, the clusters were Red Cross shelters following a hurricane in the United States. The sample of individuals required could only be identified once the clusters were chosen and individual heads of households within each shelter listed. The disadvantage of cluster sampling is that sampling error is increased and sample size has to increase accordingly.

Multi-stage sampling

This form of sampling uses more than two consecutive stages of random selection. It can combine simple random sampling, stratified random sampling and cluster sampling in some form.

Quota sampling

This is a non-probability method of sampling widely used in opinion polls. It is a form of convenience and judgement sampling, where the data collector has to recruit a number (quota) of people fitting a particular category, e.g. white males over 50, but the selection of the sample is otherwise not specified. Often the size of the quota in the sample is proportional to the number of people in that category in the target population. Bias can be introduced, however, if data collectors consciously or unconsciously avoid certain types of people, such as the homeless, or recruit in a particular area of a town. Quota sampling is not much used in health services research.

CALCULATING SAMPLE SIZE IN QUANTITATIVE RESEARCH

In quantitative research, the size of the sample aimed for should be calculated at the design stage. In intervention and comparison studies, the sample size determines the *power* of the study to detect a statistically significant difference between groups.

The *significance* of a study relates to the probability of making a type I (α) error. A type I error means finding a real (i.e.) significant difference/effect between the two groups in the sample when one does not exist in the study or target population. In other words, saying the intervention works, or a real difference between groups exists, when it does not. A type II (β) error is the probability of finding there is no effect or difference between the two groups in the sample population when one does in fact exist in the study population.

If the significance level is set at 5% and a significant result achieved, then it indicates with 95% confidence that a real difference exists. The confidence interval of 95% derives from the *probability* of obtaining the observed result due to chance alone.

Reducing the chance of making a type I error from 5% to, say, 1%, and so reducing the chance of concluding that a difference exists, when it does not, requires an increase in sample size. In general terms, the greater the *power*, the larger the sample size has to be, which then has time and cost implications. Traditionally, most studies use either 90% or 80% power. So, for example, if a study has 80% power then there is an 80% probability of detecting a real difference, if it exists. However, this also means that there is a 20% chance of missing a real difference that actually exists.

Calculating sample size for intervention or comparison studies depends on an estimation of the expected differences between groups. In choosing the outcome variables that are going to be used for the calculation, it is helpful if there is some earlier information about the likely variability of the measures selected. Calculating sample size requires a measure of the *variability* of differences, usually the standard deviation or variance, to be expected in the total population. In clinical research, the sort of clinical differences one is expecting from the intervention or between different groups that are under consideration, is required. For instance, in the study described in Research Example 12.1, the power of the study would relate to the ability to detect a real difference in the key outcome variables (drinking patterns and alcohol-related experiences) between adults in the Isle of Man and those in UK. To calculate sample size, therefore, researchers have to identify in advance the likely size of the difference in measured outcomes that is likely between the two groups and to provide a justification of the size difference selected.

147

To calculate sample size it is necessary to identify the key outcome variables being measured, the tools used to measure those variables and the expected difference between groups. To estimate the expected difference between groups it is necessary to obtain as much information as possible from previous studies or from pilot studies about the distribution of the variables across the study and target populations. Armed with this information, researchers should seek the advice of a statistician.

Studies in which the sample size is considered too small to achieve the power required to obtain a significant outcome are often deemed unscientific and not worth undertaking, because they will either produce flawed results (if significance testing is carried out) or fail to provide any new knowledge. In general, if one wishes to generalise to the target population then sufficient power is a requirement for the validity of studies. Small studies can, however, be used as pilots for larger studies in which a descriptive analysis of the findings (including percentages, means and standard deviations) of key variables across the study population may be useful for calculating the sample size required in subsequent studies. The power requirement may sometimes be waived in student research, although this is becoming less acceptable to ethics committees.

SOURCES OF BIAS IN QUANTITATIVE SAMPLING

In quantitative sampling there are two basic types of errors: random (sampling) and systematic (non-sampling). Bias is often introduced into a study through systematic errors.

Random errors create less bias as it is assumed that this type of error is evenly distributed across the sampling frame and therefore the sample, derived randomly, remains inaccurate but representative of the study population. Any errors will tend to average out across the sample and hence little or no bias is introduced. It is possible to control random errors by increasing the sample size and having an appropriate sampling technique.

Systematic errors are not reduced with increased sample size. If a study aims to recruit GPs from a particular list, for example, but certain sorts of GP practices are routinely excluded from that list (e.g. single-handed practices), then these GPs cannot be selected and the error is not random. In the example in Research Example 12.1, residents who were not registered to vote were not included in the study as their names did not appear on the electoral register. Those excluded may have been more likely to drink excessively, or be homeless, and so introduce systematic bias. No matter how much the sample size is increased, the error will not be reduced. The key to reducing sample frame bias is to use as accurate a database (or list) as possible.

In quantitative research the aim is to control as many sources of error as possible, but it is a balance. In a large sample with systematic errors, the analysis is not to be trusted. An unrepresentative sample makes it impossible to generalise to the study/target population. Sampling schemes, therefore, need to be as rigorous as possible, given the circumstances under which the researcher is working.

SAMPLING IN QUALITATIVE RESEARCH

Qualitative researchers are not so concerned with identifying the total population of people, events or settings in order to develop a sampling frame. They seek to identify key individuals, events or settings that provide a rich source of data. However, it is still important for qualitative researchers to pay attention to their sampling strategy. In assessing the rigour of qualitative research, Mays and Pope (2000) suggest the reviewer should ask the following questions.

- Did the sample include the full range of possible cases or settings so that conceptual rather than statistical generalisations could be made?
- If appropriate, were efforts made to obtain data that might contradict or modify the analysis by extending the sample (for example, to a different type of area or informant)?

In qualitative research, the problem of diversity or variation is addressed through the development of a sampling strategy designed to ensure that a range of data are identified and collected, as this increases the validity of the findings.

However, for some qualitative research the notion of selecting a sample is considered inappropriate and instead the research focuses on collecting data from a 'naturally occurring population' (Silverman 2005). Case study research may select a single case of an event or situation, such as an individual experience of healthcare (for a good example of this see Allen *et al.* 2004) or study of a single ward or hospital (Stake 2000). The populations studied, be they people, agencies or other units of study using naturalistic or case study research, are recognised by qualitative researchers to be unique. However, they share sufficient commonalities with the population from which they are drawn to be recognisable as belonging to that population group (i.e. a classroom in a school could not be mistaken for a ward in a hospital). Consequently, the study is able to inform understanding of the wider population of which the case study or naturally occurring research is an example.

Purposive sampling

A purposive sample is one where people from a pre-specified group are purposely sought out and sampled. For instance, in the example given in Research Example 12.2, the researchers purposively sampled recently qualified dietitians working in two different care settings. Purposive samples have an over-representation of people or events of interest to the researcher. This means that they are not usually representative of the whole population under study. Purposive sampling is used to justify the inclusion of rich sources of data that can be used to generate or test out the explanatory frameworks. Examples of purposive sampling given by Patton (2002) include:

- sampling extreme or deviant cases
- intensity sampling
- sampling typical cases
- sampling maximum variation in cases
- homogeneous sampling
- sampling critical cases
- criterion sampling
- confirming and disconfirming cases
- theory-based sampling

- sampling politically important or sensitive cases.

Identifying the full range of possible cases or settings again requires the qualitative researcher to at least map out potential respondents or study sites from whatever information is available before deciding who, where or what to sample. The process by which the sampling decisions are taken distinguishes purposive sampling from convenience sampling in qualitative research in that purposive sampling is done rigorously and systematically.

Theoretical sampling

Further sampling in response to data analysis is sometimes referred to as theoretical sampling. Here, the sampling strategy evolves iteratively in response to data analysis, and in particular to the conceptual and theoretical aspects of the analysis rather than the characteristics of the population. In the example in Research Example 12.5, successive interviews with participants and ongoing discussion by telephone and email after the interviews enabled analysis and data collection to be conducted in parallel, additional sampling being used as emergent ideas developed from the analysis.

As an indicator of rigour in qualitative research, Mays and Pope (2000) suggest that the researcher searches for contradictory or disconfirming sources of data or identifies exceptions to the patterns being described, in order to test out the findings from the study. These data sources can either be purposively identified at the start of the study and built into the sampling framework (purposive sampling) or identified during the course of the study in response to the analysis of the data (theoretical sampling). Either way, a sampling frame that is used to map sampling decisions is a useful way to demonstrate rigour in qualitative research.

Snowball sampling

This strategy uses human networks to gather a sample or identify informants or situations where events might be observed. For example, homeless people often know others in the same situation; similarly,

RESEARCH EXAMPLE

12.5   Theoretical and Snowball Sampling

Mills J, Francis K, Bonner A (2007) Live my work: rural nurses and their multiple perspectives of self. *Journal of Advanced Nursing* **59**(6): 583–590.

This study explored rural nurses' experiences of mentoring. A qualitative, grounded theory design was used, conducting 11 semi-structured interviews with nine nurses in rural parts of Australia. Theoretical sampling and situational analysis were used to establish rigour in the analysis, additional interviews and questions being arranged as the analysis proceeded. The study concluded that rural nurses mentor novices by developing supportive relationships and sharing their lives. Novices were protected through difficult issues and given an in-depth understanding of the communities in which they worked.

people from minority ethnic populations may be able to identify others from their population who could inform the research. Research Example 12.5 uses snowball techniques as well as theoretical sampling – each rural nurse was likely to be able to identify others in similar situations who could be invited to participate.

CALCULATING SAMPLE SIZE IN QUALITATIVE RESEARCH

Because sample size is not an intrinsic feature of the analysis in qualitative research there is very little guidance on the size of samples. In most cases, the resources available and the feasibility of obtaining the sample combine to determine the size. The rigour of the approach used is determined by the rationale given for the sampling decisions taken by the researcher within the context of available opportunities for gaining access to events or naturally occurring populations.

Grounded theory uses the concept of *saturation* to determine sample size. Here, data are collected and analysed until no new themes or perspectives are reported and it is assumed that all the component parts of the phenomenon under study have been captured. This approach creates difficulties in planning research as it is not possible to identify in advance how much data will be required to reach saturation and therefore how much resource is required to complete the study.

DePaulo (2000), in a paper designed to guide market research using qualitative methods, calculated the number of customer needs uncovered by various numbers of focus groups and in-depth interviews. Few additional needs were uncovered after 30 in-depth interviews; this was confirmed using quantitative methods. His work also indicates that if the researcher is not concerned with within-group variation, only with typicality, then a sample of 10 should suffice. Patton (2002) recommends minimum samples for planning purposes based on anticipated reasonable coverage, which can be expected to change as the research progresses. For Silverman (2005) the crucial issue is to think through theoretical priorities and to demonstrate a research design driven by those priorities. He suggests that qualitative researchers should substitute theoretical coherence for statistical representativeness.

DePaulo (2000) is mainly concerned with producing a descriptive level of analysis that maximises the range of opinions or perceptions captured. He recommends that multiple analysts review the data to maximise findings. Qualitative researchers concerned with deriving theoretical interpretations of data are not convinced by arguments for saturation or capturing maximum variation, viewing this as a search for descriptive completeness. Instead, they suggest that theory may be derived from a fragment of naturally occurring data or the in-depth study of a single case (Silverman 2005), particularly if the researcher studies that data for what is not said or done and interprets absence and omissions in the data as well as inclusions.

SAMPLING STRATEGIES USED IN QUALITATIVE AND QUANTITATIVE RESEARCH

Some types of sampling are used in both qualitative and quantitative research, although their use conforms to the principles of each type of sampling strategy as discussed above. These are discussed below.

Sampling for time, events and settings

Sampling for time, events and settings is difficult as these change over time, or vary from person to person or according to setting. Research Example 12.6 describes Meengs *et al.* (1994) quantitative observational study of hand washing in an emergency department. In this case, information for a sample of 35 participants was gathered during three-hour periods over a number of days. Estimates of hand washing then had to be totalled or averaged over standardised periods.

When undertaking this type of sampling it is important to make observations across time and space, as the pattern of event being observed, e.g. hand-washing behaviour, may change both during the day and on different days, and may vary according to how busy the department is, who is on duty and whether it is a weekday, evening, night or weekend shift.

Sampling in time and events and settings is an important feature of observational research. It is often difficult to sample events as it is not possible to know exactly when or where they are going to occur. However, the selection of situations to observe is guided by the same sampling principles used elsewhere in qualitative research and tends, therefore, to focus on naturally occurring events during different time periods and in different settings. Qualitative sampling for time, events and settings can be purposive and/or theoretical. In undertaking purposive sampling of events the researcher would seek out settings where the event might naturally occur at a time when it might be expected (see Chapter 32 for a fuller account of this process).

Convenience sampling

Novice researchers and those with few resources may select an accessible population or setting, which they believe to be typical, rather than a representative sample. Convenience may be a key feature in this decision, for example approaching nurses from a local hospital. In many ways all researchers use some form of convenience sample in the sense that the

---

RESEARCH EXAMPLE

12.6 Time and Event Sampling

Meengs MR, Giles BK, Chisholm CD, Cordell WH, Nelson DR (1994) Hand washing frequency in an emergency department. *Journal of Emergency Nursing* **20**: 183–188.

This study examined the frequency and duration of hand washing in one emergency department, and the effects of three variables: level of training, type of patient contact (clean, dirty or gloved) and years of staff clinical experience. Eleven faculty, 11 resident physicians and 13 emergency nurses were observed. Participants were informed that their activities were being monitored but were unaware of the exact nature of the study. An observer recorded the number of patient contacts and activities for each participant during three-hour observation periods. Activities were categorised as either clean or dirty according to a scale devised by Fulkerson. The use of gloves was noted and hand-washing technique and duration were recorded. A hand-washing break in technique was defined as failure to wash hands after a patient contact and before proceeding to another patient or activity.

sample must be accessible to the researcher in some form. But convenience sampling can lead to significant biases and errors if the sample used is unrepresentative of the target population, and should be avoided if possible.

CONCLUSIONS

This chapter has demonstrated that there is considerable overlap between the sampling techniques used in qualitative and quantitative research, but also some important differences. A limiting factor in undertaking quantitative research is the resources needed to undertake studies with a large enough sample to meet power requirements. Pilot work, however, is very valuable and does provide opportunities for students and less well-resourced researchers to undertake quantitative research. This chapter should have alerted readers to the idea that sampling in qualitative and quantitative research has many common factors; both are concerned to ensure rigour and this can be as difficult to achieve in qualitative research as it is in quantitative research. Expert advice from statisticians or experienced qualitative researchers should be sought before selecting a sample.

References

Allen D, Griffiths L, Lyne P (2004) Understanding complex trajectories in health and social care provision. *Sociology of Health and Illness* **26**: 1008–1030.

Bowling A, Ebrahim S (2005) *Handbook of Health Research Methods: investigation, measurement and analysis*. Berkshire, Open University Press.

DePaulo P (2000) Sample size for qualitative research: the risk of missing something important. *Quirk's Marketing Research Review* (www.quirks.com/articles).

Greenough PG, Lappi MD, Hsu EB, Fink S, Hsieh Y, Vu A *et al.* (2008) Burden of disease and health status among hurricane Katrina-displaced persons in shelters: a population based cluster sample. *Disaster Medicine* **51**(4): 426–432.

Lordly D, Taper J (2008) Assumptions lead to the devaluation of dietician roles in long-term care practice environments. *Journal of Allied Health* **37**(2): 78–81.

Mays N, Pope C (2000) Assessing quality in qualitative research. *British Medical Journal* **320**: 50–52.

Meengs MR, Giles BK, Chisholm CD, Cordell WH, Nelson DR (1994) Hand washing frequency in an emergency department. *Journal of Emergency Nursing* **20**: 183–188.

Mills J, Francis K, Bonner A (2007) Live my work: rural nurses and their multiple perspectives of self. *Journal of Advanced Nursing* **59**(6): 583–590.

Patton MQ (2002) *Qualitative Research and Evaluation Methods*, 3rd edition. Beverley Hills, Sage.

Plant ML, Miller MA, Plant MA, Ozenturk T (2007) Drinking patterns and alcohol-related experiences amongst adults on the Isle of Man: a comparison with the United Kingdom. *Journal of Substance Use* **12**(4): 243–252.

Pocock SJ (1983) *Clinical Trials: a practical approach*. London, John Wiley.

Roberts GW, Irvine FE, Jones PR, Spencer LH, Baker CR, Williams C (2007) Language awareness in the bilingual healthcare setting: a national survey. *International Journal of Nursing Studies* **44**: 1177–1186.

Silverman D (2005) *Doing Qualitative Research. A Practical Handbook*, 2nd edition. London, Sage.

Stake RE (2000) The case study method in social inquiry. In: Gomm R, Hammerseley M, Foster P (eds) *Case Study Method*. Thousand Oaks, Sage.

Further reading

Armitage P, Berry G, Matthews JNS (2002) *Statistical Methods in Medical Research*. Oxford, Blackwell Science.

Campbell MJ, Julious SA, Altman DG (1995) Estimating sample sizes for binary, ordered categorical, and continuous outcomes in two group comparisons. *British Medical Journal* **311**: 1145–1148.

Cohen J (1988) *Statistical Power Analysis for the Behavioural Sciences*, 2nd edition. Lawrence New Jersey, Erlbaum Associates.

13 Grounded Theory

Immy Holloway and Les Todres

Key points

- Grounded theory is a systematic qualitative approach concerned with generating theory from a variety of data sources. Researchers can also modify and extend existing theories. This approach is most useful when little is known about the topic or phenomenon or when a new perspective is needed on a familiar situation or setting.

- Key features of grounded theory include theoretical sampling, coding and categorisation of data through a process of constant comparative analysis.

- Researchers using a grounded theory approach need to develop theoretical sensitivity whereby they become attuned to important concepts that arise from the data. The related literature enhances theoretical sensitivity by creating awareness in the researcher of relevant and significant aspects of the data.

- The analytic process of coding and categorising is facilitated by writing fieldnotes and memos in which the development of ideas and provisional categories or theoretical ideas is recorded. The process includes the development of a core or central category.

INTRODUCTION

Grounded theory is a systematic approach within qualitative research originally developed by Glaser and Strauss (1967). It has its basis in sociology, but the data collection and analysis procedures are also used in other disciplines such as psychology, healthcare or education. It became popular in nursing in the 1980s and 1990s and is often used now.

Several informative books have been published on grounded theory, for instance *Theoretical Sensitivity* (Glaser 1978), *Qualitative Analysis for Social Scientists* (Strauss 1987) and *The Basics of Qualitative Research* (Strauss & Corbin 1990, 1998; Corbin & Strauss 2008). Strauss died in 1996 but co-authored his last two books with Corbin, a nurse academic who recently (2008) wrote its third edition. Strauss and Corbin (1997) also edited a book demonstrating the use of grounded theory in practice. Glaser and Strauss used the approach in the healthcare field and helped students to apply it, in particular in nursing and in education. One of the early books was the study by Benoliel (1973) on the interaction of nurses with dying patients. Other nurse authors have described the techniques and procedures of grounded theory, such as Schreiber and Stern and their co-writers (2001). An older but useful text for nurses was edited by Chenitz and Swanson in 1986.

In 2006 grounded theory had a new boost with the publication of the guidelines for constructivist grounded theory by Kathy Charmaz (2006). She stresses flexibility and openness for grounded theory rather than a rule-governed, rigid approach. The emphasis is also on the way participants construct their social reality on the basis of meanings shared with others. Charmaz has made her form of grounded theory very clear for beginning researchers.

THE PURPOSE AND MAIN FEATURES OF GROUNDED THEORY

There are many similarities between grounded theory and other qualitative approaches. Grounded theory is, initially at least, inductive. This means that researchers go from the specific and single instances to the general, from data to theory.

There is no hypothesis or theoretical framework prior to data collection in grounded theory. Although researchers have 'hunches' and prior ideas, of course, Strauss (1987) once said that the researcher is not *tabula rasa* – a blank sheet; the data generated by the researcher in the specific project, however, have primacy. This means that researchers need to overcome previous assumptions as they might force them into a particular direction and encourage them to follow preconceived ideas. It is dangerous, however, to disregard completely prior experiences or knowledge as these can become a useful resource for the study.

Typical research questions suitable for a grounded theory approach involve interaction, action and meaning, and focus on process. Examples might be:

- What is happening in this setting?
- How do people behave and interact in this situation?
- How do the participants make sense of their experience?
- How do things change over time in the setting to be studied?
- What are the phases or stages of the experience, treatment or condition?

Grounded theory can be distinguished from other qualitative approaches. The main purpose of grounded theory is the generation of concepts and theory from the data, although Strauss and Corbin (1998) suggest that existing theory may be modified or extended. Theory production is possible in other qualitative approaches, but essential in grounded theory; this theory is always rooted in the data. It shows links and relationships between concepts, and the researcher gives not only an overview but also an explanation for the phenomenon under study. The theoretical ideas have to be applicable to a variety of similar settings and contexts.

Distinct features of grounded theory are the interaction between data collection and analysis, and the procedure of theoretical sampling (see later in this chapter). While many other qualitative approaches describe a phenomenon, grounded theorists go further than generating description by producing theory that has explanatory power. Like most other qualitative research methods, it is person-centred and focuses on the experience, behaviour and perspectives of participants.

THE RELEVANCE OF GROUNDED THEORY IN NURSING RESEARCH

The findings of grounded theory research in nursing will generally have implications for practice as they identify how participants make sense of their experiences. Nurses can take account of the findings of the research. In the past, nurse researchers used traditional methods of inquiry to generate knowledge. They focused on hypothesis testing, using deductive rather than inductive approaches.

More recently nurses have utilised qualitative forms of inquiry, as they produce rich and deep data. This has a number of advantages for nursing.

- Nurses will be able to understand patients' behaviour and emotions better, and this has implications for professional care and treatment.
- Nurses study interactions between patients and health professionals, which is important for

professional action; solutions to clinical problems might be found more quickly.

- Nurses learn to understand their professional world in more depth when studying the perspectives of their own and other professions as well as students' perspectives. Solutions to clinical problems might be more easily found.
- Through qualitative evaluation, programmes and processes can be improved.
- Nurses have learnt during their education to be structured and systematic in their approach to work; hence the structured and systematic approach of grounded theory has a particular appeal for them.
- Flexibility and openness is demanded of nurses in clinical practice and nurse educators. Nurses are able to apply these skills to grounded theory.

Holloway (2008) reiterates that much qualitative research, including grounded theory, examines cultural practices and behaviours, of both patients and professionals. Sick people's illness and suffering, and their perspectives on this, can be understood more clearly, and a greater understanding of this will lead to better care. Most important of all, however, as Suddaby (2006) explains, grounded theory focuses on processes of meaning making in interaction.

THE THEORETICAL BASIS OF GROUNDED THEORY: SYMBOLIC INTERACTIONISM

Grounded theory has its roots in the movement of symbolic interactionism, a theoretical perspective initially developed by George Herbert Mead in the 1920s and 1930s. He saw the use of symbols in interaction as a major feature of human life (Mead 1934). In Mead's view, individuals develop their own action on the basis of those of others; they take account of each other's behaviour, interpret and respond to it. In the light of change, the meanings are re-interpreted. The emphasis is on the process of interaction between

people and the way they understand social roles. The self thus is a social rather than a psychological phenomenon. Interactionists contribute to grounded theory the idea that human beings are active agents in their own experience through interpreting this experience and acting according to their interpretations.

Other people affect the development of a person's social self by their expectations and influence. When they start life, human beings develop through interacting with the important people in their lives – significant others. They learn to act according to others' expectations, thereby shaping their own behaviour through the process of socialisation. At a later stage, individuals as members of society analyse the symbols of others, such as language, gestures, mime and appearance, and interpret them. People share the attitudes and responses to particular situations with members of their group. The observation of these interacting roles and responses to each other is a source of data in grounded theory.

To understand action and interaction researchers look at the meanings human beings give to it. In grounded theory, researchers explore these meanings and 'the definition of the situation' by those observing and living in it. Thomas (1928) claimed:

'If men (*sic*) define situations as real, they are real in their consequences' (Thomas 1928: 584)

He suggested that individual definitions of reality and meanings they give to it shape perceptions and actions. Participant observation and interviewing help understand this process.

Human beings are creative individuals who plan, project and revise their thoughts and behaviour in relation to others within a particular context. Their conduct can only be understood in context. Grounded theory, therefore, stresses the importance of the context in which people function and share their social world with others.

Symbolic interactionism is sometimes criticised for neglecting society and its structure. This criticism is not wholly appropriate. Symbolic interactionism does see the individual in context, in relation to others and in their social situation.

DATA COLLECTION AND INITIAL SAMPLING

Researchers use a variety of data sources for grounded theory research, including interviews, observation and documents such as patient diaries, letters or professional notes. Morse (2001), however, advises against collecting data by focus group interviews when carrying out grounded theory; she maintains that the 'snippets of data' obtained are not appropriate, as process cannot be easily uncovered in focus group interviews. In-depth or narrative interviews are more useful. Unstructured and semi-structured interviews are the favoured methods of data collection, but grounded theorists stress the value of participant observation.

It must be emphasised that data collection and analysis proceed at the same time, and interact at each stage. Memos or fieldnotes are written throughout so that nothing of importance is forgotten. Researchers decide on the basis of the early collection and analysis what data to obtain next. Subsequently, concepts are followed up and the research becomes progressively focused on particular issues that are important for developing the theoretical ideas, for the participants and for the researcher's agenda. It means that researchers formulate 'working propositions', which they can then test through further data collection and analysis. In this sense, grounded theory, unlike other qualitative research approaches, has deductive elements as researchers develop ideas gained from working hypotheses. Grounded theory is mainly seen as starting with induction; however, once working propositions are established, Corbin and Strauss (2008) maintain that it is also deductive.

This has implications for sampling. The early sample might include a variety of participants, and concepts emerge from the very beginning in the inductive phase. Depending on the findings during the early stages of data collection and analysis, more people may be added to the sample. Others can be interviewed more than once to follow up later findings and to lead to saturation. This means that the number of participants at the beginning may differ from the number at the end of the research. For instance, if a researcher finds during early stages that the young feel differently from older people about a particular issue or problem, more young people (or older individuals) can be added to the sample.

Theoretical sampling

Glaser and Strauss (1967) developed the process of theoretical sampling. In this, grounded theory is distinct from other approaches, although other methods also use this type of sampling occasionally. Theoretical sampling is guided by concepts and constructs that have significance for the developing theory. At the beginning of the study initial sampling decisions are made regarding specific individuals or groups of people who have knowledge and information about the area of study. When the initial data have been analysed, particular concepts arise and are followed up by a choice of further participants, events and situations; this process can further illuminate the initial findings (see Research Example 13.1). The researcher can continue doing this, choosing a variety of settings or a particular age group to extend the conceptualisation. Certain concepts may be found initially, and during the analytic phase these will be tested out with a further search of these concepts. Theoretical sampling continues until the point of saturation. Although theoretical sampling has its roots in grounded theory, it is used in other qualitative research approaches such as ethnography. In theoretical sampling the research process is determined by the ideas that emerge. Draucker *et al.* (2007) developed a useful theoretical sampling guide.

The main differences between this and other types of sampling are time and continuance. Unlike other types of sampling, theoretical sampling is not planned from the outset but proceeds throughout the study. However, the fact that details of the sample and interview questions are not fully known beforehand may raise challenges during the process of ethical review.

Theoretical sensitivity

Grounded theory, and in particular theoretical sampling, needs theoretical sensitivity. Glaser (1978) first used the term to help the researcher develop theory. Theoretical sensitivity means that the researcher

13.1 Theoretical Sampling

Gass J (2008) Electroconvulsive therapy and the work of mental health nurses: a grounded theory study. *International Journal of Nursing Studies* **45**(2): 191–202.

In research on the work of mental health nurses, Gass (2008) observed and interviewed participants who used electroconvulsive therapy. He initially used purposive and then theoretical sampling based on previous findings and following up concepts that emerged. For instance, he found that *Selling ECT* became an important concept in his research and followed this up by examining nurses' roles. Ideas about nurses' interactions and relations with patients were pursued by theoretical sampling in the late stages of the research. He recruited and added new participants depending on the developing concepts.

becomes aware of important concepts or issues that arise from the data. Paying attention to detail and immersion in the data are essential in becoming sensitive. Not only do personal and professional experiences guide researchers, but reading the relevant literature throughout the process of research is also a useful tool in recognising important concepts. There are, however, dangers inherent in having theoretical sensitivity as it might mean reliance on prior assumptions or research developed by others. Hence the grounded theorist needs to take care not to be directed to certain issues.

In summary, sensitivity derives from personal and professional experience; it needs a continuous dialogue with the data and knowledge of the relevant literature.

DATA ANALYSIS

Data analysis in grounded theory is iterative and interactive. Iteration means that researchers go backwards and forwards during the course of the research, returning to previous data and the issues contained in them. Constant comparison and theoretical sampling go on throughout the research and decisions are not made once and for all but are provisional.

Data analysis includes the following procedures:

- constant comparison
- coding the data
- reducing the codes and developing categories

- linking the categories and finding patterns
- discovering the core category
- discovering or building the theory.

Constant comparison

Grounded theory is characterised by the *constant comparative method*. Constant comparison means that researchers take a series of iterative steps in which they compare incidents in, and sections of, the data. Glaser and Strauss (1967) explain that researchers not only compare qualitative data from interviews, documents and observations, but also related information found in the literature. Differences and similarities across incidents in the data are explored. Ideas that develop within a category are compared with those that previously emerged in the same category. Through comparison, properties and dimensions (characteristics) of categories can be produced and patterns established which enhance the explanatory power of these categories and help in the development of theory.

Computer software may be used to assist in data analysis. Qualitative software packages, for example NVivo or Atlas/ti, are intended for in-depth inductive analysis and allow for theory-building models and diagrams. There are limitations to the use of computers, particularly for novice researchers. Where researchers are deeply involved with the participants and need sensitivity, computer analysis might have a distancing effect (Charmaz 2000).

Coding and categorising

Initially the data will be coded line by line or sentence by sentence. Coding is the process by which the researcher identifies and names concepts. The first step is *open coding*. This involves breaking down and conceptualising the data and starts as soon as the researcher has collected the first group of data. It includes *in-vivo* coding, when the researcher examines phrases that the participants themselves have used. For instance, a patient might say 'nurses treat you with kindness'. 'The kindness of nurses' is then an *in-vivo* code. Box 13.1 provides an example of open coding.

The researcher generates a great number of open codes in the first stage of analysis and then has to collapse or reduce them. This process is called categorising. Categories tend to be more abstract than initial codes and group open codes together. Box 13.2 provides an example of a category developed from three open codes.

Categories are provisional in that new ideas can be integrated. Also their characteristics (properties and dimensions) should be uncovered, as well as the conditions under which they occur and the consequences that they have. For instance, the analysts might explore the specific conditions and consequences around the category *Being in Control*. What are the conditions that determine whether patients see themselves as 'in control'? What are the consequences of 'being in control'? Strauss and Corbin (1998: 224) give the properties and dimensions of *the pain experience* as an example; properties refer to intensity, location and duration.

Relating categories and linking them with their characteristics and 'subcategories' is important for the emerging theory. Relationships and links are connected with the 'when, where, why, how and with what consequences an event occurs' (Strauss & Corbin 1998: 22). Strauss and Corbin call this type of categorising *axial coding*. Research Example 13.2 provides an illustration of axial coding.

The next stage involves the search for patterns. At this stage data are combined. The constructs developed are major categories formulated by the researchers and rooted in their nursing or academic knowledge.

Box 13.1 Open coding

Lines	Codes
1 I was frightened when I had my first test	1 Fear of the unknown
2 I felt I was thrown in at the deep end but ...	2 Thrown in at the deep end
3 The nurse told me I was OK	3 Feeling reassured

Box 13.2 Category development

Initial code	Category
Being lonely Lack of attention Missing visits	Feeling abandoned

RESEARCH EXAMPLE

13.2   Axial Coding

Fenwick J, Barclay L, Schmied V (2008) Craving closeness: a grounded theory analysis of women's experiences of mothering in the special care nursery. *Women and Birth* **21**(2): 71–85.

Fenwick *et al.* (2008) demonstrated axial coding in their Australian grounded theory study which aimed to expand the knowledge of health professionals about first time motherhood. The research was carried out in the neonatal nursery and showed that the quality of interaction between mothers and nurses is crucial in the process of learning to be a mother. While level one of the data analysis consisted of open coding by identifying ideas, grouping and labelling them, in the second level of analysis researchers developed relationships between categories, found relationships between them and attempted connecting them in new ways, thereby carrying out axial coding.

These constructs contain emerging theoretical ideas and through developing them, researchers reassemble the data. There is no reason why researchers cannot occasionally use the categories that others have discovered. Constant comparison of new data, incidents, codes and categories is needed throughout, but especially at this stage.

The last phase of the analysis is *selective coding*. Selective coding involves integrating and refining the categories, and identifying the story line. This means that the theory is starting to emerge; the categories are grouped around a central or core concept – or occasionally concepts – which have explanatory power.

Developing the core category

Through finding relationships between categories, the researcher discovers the core category from the data. Glaser (1978) and Strauss (1987) identify the characteristics for the core category.

- It is a central phenomenon in the research and should be linked to all other categories so that a pattern is established.
- It should occur frequently in the data.
- It emerges naturally without being forced out by the researcher.
- It should explain variations in the data.

- It is discovered towards the end of the analysis.

The core category is the basic social-psychological process involved in the research that occurs over time and explains changes in the participant's behaviour, feelings and thoughts. Research Example 13.3 provides an example of a core category.

Theoretical saturation

Saturation is a particular point in category development. It occurs when no new relevant concepts can be found that are important for the development of the emerging theory. Sampling goes on until categories, their properties and dimensions, as well as the links between the categories are well established. The theory will not be wholly adequate unless saturation has been established. When time is limited, researchers may not have sufficient data to reach saturation or may stop without fully analysing the data; this is known as premature closure (Glaser 1978).

New researchers do not always understand what saturation means. Sometimes it is thought that saturation has taken place when a concept is mentioned frequently and is described in similar ways by a number of people, when the same ideas arise over and over again or when the main concepts have been examined in depth. It is difficult, however, to decide

RESEARCH EXAMPLE

13.3   Core Category

Larsson IE, Sjöström B, Plos KLE (2007) Patient participation in nursing care from a patient perspective: a grounded theory study. *Scandinavian Journal of Caring Sciences* **21**(3): 313–320.

Larsson *et al.* (2007) studied the factors that affect patients' participation in their own care. The aim of the study was to explore the meaning of participation in nursing care from the patient perspective through in-depth interviews. The research demonstrated that insight, based on patients' own experiences, contributes to participation in nursing care. The core category in this grounded theory emerged from four main categories and subthemes: *obliging atmosphere*, *emotional response*, *concordance* and *rights*; the researchers called it *insight through consideration*.

when saturation has occurred. It happens at a different stage in each project and cannot be predicted at the outset.

THE THEORY

Categories in grounded theory are more abstract than initial codes and assist in building theory. A theory must have 'grab' and 'fit'; it should be recognised by other people working in the field and grounded in the data. Strauss and Corbin (1998) demand that:

- theory shows systematic relationships between concepts and links between categories
- variation should be built into the theory, that is it should hold true under a number of conditions and circumstances
- the theory should demonstrate a social and/or psychological process
- the theoretical findings should be significant and remain important over time.

Glaser and Strauss distinguish between two types of theory, substantive and formal. While substantive theory is derived from the study of a specific context, formal theory is more abstract and conceptual. For instance, a specific theory of negotiating between patients and nurses about pain relief would be substantive theory. A theory about the concept of negotiation in general that can be applied to many different settings and situations becomes formal theory. Most researchers, particularly novices, produce substantive theories that are specific and can be applied to the situation under study or similar settings.

Strauss and Corbin consider the applicability of theoretical ideas to other settings and situations. For instance the concept of 'transition' or 'status passage' may be applied to a variety of situations, such as 'becoming a mother' or 'seeking a diagnosis'. Indeed, a theory and theoretical ideas can be re-contextualised in a number of situations and verified in a variety of settings.

WRITING MEMOS

In the early stages of a study important ideas may emerge, and as the work progresses the researcher becomes increasingly aware of theoretical perspectives. These thoughts need to be recorded in a field diary and memos. Memos are, according to Corbin and Strauss (2008: 117), 'written records of analysis'. They might be physical descriptions of the setting or theoretical ideas. The researcher should date them, as well as supply detail.

Memos are meant to help in the development and formation of theory. Initially they are simple, but become progressively more theoretical. In theoretical memos, researchers develop ideas and occasionally working propositions, compare findings and record their thoughts. Strauss (1987) provides examples of different types of memo that might be written. Diagrams may be used in memos to help the researcher capture ideas. They can guide the researcher to base abstract ideas in the reality of the data (Holloway & Wheeler 2010).

THE USE OF LITERATURE IN GROUNDED THEORY

Grounded theory research is generally carried out where little is known about the phenomenon to be studied. Researchers need to identify a gap in knowledge that their research questions will address. They should read around the topic, as this can generate questions and some initial concepts. However, if researchers are steeped in the literature from the very beginning, they might be directed to certain issues and constrained by their expectations developed from previous reading, rather than developing their own ideas. Corbin and Strauss (2008) repeat their earlier warning and state that researchers might become rigid and stifled through reading too much. Indeed, a full search of the literature would not be appropriate for grounded theory. Of course, there is a need to review the literature on the research topic, but researchers should enter the arena without major preconceptions.

Nurse researchers generally start their research with certain assumptions, as they often have some knowledge of the field they wish to explore. Moreover, their professional experience and reading of the literature can enhance their research as it generates theoretical sensitivity to concepts and issues that are important for the developing theory. Researchers do need to be explicit, however, and uncover their own preconceptions.

As a grounded theory study progresses, categories and theoretical concepts are developed. The literature relating to these concepts is reviewed and a dialogue takes place between the literature and the researcher's emerging ideas. The researcher's data have priority over those of other studies in the same topic area. Concepts arising from the research can be compared with those emerging from other studies. In this sense,

the literature can become a potential source of data. As categories are identified, researchers trawl the literature for confirmation or refutation of these categories. Grounded theorists examine what other researchers have found and whether there are any links to existing theories. In the dialogue with the literature, researchers should explore why other studies come up with similar or different findings, and the reasons for any discrepancies. This interaction with the literature, and the debate about it, is integrated into the discussion section of the research report.

THE CHOICE BETWEEN GLASERIAN AND STRAUSSIAN GROUNDED THEORY

Glaser and Strauss started together on the path of developing grounded theory but subsequently diverged from each other. Glaser (1992) criticised Strauss and Corbin (1990), accusing them of distorting the procedures and meaning of the grounded theory approach. A full discussion of the differences between the two perspectives can be found in MacDonald (2001). Glaser and Strauss (and Corbin) differ mainly on the following points.

The research topic

Glaser suggests that researchers approach the topic without preconceptions and have a research interest rather than a research problem. While Strauss and Corbin advise researchers to identify a phenomenon to be studied at the beginning of the study, Glaser claims that this would arise naturally during the process of the research. This has implications for the initial literature review, which would be somewhat more detailed for Strauss and Corbin, while Glaser believes that it might 'contaminate' the participants' data, although he too suggests that the literature should be integrated into the developing concepts. Annells (1997) suggests that Strauss and Corbin see theory as a construct 'co-created by the researcher and the participants', while Glaser sees it as emerging from the data.

Coding and categorising

Coding is mentioned by both Glaser and Strauss but seems to have slightly different meanings. Although Glaser does not like the term axial coding, his 'theoretical coding' seems very similar to axial coding.

Verification

One of the main factors that distinguish the ideas of Glaser and Strauss is the issue of verification. Strauss and Corbin suggest that working propositions are examined and provisionally tested against new data (as, indeed, the original text by Glaser and Strauss had suggested). Glaser believes that these hypotheses should not be verified or validated at this stage by the researcher, and new data should be integrated into the emerging theory.

The process of generating theory

While Strauss and Corbin advocate the building of theory through axial coding, Glaser suggests that the theory will eventually emerge naturally, as long as the researcher continuously engages with the data, and they are analysed adequately and in depth. There are also differences of opinion regarding the generalisability of grounded theory. Strauss and Corbin consider that grounded theory is generalisable, whereas Glaser considers this not to be the case.

Which approach?

Both approaches are viable forms of grounded theory research so researchers have to decide for themselves which one to adopt. The more prescriptive and formulaic approach of Strauss and Corbin (1990, 1998) may be easier for novices, while experienced researchers might find the Glaserian perspective (which he calls 'classic grounded theory') more appropriate and flexible. Researchers can modify the approach to fit their own purposes; Charmaz (2008) advises, however, that they should be thoroughly familiar with the original approach to justify their modification and deviation from it. She stresses that Anselm Strauss was a pragmatist and that grounded theorists should stay pragmatic and not become rigid in their approach.

PROBLEMS AND STRENGTHS OF GROUNDED THEORY

Grounded theory has been criticised for its neglect of social structure and culture, and the influence of these on human action and interaction. Indeed, Glaser and Strauss (1967) advise researchers not to research topics linked to structure and culture. Symbolic interactionism as the basis of grounded theory is also more concerned with interaction, action and meaning rather than macro-issues such as societal factors.

Layder (1982), in particular, criticised the lack of emphasis on such concepts as power, gender and ethnicity. MacDonald (2001) also develops these points in a critique of grounded theory and symbolic interactionism.

Researchers who use other qualitative approaches also stress process and human agency rather than society and structure. One might argue, however, that there is no rule stating that these approaches cannot be used in the discussion of macro-issues. After all, processes change. Layder wrote more than two decades ago, and early writings by Strauss and Glaser have been superseded by later texts. A large number of grounded theory studies have been carried out, some of which do centre on macro-issues such as gender and power, in particular work by feminists. Others, focusing on policy or health education and promotion cannot help but consider structural, cultural and societal factors.

Nevertheless, it should be stressed that most qualitative approaches, including grounded theory, are used for the exploration of micro- rather than macro-issues. They are designed to focus on the meanings people give to their experience and behaviour.

Some problems with grounded theory are not connected with style or procedures but with the inexperience of researchers. Many novice researchers end up with a conceptual description rather than a theory. There is nothing wrong with dense, conceptual (sometimes called 'analytic') description, but this alone cannot be called grounded theory.

CONCLUSIONS

Grounded theory is a systematic and processual approach to collecting and analysing data. Good grounded theory produces a theory that has explanatory power, or modification of a theory that already exists. Such theory generation is unique within qualitative research.

There are some major elements that are always present in this type of research.

- Data collection and analysis are in constant dialogue and interaction with each other.
- Constant comparison of data occurs throughout the research process.
- The researcher uses theoretical sampling by following up concepts.
- The data are analysed through coding and categorising.
- The researcher discovers the core category through links between other categories.
- The theory or the theoretical ideas that are generated should always have their basis in the data themselves.

References

Annells M (1997) Grounded theory method, part 2: options for users of the method. *Nursing Inquiry* **4**: 176–180.

Benoliel JQ (1973) *The Nurse and the Dying Patient*. New York, Macmillan.

Charmaz K (2000) Grounded theory: objectivist and constructivist methods. In: Denzin NK & Lincoln YS (eds) *Handbook of Qualitative Research*, 2nd edition. Thousand Oaks, Sage, pp 509–536.

Charmaz K (2006) *Constructing Grounded Theory: a practical guide through qualitative analysis*. London, Sage.

Charmaz K (2008) Advancing qualitative research through grounded theory. Paper presented at the 7th Qualitative Research Conference, Bournemouth University, September.

Chenitz WC, Swanson JM (eds) (1986) *From Practice to Grounded Theory: qualitative research in nursing*. Menlo Park, Addison-Wesley.

Corbin J, Strauss A (2008) *Basics of Qualitative Research: techniques and procedures for developing grounded theory*, 3rd edition. Los Angeles, Sage.

Draucker CB, Martsolf DS, Ross R, Thomas TB (2007) Theoretical sampling and category development in grounded theory. *Qualitative Health Research* **17**(8): 1137–1148.

Fenwick J, Barclay L, Schmied V (2008) Craving closeness: a grounded theory analysis of women's experiences of mothering in the special care nursery. *Women and Birth* **21**(2): 71–85.

Gass J (2008) Electroconvulsive therapy and the work of mental health nurses: a grounded theory study. *International Journal of Nursing Studies* **45**(2): 191–202.

Glaser BG (1978) *Theoretical Sensitivity*. Mill Valley, Sociology Press.

Glaser BG (1992) *Basics of Grounded Theory Analysis*. Mill Valley, Sociology Press.

Glaser BG, Strauss AL (1967) *The Discovery of Grounded Theory*. Chicago, Aldine.

Holloway I (2008) *A–Z of Qualitative Research in Healthcare*. Oxford, Blackwell.

Holloway I, Wheeler S (2010) *Qualitative Research in Nursing*, 3rd edition. Oxford, Wiley-Blackwell.

Larsson IE, Sjöström B, Plos KLE (2007) Patient participation in nursing care from a patient perspective: a grounded theory study. *Scandinavian Journal of Caring Sciences* **21**(3): 313–320.

Layder D (1982) Grounded theory: a constructive critique. *Journal for the Theory of Social Behaviour* **12**: 102–123.

MacDonald M (2001) Finding a critical perspective in grounded theory. In: Schreiber RS, Stern PN (eds) *Using Grounded Theory in Nursing*. New York, Springer Publishing, pp 113–136.

Mead GH (1934) *Mind, Self and Society*. Chicago, University of Chicago Press.

Morse JM (2001) Situating grounded theory within qualitative inquiry. In: Schreiber RS, Stern PN (eds) *Using Grounded Theory in Nursing*. New York, Springer, pp 1–15.

Schreiber RS, Stern PN (2001) The 'how to' of grounded theory: avoiding the pitfalls. In: Schreiber RS, Stern PN (eds) *Using Grounded Theory in Nursing*. New York, Springer, pp 55–83.

Strauss AL (1987) *Qualitative Analysis for Social Scientists*. New York, Cambridge University Press.

Strauss AL, Corbin J (1990) *Basics of Qualitative Research: grounded theory procedures and techniques*. Newbury Park, Sage.

Strauss AL, Corbin J (eds) (1997) *Grounded Theory in Practice*. Thousand Oaks, Sage.

Strauss AL, Corbin J (1998) *Basics of Qualitative Research: techniques and procedures for developing grounded theory*, 2nd edition. Thousand Oaks, Sage.

Suddaby R (2006) From the editors: What grounded theory is not. *Academy of Management Journal* **49**(4): 633–642.

Thomas WI (1928) *The Child in America*. New York, Alfred Knopf.

Further reading

Bryant A, Charmaz C (eds) (2007) *The Sage Handbook of Grounded Theory*. London, Sage.

Cutcliffe JR (2000) Methodological issues in grounded theory. *Journal of Advanced Nursing* **31**: 1476–1484.

Glaser BG (2001) *The Grounded Theory Perspective: conceptualization contrasted with description*. Mill Valley, Sociology Press.

Morse JM, Stern PN, Corbin J, Charmaz KC, Bowers B, Clarke A (eds) (2009) *Developing Grounded Theory: the second generation*. Walnut Creek, Left Coast Press.

Website

www.groundedtheory.com – Grounded Theory Institute is dedicated to helping people learn about Glaserian Grounded Theory (also known as Classic, or Orthodox Grounded Theory).

14 Ethnography

Immy Holloway and Les Todres

Key points

- Ethnography is concerned with the study of a culture or subculture – in nursing, for instance, the study of specific groups or settings. Large-scale (macro) ethnographies examine a culture with its institutions, communities and value systems. Micro-ethnographies investigate a single social setting such as a ward or small group of staff.

- Data collection involves immersion in the setting by means of participant observation and interviews with key informants.

- The researcher seeks to uncover the *emic* or 'insider view' of the members of the particular culture being studied.

- 'Thick' description is used to provide a detailed account that makes explicit the patterns of cultural and social relationships and puts them into context.

INTRODUCTION

Ethnography is distinct from other qualitative research approaches in that it focuses on culture or social group. It can be seen as a process that includes the methods of research – and a product, which is the written story as the outcome of the research. Researchers 'do' ethnography; they study a culture by observing cultural members' behaviours and ask questions about their actions, interactions, experience and feelings. They also write 'an ethnography', a narrative account in which they give a portrayal of the culture they study. Ethnography is both 'doing science' and 'telling stories'.

Serrant-Green (2007) claims that 'ethnography' is not a single research method but consists of many activities; it encompasses many viewpoints. It is

sometimes used synonymously with 'qualitative research', but in this chapter we adopt the original meaning of the term: an approach within anthropological/sociological traditions that can also be applied to our own society.

The term 'ethnography' means 'writing culture' or 'writing people', and comes from the Greek. The major traits of ethnography include the researcher's first-hand experience of the 'natural setting' that the informants inhabit, the culture or community that is being studied. Ethnographers can utilise both qualitative and quantitative procedures. In this chapter the qualitative approach will be discussed, as this is most often used in nursing. Ethnography is probably the oldest of the research approaches, as even in ancient times travellers to a country other than their own studied and described foreign cultures and wrote about their experiences. It was particularly popular in the 19th and 20th twentieth centuries, when the approach became more systematic in the writing of anthropologists such as Malinowski (1922) and Boas (1928). They gave detailed descriptions of the cultures in which they immersed themselves for many years. Initially anthropologists explored only foreign cultures, often adopting a colonialist and ethnocentric stance. Today, anthropologists are less ethnocentric, that is, they are less inclined to view other groups from their own (Western) perspective.

From 1917 to the early 1940s the Chicago School of Sociology influenced later ethnographic methods because its members examined marginal cultures such as ghettos, urban gangs and slums of the city. Researchers subsequently explored their own cultures, researching that with which they were already familiar. These studies were carried out by members of many disciplines apart from anthropology, for example by sociologists, educationists and nurses. Janice Morse, the best-known nurse anthropologist and author of qualitative research texts, has discussed this approach in nursing for several decades (see the history of ethnographic research in Gobo 2008).

Like most other qualitative approaches, ethnographic research is inductive, at least initially. This means that it proceeds from the specific to the general, and that initially no preconceptions or hypotheses guide the researcher towards the outcomes of the inquiry. In ethnography, as in other forms of qualitative inquiry, the researcher is the main research tool.

Ethnography is distinct from other qualitative approaches in that it generates descriptions of a group in its cultural context, and focuses mainly, though not exclusively, on the routine activities and customs in the culture, as well as on the location of the people within it.

THE CHARACTERISTICS OF ETHNOGRAPHY

Roper and Shapira (2000) state that:

'ethnography is a research process of learning *about* people by learning *from* them' (their italics) (Roper & Shapira 2000: 1)

The main features of ethnography are:

- immersion in a setting and a focus on culture
- the emic (insider's) dimension from the participants, in particular key informants
- 'thick', dense or analytic description.

The focus on culture

Fetterman (1998) suggests that the interpretation of a culture (or subculture) is the main aim of ethnography. Culture can be defined as the way of life of a group, the learnt patterns of behaviour that are socially constructed and transmitted. This includes a shared communication system in language, gestures and expressions – the messages that most cultural members understand and recognise. Individuals in a culture often share values and ideas acquired through learning from other members of the group. Researchers need to be aware, however, that a culture is not necessarily homogeneous, and that the value system of people within it is influenced by their social location.

Learning group values and behaviour is referred to as socialisation. For instance, members of the nursing profession have been socialised into the values and perspectives of their own group through their education and training. The perspectives of the group, the actions and interactions of group members, and the meaning they place on their own and others' behaviour, are legitimate areas of research for the ethnographer. Adopting an ethnographic approach to a familiar culture helps researchers to avoid assumptions about their own cultural group or take its working for granted.

Knowledge that the members of a culture share but do not articulate to each other is referred to as 'tacit knowledge'. Social behaviour and interpretations of the social world are based on this. Ethnographers uncover tacit knowledge and make it explicit. They also reveal some of the hidden meanings in the routines and rituals of a group and place.

Ethnographers have recently changed their perspective from a monolithic understanding of culture where all individuals share values, beliefs and perceptions, to a focus on cultural diversity (Holloway & Todres 2003). They demonstrate how cultural members are located within their setting and how they can only be understood within the specific context. For instance, although nurses and doctors in an orthopaedic department might have certain perceptions in common (particularly about their patients), there are other elements where their beliefs and ways of working are in conflict with each other.

Important research questions are linked to culture or subculture within a healthcare setting. For example, a researcher might observe the subculture of nursing students, the culture of a nursing home or a children's hospital.

Emic and etic perspectives

The term *emic* perspective is often used in ethnographic research. Although the concept has a variety of interpretations, in its simplest form it means 'insider view'. The emic perspective is the perception of those who are members of a particular culture or group, or, in anthropological terms, the 'native' point of view. The linguist Pike coined this phrase, but it was used more extensively and with a different meaning by the anthropologist Harris (1976) and most ethnographers since. Members of a culture have special knowledge of this culture and can share this with the researcher. For instance, nurses in the A&E department know about the special problems facing members of the department, but they would also be able to narrate the dramatic events that might make this type of work exciting.

Insiders give meaning to their experiences and generate knowledge about the reasons for their actions. They know the rules and rituals of their group or subculture. The emic perspective is thus culture-specific. Outside observers would find it difficult to gain the same familiarity and intimacy with this setting as insiders do.

In contrast, ethnographers also speak of the *etic* perspective, which is the view of the outsider who may or may not be a member of the culture being studied. As an example, an A&E nurse might wish to research the culture of A&E departments. In this sense they are a 'native' of the group. Nurses are also researchers, however, and in this particular sense they are outsiders and they need to produce scientific knowledge about

what they see and hear, which means taking an etic view. Thus the emic perspective is the subjective view of insiders that has to be retold by the researchers in the account of the research. Indeed the A&E nurse researchers in the earlier example have to attempt to become 'naive' observers or interviewers, taking the view of a 'cultural stranger' to the setting. The etic perspective is needed to transform the story into an ethnography with its roots in social science. Harris (1976) explains that etics are scientific transformations of the empirical data by the researchers who adopt an approach to the data that is more theoretical and abstract than that of the insiders.

Thick description

The concept of thick description has its origin in the work of the philosopher Ryle and was taken on by the anthropologist Geertz (1973), who applied it to ethnography. He suggests that it is a detailed account that makes explicit the patterns of cultural and social relationships and puts them in context. It is a result of observations and interviews in the field. The notion of thick description is sometimes understood as a detailed description of a culture or group, but this does not suffice. It must be theoretical and analytical, in that researchers concern themselves with general patterns and traits of social life, and it gives the reader of the ethnographic text a sense of the emotional experience of the participants in the study. Thick description builds up a clear picture of the individuals and groups in the context of their culture, and encompasses their meanings and intentions. On the other hand, thin description is superficial and factual and does not explore the underlying meanings of cultural members (Denzin 1989). It does not lead to a good ethnography.

THE USE OF ETHNOGRAPHY IN NURSING

Many cultures and subcultures exist within nursing. One might think, for instance, of the culture of a hospital or the subculture of an orthopaedic ward. Ethnographic research is therefore helpful in:

- studying cultures linked to nursing with their rules and rituals and routine activities – this includes transcultural research, which examines different ethnic groups, their interactions and meaning creation
- discovering the 'insider view' of patients and colleagues
- explaining phenomena related to nursing
- examining the conflicting perspectives of professionals within the organisational culture.

Nurse researchers contextualise the perspectives, actions and emotions of their patients or colleagues and those of other health professionals through ethnographic methods. They become culture-sensitive and learn to identify the influences of the environment on the person. The aim of nurse researchers, however, is different from that of other anthropologists. They do not merely generate knowledge, which is seen as the goal of ethnography (Hammersley & Atkinson 2007), but they also wish to change and improve professional practice through understanding the culture they study.

Leininger (1985) has coined the term 'ethnonursing' to refer to the use of ethnography in nursing. She describes this as an adaptation and extension of ethnography. Ethnonursing, she suggests, is concerned with studying groups and settings linked to nursing, but is also specifically about nursing care, produces nursing knowledge and explains or demonstrates nursing phenomena.

Nurse ethnographers do not always investigate their own cultural members. In Britain, nurses care for patients from a variety of ethnic groups and need to be knowledgeable about different cultures. Indeed, all nurses and patients belong to ethnic groups, and sometimes they come from different countries and have a variety of religions. Awareness of cultural differences is important because both nurses and patients are products of their group. DeSantis (1994) suggested that at least three cultures are involved in nurses' interactions with patients: the nurses' professional culture, the patients' culture and the context in which the interactions take place.

Nurse researchers usually proceed in the following way.

- They describe a problem in the group under study and, through this, they come to understand the causes of the problem and may be able to prevent it.
- They help patients to identify and report their needs.
- They give information to the readers of their accounts – their colleagues and other health professionals – to effect change in clinical and professional practice.

When undertaking research with colleagues or students, nurse researchers proceed through similar phases. The ultimate goal of their research is to improve professional practice.

Savage (2000) draws certain parallels between ethnography (in particular participant observation) and clinical practice:

- the physical involvement with the setting is common to nursing and research
- the claims nurses and researchers make about knowledge through experience
- the assumptions they share as nurses and observers.

Savage suggests that nurses and ethnographers should be concerned with the links between their own experience of the setting and that of their patients. Nurses and researchers also attempt to translate the understanding they gain of patients to others.

DESCRIPTIVE AND CRITICAL ETHNOGRAPHY

There are two main approaches to ethnography: descriptive and critical ethnography. Thomas (1993) states the difference:

'Conventional ethnographers study culture for the purpose of describing it; critical ethnographers do so to change it' (Thomas 1993: 4)

It should be noted, however, that most of the nursing research carried out has implications for practice. While descriptive ethnography centres on the description of cultures or groups (see Research Example 14.1), critical ethnography involves the

14.1 Descriptive Ethnography

Hunter CL, Spence K, McKenna K, Iedema R (2008) Learning how to learn: an ethnographic study in a neonatal intensive care unit. *Journal of Advanced Nursing* **62**(6): 657–664.

This example is an Australian study that included observation and interviews in a neonatal intensive care unit. The observational element was particularly important in the research. Hunter *et al.* (2008) investigated how nurses, especially new staff, learn from each other in the clinical setting. The research centred on the interaction of the professionals with each other. It was found that, apart from formal learning, incidental and informal learning also takes place. The analysis of workplace learning points to the way in which professionals learn and from whom, as well as where they gain professional knowledge. It was also shown that an allocation of time is important for multiple types of learning to take place.

14.2 Critical Ethnography

Caldwell PH, Arthur HM (2008) The influence of a culture of referral of access to nursing care in rural settings after myocardial infarction. *Health and Place* **14**(1): 180–185.

In a critical ethnography, Caldwell and Arthur (2008) explored the referral system for women with myocardial infarction and found that this had an 'urban-centric' focus to the provision of care for these women. The authors based their work on the ideas of Thomas (1993), who discusses this approach in terms of power relationships and social change. It was demonstrated how sociocultural factors and the medical hierarchy influence access to care. The implications of the study were that support systems and the way patients were referred needed to change.

study of macro-social factors such as power and control, and examines commonsense assumptions and hidden agendas in this arena (Holloway & Wheeler 2010); it therefore has political elements or focuses on power relationships (see Research Example 14.2).

Nurse researchers often use critical ethnography because women form the majority of these professions and power relations are part of the complex factors influencing interaction between nurses and doctors or nurses and patients. Penney and Wellard (2007) speak of the need to change practice, which is one of the aims of critical ethnography. (See also Hardcastle *et al.* 2006 on Carspecken's critical ethnography.)

While ethnographers undertaking descriptive and critical ethnographies use the same data collection and analysis procedures, those undertaking critical ethnographies aim to highlight the power dimensions of interaction and are often more reflexive of their own involvement in the research.

SELECTION OF SAMPLE AND SETTING

Ethnographers use purposive or criterion-based sampling, i.e. they adopt specific criteria to select their informants and setting, such as patients undergoing orthopaedic surgery, children with diabetes, nursing students or a maternity unit. The criteria for sample selection must be explicit and systematic (Hammersley & Atkinson 2007) to ensure that participants are representative of the group under study. The participants in ethnographic research are usually called informants, because they inform the researcher about issues in their world. Alternative terms include participant, cultural member or key actor. Key informants are those participants whose knowledge of the setting is intimate and long-standing. Patients are often the main informants in nursing ethnography. They tell of their experience and the meanings they attach to it, and of the expectations and health beliefs that form part of their perspective (DeSantis 1994). Informants might be interviewed formally or participate by talking informally about the cultural beliefs and practices as well as ways of communicating. They become active collaborators in the research rather than passive respondents (hence the term 'informant'). Nurses can compare their own interpretations of the group with those of key informants through the process of member-checking, whereby they ask informants to check the script and interpretation (Lincoln & Guba 1985).

DATA COLLECTION

Ethnographers have three major strategies for collecting data (Roper & Shapira 2000):

- they observe what is going on in the setting while participating in it
- they ask informants from the cultural group they are studying about their behaviour, experiences and feelings
- they study documents about and in the setting, in order to familiarise themselves with it.

Observation takes place through engagement and immersion in the setting, interviews are the accounts of the insider experience and documents are added sources for studying the culture. Indeed, often researchers supplement interviews and observation by taping oral histories from the cultural members whose world they study, or they examine photographs or pictures of the group and the setting.

Observing

Participant observation, the type of observation most commonly used, means that the researchers are immersed in the setting and become familiar with it. Prolonged observation produces more in-depth

knowledge of a culture. Occasionally, researchers need to withdraw from the setting, to stand back and take stock. They also need to try to put aside their assumptions, come to the setting as 'cultural strangers' and keep an open mind in seeking the emic perspective, the view of the inhabitant of the world they study. Ethnographers observe the setting and situation, the way people act and interact, the use of space and time, but they also observe critical incidents that may occur and the way rules are followed and rituals are carried out.

Spradley (1980: 78), a well-known ethnographer, identifies the dimensions of the social settings that ethnographers study. These include the following.

Space	location of the research
Actor	the people who take part in the setting
Activity	the actions of people
Object	things located in the setting
Act	single actions of participants
Events	what is happening in the setting
Time	sequencing of activities and time frame
Goals	what people aim to do
Feeling	emotions that participants have

The observation setting can be open or closed. Open settings can be highly visible public spaces such as a reception area or a corridor, whereas closed settings have to be more carefully negotiated and could be hospital wards or meeting rooms. In nursing settings, observation is normally overt, where the researcher makes explicit their intention to observe the social setting. Covert observation, where participants do not know that they are being observed, is usually seen as unethical. Indeed, participant observation is a challenge to the researcher, as ethical issues might become problematic in this type of open setting where the participants' behaviour can be observed throughout. There is a fine line between disclosure for the purpose of the researcher's agenda and confidentiality or anonymity of the participants.

Observations are initially unstructured, although they become progressively more focused as important features emerge that might be of significance for the study. Observations inform the researcher's interviews with key informants. Incidents or issues that are puzzling or problematic are explored with participants.

The ethnographic interview

During and following observations researchers ask questions about the meaning of behaviour, language and events. This happens initially through informal conversations with participants. There are several consequences of these conversations: researchers familiarise themselves with the arena, bond with participants and acquire cultural knowledge from the informants.

In-depth interviews are commonly used to allow informants the opportunity to explore issues within the culture that they see as important. Although the researcher has an agenda, participants have control within certain boundaries. The researchers follow up the issues and ideas that the informant sees as significant, without neglecting their own research agenda. The interviews may be formal or informal, in-depth, unstructured or semi-structured (see Chapter 28).

Spradley (1979) distinguishes between grand-tour and mini-tour questions. While the former questions are broad, the latter are more specific. An example of a grand-tour question might be: 'Can you describe your life as an orthopaedic nurse?' A mini-tour question might be: 'Tell me about the pain you had after your operation.' Researchers often start an interview with a broad question and the interview becomes more focused, following up participants' answers (see Box 14.1).

These questions are then followed up, depending on the participants' answers. If something important emerges, gentle prompts can be used, such as 'Can you tell me more about that, please?'

Ethnographers also listen to naturally occurring talk in the setting, for example people communicating with each other on the ward, in meetings, or in the classroom. These conversations may be analysed in the same way as interviews. To make sure that data are not lost, interviewers generally record participants' words, whereas detailed fieldnotes are made of conversations.

Box 14.1 Examples of general and focused questions for ethnographic interviews

General questions

- Tell me about your experience of your (condition)?

Focused questions (following the participants ideas)

- What were your visits to the hospital like?
- What was the reaction of your family to this?

General questions

- Can you describe your stay in hospital?

Focused questions

- Tell me about the care of the nurses?
- You said that the nurses always have time for patients, please can you elaborate?

FIELDWORK AND FIELDNOTES

The field, fieldwork and fieldnotes are well-known concepts used in ethnography. The field is the location in which the research is taking place and in which the researcher has a presence (Gobo 2008). It may be a ward, a hospital or a specific community of people. The term fieldwork refers to the work undertaken in an ethnographic study such as collecting data from various sources. Fieldwork also includes the description and interpretation of cultural behaviour, the meaning people give to their actions and the setting in which the study takes place. This is an ongoing process in the research.

Researchers keep a field journal or diary in which they jot down their thoughts about their experiences and make theoretical comments. These fieldnotes or 'ethnographic record' (Gobo 2008) are used at a later stage to help remember important issues, questions or solutions to problems. They have their basis in the observations and interviews undertaken in the setting. Initially, fieldnotes are only for the eyes of the ethnographer, but ultimately excerpts are used as data or extended descriptions in ethnographic writing. At first, fieldnotes tend to be simple but become more complex as the study progresses, and may become notes about analysis and interpretation.

Spradley (1979) identifies different types of fieldnotes in terms of condensed and extended accounts. Condensed accounts are short descriptions made in the field during data collection, while expanded accounts extend the descriptions and fill in detail. Short fieldnotes are extended as soon as possible after a period of observation or interview if it was not possible to record the full detail during the data collection. Ethnographers also note their own biases, reactions and problems during fieldwork. They may use additional ways to record events and behaviour such as audiotapes, video film or photos, flowcharts and diagrams.

MACRO- AND MICRO-ETHNOGRAPHIES

Spradley (1980) identifies macro- and micro-ethnographies, which can be viewed on a continuum of scale. At one end of this continuum are large-scale studies examining a complex society, one or more communities or social institutions (*macro-ethnography*); at the other are small-scale studies into a single social situation (*micro-ethnography*).

A macro-ethnography examines a large culture with its institutions, communities and value systems. In nursing, this might be the wider culture of nursing. Such studies are rarely carried out by a single researcher. Both macro- and micro-ethnographies proceed in similar ways and produce an account of the culture being studied. The type of study depends on the focus of the investigation, the researcher's own interests or the interests of those who fund the research.

Novice nurse researchers often choose a micro-ethnography as it makes fewer demands on their time than macro-ethnography and seems more immediately relevant to the world of the nurse. Micro-ethnography focuses on small settings or groups, such as a single ward or a group of specialist nurses. Research Example 14.3 provides an example of a micro-ethnography.

DATA ANALYSIS AND INTERPRETATION

Analysis involves interaction with the data. The data are scanned and organised from the start of the research, and the focus on particular issues becomes clearer as the research progresses. Analysis and interpretation proceed in parallel. The analytic process is not linear but iterative; this means that researchers go back and forth, from the data collection and reading and thinking about them, to the analysis. They then return to collecting new data and analysing them. This process continues until the collection and analysis are complete.

The main steps in data analysis include:

- bringing order to the data and organising the material
- reading, re-reading and thinking about the data
- coding the data
- summarising and reducing the codes to larger categories

14.3 A Micro-ethnography

Happ MB, Swigart VA, Tate JA *et al.* (2007) Patient involvement in health-related decisions during prolonged critical illness. *Research in Nursing and Health* **30**: 361–372.

The authors Happ *et al.* (2007) collected data during prolonged mechanical ventilation through observation of the situation and interviews – that is, patterns of communication. Patients participated in decision making about their care and other critical issues, such as artificial feeding and financial and legal issues. This study was restricted to a particular setting, a detailed view of a small unit, namely a 20-bed ICU and an adjacent unit with eight beds in which decisions were made about life-supporting treatment and daily care. Although patients did not demand to be involved in the decision-making processes, there was consistent involvement and shared decision making in these units through questions and non-verbal and verbal answers of patients.

The study is a micro-ethnography in that it was conducted in only one hospital and two small units. Obviously the results cannot be generalised to other settings, although some of the ideas can be applied.

- searching for patterns and regularities in the data, sorting these and recognising themes
- uncovering variations in the data and revealing those cases that do not fit with the rest of the data, and accounting for them
- engaging with, and integrating, the related literature.

When the audiotapes have been listened to and transcribed, and the observation notes ordered, the transcripts of interviews and observation notes are read several times. The researcher thinks about the data and their meaning. The next step is coding, the process of breaking down the data and giving each important section a descriptive label. For instance, the sentence from an informant: *I really was sick of all the grand words and could not understand anything that was going on*, might be labelled 'feeling frustrated' or 'lack of information', depending on the context. An observation note that reads: *The nurse comforted the critically ill patient*, could be labelled 'being there'. The names given to codes are determined by the individual researcher.

Once coding has been completed, codes with similar meaning or themes linked to the same area of analysis are grouped together into larger and more abstract categories. For instance, the codes: *need for*

independence, wanting to be in control, reluctance to be helped, rejecting care from others might be reduced to the category *the wish for self-determination* or *being empowered*. Thematically similar sets of categories are grouped together, with links and relationships established between them. Broad patterns of thoughts and behaviour emerge at this stage, and major 'constructs' or themes are developed. The ethnographer needs to check that there is a fit between the data and the analytic categories and themes.

While ethnographers sometimes produce theories, they often generate typologies. This means developing a classification system that points to variations in the data. For example, an ethnographer might find two types of nurse in a particular ward, those who take control and make firm decisions, and others who generally ask their colleagues and doctors for advice and rarely make difficult decisions. The ethnographer might call these types *decision makers* and *advice takers*. As in all typologies, these are types at the end of a continuum. At some point on the continuum these types overlap.

Interpretation of the data or 'going beyond the results' (Roper & Shapira 2000) means that researchers uncover the meaning of the patterns and themes that they developed. It allows them to answer the research question and to reveal elements of the cultural phenomena studied. Interpretation starts in early data collection and proceeds throughout, but data are often reinterpreted at a later stage. While interpreting the data, researchers make inferences and discuss the possible meanings of the data. Interpretation, although linked to the analysis, is more speculative, involving theorising and explaining. Interpretation links the findings of the project, derived from the analysis, to previously established theories through comparing other researchers' work with one's own. At this stage, the research literature related to the themes and patterns will be considered. It might confirm or 'disconfirm', that is, challenge the findings of the study. The researcher discusses this in a critical and analytical way. The processes of analysis and interpretation are stages in which a phenomenon is broken down, divided into its elements and 'reassembled in terms of definitions or explanations that make the phenomenon understandable to outsiders' (LeCompte & Schensul 1999: 5). Thus researchers build a holistic portrait of a culture from a number of building blocks.

RELATIONSHIPS AND PROBLEMS IN THE SETTING

Ethnography is an appropriate approach when addressing questions about culture and subcultures or a particular group with common traits. However, problems do exist for nurses who wish to carry out ethnographic research. Ethnography needs prolonged engagement and immersion in the setting under study. Gaining admittance to the group and establishing rapport takes time and commitment. Many nurse researchers who study groups other than their own are unable to undertake participant observation over a long period of time, such as a year or more. Hence some nursing ethnographies are not as fully developed as they might be.

Insider researchers also experience problems. They must attempt to see familiar events with new eyes (DeWalt & DeWalt 2002). Nurses who carry out research in their own setting may be seen as health professionals and not as researchers, and this might prevent their colleagues, who are participants in the

research, from making themselves explicit. They might have preconceptions and make assumptions about the setting under study and miss nuances or fail to observe important details. Patients, too, might see them as carers who know them well and may be reluctant to disclose their thoughts for fear that this might prejudice their treatment. Nurse ethnographers often experience conflict between their role as researcher and their nursing role. This was demonstrated by Cudmore and Sondermeyer (2007), who reported on the difficulties of doing ethnography in one's own setting. On the other hand, it is easier to gain access and develop rapport with the research participants as an insider. Holloway and Wheeler (2010) identify a further problem. Nurses have a background in the natural sciences and learn to approach their clinical practice systematically. This means that they might find it difficult to deal with ambiguity. Social inquiry is always provisional and rarely unambiguous. It is better, however, to admit to uncertainty than to make unwarranted claims about the research. Findings can be re-interpreted at a later stage in the light of reflection or new evidence.

Key informants might have their own preconceptions of the setting and let this guide their own observations or discussions about the culture under study. This means that researchers need to compare the informants' accounts with the observed reality (which is, of course, that of the researcher). There is also the risk that participants might tell only what they think researchers wish to hear. This danger is particularly strong in healthcare, as patients (and also nursing students) often want to please those who care for them or deal with them in a professional relationship. However, immersion in the culture by the researcher, and the prolonged relationship of researcher and informants, helps to overcome this.

THE ETHNOGRAPHIC REPORT

Ethnography is not only 'analytic' description but also interpretation. Ethnographers describe what they observe and hear while studying cultural members in context; they identify the main features of the group and the setting, and uncover relationships between separate and varied data through analysis; they also interpret the findings by asking for meaning and inferring such meaning from the data. It is important that the participants in the study recognise their own social reality and the traits of their culture and group in the final account, and also that the readers of the study grasp the perspective of the participants.

The ethnography – the account of an ethnographic study – usually takes the form of a narrative and includes quotes from the interviews with participants and excerpts from fieldnotes that illustrate the descriptions and explanations. Thick description is one of the features of the report. An ethnography should be a clearly written text that engages its readers.

CONCLUSIONS

Ethnography is the method of choice when the researcher wants to investigate a culture. The complete ethnography paints a detailed, yet holistic, portrait of the culture that has been studied. Ultimately, a nursing ethnography contributes not only to nursing knowledge but also assists in applying that knowledge for the improvement of nursing practice.

Some of the main features of ethnography include the following.

- An ethnography is the description of a culture, a subculture or group.
- The data sources are mainly participant observation by immersion in the setting and interviews with key informants.
- The researcher uncovers the emic view.
- Thick description is used to make the study come alive and to give both an empirical and a theoretical perspective.

References

Boas F (1928) *Anthropology and Modern Life*. New York, Norton.

Caldwell PH, Arthur HM (2008) The influence of a culture of referral of access to nursing care in rural settings after myocardial infarction. *Health and Place* 14(1): 180–185.

Cudmore H, Sondermeyer J (2007) Through the looking glass: being a critical ethnographic researcher in a familiar setting. *Nurse Researcher* 14(3): 25–35.

Denzin NK (1989) *Interpretive Interactionism*. Newbury Park, Sage.

DeSantis L (1994) Making anthropology clinically relevant to nursing care. *Journal of Advanced Nursing* 20: 707–715.

DeWalt KM, DeWalt BR (2002) *Participant Observation*. Walnut Creek, Altamira Press.

Fetterman DM (1998) *Ethnography Step By Step*, 2nd edition. Thousand Oaks, Sage.

Geertz C (1973) *The Interpretation of Cultures*. New York, Basic Books.

Gobo G (2008) *Doing Ethnography*. Los Angeles, Sage.

Hammersley M, Atkinson P (2007) *Ethnography: principles in practice*, 3rd edition. London, Routledge.

Happ MB, Swigart VA, Tate JA, Hoffman LA, Arnold RM (2007) Patient involvement in health-related decisions during prolonged critical illness. *Research in Nursing and Health* 30: 361–372.

Hardcastle M, Usher K, Holmes C (2006) Carspecken's critical qualitative research method: an application to nursing. *Qualitative Health Research* 16(1): 151–161.

Harris M (1976) History and significance of the emic/etic distinction. *Annual Review of Anthropology* 5: 329–350.

Holloway I, Todres L (2003) The status of method: flexibility, consistency and coherence. *Qualitative Research* 3: 345–357.

Holloway I, Wheeler S (2010) *Qualitative Research in Nursing*, 3rd edition. Oxford, Wiley-Blackwell.

Hunter CL, Spence K, McKenna K, Iedema R (2008) Learning how to learn: an ethnographic study in a neonatal intensive care unit. *Journal of Advanced Nursing* 62(6): 657–664.

LeCompte MD, Schensul JJ (1999) *Analyzing and Interpreting Ethnographic Data*. Walnut Creek, Altamira Press.

Leininger M (ed) (1985) *Qualitative Research Methods in Nursing*. Philadelphia, WB Saunders.

Lincoln YS, Guba EG (1985) *Naturalistic Inquiry*. Newbury Park, Sage.

Malinowski B (1922) *Argonauts of the Western Pacific: an account of native enterprise and adventure in the archipelagoes of Melanesian New Guinea*. New York, Dutton.

Penney W, Wellard SJ (2007) Hearing what older consumers say about participation in their care. *International Journal of Nursing Practice* 13(1): 61–68.

Roper JM, Shapira J (2000) *Ethnography in Nursing Research*. Thousand Oaks, Sage.

Savage J (2000) Participant observation: standing in the shoes of others. *Qualitative Health Research* **10**: 324–339.

Serrant-Green L (2007) Ethnographic research. *Nurse Researcher* **14**(3): 4–6.

Spradley JP (1980) *Participant Observation*. Fort Worth, Harcourt Brace Jovanovich College.

Spradley JP (1979) *The Ethnographic Interview*. Fort Worth, Harcourt Brace Jovanovich College.

Thomas J (1993) *Doing Critical Ethnography*. Newbury Park, Sage.

Further reading

Angrosino M (2007) *Doing Ethnographic and Observational Research*. London, Sage.

Savage J (2006) Ethnographic evidence: the value of applied ethnography in health care. *Journal of Research in Nursing* **11**(5): 383–393.

Schensul SL, Schensul JJ, LeCompte MD (1999) *Essential Ethnographic Methods: observations, interviews and questionnaires*. Walnut Creek, Altamira Press.

15 Phenomenological Research

Les Todres and Immy Holloway

Key points

- The phenomenological researcher uses descriptions and/or interpretations of everyday human experiences (the lifeworld) as sources of qualitative evidence.

- The purpose of phenomenology is to find insights that apply more generally beyond the cases studied.

- Descriptive phenomenology uses 'bracketing' of preconceptions and attempts to arrive at the 'essences' of experienced phenomena.

- Hermeneutic phenomenology uses interpretation and personal or theoretical 'sensitising' to highlight important themes. It seeks to enhance understanding in readers by presenting 'plots' or stories.

INTRODUCTION

Phenomenology as a discrete philosophical research tradition emerged in the early part of the 20th century. Although Edmund Husserl (1859–1938) is credited as the central founder of this tradition (Spiegelberg 1994), he built on earlier philosophers who wished to describe human experience as the valid starting point of philosophy. This grabbed the attention of researchers who were looking for ways to study human experience on its own terms without reducing it to language that comes from other sciences such as chemistry or physiology. The promise of phenomenology was that human beings could be understood from 'inside' their subjective experience, which could not be adequately replaced by any external analysis or explanation. A view from within a person's perspective is needed for any comprehensive understanding of human behav-

iour. Phenomenologists thus emphasise the value of describing and interpreting human experience and seek to do this in credible and insightful ways. This chapter will outline the main principles of phenomenology and illustrate some of the practical ways it is used in research. Some illustrations from published studies will be used to demonstrate particular principles or concepts. In some cases, only a brief excerpt of the study will be presented. In other cases, more detail and context will be given so that readers may get a sense of the research study as a whole.

THE PURPOSE OF PHENOMENOLOGICAL RESEARCH

Phenomenological research begins with gathering examples of everyday experiences, describing them and reflecting on them. Husserl called these everyday experiences the 'lifeworld', while other phenomenologists have used the term 'lived experience'. So lived experiences such as 'having a baby' or 'the experience of back pain' are chosen as phenomena to be described and studied in depth. The purpose of focusing on such named experiential phenomena is: *to find insights that apply more generally beyond the cases that were studied in order to emphasise what we may have in common as human beings.* Husserl called such common themes 'essences'; they are also known as 'essential structures'.

One may find universal 'essences' in nature. For example, gravity can be described as the essence of all falling objects to earth. However, when it comes to human beings, one seldom finds common themes that are universal across all cultures and circumstances. Rather, one finds common themes that are typical within a context such as a particular culture or time in history. The other thing about 'essences' in relation to human experience is that the essential themes relate to other themes, like *in* a story. So when

phenomenologists present their findings, they usually express this in such a way as to show how a number of common themes are related. This is referred to as 'the essential structure' of the phenomenon. The example in Research Example 15.1 provides insight into how an essential structure is like a story: it has a general plot that brings the essential themes together in an understandable way.

Another important concept in phenomenological research is the idea of 'bracketing', in which phenomenological researchers attempt to suspend (or bracket) their preconceptions so that they can approach the phenomenon to be studied with 'fresh eyes'. Husserl called this suspension of preconceptions 'the phenomenological reduction', where a certain open-mindedness is achieved. In such 'openness', something new can be discovered that is not tainted by previous theory or taken-for-granted assumptions. In practical terms, this involves a certain self-discipline similar to true listening in which one lets the information and data 'speak' more fully before imposing one's own understanding or interpretation.

RESEARCH EXAMPLE

15.1   A Section of an Essential Structure: Women's Experience of Self-harm through Self-cutting

Robinson FA (1998) Dissociative women's experiences of self-cutting. In: Valle R (ed) *Phenomenological Inquiry in Psychology: existential and transpersonal dimensions*. New York, Plenum Press, pp 209–225.

'Emotional states prior to cutting include feelings of being trapped, inner emotional chaos and noise, intolerable emotional pain, intense anger and feelings of separation from significant others. Cutters want a release of tension, a relief from their enduring pain and a quieting of the chaos and the noise. They reach a place where it feels as if they will explode or die or where they are feeling out of control and desperate. It feels as if physical pain could take away their emotional pain.

   Alters emerge who seem responsible for the cutting ...

   Cutters shift into an altered mental state. They find a pleasurable place where they are feeling in total control of their life. The pain subsides ...

   The sight and feel of flowing blood has much symbolism for cutters. It represents life, the possibility of death, release of things trapped in the body and survival ...

   Cutters experience much fear and shame after cutting. Their good feelings and relief are always temporary. They feel sad knowing cutting brings their greatest comfort and meets their love and nurturing needs ...'

Here is an example of 'bracketing' as an ongoing discipline during the research:

> Imagine an interview situation where something is said which reminds the interviewer of something they have read about. They then need to be careful not to influence the interview in the direction of what has been read. Also, when analysing the interview, the researcher needs to be careful not to impose the ideas from their reading on to the analysis. This can be done later in a discussion section, but descriptive phenomenology seeks to stay very close to the data when formulating meaningful themes.

THE USE OF PHENOMENOLOGY IN NURSING

Phenomenological studies have become an increasingly important qualitative approach in nursing. Topics have included the lived experience of caring for a partner with Alzheimer's disease (Todres & Galvin 2006), experiences of care in relation to the physical environment of an oncology centre (Edvardsson *et al.* 2006), experiencing aphasia and the struggle to regain the ability to communicate (Nyström 2006) and the lived experience of waiting for colorectal surgery (Moene *et al.* 2006). By way of illustration, Research Example 15.2 provides a summary of a phenomenological study examining the lived experience of patients in a critical care setting.

A strong indication that phenomenological attention to lifeworld descriptions is entering mainstream healthcare is evidenced by the UK's National Health Service modernisation agency, which is adopting a methodology of 'discovery interviews'. Here, detailed guidance is given to healthcare practitioners of how to elicit experiential descriptions from service users so that those services may be improved (Wilcock *et al.* 2003). This approach, whereby users are asked to describe significant experiences of care, is proving to be much richer than surveys that are based on preconceived questions.

This kind of knowledge of 'what it may be like' is particularly useful for helping nurses to imagine what the patient is going through. Such understanding can provide a kind of empathy that is an important foundation for making ethical judgements about care.

As an adjunct to technical proficiency, this kind of knowledge may be action-oriented in the way, for example, that a nurse having considered the reflection in Research Example 15.2 about being weaned from an intubator, now begins to welcome a patient's protest, and is flexible in attuning themself to the patient's ambivalent struggles regarding dependence and independence.

Such kinds and levels of knowledge may also be important in designing nursing education, where a grasp of the 'world of the patient' may help to underpin the development of more uniquely tailored, person-centred practice. Such lifeworld-led education may increasingly expand the horizons of evidence-based education to include qualitative evidence about the world from the patient's point of view.

MAIN FEATURES

Phenomenological research as used by nurses is generally divided into two types: descriptive phenomenology and interpretive or hermeneutic phenomenology. Descriptive phenomenology stays close to Husserl and has been translated into an empirical research approach by Amedeo Giorgi, his colleagues and students (Giorgi 1970, 1997; Giorgi & Giorgi 2004). Interpretive or hermeneutic phenomenology stays close to Heidegger, Gadamer and Ricoeur, and their philosophical insights are used in various ways to underpin qualitative research. Hermeneutic phenomenologists do not believe that researchers can be very successful in suspending their preconceptions. Rather, they should use their preconceptions positively, making them more explicit so that readers of the research can understand the strengths and limitations of the interpretations that the researcher makes. So, for example, a hermeneutic phenomenologist may use 'feminism' as an interpretive framework and demonstrate how this perspective may throw some new light on the phenomenon studied. Hermeneutic phenomenologists are also very cautious about finding common essences, as they wish to emphasise uniqueness and diversity.

RESEARCH EXAMPLE

15.2   The Experience of a Patient in an Intensive Care Unit

Todres L, Fulbrook P, Albarran J (2000) On the receiving end: a hermeneutic-phenomenological analysis of a patient's struggle to cope while going through intensive care. *Nursing in Critical Care* **5**(6): 277–287.

Consider a patient in an intensive care unit. What kind of endurance does this require? What are the experiential tasks and stages that such a patient may be negotiating? What do nurses need to understand about the totality of this experience that could help them in their caring tasks? In such a phenomenological study, Todres *et al.* (2000) were able to provide insight into, for example, a challenging form of endurance at one of the stages of the intensive care experience: how, in relation to intubation, the body wants to resist what feels alien and unnatural, while the person understands at the same time that such 'intrusion' is not only *help* but *lifesaving help.* In articulating this structure, one may see how this could be a plausible transferable theme for other patients as well. Different patients may respond to this meaningful structure differently, but the structure helps us to understand these variations in terms of the central issue at stake, that is having to accept bodily-repulsed intrusion as *help.* They were also able to articulate other stages of the experience, such as entering a 'twilight world', the frustration of not being understood, ambivalent feelings during the weaning process and the importance of having someone to advocate on one's behalf, among other themes. It may be helpful for nurses to understand, for example, the transitions that a patient may be experiencing when being weaned from the ventilator after some time. Here is one of the essential structures that was formulated on the basis of an interview.

'Adapting to breathing again on her own marked a transition from the twilight world where she drifted between life and death, between technological and human support, between caring and not caring, between fight and flight. Anne's hand was now not just looking for human contact and reassurance, but beginning to become again what it used to be: a power towards personal competence and self-support. Issues in the social world again became relevant and particularly focused on the beginnings of power struggles between herself and others. Though she was still unpractised in negotiating interpersonal power, and even confused and ambivalent about this, she recognised that her growing self-assertion was a good thing. In "being weaned" one re-enters again the world where saying yes and no is granted more meaning: clarifying the ambiguity of where dependence is still needed and where a degree of independence is possible, is both a personal and interpersonal task. Both patient and caregiver need to recognise and adjust to this transition. Its inconvenience and ambiguity needs to be welcomed. It is a *welcome back* like the protest and cry of a baby first gasping for breath. As such, protest is the beginning of choice and personal competence' (Todres *et al.* 2000: 284)

In the authors' view, the distinctions between descriptive and hermeneutic phenomenology have been overemphasised. Both these types of phenomenology share the following features: starting from 'lifeworld' descriptions, the use of 'bracketing' or sensitising as a reflective analytic method and arriving at 'essences' or 'fusion of horizons' to characterise the experienced phenomena.

Starting from 'lifeworld' descriptions

Both descriptive and hermeneutic phenomenologists use the term 'lifeworld' instead of using the traditional term 'data'. This is because they are not gathering separate pieces of information but rather interrelated themes or stories. Individual experiences are the starting point for inquiry. This approach moves from the specific to the general. In other words, it uses specific examples of concrete, everyday experiences (lifeworld experiences) as a starting point for further analysis and reflection. With insight and reflection, more general insights across cases can then be formulated. So the phenomenological researcher studies 'experiential happenings', and one often finds that fresh insights are 'in the details'. The findings of a good phenomenological study can resonate at a feeling level and richly describe experiences that human beings can identify with, or alternatively, they can help them to understand something more about the differences from their own experience.

The use of 'bracketing' or 'sensitising' as a reflective analytic method

Descriptive phenomenology uses the term 'bracketing', while hermeneutic phenomenology is more likely to use the term 'sensitising'. Descriptive phenomenologists do not wish to start out with a hypothesis or preconceived idea or theory which they then try to prove or disprove. Rather, they wish to be open-minded about what they may discover and therefore try to suspend preconceptions and theories as much as possible. This attitude has been called the 'phenomenological reduction', whereby fresh meanings can be seen and expressed in language. Both descriptive and hermeneutic phenomenologists would agree that the possibility of 'seeing something' freshly, differently or from a new perspective, is a crucial dimension of phenomenology's discovery-oriented approach. But hermeneutic phenomenological researchers may use existing preconceptions as a way of 'sensitising' themselves to what is missing or different. For example, as a researcher, Finlay (Fitzpatrick & Finlay 2008) reflected on her own personal experience of struggling with a severe shoulder injury and how this 'sensitised' her to the impact of pain for patients undergoing the rehabilitation phase following flexor tendon surgery. She notes that such an empathic awareness of 'what it may be like' helped her to 'see' the pain in patients' movements during rehabilitation, something that may have been left implicit without such sensitivity. However, she also acknowledges how important her co-researcher was in helping her to

check such personally informed insights against the stories of the participants. Their study is a good illustration of how personal sensitivity can bring 'humanity' to the study, while 'bracketing' can bring a certain discipline and rigour that realises fresh insights beyond the preconceptions of the researchers.

The findings of phenomenological research: essences or 'fusion of horizons'

Descriptive phenomenology uses the term 'essence' or 'essential structure', while hermeneutic phenomenology is more likely to use the term 'fusion of horizons'. Learning about and communicating the meaning and significance of an experienced phenomenon is a qualitative and literary effort. Husserl, in representing the descriptive emphasis, was interested in finding qualitative features that define what a phenomenon is most generally. For example, one defining feature of many different examples of anger may be the quality of wanting to change another person or something in the world. When formulating 'essences' from a number of cases of an experience one notices and tries to put into words what is common, but also what varies or is different between cases studied. So, the findings of phenomenological research should make sense of both the unique details and the commonalities between the experiences studied. This has been referred to as the 'essential structure' of the phenomenon and is expressed in a narrative way that points out how everything fits together. Hermeneutic phenomenologists are also interested in communicating the meaning and significance of experience, but express this differently. Meaning is 'pointed out' in multiple ways and relies on personal insight as well as helpful theories that may be relevant. It is less concerned than descriptive phenomenology to come to a specific conclusion, and may evoke deeper understandings in a similar manner as that of a good film-maker or novelist, who 'paints a picture' from various angles.

This kind of writing requires an artistic capability. Even though the different phases and parts of this writing may not be conclusive, they are aimed at forming a coherent picture so that they can offer the reader a place of 'meeting' and understanding about

15.3 Burn Injury Patients: Challenges of Adjustment

Moi LA, Vindenes HA, Gjengedal E (2008) The experience of life after burn injury: a new bodily awareness. *Journal of Advanced Nursing* **64**(3): 278–286.

Moi and colleagues undertook a descriptive phenomenological study to explore patients' experiences of life after a major burn injury. In-depth interviews were undertaken with 14 patients conducted on average 14 months after the injury had taken place. The interview began with a request to describe what had happened in their lives from the time of the accident to the time of the interview. Beyond this, the interview was unstructured, and non-leading questions were asked to encourage participants to express their experiences in their own words. The researchers sought to bracket previous knowledge about the phenomena encountered so that it would not influence the interviews or subsequent analysis. The transcribed interviews were analysed using Giorgi's method for formulating essential meanings. Transferable themes between cases were finally expressed in an extensive narrative that highlighted both the common themes as well as some of the unique and different ways in which patients responded. Some of the general themes included:

- how patients came to terms with the fact that, in some respects, their bodies had changed in irrevocable ways
- how significant others played an important role in helping them live with changes in appearance and functioning
- the ways in which patients compensated for restricted functioning by finding alternative solutions.

In-depth description of each of these and other themes were elaborated on by drawing on quotations from selected patients to elucidate the themes. The value and relevance of these insights for clinical practice were discussed at the end of the article, with specific emphasis on how nursing practice could benefit from an understanding of the kinds of insecurity these patients experience over an extended period of time regarding their self-image and functioning.

the topic. Gadamer, a hermeneutic phenomenologist, used the term 'fusion of horizons' to mean how different people's understandings could come together, thus achieving broad shared insights that, nevertheless, tolerate some freedom in how readers interpret the significance of findings for their own lives or situations. By this, he was pointing out that the validity of phenomenological findings are not based on their ability to correspond perfectly to all cases, but rather that they have sufficient coherence to be applied meaningfully in similar situations.

Whether the researcher adopts a descriptive emphasis or a hermeneutic emphasis, we would argue that a coherent phenomenological study would include all three features discussed above. Moi *et al.* (2008) provide an account of how these features were applied

in a study of patients' experiences of adjusting to life following a major burn injury (see summary in Research Example 15.3). We now turn to the more practical details of fieldwork and analytical procedures. We can only be indicative here as the practice of these principles varies.

FIELDWORK

It has been suggested that researchers adopting a phenomenological approach should read very little relevant literature about the research topic before starting so that they are not influenced by preconceptions. However, the research questions do need to be informed by what has already been done, and what the gaps are. 'Bracketing' is not about pretending that prior knowledge does not exist, but about looking freshly at the area of study and questioning the assumptions that may be in the literature. So, for example, in a study on therapeutic self-insight, one of the authors was aware of the literature and research that referred to therapeutic self-insight using different theories and terms such as 're-organising psychic energy', 'cognitive re-structuring' and 'transcending developmental fixations' (Todres 2002). This made the author more interested in describing what was occurring without these theoretical ideas by going back to people's specific experiences and letting the concepts come 'from there'.

The kind of data that need to be gathered in phenomenological studies are from people who can give examples of experiences they have personally lived through. It is not enough that they just have general opinions or views about the topic. They must be able and willing to give descriptions of their own personal experiences. So it is often useful as a starting point to ask: 'Have you had something like this kind of experience?' Sometimes this is obvious and may not need to be asked, such as in approaching fathers about their experience of becoming a father for the first time. But at other times it is less obvious, such as in a study of the experience of phantom limb pain. This kind of sampling has been called purposive sampling, in that selection of informants is made on the basis of a particular purpose. In the case of phenomenological research, such purpose is that the research participants included in the study can provide good personal accounts of the experience to be studied. It is also important to gather as much relevant context about the person and the experience as possible. This contextual information helps the researcher to not only make sense of the experience, but also to specify the nature of the examples on which the reflections are built.

Phenomenological research can generate valuable transferable insights based on an in-depth analysis of only one case study, but value may be increased by studying a number of cases. Phenomenological research, in the authors' experience, has achieved the most profound insights with in-depth reflections on about six to 12 cases as 'windows' to, and illustrations of, a phenomenon. There is a danger in choosing a sample that is too large. A number of journal reviewers have commented that, in such cases, depth and thoughtfulness in the analysis is sacrificed. One then wonders why an alternative research design was not chosen that is better able to capture the quantitative incidence of themes.

In phenomenological research, cases of relevant experiences have been gathered from written descriptions, autobiographical texts, journals and dialogues. Most phenomenological studies are, however, interview based. This may be because an in-depth interview is able to focus on the complexity of the experience, as well as provide a clear focus for exploration.

A phenomenological interview that gathers lifeworld descriptions of experiences is similar to, but different from, other types of non-structured, open-ended interview. It begins with a request that an interviewee describe a relevant experience as fully as possible. This request is generally similar for all respondents. Instructions are sometimes given which may help the respondent to focus on the details of the experience. One can study lived experience in retrospect because it still has meaning for the person, even though the event may have taken place a while ago. An account of an experience usually begins with some of the factual details, but also includes what they meant to the person, the feelings and attitudes. However, the richness of the account is often better when it is closer to the experience in time. The interviewer then helps the interviewee to 'tell the story' as fully and concretely as possible, eliciting examples of the experience and what it was like for the respondent. The logic of the interview is: 'Have you had this kind of experience, and if so, how did it occur for you and what was it like for you?' The interview is open-ended, but the interviewer at times may become more focused on attempting to clarify in greater depth the nature of the phenomenon being studied. This often requires a sensitivity and timing so that the interviewee feels understood and comfortable about the interaction. Box 15.1 provides an example of an interview designed to obtain a lifeworld description.

ANALYTICAL PROCEDURES

After gathering lifeworld descriptions of personal experiences, each account becomes a 'text' that is

183

Box 15.1 Using interviews to obtain 'lifeworld descriptions'

Imagine that we wish to better understand what happens when a patient is given a diagnosis they were not expecting. Using a phenomenological approach that focuses on their lifeworld, we would ask patients who have had this experience to describe as fully as possible the story of the happening, the events in sequence, the interactions, the 'before' and 'after', their thoughts, feelings and actions – all that goes into the meaning of the experience for them. The value of such lifeworld description is that it provides sources of information that may have been unanticipated by both the respondent and researcher. It does not depend on the ability of the respondent to come up with already formulated views or articulate generalisations.

Box 15.2 Example of expressing 'meaning units' in more transferable and general ways: responding to a loved one's memory loss through Alzheimer's disease

Interviewee's narrative (one meaning unit divided from the rest of the text)	Transferable, more general meaning
In retrospect, the earliest indication that there was a problem with Betty's memory loss was when we purchased our new car. Betty had extreme difficulty in the use of fifth gear. Indeed teaching her how to drive the new car was slow and tedious. It should be noted that at this time, Betty was very cognitive and was enjoying secretarial duties	The earliest indication of him becoming aware of Betty's memory loss was her difficulty in learning an operational task that was, in his view, not in keeping with her usual competent functioning

ready for the analysis of meanings, and for the formulation of these meanings into a coherent story of interrelated themes and insights. The analysis is different from procedures in other qualitative research, such as coding and qualitative content analysis. The articulation and clarification of the meanings in the text, both explicit and implicit, requires a 'reading' or strategy that entails a back-and-forth movement between particular expressions and details within the text and a sense of the meaning of the text as a whole (see Box 15.2 for an illustration of this process). It is only the whole of the text and its context that can make sense of the details within the text. On the other

hand, the details contribute to, and refine, the process of formulating and synthesising meanings into a coherent overall structure as a whole. The danger of computer-aided analysis packages is that they can divert attention in a way that overemphasises a concern with 'parts', and this can obscure an understanding of the text as a whole.

There has been some controversy about how much to use a systematic method of analysis in phenomenology. Giorgi and colleagues (Giorgi 1985; Giorgi & Giorgi 2004) have recommended and demonstrated a systematic procedure which includes:

- reading to get a narrative sense of the text as a whole
- dividing the text into 'meaning units' that discriminate changes in meaning
- expressing the meanings in more transferable and general ways
- formulating a narrative structure that highlights and integrates the essential meanings of the experiences across cases
- illustrating the common themes in greater detail by elaborating further, and also by using quotations from research respondents' original descriptions. This phase also indicates some of the different and unique ways that different people 'lived out' the essential meanings of a phenomenon.

Other phenomenologists such as Van Manen (1994) take a less systematic approach and are more concerned with the insightful art of writing that is grounded in lifeworld experiences. Van Manen follows some of the thoughts of Gadamer, who feels that no method can ensure insight. Insight emerges through the way researchers interpret the experiences in the act of writing. Narrative writing is used as a method in itself for reflecting further in order to integrate the different strands of meanings that may be implicit in people's descriptions. Van Manen provides some guidance for writing, which includes:

- involving the readers by writing in a compelling way
- building a plot-line with subplots
- providing enough details and concrete examples to illustrate the themes
- offering new insights that come out of the analysis.

An illustration of this approach is given in Research Example 15.4, which provides an example of a hermeneutic phenomenological study exploring the experiences of patients who have been diagnosed with exhaustion disorder.

As in other forms of qualitative research, the findings of phenomenological research are finally considered in dialogue with the literature and current research in order to offer critique, possible applications and further directions for research.

STRENGTHS AND LIMITATIONS

The central strength of a phenomenological approach is that it provides both philosophical and methodological support in attempting to capture and express the meaning of significant human experiences in a rigorous manner. When done well, this gives others deeper insight into what an experience or lived situation is like. Such forms of knowledge humanise our understanding, and this may be crucially important as a basis for ethical practice. The narrative product of phenomenological studies seeks to express insights in such a way that it may evoke a sense of recognition and understanding in readers. This kind of narrative knowledge is also interpersonal knowledge in that it describes 'people in situations' in holistic and interactive ways, guarding against viewing humans as objects like other objects. This may be why the humanistic school of psychology has adopted phenomenology as one of its core methodological approaches. It is also resonant with some feminist contributions to psychology (Gilligan 1982) and sociology (Oakley 2000).

The central limitations of a phenomenological approach in our view are three-fold.

- The use of observation is problematic in phenomenological research. Because phenomenology wants to get the inner perspectives of people from their own point of view, it is reluctant to judge behaviour from an external perspective. Critics of phenomenology have noted that descriptions of the world from an 'insider' perspective may be inadequate as an account of human behaviour. Such critics would say that it is not people themselves who can best explain their behaviour, as their behaviour may be caused by forces that are more appropriately analysed in other ways with reference to social, political or chemical analyses.
- Descriptions of lifeworlds depend on full and rich verbal accounts by people who are articulate. This raises challenges for phenomenological methodology, for example when studying children. There are some ways forward in this regard, such as using photographs or drawings as prompts for people to talk about a particular topic.

RESEARCH EXAMPLE

15.4 Pervasive Life Changes in Exhaustion Disorder

Jingrot M, Rosberg S (2008) Gradual loss of homelikeness in exhaustion disorder. *Qualitative Health Research*. **18**(11): 1511–1523.

These researchers conducted a hermeneutic-phenomenological study influenced by the philosopher Hans-Georg Gadamer. Gadamer had written about how illness took one away from the feeling of being at home in one's body and in one's life. The researchers drew on these ideas when interpreting their research data. The phenomenon studied was the lived experience of suffering from exhaustion disorder as medically defined. The study explored the experiences of 11 individuals on sick leave for at least six months because of a diagnosis of exhaustion disorder. In open-ended interviews, research informants were asked to describe their experience of the illness, their life situation, work and future. Each interview was transcribed and analysed before the next one was conducted, and the emerging understandings were used to sensitise the dialogue with the remaining research participants. The analysis of the texts involved a variation on the idea that the researchers go back and forth between their sense of the meaning of the text as a whole and an attention to the detailed meanings in the parts of the text. In addition, the concept of 'unhomelikeness' was used to make sense of the findings in an interesting way. By means of this interpretive lens, the researchers were able to identify a gradual process whereby patients experienced an increasing detachment from their body and world. The findings were formulated in terms of five stages of 'unhomelikeness' that progressively characterised the lifeworlds of patients living with exhaustion disorder. These stages included increased bodily preoccupation and withdrawal from 'normal' life, a loss of a sense of continuity (even memory loss), everyday life as weary struggle and a sense of 'uncanniness' in which there was a frightening feeling of detachment from the body and the world. The clinical significance of this study was highlighted: the importance of early interventions designed to help the patient regain a sense of 'homelikeness' in the body and the world through body-awareness exercises and normalising routines.

■ It can be elitist in that there is an artistic-literary capability required of the researcher when reflecting and writing. The 'method' does not guarantee the quality of the narrative coherence achieved in the writing of the final stages of the research product. This can be said to some degree of all research, but phenomenology is on the literary side of the scientific–literary continuum.

CONCLUSIONS

Phenomenology is a discrete qualitative research approach that is embedded in the philosophical traditions of the early part of the 20th century. Phenomenologists emphasise the value of describing and interpreting human experience and seek to do this in credible and insightful ways that apply more generally beyond the particular cases studied. The phenomenological researcher uses descriptions and/or interpretations of everyday human experiences (the lifeworld) as sources of data. When undertaking descriptive phenomenology the researcher seeks to bracket any preconceptions and attempts to arrive at the essences of experienced phenomena. By contrast, hermeneutic phenomenology uses interpretation and personal or theoretical sensitising to highlight important themes. It seeks to enhance understanding in readers by presenting plots or stories in a narratively coherent way.

References

Fitzpatrick N, Finlay L (2008) 'Frustrating disability'. The lived experience of coping with the rehabilitation phase following flexor tendon surgery. *International Journal of Qualitative Studies on Health and Well-being* **3**(3): 132–142.

Edvardsson D, Sandman PO, Rasmussen B (2006) Caring or uncaring – meanings of being in an oncology environment. *Journal of Advanced Nursing* **55**(2): 188–197.

Gilligan C (1982) *In a Different Voice: psychological theory and women's development*. Cambridge, MA, Harvard University Press.

Giorgi A (1997) The theory, practice and evaluation of the phenomenological method as a qualitative research procedure. *Journal of Phenomenological Psychology* **28**: 235–260.

Giorgi A (1985) *Phenomenology and Psychological Research*. Pittsburgh, Duquesne University Press.

Giorgi A (1970) *Psychology as a Human Science: a phenomenologically based approach*. New York, Harper and Row.

Giorgi A, Giorgi B (2004) The descriptive phenomenological psychological method. In: Camic PM, Rhodes JE, Yardley L (eds) *Qualitative Research in Psychology: expanding perspectives in methodology and design*. Washington, DC, American Psychological Association (APA), pp 243–274.

Jingrot M, Rosberg S (2008) Gradual loss of homelikeness in exhaustion disorder. *Qualitative Health Researh* **18**(11): 1511–1523.

Moene M, Bergbom I, Skott C (2006) Patients' existential situation prior to colorectal surgery. *Journal of Advanced Nursing* **54**(2): 199–207.

Moi LA, Vindenes HA, Gjengedal E (2008) The experience of life after burn injury: a new bodily awareness. *Journal of Advanced Nursing* **64**(3): 278–286.

Nyström M (2006) Aphasia – an existential loneliness: a study on the loss of the world of symbols. *International Journal of Qualitative Studies on Health and Well-being* **1**(1): 38–49.

Oakley A (2000) *Experiments in Knowing: gender and method in the social sciences*. London, Blackwell.

Robinson FA (1998) Dissociative women's experiences of self-cutting. In: Valle R (ed) *Phenomenological Inquiry in Psychology: existential and transpersonal dimensions*. New York, Plenum Press, pp 209–225.

Spiegelberg H (1994) *The Phenomenological Movement: a historical introduction*, 3rd revised edition. Dordrecht, Kluwer Academic Publisher.

Todres L (2002) Humanising forces: phenomenology in science; psychotherapy in technological culture. *Indo-Pacific Journal of Phenomenology* **3**: 1–16.

Todres L, Fulbrook P, Albarran J (2000) On the receiving end: a hermeneutic-phenomenological analysis of a patient's struggle to cope while going through intensive care. *Nursing in Critical Care* **5**(6): 277–287.

Todres L, Galvin K (2006) Caring for a partner with Alzheimer's disease: intimacy, loss and the life that is possible. *International Journal of Qualitative Studies on Health and Well-being* **1**(1): 50–61.

Van Manen M (1994) *Researching Lived Experience: human science for an action-sensitive pedagogy*. London, Ontario, Althouse Press.

Wilcock PM, Brown GCS, Bateson J, Carver J, Machin S (2003) Using patient stories to inspire quality improvement within the modernisation agency collaborative programmes. *Journal of Clinical Nursing* **12**: 1–9.

Further reading

Holloway I, Wheeler S (2009) *Qualitative Research in Nursing*, 3rd edition. Oxford, Wiley-Blackwell.

Rapport F (2005) Hermeneutic phenomenology: the science of interpretation of texts. In: Holloway I (ed) *Qualitative Research in Healthcare*. Maidenhead, Open University Press, pp 125–246.

Thomas SP, Polio HR (2002) *Listening to Patients: a phenomenological approach to nursing research and practice*. New York, Springer.

Todres L (2007) *Embodied Enquiry: phenomenological touchstones for research, psychotherapy and spirituality*. Basingstoke, Palgrave Macmillan.

Todres L (2005) Clarifying the lifeworld: descriptive phenomenology. In: Holloway I (ed) *Qualitative Research in Healthcare*. Maidenhead, Open University Press, pp 104–124.

Websites

http://phenomenology.utk.edu/ – the Center for Applied Phenomenological Research represents a group of scholars from a variety of departments at the University of Tennessee.

www.phenomenologyonline.com/ – Phenomenology online. This site provides public access to articles, monographs and other materials discussing and exemplifying phenomenological research.

16 Narrative Research

Dawn Freshwater and Immy Holloway

Key points

- Narrative research is a qualitative approach that relies on participants' stories about their experiences.

- The stories can be obtained through a number of means, such as narrative interviews or oral stories, diaries, autobiographies or even visual images.

- Through narratives, people give meaning to their experience and life condition. In nursing, telling stories can help ill and vulnerable individuals to adapt to their situation.

- Different ways of narrative analysis can be used to make sense of these stories.

INTRODUCTION

Narratives, or stories, permeate our everyday lives. It is widely accepted that we are all storytellers and interpret the world, defining ourselves through the diverse stories we tell. Narrative research is, of course, inquiry based on narratives, but the definitions of 'narrative' itself are also diverse, perhaps surprisingly so given the nature and context of research and research methods. In the human sciences, narrative, in its simplest form, means storytelling, a recreation of experiences and events in people's lives, either by themselves or others. (We shall not follow up the potential distinction between story and narrative; in this chapter the terms are used interchangeably. An extensive analysis can be found in Holloway and Freshwater 2007, Frid *et al.* 2000 and Riessman 2008, for the interested reader.) Narratives

give meaning to experiences and life course events, and through narrative people make sense of what has happened to them. Holloway and Freshwater (2007) share the beliefs of other narrative researchers, viewing storytelling as a natural way of communicating between human beings who wish to transmit to others what they live through, think and feel. Indeed Bruner sees 'no other way of describing "lived time" save in the form of a narrative' (Bruner 2004: 692). The term 'narrative research' or 'inquiry' is described here as an independent approach within qualitative methods, although other approaches, such as ethnography and, in particular, phenomenology, also use narratives. In this chapter, narratives are the accounts of people, by people and about people. They are about events and refer to people's own and others' behaviour, their motives and feelings as well as interpretations of the actions of others. These are stories that are coherent and reflective; both the identities of the participants and their culture are embedded in these stories, that is to some extent they are culturally and personally specific, although universal patterns can be uncovered in the accounts of those who share the experience of being human.

There exists a long tradition of storytelling in literature, where stories are generally fictional, while the narratives of participants in research are seen as the perspectives on their experience. They, too, may be imagined or invented (see later in this chapter) but demonstrate the participants' *take* on events and experience. Fairy tales, as well as religious and historical texts, contain stories and further generate new and adapted stories. Narratives have been used in autobiography, life story or oral history in either spoken or written words. Even in ancient times people told stories of events and incidents, relating what had happened to them. Linguists and literary theorists expanded and followed the narrative tradition. In recent decades, narrative works by educationists such as Labov and Waletzky (1967), and Clandinin and Connelly (2004) (which culminated in the edited text by Clandinin (2007)), have been published. Psychologists such as Polkinghorne (2007), Bruner (1986) and Riessman (1993, 2008) have also been active in doing and writing narrative research. Polkinghorne (2007) states that 'the storying process' is now common in social science, philosophy, history, organisational theory and other areas. In nursing, Sandelowski wrote on narrative in 1991. Since then Frid *et al.* (2000) have published their article on narrative inquiry in nursing, and articles as well as chapters have appeared in a variety of journals and books. In 2007, Holloway and Freshwater wrote a text on narrative research in nursing. This type of research in the caring professions has mostly been based in illness narratives – the stories sick people tell (though stories from professionals and students are also analysed). The most well known of books on illness narratives is probably that of Kleinman (1988). Outside of this definitive text, Mattingly and Garro (2000) as well as Brody (2003) and others have written about illness narratives or stories of sickness. Hurwitz *et al.* (2004) also edited a book on narrative research in health and illness among their other writings on narrative.

THE NATURE AND PURPOSE OF STORIES

As mentioned above, narratives are stories that people tell, usually with a beginning, a middle and an end; they may take many forms, usually orally or in written form and include a plot, a cast of actors and a problem that needs solving. For stories to be heard they need to be interesting to the listener. Emplotment and temporality are central to a story (Ricoeur 1991). Emplotment is an act that links diverse events to form a plot, which generates a coherent story; it is the structure through which sense is made of events and the way in which things are connected (Czarniawska 2004; Freshwater & Rolfe 2004). Ryan (1993) points out that while what is happening in the story (the chronicle) and how the story is painted to the listener or reader are important dimensions of the way a story is constructed, it is in fact the emplotment that is the real challenge and, as we interpret, the craft. That is what links the events into a meaningful sequence and structure. It is natural, of course, for the audience, whoever they may be, to want to create their own emplotment in response to the story. Plot then, is a device of narrative. Temporality is discussed a little later in this section.

Despite the emphasis on time and space in narrative, Czarniawska (2004) reminds us that temporal and spatial connections are not sufficient to act as a plot. She notes that:

> 'To become a plotted story, the elements, or episodes, need also to be related by *transformation*' (Czarniawska 2004: 125)

This could be related to linking of narrative, plot, authority and reflexivity in 'the event of a narrative', which does not explicitly refer to transformation, rather they emphasise the notion of power and freedom afforded through narrative to expose the limitations and constraints of old meanings and old plots (Freshwater & Rolfe 2004).

Greenhalgh and Hurwitz (1998) suggest a difference between a simple story and a plot, taking their suggestion from EM Forster's explanation that a simple story continues in a chronology '… and then … and then …', while the plot suggests 'why'. Plot is the sequential element and the essential structure of narrative (Cortazzi 1993), as we have suggested. Plotlines, however, are not always linear; they may be circular, iterative and can be revised or 'edited' in their retelling. Going back and forth is quite common among narrators, but the listener is still left with the essential features of the story. Researchers attempt to find the 'narrative thread' to grasp the whole story and give it coherence.

A narrative is a journey or pathway through time, which is told by its author, who tells the listener what happens on the way. The narrator takes a reflective stance on events and processes on the journey. However, narrators do not merely communicate a simple story to the listener; they also clarify and reflect on the past, justify their past behaviour and link the past to their present thinking and actions. Brody adds another element to these features of narrative: the story has to be special, that is 'worthy' of narration. It does not rely merely on everyday sequences of events: 'I took the car; I drove to work; I talked to my friends'. Instead, it relies on dramatic and critical events and behaviour when critical events or situations are discussed, such as an unusual condition, an illness or an 'epiphany' where some thing or person is illuminated by a sudden insight: 'I was digging in the garden, and all of the sudden I felt a snap in my back. The pain was excruciating …'

As already mentioned the term emplotment describes the way a story is organised. Cortazzi (1993) describes three major elements in a plot:

- temporality (how time is framed within the story)
- causation (relationship between events in the story)
- human interest (how the story interacts with the audience).

Temporality

Temporality is a complex term in philosophy about the nature of time (used by Ricoeur (1984) in relation to narrative) and how human beings are bounded in time. Sequencing over time and the links between events provide continuity – 'this happened and then …'; the plot includes causality – '*why* this happened, *how* this happened'. Everything is seen in relation to

everything else. Holloway and Freshwater (2007) state that the narrative is a journey through time in which narrators share their experience, justify their actions and link the present to the past and the future. The story involves a group of characters who act or who are experiencing the actions of others. Narrators tell personal as well as social/cultural stories, which means that these tales are not only unique to the participants, but also present the cultural context in which they are located and thus have commonalities within a particular context.

Temporality implies that the story evolves more or less sequentially (although this could be disputed). It means that there are three linked sequences:

- when the story is set up and opens up towards the future – the beginning
- when the story unfolds – the middle
- when the story is resolved – the end.

The listener can hear that the story has coherence because the narrator links past, present and future. Indeed, even in a dramatic and chaotic story, the listener can detect plot and coherence, though Freeman (2003) suggests that narratives are more chaotic than is sometimes assumed as lives themselves are not necessarily coherent and structured.

Causation

A story often contains causal relationships, which the listeners and readers generally perceive, even though it is often assumed by them.

As human beings we are constructed in such a way that we continually search for the causes of things. Story, and its inherent linearity, provides a powerful experience of causation, gratifying this basic need. Porter-Abbott (2002) suggests that:

'Narrative itself, simply by the way it distributes events in an orderly, consecutive fashion, very often gives the impression of a sequence of cause and effect' (Porter-Abbott 2002: 37)

Forster (1927) in his definitive text *Aspects of the Novel* gives some practical examples of the way in which readers do not always need causation to be obvious in a text in order to think causally. In other words, human beings have a tendency towards a narrative logic, in which things that follow other things are caused by those things.

Human interest

Human interest is another element in the story. If no one has an interest in the story, then there is no listener and no narrative. Often a story of experience includes crises and turning points as well as justification for the storyteller's actions and behaviour that is a response to the interpretation of experience. Researchers construct a plot in which they involve separate events forming a coherent whole.

It can be seen that people do not only develop stories to communicate with others, but also to make sense of their own lives, and in particular of problematic and tragic circumstances. There are thus commonalities for the cultural context (and indeed commonalities of human experience in general) and distinctions between different narrators.

There are, as already alluded too, many reasons for storytelling, some of which are listed below.

- People try to interpret their experience and make sense of it.
- They communicate with others through stories.
- They organise events and happenings by narrative.
- They justify their own actions and feelings.
- They attribute praise and blame to others and themselves.

(See also Holloway & Freshwater 2007.)

There may be a number of reasons why vulnerable people in particular wish to tell their stories. Common to all of these is the idea that storytelling provides the narrator with a distance from the (often threatening) experience of vulnerability, in other words storytelling can be useful as a coping strategy for vulnerable persons to manage the psychosocial and emotional aspects of their predicament. Moreover, once the story is in the process of being narrated, it enables the narrator to gain a different perspective on the experience.

Stories therefore can be useful devices for individuals that enable them come to terms with their vulnerability, make sense of their lives and construct their versions of reality and identity through social discourse. According to Ricoeur's (1984) notion of temporality, through storytelling people are able to locate their 'now' experience in a context of 'back then' and 'not yet'. For instance, a vulnerable person might connect an experience in the past with the cause of condition in the 'here and now', or might justify present thought and action, or future behaviour, using a story from the past. Garro (2000) maintains that 'people make sense of the past from the perspective of the present' (Garro 2000: 71); memory helps reconstruct past experiences and connects these to the present and to expectations of the future. This is evident in stories. Fundamental to the process of storytelling, then, is the imposition of narrative form and sequencing, such that the movement between beginning and end point enacts a relationship to time. Even when this storytelling loses its thread and the temporal sequencing is disrupted, people still confirm their identity through stories. Research Example 16.1 gives an example of autobiographical narrative where this is illustrated.

Of course, stories are not necessarily factual constructions and are often evaluated for their credibility or authenticity. Researchers usually accept the participant's story as true, though they know that storytellers sometimes do not remember well, are confused, or over-dramatise for effect (Rolfe 2005; Holloway & Freshwater 2007). In any case, plausibility does not guarantee authenticity. However, storytellers in nursing research rarely seem to tell 'lies', and even when not telling the truth – consciously or otherwise – they demonstrate their intentions and motivations. The knowledge individuals share may include implicit and 'tacit' knowledge, which researchers have to uncover.

NARRATIVE INQUIRY IN NURSING

Narrative as a form of inquiry differs somewhat from other qualitative approaches in that it generates coherent stories rather than 'fractured text' (Riessman 1993). It is important that the researcher listens, does not ask too many intrusive questions and empowers

16.1 Autobiographical Narrative

Hydén LC, Örulv L (2009) Narrative and identity in Alzheimer's disease: a case study, *Journal of Aging Studies* doi:10.1016/j.jaging.2008.01.001.

Research about the link between narrative and identity of people with Alzheimer's disease was carried out by the Swedish researchers Hydén and Örulv in 2009. The researchers suggest that identity and a sense of self is often confirmed through narratives. In this study, the researchers use a particular 'case' to illustrate the value of storytelling in old age for people with Alzheimer's and other forms of dementia. Even though the usual temporal continuity of the story is disrupted, a sense of identity is maintained. This research shows the use of autobiographical work in nursing research.

16.2 Narrative Research from the Nursing Literature

Brown J, Addington-Hall J (2008) How people with motor neurone disease talk about living with their illness: a narrative study. *Journal of Advanced Nursing* **62**(2): 200–208.

Brown and Addington-Hall (2008) obtained the stories of the experiences of people with motor neurone disease, who lived in care homes or in their own place. The sample consisted of 13 patients recruited through purposeful sampling. The form and content of stories were analysed. This study relied on narrative interviews; participants were able to tell their stories in consecutive meetings with the researchers. Four types of narrative were identified: living life as well as possible through keeping active and engaged, living in insurmountable situations, fear of the future, survival. These were seen as the sustaining, enduring, fracturing and preserving narrative storylines. The stories aimed to help nurses to understand the patients in order to engage with them more effectively.

the participants to be in control of their tales. Narratives are sources of data for researchers in many areas of nursing, for instance stories of caring for patients, of interaction with other professionals, of learning and education. Nursing stories, according to Kelly and Howie (2007), are a means of sharing nursing knowledge and they help researchers to understand professional practice and the perception of professional roles. Most frequently, however, nurse researchers elicit the stories of patients, and illness narratives – a term made known particularly by Kleinman (1988) – become the focus of their research. Patients tell these stories because they want to make sense of their suffering and share their thoughts and feelings with others. (In this chapter we are focusing on narratives that are elicited by few interview questions and where people have the chance to tell stories without much interruption, rather than biographical interviews where the researcher often interrupts.) Research Example 16.2 gives an example of narrative nursing research using stories of people living with motor neurone disease.

ILLNESS NARRATIVES OR STORIES OF SICKNESS

We have already referred to the reasons why vulnerable people might engage in storytelling. Now we turn our attention to those stories of sickness and vulnerability, sometimes known as illness narratives. Illness narratives have been told over centuries; nurses have listened to these stories so they can help their patients. Only in recent decades have they become a focus of research. Illness in these stories is perceived as a 'biographical disruption' (Bury 1982), not only as a significant life event but one that might change the identity of the storyteller, who often wishes to regain their former self and return to normality (see restitution narrative below). Frank (1995) discusses stories of sickness in his classic, *The Wounded Storyteller*. The three types of narrative that he proposes are 'the restitution narrative', 'the chaos narrative' and 'the quest narrative'. He suggests that these types have fit with the stories people tell, though they often overlap.

The most frequent of story types is the *restitution narrative*, with the inherent plot stressing a future of normalisation and the regaining of the old identity. The restitution narrative is one that is not only favoured by ill patients but also by health professionals. For acute illness this is often the general outcome, as patients see themselves regaining their health and their former selves, although the chronically ill also wish to reclaim at least some sort of normality. (In relation to this Frank (1995) also discusses the concept of 'sick role' in Chapter 4.) The *chaos narrative* contains a plot of not getting better. Stories of terminal cancer are chaos narratives, and some tales of chronic illness with its ups and downs of suffering and pain can contain disorder, disruption and chaos. Nurses and doctors feel impotent in the face of people who tell these types of tale. We found that chaos narratives are the least welcome and not as often used in research. *Quest narratives* contain the missionary spirit of the storyteller who accepts, uses and confronts illness to gain something in the process; often they wish to be a model or example to others. Frank claims that quest narratives are the most commonly told in public. He suggests that they often include a call for social action; many of us have heard stories from the media where narrators use their experiences in the health system 'so that this will never happen again', with people showing their scars to give testimony to suffering. Stoicism and heroism are part of the plot.

Smith and Sparkes (2004) give examples of these types of narrative in their article on disabled sportsmen and show the ways individuals use metaphors to illuminate their experience such as, for example, equating the disability to a battle or likening the stages to a journey.

ETHICAL ISSUES IN NARRATIVE RESEARCH

Elliott (2005), in her writings on ethics in narrative research, divides the discussion for the sake of clarity, dealing first with ethics and then with political issues. The ethical dimension is defined as issues relating to the relationship between the researcher and participant, and the impact of the research process on individuals directly involved in the research. The political dimension is defined as being the broader implications of research, namely the impact on society or subgroups in society.

In more detail, Elliott (2005) suggests that the researcher enters into a personal and moral relationship with the participant during data collection, analysis and dissemination. She focuses her attention on the full research process – data collection, informed consent, the potential impact of the research encounter on the participant and additionally on the implications of using narrative with regard to confidentiality and anonymity during analysis and dissemination. The processes can be quite complex.

Narrative interviewing brings with it a range of interesting but challenging issues for consideration. While commendable, the move over the past two decades away from structured interview techniques and towards providing participants with the opportunity to relate narratives about aspects of their lives and experiences as a means of empowering the participant, does raise questions regarding the nature of the research relationship, specifically the blurring of boundaries between the expert (i.e. researcher) and the storyteller.

Issues concerning the exploitation of the research relationship (specifically related to the power dynamic) have been the topic of debate for many years. Narrative research does have the potential to

193

provide the opportunity for the participant to have a form of control over the data collected. Rather than the researcher asking the questions they want to ask, the participants are both the 'subjects and objects in the construction of sociological knowledge' (Finch 1984: 118). Ochberg (1996) argued that questionnaires provide a narrow menu of selected foci, but that narrative lets participants choose the events that matter to them. Although this is theoretically true, there is still a potential for exploitation and, as with all research, the assumption of equality and reciprocity cannot be taken for granted or assumed.

Finch (1984) discusses the ethics of interviewing groups of women in their own homes in which the research took on an informal, intimate character. Although this form of data collection is effective, it can leave the participant open to exploitation as narrators often disclose confidential and intimate information, where the researcher can only provide fairly 'flimsy' guarantees of confidentiality. In addition, when working with participants in their own homes, it is inevitable that the researcher learns much more than what is said in words.

Any research experience could prove positive or negative for the participant. In narrative research there is the possibility that by sharing a narrative on an unpleasant situation (and/or unresolved situation), raw emotions may arise; however, an informal, intimate conversation could also provide a safe and positive opportunity for the participants to tell someone who is interested, and listening, about their experience. From the latter viewpoint, narrative encounters can be healing and provide a therapeutic environment within which a transformation can begin or be supported.

COLLECTING AND ANALYSING NARRATIVE DATA

The initial research question (not to be confused with interview question) needs to be broad to fit with a narrative approach. Narrative inquiry has sampling strategies and data sources that are similar to those of other forms of qualitative inquiry, such as interviews or diaries, even occasionally visual sources. However, narrative researchers usually use fewer questions in their interviews, generally starting with an open and general question about their experience, which elicits a full story. On completion of this, researchers might pursue issues that they do not understand or that are unclear. These questions could enhance the relationship between the researcher and the participant. Box 16.1 gives some examples of starter questions for narrative research.

Box 16.1 Example of starter questions for narrative research

General questions

- Tell me the story of your illness?
- Tell me how it all started

Follow-up questions if necessary (following the participants ideas)

- What happened then?
- And the story of your stay in hospital?
- How did your treatment proceed?

It is important to remember that these questions are questions that aim to facilitate the storytelling process.

In narrative inquiry a number of models of analysis exist and different researchers adopt a particular stance or orientation. There are various ways to analyse narrative data; whatever model the researchers choose, they need to be analytic and theoretical and take the stories to a new level as narrative research is more than retelling or even reformulating the participants' tales. Riessman (2008) gives four models of narrative analysis.

Riessman's first type of analysis, *thematic analysis*, focuses on the content of stories, and researchers proceed in the same way as other qualitative researchers do. They organise, label and group related data together in themes and illustrate their accounts with quotes from the participants and short vignettes of the individuals involved. Hence, the researcher centres on 'what' is said. Less attention is given to 'how is the story told?', 'who is the narrator?' and 'to whom is it addressed?'. Accounts of experience first looked at the plot as a whole without breaking the text into its structure. The 'voice' of the narrator is heard throughout. Riessman states that this type of analysis neglects context; we would claim, however, that context, knowledge of culture and circumstance are essential for understanding the contents of these stories.

Riessman states that *structural analysis* focuses on the language and analyses how the story is told, not just on the storyline. This type of analysis has its origin in the work of Labov and Waletzky (1967) and resembles conversation analysis because of the emphasis on text. They analyse how language is used in stories. The text is broken down into a variety of elements. It could be argued, however, that narrative needs a holistic rather than a structural account. In structural analysis, the researcher takes account of six major features according to Labov and Waletzky.

- *Abstract* – summary, the point of the story.
- *Orientation* – towards location, characters and time, for instance.
- *Complicating action* – the plot, which includes crisis point and sequence.
- *Evaluation* – the narrator takes stock of what has been said.
- *Resolution* – the outcome of the story.
- *Coda* – an end to the story, which rounds it off.

In other words, the story is organised into ideas and units, which rely on the spoken narrative and not on its content. This micro-analysis of text seems inappropriate for stories, which, after all, are told as a whole, and the storytellers wish them to be understood as wholes.

Riessman discusses three more types of analysis: interactional, dialogic/performance and visual analysis. The first two focus on interaction of researcher and storyteller and the research situation as a dialogue and seem to be the same as other dialogic research in qualitative inquiry. Visual analysis is based on the non-language-based sources of data such as pictures, photographs, films and other images which complement the story or the written account. It should be stressed, however, that no definitive type of narrative analysis exists.

CRITICAL ISSUES IN NARRATIVE INQUIRY

Narrative research has been criticised by several insiders such as Atkinson (1997) and Atkinson and Delamont (2006). These writers suggest a preoccupation of qualitative researchers with narratives, and maintain that narrative research is not privileged over other forms of research and needs analytic rigour. They emphasise that narrative research does not consist of the retelling of stories in an uncritical and non-analytic way. In particular, Atkinson and Delamont regret that narratives are often used in an unreflective way and not contextualised. Nevertheless, analytic and reflexive narrative research gives voice to people who might not have been heard before, as well as opening up the stories of more powerful groups, while at the same time reflecting cultural and social location.

Storytelling can include imagination or even distortion, thus storytellers do not always tell the truth. If people tell stories to make sense of their experiences, even unconscious 'untruths' are important, as these are based on the tellers' perceptions and they are likely to act upon them (it is rare that narrators tell deliberate lies to the researcher). As Lorem (2008) says, in these stories, patients reconcile themselves with their experience and justify their own and others' behaviour. What is revealed will include the elements in the story that the narrators wish to show as central to their experience, even if it is not true historically. Polkinghorne (2007) maintains that 'storied texts serve as evidence for personal meaning, not for the factual occurrence of the events reported in the stories' (Polkinghorne 2007: 479) Furthermore, the validity of the research does not depend on the 'truth telling' of the participants but on the credibility of the researcher's account of their perspectives. The research report needs reflexivity on the part of the researcher, it needs an audit trail – or enough evidence from the study that the claims made by the researcher are credible.

When judging the usefulness, quality and appropriateness of narrative inquiry, its readers search for and use various ways to evaluate. Most qualitative researchers set up criteria different from those used in quantitative research, although 'criteriology' has recently been criticised by Seale (1999) and Parker (2004) in particular. Parker extends Salmon's argument for qualitative research that some of the most innovative research in quantitative inquiry has been carried out by those who broke the rules of accepted criteria; only in this way can progress be made. Criteria, so Parker argues, should be flexible guidelines in any case, not rigid rules and conventions. Nevertheless, if narrative researchers wish to demonstrate the quality of their research to the readers of their work, whether they have quantitative or qualitative orientations, they have to develop a framework by which narrative research can be judged.

Thus the standards for establishing validity and reliability in narrative research are different to most other approaches. As Freshwater and Rolfe (2004: 532) state, this consists of three principal criteria.

- Detailed writing ('thick description'), which makes both the research process and the context of the research transparent. For instance, the final write-up should include reference to how the initial formulations have been deconstructed and rewritten during the process of the research and how the researcher has developed an understanding of their limitations.
- Exposure of the researcher's bias (or 'interest'). Once again the final draft should refer to the

way in which the researcher has come to an awareness of the underlying 'plots' in their developing narrative and how, as a result of the research process, they have raised their awareness of the limitations and biases that were inherent in both the initial formulations and the final write-up.
- The way in which the professional community view the research (which should also be included in the final write-up). Ideally this should include reference to peer response to any published work. If this is not possible the researcher should include an account of the results of their dialogic engagement with peers, supervisors and any other professional who has read a draft in the final report. If necessary, the researcher should set up peer groups with the express purpose of critically engaging with the work.

Other questions that may guide the evaluation of narrative research findings can be found in Holloway and Freshwater (2007); however, the main judgement depends on its appropriateness, relevance, holism, credibility – and readability.

WRITING AND REPORTING NARRATIVE RESEARCH

In narrative research in particular, writers need to develop a good *title*, because the title sets the scene for the whole of the report and arouses the reader's interest.

Box 16.2 gives examples of titles from published narrative research.

The *abstract* is a summary of the research, including a short description of the topic, the aim, the methodology including design and approach, procedures and sample. A summary of the main findings is also given.

Usually the tale proceeds in the following way.

1 Authors explain the background of the study, give a rationale for the research, describe the setting and context in which it takes place (introduction).

Box 16.2 Examples of titles for narrative research

Challenging 'ordinary pain': narratives of people who live with pain (Becker 2001)
Narrative representations of chronic illness experience: cultural models of illness, mind, and
   body in stories concerning the temporomandibular joint (Garro 1994)
Recovering bodies: illness, disability and life Iriting (Mairs & Couser 2006)

---

2 They set out critically what others have found while exploring the same phenomenon and point to the gap in the state of knowledge and show how they plug the gap (literature review).

3 They describe and justify the approaches and strategies they adopted to investigate the phenomenon they wished to research (research design, which includes methodology and strategies).

4 They describe what they found (findings).

5 They interpret the findings, set out their arguments and enter into a dialogue with the literature that confirmed or challenged what they found (discussion).

6 They tell the reader what they have learnt from their research (conclusion).

7 They describe its significance for professional or academic practice (implications).

8 They reflect on the journey that they have taken as researchers (reflexivity and reflectivity).

CONCLUSIONS

This chapter has outlined some of the main tenets of narrative research, referring to the 'narrative turn' in the human sciences. The basic concepts of narrative, story, plot and emplotment have been described; however, we also acknowledge that the concept of narrative is open to multiple interpretations. What is clear is that narrative and storytelling are part of human nature; narrative research is closely associated with understanding people's lives rather than abstract principles and, as such, it is aligned with the philosophy and practice of the healthcare professions and indeed the art and science of nursing.

References

Atkinson PA (1997) Narrative turn or blind alley? *Qualitative Health Research* **7**(3): 325–344.

Atkinson P, Delamont S (2006) Rescuing narrative from qualitative research. *Narrative Inquiry* **16**(1): 164–172.

Becker B (2001) Challenging ordinary pain: narratives of older people who live with pain. In: Kenyon G, Clark P, de Vries B (eds) *Narrative Gerontology: theory, research and practice*. New York, Springer, pp 91–112.

Brody H (2003) *Stories of Sickness*, 2nd edition. New York, Oxford University Press.

Brown J, Addington-Hall J (2008) How people with motor neurone disease talk about living with their illness: a narrative study. *Journal of Advanced Nursing* **62**(2): 200–208.

Bruner J (2004) Life as narrative. *Social Research* **71**(3): 691–710.

Bruner J (1986*) Actual Minds, Possible Worlds*. Boston, Harvard University Press.

Bury M (1982) Chronic illness as biographical disruption. *Sociology of Health and Illness* **4**(2): 167–182.

Clandinin DJ (ed) (2007) *Handbook of Narrative Inquiry: mapping a methodology*. Thousand Oaks, Sage.

Clandinin DJ, Connelly FM (2004) *Narrative Inquiry: experience and story in qualitative research*. San Francisco, Wiley.

Cortazzi M (1993) *Narrative Analysis*. London, Falmer Press.

Czarniawska B (2004) *Narratives in Social Science Research*. London, Sage.

Elliott J (2005) *Using Narrative in Social Research: qualitative and quantitative approaches*. London, Sage.

Finch J (1984) It's great to have someone to talk to: the ethics and politics of interviewing women. In: Bell C, Roberts H (eds) *Social Researching*. London, Routledge and Kegan Paul, pp 70–87.

Forster EM (1927) *Aspects of the novel*. London, Penguin.

Frank AW (1995) *The Wounded Story Teller: body, illness, and ethics*. Chicago, The University of Chicago Press.

Freeman M (2003) Identity and difference in narrative inquiry. *Narrative Inquiry* **13**(12): 331–346.

Freshwater D, Rolfe G (2004) *Deconstructing Evidence Based Practice*. London, Routledge.

Frid I, Ohlén J, Bergbom I (2000) On the use of narratives in nursing research. *Journal of Advanced Nursing* **32**(3): 695–703.

Garro LC (2000) Cultural knowledge as a resource in illness narratives: Remembering through accounts of illness. In: Mattingly C, Garro LC (eds) *Narrative and the Cultural Construction of Illness and Healing*. Berkeley, University of California Press, pp 70–87.

Garro LC (1994) Narrative representations of chronic illness experience: cultural models of illness, mind, and body in stories concerning the temporomandibular joint. *Social Science and Medicine* **38**(6): 775–788.

Greenhalgh T, Hurwitz B (1998) Why study narrative? In: Greenhalgh T, Hurwitz B (eds) *Narrative Based Medicine: dialogue and discourse in clinical practice*. London, Routledge, pp 3–16.

Holloway I, Freshwater D (2007) *Narrative Research in Nursing*. Oxford, Blackwell.

Hurwitz B, Greenhalgh T, Skultans V (eds) (2004) *Narrative Research in Health and Illness*. Oxford, Blackwell.

Hydén LC, Örulv L (2009) Narrative and identity in Alzheimer's disease: a case study. *Journal of Aging Studies* doi:10.1016/j.jaging.2008.01.001.

Kelly T, Howie L (2007) Working with stories in nursing research: procedures used in narrative analysis. *International Journal of Mental Health Nursing* **16**(2): 136–144.

Kleinman A (1988) *The Illness Narratives: suffering, healing and the human condition*. New York, Basic Books.

Labov W, Waletzky J (1967) Oral versions of personal experience. In: Helm J (ed) *Essays on the Verbal and Visual Arts*. Seattle, University of Washington Press, pp 12–44.

Lorem GF (2008) Making sense of stories: the use of patient narratives within mental health care research. *Nursing Philosophy* **9**(1): 62–71.

Mairs N, Couser GT (2006) *Recovering Bodies: illness, disability and life writing*. Madison, University of Wisconsin Press.

Mattingly C, Garro LC (2000) *Narrative and the Cultural Construction of Illness and Healing*. London, University of California Press.

Ochberg RL (1996) Interpreting life stories. In: Josselson R (ed) *Ethics and Process in the Narrative Study of Lives*. Thousand Oaks, Sage, pp 259–263.

Parker I (2004) Criteria for qualitative research in psychology. *Qualitative Research in Psychology* **1**(2): 95–106.

Polkinghorne D (2007) Validity issues in narrative research. *Qualitative Inquiry* **13**(4): 471–486.

Porter Abbott H (2002) *The Cambridge Introduction to Narrative*. Cambridge, Cambridge University Press.

Ricoeur P (1991) Life in quest of narrative. In: Wood D (ed) *On Paul Ricoeur: narrative and interpretation*. London, Routledge, pp 29–33.

Ricoeur P (1984) *Time and Narrative* (Vols 1–3). Chicago, University of Chicago Press.

Riessman CK (2008) *Narrative Methods for the Human Sciences*. Los Angeles, Sage.

Riessman CK (1993) *Narrative Analysis*. Newbury Park, Sage.

Rolfe G (2005) Evidence, memory and truth: towards a deconstructive validation of reflective practice. In: John C, Freshwater D (eds) *Transforming Nursing through Reflective Practice*, 2nd edition. Oxford, Blackwell, pp 13–26.

Ryan ML (1993) Narrative in real time: chronicle mimesis and plot in baseball broadcast. *Narrative* **1**(2): 138–155.

Sandelowski M (1991) Telling stories: narrative approaches in qualitative research. *Image, Journal of Nursing Scholarship* **23**(3): 161–168.

Seale C (1999) *The Quality of Qualitative Research*. London, Sage.

Smith B, Sparkes A (2004) Men, sport, and spinal injury: an analysis of metaphors and narrative types. *Disability and Society* **19**(6): 513–626.

Further reading

Andrews M, Squire C, Tamboukou M (2008) *Doing Narrative Research*. Los Angeles, Sage.

Gubrium JF, Holstein JA (2009) *Analyzing Narrative Reality*. Thousand Oaks, Sage.

17 Experimental Research

Andrea Nelson, Jo Dumville
and David Torgerson

Key points

- Experimental research makes a useful contribution to nursing research as it is a powerful design able to distinguish between cause and effect.

- There are many different types of experimental design used in healthcare research.

- The randomised controlled trial is particularly valued for its ability to test rigorously the effectiveness of treatments and interventions.

- Experimental research seeks to minimise all possible sources of bias and confounding.

- Strengths and weaknesses of the experimental design for different research questions and contexts must be acknowledged.

BACKGROUND

Well-designed and executed experimental research can contribute to theoretical understanding and to nursing practice. There are several different types of healthcare interventions, including screening, drugs, information giving and education, and different ways of delivering care (e.g. walk-in clinics) that are amenable to experimental research as a way of testing their effectiveness. Since the thalidomide disaster, drugs must be evaluated in large randomised controlled trials (RCTs) before they are licensed for use. However, other types of interventions are not routinely evaluated in this way, with some commentators arguing that RCTs are of limited use in evaluating nursing interventions.

EXPERIMENTAL VERSUS OBSERVATIONAL STUDIES

True experimental studies are more powerful than observational studies in determining the cause of an observed outcome. Using an observational design, an association may be found between two variables, but it is difficult to be certain about the direction in which the causal effect is operating. For example, women who give up breast feeding soon after birth use dummies more often than women who maintain breast feeding. An RCT of discouraging dummy use found no effect on breast-feeding rates (Kramer *et al.* 2001). In fact, the association between dummy use was observed because women who were going to give up breast feeding (for whatever reason) tended to use dummies more. Cessation of breast feeding led to increased dummy use, not the other way around.

It may be tempting to address questions about the effects of interventions by surveying a large number of people. This approach can also be misleading as the intervention a person receives may be related to another factor. For example, in a study of the impact of support group meetings for people with angina on their quality of life, it may happen that those people who attended the support group report a higher quality of life, but this could be because the most active patients attend the group. Concluding that support groups lead to a higher quality of life *on the basis on this evidence alone* would be inappropriate.

Results from observational studies should be used to generate further questions for study, rather than to give the definitive answer. Treatments with plausible modes of action, and some limited support through anecdotal evidence, may in fact be ineffective or harmful. This means that robust evaluation of interventions sometimes gives 'surprising' results (see Table 17.1).

CHARACTERISTICS OF EXPERIMENTAL DESIGN

In an observational study, the researcher describes a number of variables. Conversely, in an experimental study the researcher (or someone else, e.g. the government) manipulates some aspect of the phenomenon under study, and researchers then observe what happens.

An experiment is carried out to test a hypothesis or research question. An example might be:

'Does patient-controlled analgesia (PCA) reduce postoperative pain better than intra-muscular analgesia (IMA)?'

Formally, hypotheses are usually expressed as a statement rather than a question, for example:

'PCA is more effective than IMA at reducing pain scores in the 48 hours after major surgery'

It is important to specify the components of the hypothesis precisely, for example the population

Table 17.1 'Surprising' results of treatments

Question	Impact of intervention	Reference
Are occlusive dressings better than gauze-based dressings for surgical and traumatic wounds?	Occlusive dressings were associated with higher total costs and had longer hospital stay than the gauze dressing group. Groups did not differ for complete wound healing, time to wound healing or pain	Ubbink *et al.* 2008
Do honey-impregnated dressings help the healing of venous ulcers or reduce infection rates?	There was no significant difference in the number of infections or ulcer healing rate between people who had honey dressings and those who had a dressing chosen by their nurse. People treated with honey dressings had more pain and withdrawals	Jull *et al.* 2008
Does providing an automated external defibrillator (AED) in the home in patients at risk of sudden cardiac arrest reduce deaths?	There was no difference in mortality between patients given an AED for home use and a control group that received CPR training and usual access to emergency services from home	Bardy *et al.* 2008
Does using larval therapy (maggots) clean sloughy venous ulcers quicker than a hydrogel, and does it lead to quicker healing and reduced infection rates?	Larval therapy reduced time to removal of slough tissue in venous ulcers but had no impact on time to healing when compared with a simple hydrogel dressing	Dumville *et al.* 2009

being studied, the variable being changed (the independent variable) and the variable being measured (the dependent variable).

It is common to express the hypothesis as a null hypothesis (Ho), a statement that there is no relationship between the variables under investigation, for example:

> 'There is no difference between IMA and PCA with respect to pain scores in the 48 hours after major surgery'

Statistical testing is commonly set up with the assumption that the null hypothesis is true until there is enough evidence to reject it (see Chapter 36 for further information on null hypotheses). More recently there has been a resurgence of interest in statistical methods that do not assume that the null hypothesis holds, e.g. Bayesian analysis. These methods are complex and beyond the scope of this book.

In the PCA example, the independent variable is the type of analgesia (IMA, PCA) and the pain score is the dependent variable. Increasingly, the terms participant/population, intervention, comparator and outcomes (PICO) rather than independent and dependent variables are used when reporting experiments. The relationship between these terms can be seen in Box 17.1. PICO helps clinicians to frame questions by defining the elements of a patient problem (population), intervention, comparator and outcomes. As with all research the characteristics of the study population, the type of interventions used and the outcome(s) of interest must be defined.

PRE-/POST-TEST STUDIES

There are a number of forms of experiment used in healthcare. The simplest type of experiment uses a pre-/post-test design (before and after study). Figure 17.1 shows a representation of this design.

This design reports a change in an outcome following a change in an intervention. It does not, however, allow us to confidently state that the change occurred *because of* the intervention, i.e. it does not allow us to ascribe cause and effect. Three reasons that a change in the outcome might not be due to the intervention are temporal effects, testing effects and regression to the mean.

Temporal effects

A change in an outcome over time might be due to changes over time, rather than the intervention. In our example, a reduction in pain scores after use of the PCA device might be due to the reduction in pain levels that would be observed anyway in the first few days after surgery.

Testing effects

A change in outcome may occur because the initial measurement highlighted to the participants that they should pay attention to particular phenomena, or it showed up deficits in knowledge. These may affect the robustness of pre-/post-test designs, particularly in studies of educational interventions, as the initial testing may affect the outcomes, e.g. see Research Example 17.1 (Jones & Nelson 1997).

Box 17.1 Terms used to describe elements of an experiment

Population	Independent variable	Dependent variable
Population, e.g. people undergoing surgery	Intervention, e.g. analgesia administered via a patient-controlled device	Outcome, e.g. pain levels

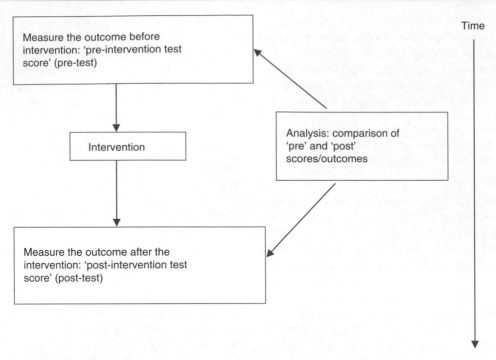

Time

Figure 17.1   Diagrammatic representation of a simple experiment: pre-/post-test study

RESEARCH EXAMPLE

17.1   The Possible Testing Effect on Outcome

Jones JE, Nelson EA (1997) Evaluation of an education package in leg ulcer management. *Journal of Wound Care* **6**(7): 342–343.

A before-and-after study to assess the impact of an educational intervention on the knowledge of nurses managing venous ulcers.

   Community nurses involved in leg ulcer care attended two study days. On the first day they attended lectures and workshops and were given an open learning pack and a video on compression bandaging. Between the first and second days they had a supported visit from a local expert in leg ulcer care to address any issues in practice. On the second day there were more lectures and workshops. Knowledge on leg ulcer aetiology and management was tested by means of a self-administered questionnaire at the start of the first study day, repeated at the end of the second study day. The number of correct responses was compared. The number of correct responses increased, but this may not have been due to the study day content, as the questionnaire itself may have helped nurses identify gaps in knowledge and prompted further study.

Regression to the mean

Regression to the mean describes a phenomenon that occurs when a variable is measured in a group of people more than once. In our example, the researchers recorded pain scores from a number of people, introduced PCA and then recorded pain scores for a second time. In the baseline pain scores, a few people had very high pain scores, a few had low pain scores and the majority had pain scores that clustered around the average (mean). If the pain scores are measured again, the people with low pain scores will tend to 'regress' upwards towards the mean, and the people with very high pain scores will tend to 'regress' down towards the mean due to measurement error. This phenomenon means that if an intervention is tested on people with a high pain level, then as a group, their pain scores will decrease whether or not the intervention is actually effective (Bland & Altman 1994).

One approach to addressing the limitations of the pre-test/post-test design is to monitor the outcomes over long periods before and after the introduction of the intervention. An alternative is to form a group that is not given the intervention being studied but still followed. The former is called an interrupted time series, the latter a controlled trial.

INTERRUPTED TIME SERIES

The stability of the outcome can be assessed both before and after use of the intervention by measuring it several times prior to and after the intervention's introduction. This design might be used when it is impossible to allocate people to different groups, e.g. if there are ethical barriers to randomisation or if it is not possible to control the release of the intervention, for example advice from government. Sheldon *et al.* (2004) monitored the rates of various procedures before and after guidance by the National Institute for Health and Clinical Excellence (NICE) on interventions, e.g. prophylactic extraction of wisdom teeth.

CONTROLLED BEFORE AND AFTER STUDIES

The simplest way to evaluate the effect of an intervention is to administer it to one group and compare this with a similar group who happened not to receive it. Both groups must be similar at baseline, and data collection should have happened contemporaneously, reducing testing and temporal effects. Controlled before and after (CBA) studies, sometimes called quasi-experimental studies, are often used in evaluating public health interventions as it is often not possible to allocate people or groups to different interventions. Christie *et al.* (2003) evaluated the effect of mobile speed cameras by comparing the number of crashes at road sites before and after the use of mobile speed cameras, versus similar sites without cameras. CBA studies are limited by threats to internal validity such as having similar groups at the baseline for both known and unknown characteristics, as well as problems identifying similar groups and high-quality data.

CONTROLLED TRIALS

In a controlled trial, a group (the control group) is formed to act as a comparison to assess whether changes in outcomes are unrelated to the intervention under study. Outcomes from the intervention group are then compared with outcomes from the control group. The design is similar to that shown in Figure 17.1 but has at least two groups so that you can be confident that any changes in outcome were not due to temporal effects (see Figure 17.2).

If the two groups have different outcomes it might be concluded that the differences were due to the experimental treatment being given to the first group (i.e. ascribing cause and effect). However, this is only the case *if the groups were similar at the outset*. If people self-selected their treatment group, or if clinicians chose treatments, then the groups are likely to be systematically different at the outset due to this selection bias, and therefore likely to have different outcomes regardless of the intervention received.

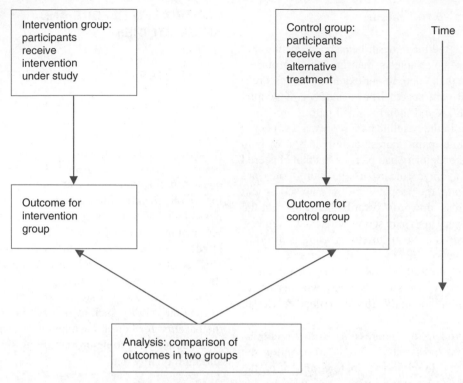

Figure 17.2 Diagrammatic representation of a controlled trial

Essentially, controlled trials allocate people to groups so they form similar cohorts (rather than simply observing similar groups as in a CBA study). 'Matching' patients with important characteristics is one approach, e.g. medical history, but this can only 'match' for those variables already known to be prognostic. There are unknown factors that predict outcomes (such as genetic make-up), hence 'matched' groups might still be quite different in some important aspects, such as compliance. To address this problem, the most powerful way of allocating people to groups is to allocate them 'randomly'. People are allocated to the groups in a purely random manner, with no way of predicting which group the next person will be allocated to. A controlled trial in which the participants are allocated to the intervention groups at random is a randomised controlled trial (RCT) (see Figure 17.3).

In a quasi-randomised trial, researchers allocate people using methods that are not strictly random, for example according to case note number (e.g. odd/even), date of randomisation, week of admission or ward/clinic. Meyer *et al.* (2008), for example, allocated smokers to one of three groups: personalised letters, brief counselling by GP or no intervention. The aim was to assess whether there was any impact on quit rate. Patients were allocated according to the week of visit to GP practice (1, 2 or 3), hence the three groups may not be completely comparable, as holidays may mean that patients seen in these periods may be different.

THE RANDOMISED CONTROLLED TRIAL (RCT)

In addition to assessing the direction of causal effects and removing temporal effects, the RCT reduces the possibility of selection bias. Most commonly, people are randomised to a treatment group, in which they remain until the end of follow-up: an individually randomised, parallel group trial. Other designs build on the simple RCT and are described below.

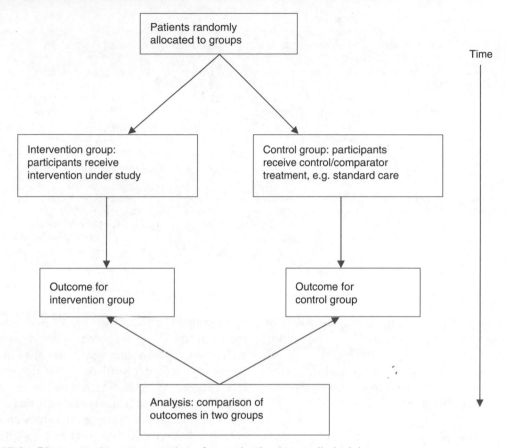

Figure 17.3 Diagrammatic representation of a randomised controlled trial

Randomisation

To ensure that such selection bias does not take place, the process of random allocation should be concealed from the person(s) recruiting participants into the study if possible. Methods of randomisation that minimise selection bias have two components: randomly generated number sequences and blinded (or masked) allocation, either via remote telephone randomisation or sealed, sequentially numbered, opaque envelopes. Failure to adequately mask allocation has led, in some studies, to inflated estimates of effectiveness of interventions (Schulz & Grimes 2002).

Comparator/control intervention

The control group in an RCT consists of people from the same population who are treated identically to the treatment group, except they receive a different intervention to that being tested. The choice of a comparison treatment may be 'standard care', a placebo or nothing at all, depending on the clinical question and state of knowledge. A placebo treatment is identical to the active treatment in every respect, except that it does not contain the proposed therapeutic benefit of the active intervention. Placebo controls are easier to develop and use in pharmaceutical trials (e.g. a sugar pill) compared with many nursing trials, but the lack of a placebo does not preclude the design of RCTs with meaningful comparison interventions. Table 17.2 illustrates the different types of comparison that can be used.

If there is an accepted standard of care, then this should be used as the comparison, as failure to use this means the trial cannot be used to determine if a change in policy from current practice to the new

Table 17.2 Examples of control groups

Population	Intervention	Outcome	Control 1	Control 2	Comment
Young people with asthma	New low-allergy bedding	Reducing asthma attacks (number and severity)	Standard treatment – old bedding	Placebo – new 'non-allergenic' bedding	If one uses old bedding, then any reduction in asthma attacks may be due to the fact that newer bedding has fewer allergens. If new 'non-allergenic bedding' is used, and participants are not told which group they are in, then the control bedding is a placebo
People with diabetic foot ulcers	Growth factor	Healing foot ulcer	Standard care – e.g. semi-occlusive dressings	Placebo – the gel 'vehicle' without the growth factor	If one uses a standard care comparator, then any improvement in healing with the growth factor gel may be due to the gel or growth factor or both

system would be beneficial. For example, an RCT of compression bandages compared a multi-layered system with non-compressive technologies for venous ulcers (O'Brien *et al.* 2003). As we already know that compression is better than no compression, this trial simply reaffirms what was already known.

RANDOMISED CONTROLLED TRIALS AND THE REDUCTION OF BIAS

RCTs are designed to reduce an important source of bias – selection bias – where people in the different treatment arms of a study have been selected in some way such that their chances of experiencing the outcome differ from the very start of the study. The results cannot therefore be attributed to the intervention. However, there are other forms of bias that may lead to systematic error in the results of an RCT, and well-designed and executed RCTs will seek to minimise these.

Performance bias/confounding

In an RCT, if people are treated in different ways other than the treatment of interest, for example one group gets an 'active' treatment plus extra attention such as more visits, then that group may fare better because of the effect of the extra 'care' rather than the treatment being evaluated. Where interventions are complex, in that they have more than one component that could contribute to the intervention's effectiveness, researchers should ensure they have an understanding of the various elements that make up the intervention. For example, in a study comparing cognitive behavioural therapy (CBT) with drugs for depression in primary care, it needs to be recognised that the CBT group would also receive, potentially, increased frequency and duration of contact with health professionals. Both may contribute to improvement in depression as well as the CBT. An RCT might take account of this by having a control group in which people received extra attention and contact but not CBT.

Attrition bias

Attrition bias refers to differences between the comparison groups due to the loss of participants from the study. These can be described as withdrawals, dropouts or protocol deviations, and the way in which they are handled has potential for biasing the results of an RCT. This is because the reasons for 'withdrawing' from a trial might be related to the intervention or outcomes.

Having a significant minority of people without any final outcome data can threaten the validity of the results of an RCT as it is not known whether the missing people on the treatments fared well or badly. People who were 'lost to follow-up' should not be ignored in the results and analysis, as this would undermine what was achieved by using randomisation.

Figure 17.4 explains this. Two treatments, A and B, are being evaluated in a trial of 100 people (50 in each group), and in each group 10% of people are lost to follow-up. The remaining two groups, of 45 people each, may differ in a systematic way, because people leave trials for reasons that may be related to their condition or the treatment; one cannot assume these withdrawals are random events. If one assumes that treatment A was ineffective, then it may be that five people lost to follow-up in that group had not improved and were demoralised, so did not return for follow-up. By contrast, let us assume that treatment B was mildly effective and the five people lost to follow-up did not return because they had experienced a complete cure. The 45 people remaining in group A would consist of people with mild to moderate disease (the more severe cases dropped out), whereas the people remaining in group B would be people with moderate to severe disease (the least severe cases having been cured). Making a comparison between the two groups on the basis of the 90 people remaining would not maintain the comparable groups obtained through randomisation, and could mislead.

An analysis in which all randomised participants are included, regardless of whether they received the intervention or not, or had any follow-up data is called an 'intention to treat' (ITT) analysis. Analysing data only from those people who received the intervention and attended follow-up is called a 'per protocol' analysis, and these tend to be less conservative than an ITT analysis. Note that articles may state that they undertook an ITT analysis, but did not (Hollis & Campbell 1999).

To prevent RCTs being threatened by loss to follow-up, they should be designed and conducted to maximise follow-up. In some studies, e.g. cancer RCTs, it may be possible to determine eventual outcomes by 'flagging' patients in national registers.

Measurement bias

Outcome data should be collected in the same way, and with the same rigour, for all the study groups. To facilitate this, where possible, participants, health professionals and outcome assessors may remain unaware of the intervention being received. Such blinding (also called masking) aims to prevent knowledge of the participant's treatment group consciously or unconsciously influencing the measurements made in the study (see Research Example 17.2).

RESEARCH EXAMPLE

17.2   Measurement Bias

Reynolds T, Russell L, Deeth M, Jones H, Birchall L (2004) A randomised controlled trial comparing Drawtex with standard dressings for exuding wounds. *Journal of Wound Care* **13**(2): 71–74.

In a randomised controlled trial in wound care, a new dressing was compared to standard care. Both patients and nurses were aware of the allocation. The outcomes were assessed in two ways: by asking the nurse treating the patient if the wound was improving/deteriorating/static, and by taking photographs of the wound to be assessed by someone unaware of the dressing being used. When nurses knew which group the patients belonged to they rated the new dressing as being better than standard care. This apparent benefit associated with the new dressing disappeared when the wounds were assessed by blinded assessors looking at the photographs.

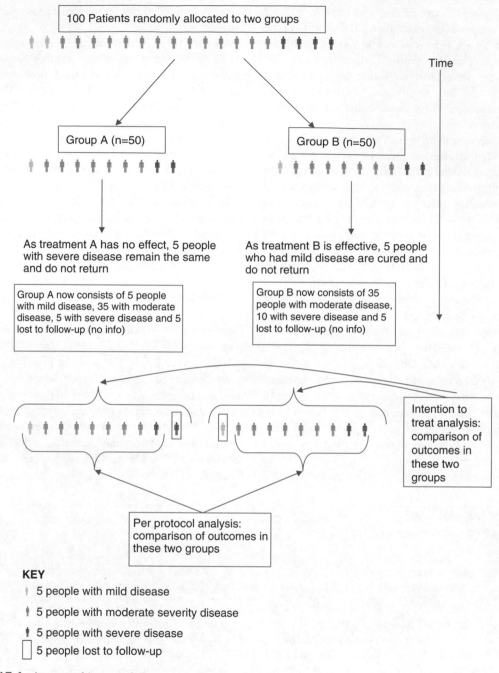

Figure 17.4 Impact of loss to follow-up on results of trials

Blinding can be especially important if the outcome measure has a subjective aspect to it. Various people may be 'blinded' to the allocation, for example, the person randomising the patients, the patient, the person delivering care, the outcome assessor and the statistician analysing the results. 'Single-blind' studies usually mean that the patient is unaware of the group to which they have been allocated. In 'double-blind' studies both the patient and their clinician are unaware of treatment allocation. It is always possible to mask allocation and the person conducting the analysis. It is usually possible to mask the person performing the outcome assessment, and it is sometimes possible to mask the patient and their clinician.

Hawthorne effect

Franke and Kaul (1978) described the effect of being observed and studied on workers in the Hawthorne factory. A series of experiments were designed to assess if environmental changes, e.g. lighting, improved productivity. It was found that at each change in environment, productivity rose. Strangely, productivity even rose when there was no actual change in environment, as the participants (factory workers) knew they were being studied and the effect of being studied changed their behaviour. The Hawthorne effect emphasises the need for control groups in experimental research.

OTHER EXPERIMENTAL DESIGNS

Cluster RCTs

In the trials described above, individuals were randomised to two or more interventions. An alternative is for natural groups of people (clusters) to be randomised, for example hospital wards or geographical areas. By allocating a cluster of people to an intervention, it is possible to be more confident that there will be no contamination between groups. For example, if testing the impact of advanced training for nurses to recognise and treat depression in primary care, it would not be appropriate to randomly assign indi-vidual patients to nurses, as one could not expect nurses with this additional training not to assess or treat a patient. One would allocate whole practices to 'advanced nurse training' or not, and compare the outcomes across the clusters. The reporting and analysis of cluster RCTs must take into account that people in clusters have shared characteristics and therefore cannot all be regarded as independent from each other.

Factorial RCTs

The majority of RCTs seek to test out the effect of changing just one element of treatment at a time. Factorial trials, by contrast, evaluate the effect of multiple interventions at the same time. These RCTs, therefore, may reflect clinical practice where multiple treatments are introduced, e.g. wound management or lifestyle changes. For example, with a factorial trial the effects of two wound dressings and two compression bandages for venous leg ulcers can be compared at the same time.

In a '2 by 2' factorial RCT there are two comparisons of two interventions being made, e.g. two bandages and two dressings. Half the people would get dressing 1 and half would get dressing 2; half would get bandage 1 and half would get bandage 2. Figure 17.5 shows a diagram of a factorial trial making this comparison for venous leg ulcers (Nelson *et al.* 2007).

To evaluate the two dressings the healing rates in the columns are compared, and to evaluate the two bandages the healing rates in the rows are compared. As people were randomly allocated to the dressings and to the bandages, the two dressings groups are assumed to be balanced for bandages, in the same way that age, sex, ulcer size, etc., are balanced across trial groups by randomisation.

One strength of a factorial trial is that it allows researchers to undertake more than one trial at a time, reducing the cost and increasing efficiency. The sample size needed is usually the same as for a simple trial, so two trials can be completed in the same time and at almost the same cost as a single treatment trial (as long as there is no interaction between treatments). The other advantage of the factorial

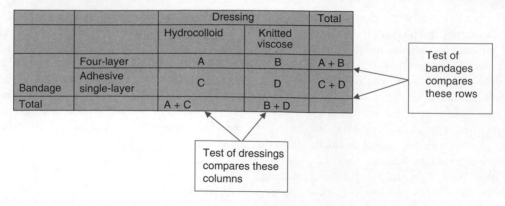

Cell A: patients receive four-layer bandage with hydrocolloid dressing

Cell B: patients receive four-layer bandage and knitted viscose dressing

Cell C: patients receive adhesive single-layer bandage with hydrocolloid dressing

Cell D: patients receive adhesive single-layer bandage and knitted viscose dressing

Figure 17.5 A '2 by 2' factorial trial

trial is that it allows determination of whether the interventions being evaluated have a synergistic (additive) or an antagonistic (working against each other) effect.

Crossover trial

One of the reasons control groups are used is to determine whether any change in outcome is part of the pattern of the disease process or whether it is due to the intervention. However, if studying the impact of an intervention in a very stable health condition, i.e. ones in which there is unlikely to be rapid resolution or deterioration, it is possible to perform *some* evaluations with patients acting as their own control. Essentially, the effect of a treatment is evaluated over a period of time and then the participant is given an alternative treatment (the crossover). The outcomes at the end of each period are compared for each patient to see whether there is any systematic difference in outcomes. To check that any change in outcome is due to the intervention being evaluated rather than temporal changes in outcomes, it is usual to randomise participants to either start on treatment A and cross over to B, or start on B and cross over to A (see Figure 17.6). This also allows determination of whether there is an 'order effect', whereby treat-

ment B performs differently if preceded by treatment A than if B is given first.

Treatments should not have a prolonged effect, as otherwise their effects may not be seen until the second period of the crossover and therefore the effectiveness would be wrongly attributed to the second treatment used. The analysis of these trials also requires care, as the crossover design needs to be accounted for. Behavioural or educational interventions cannot be evaluated in this way as it is not possible to 'take away' the knowledge or behaviour from the first period.

SINGLE-CASE EXPERIMENTAL DESIGN (N OF 1 TRIAL)

In the face of incomplete evidence to guide a decision about selecting a treatment for a chronic condition, or if a patient does not get relief from those treatments recommended in guidelines, there is a systematic alternative approach to 'trying things out'. In an 'n of 1' trial, the clinician and patient work together to evaluate which of the treatments result in consistent benefit. As in the crossover trial, the condition of interest should be a relatively stable one, e.g. arthritis, so that attributing the effect of the treatment to any

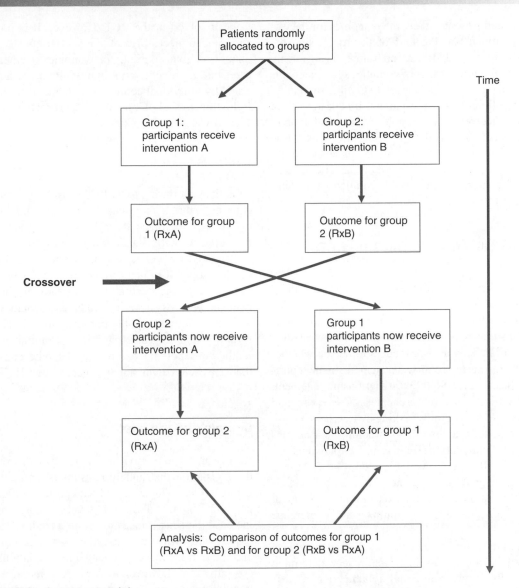

Figure 17.6 A crossover trial

improvement or deterioration is a robust conclusion and not undermined by any natural change in the underlying severity of the condition over time. For example, in an 'n of 1' trial of two treatments for osteoarthritic knee pain, the clinician would draw up a randomly selected schedule of options being investigated, e.g. a magnetic or heat wrap. The patient would keep a pain and stiffness diary and agree to use one of the treatments for a specified time, before swapping to the alternative, and then back again, possibly a few times. Evaluating the two treatments over a number of swap-overs allows the researcher to be more confident that any difference in pain or stiffness is due to the treatment rather than temporary changes in arthritis. If a drug is being evaluated in this way, the clinician may even arrange with a pharmacist to supply the preparation in a masked container so that the patient is 'blinded' to the effective treatment. The

211

clinician and patient review the outcomes for the different treatments at the end of the trial, using the patient's diary, and decide on future management. Given the limited number of conditions for which this is relevant, and the need for relatively intensive input from the clinician and the patient, this design is not common. However, it may be a powerful tool to distinguish between the placebo effect and true effects of treatment for individual patients. Nikles *et al.* (2006) provide an example of an 'n of 1' trial examining the effectiveness of stimulants for attention deficit disorder.

REPORTING AND READING OF RCTS

Given the important role RCTs have in informing clinicians of the effects of interventions, and the number of potential threats to their validity, it is important that researchers report exactly what they did in a trial. This allows readers to decide whether the study results are robust. A statement on the reporting of trials (CONSORT) (www.consort-statement. org) describes what researchers should report, and journals are increasingly asking researchers to use the CONSORT framework to structure their articles on RCTs for publication (Begg *et al.* 1996). Extensions to CONSORT are available for cluster trials, non-inferiority and equivalence trials, herbal medicinal interventions, non-pharmacological treatment interventions, harms, and journal and conference abstracts.

There are a number of critical appraisal checklists and tools available to help the reader determine whether RCTs are valid and reliable (e.g. CASP, www.phru.nhs.uk/Pages/PHD/resources.htm).

IMPORTANT CONSIDERATIONS IN USING RCTS

Securing ethical approval

To gain ethical approval an RCT must conform to the procedures discussed in Chapters 3 and 10. Participants must usually give their informed consent

to be involved in the RCT. However, it is possible, and indeed necessary, to conduct trials in people unable to give consent, for example in emergency care, but approaches for obtaining consent are governed by individual country arrangements in the UK, following the EU Clinical Trials Directive and the Mental Capacity Act (2005).

Equipoise

Clinicians recruiting to an RCT must be in collective equipoise, that is they must believe that the question of whether treatment A or B is better needs to be answered. If there is a clear preference for one intervention over another, then it is not appropriate to conduct an RCT in that area, as researchers would be asking clinicians to administer a treatment that they believed was less beneficial than an alternative.

There is a window of opportunity for RCTs, therefore, in evaluating interventions that clinicians think might be beneficial before they become convinced that it is better than standard care, when RCTs will not be possible.

Complexity and cost

RCTs can be expensive to carry out. Adherence to the legislation that underpins trials (such as the EU Clinical Trials Directive and data protection) and the need for ethical and research governance approval all increase the time it takes to set up a trial. RCTs also require the infrastructure to support randomisation and data collection and management. Trials may be cost-effective, however, if they demonstrate that a treatment is no more effective than standard care, or is better at a very high cost, and therefore inappropriate for many cases. Health economists study the cost-effectiveness of treatments within RCTs, comparing the cost of a treatment with its benefit to participants, to ensure that limited healthcare resources are used most efficiently. They can also assess the likely benefit of trials to determine which should be prioritised so that greater value for money can be obtained. An example of such an RCT is used throughout Chapters 35 and 36, and is summarised in Box 35.1.

STRENGTHS AND LIMITATIONS OF RCTS

Strengths

An RCT is the best way to determine, with certainty, whether an intervention works. It controls for those variables we know might influence outcome, such as concordance, age and disease severity, but crucially, for those factors that affect prognosis, but which are not measurable or are as yet unknown. Results from well-conducted RCTs are the most reliable research source for informing medical practice about the clinical effectiveness of treatments and interventions, and as such are regarded as the 'gold standard' for answering questions of effectiveness in evidence-based practice.

Limitations

Poorly designed and conducted RCTs can mislead, as often the sizes of effect observed in healthcare are small, and the potential problems with designing and doing trials well can introduce biases and errors that swamp the treatment effect between groups.

Learning curve for technologies

Designing, implementing and completing an RCT can take a long time – if an intervention is changing the trial evidence may prove to be irrelevant.

If there is likely to be a 'learning curve', it is important to consider when an RCT was conducted. If a trial is done when few people know how to deliver the intervention effectively, then the trial may conclude no benefit, when in fact there might be benefit if a trial was done in the middle or top of the learning curve, when more people were using it appropriately, for example skills such as compression therapy or endoscopy.

Explaining the results of trials

Experiments only answer the question of whether something works, not why it does so. For example, a few RCTs of hip-protector pads to prevent fractured hips on falling, have found that they do not work and that many people did not wear them. The reasons why the participants did not wear them, or why, in those who did fall, the hip protectors did not reduce fracture rates are not explored. Qualitative studies are increasingly nested within RCTs to help explain the findings.

Poor choice of control groups

If a study has stated it intends to evaluate the effectiveness of a new treatment but compares it against a treatment not in current use, e.g. a sub-therapeutic dose of the standard care regimen, then it is likely to conclude that the new therapy was effective even if it offers no benefit over current best practice.

Surrogate/interim outcomes

Some RCTs may report outcomes that are easier or quicker to assess than the actual outcome of interest for patients and clinicians. For example, in an RCT investigating rehabilitation after myocardial infarction to determine the effect on life expectancy, a long-term follow-up would be needed. But to avoid having to follow up participants for decades, researchers might report a surrogate outcome instead, e.g. treadmill walking distance. They may assume that improvements in the physiological outcomes will mirror longer life expectancy. Such use of surrogate outcomes relies on their association with the more relevant, patient-oriented outcomes, such as incidence of disease or survival. Surrogate outcomes commonly mislead, and if they are used, there should be clear evidence of their ability to predict long-term outcomes.

Patient-reported outcomes

As well as reporting objective outcomes such as infection rates, wound healing, death, falls, pressure ulcers or resource use (number of GP visits, hospital stay), it is increasingly important for decision makers to have information on patient perspectives derived not only from single-domain scales (e.g. for pain, anxiety), but also from quality-of-life tools, as they assess the effect of changes in the condition being treated and the impact of the treatment.

CONCLUSIONS

Given the ever-increasing pressure on healthcare systems to make efficient use of the limited resources available, the question of 'what works' needs to be answered by high-quality studies with minimal potential to mislead and thereby waste resources. For evidence of effectiveness, RCTs are often described as 'the gold standard' as they seek to minimise confounding and selection bias, which may make the results of other comparative studies unreliable. There are a number of biases that may threaten the results of studies, including RCTs, therefore decision makers need to be able to understand how these may threaten the validity of studies, and to identify and appraise such studies to inform their decision making.

References

Bardy GH, Lee KL, Mark DB *et al.* (2008) Home use of automated external defibrillators for sudden cardiac arrest. *New England Journal of Medicine* **358**: 1793–1804.

Begg C, Cho M, Eastwood S, Horton R, Moher D, Olkin I *et al.* (1996) Improving the quality of reporting of randomized controlled trials. *Journal of the American Medical Association* **276**: 637–639.

Bland JM, Altman DG (1994) Regression towards the mean. *British Medical Journal* **308**: 1499.

Christie SM, Lyons RA, Dunstan FD, Jones SJ (2003) Are mobile speed cameras effective? A controlled before and after study. *Injury Prevention* **9**: 302–306.

Dumville J, Worthy G, Bland JM, Cullum N, Dowson C, Iglesias C *et al.* (2009) Larval therapy for leg ulcers (VenUS II): randomised controlled trial. *British Medical Journal* **338**: b773.

Franke RH, Kaul JD (1978) The Hawthorne experiments: first statistical interpretation. *American Sociological Review* **43**: 623–643.

Hollis S, Campbell F (1999) What is meant by intention to treat analysis? Survey of published randomised controlled trials. *British Medical Journal* **319**(7211): 670–674.

Jones JE, Nelson EA (1997) Evaluation of an education package in leg ulcer management. *Journal of Wound Care* **6**: 342–343.

Jull A, Walker N, Parag V, Molan P, Rodgers A (2008) Randomized clinical trial of honey-impregnated dressings for venous leg ulcers. *British Journal of Surgery* **95**: 175–182.

Kramer MS, Barr RG, Dagenis S, Yang H, Jones P, Ciofanis L, Jane F (2001) Pacifier use, early weaning, and cry/fuss behaviour. *Journal of the American Medical Association* **286**: 322–326.

Meyer C, Ulbricht S, Baumeister SE, Schumann A, Ruge J, Bischof G *et al.* (2008) Proactive interventions for smoking cessation in general medical practice: a quasi-randomized controlled trial to examine the efficacy of computer-tailored letters and physician-delivered brief advice. *Addiction* **103**(2): 294–304.

Nelson EA, Prescott RJ, Harper DR, Gibson B, Brown D, Ruckley C (2007) A factorial, randomized trial of pentoxifylline or placebo, four-layer or single-layer compression, and knitted viscose or hydrocolloid dressings for venous ulcers. *Journal of Vascular Surgery* **45**(1): 134–141.

Nikles CJ, Mitchell GK, Del Mar CB, Clavarino A, McNairn N (2006) An *n*-of-1 trial service in clinical practice: testing the effectiveness of stimulants for attention-deficit/hyperactivity disorder. *Pediatrics* **117**: 2040–2046.

O'Brien JF, Grace PA, Perry IJ, Hannigan A, Clarke Moloney M, Burke PE (2003) Randomized clinical trial and economic analysis of four-layer compression bandaging for venous ulcers. *British Journal of Surgery* **90**: 794–798.

Reynolds T, Russell L, Deeth M, Jones H, Birchall L (2004) A randomised controlled trial comparing Drawtex with standard dressings for exuding wounds. *Journal of Wound Care* **13**(2): 71–74.

Schulz KF, Grimes DA (2002) Allocation concealment in randomised trials: defending against deciphering. *Lancet* **359**: 614–618.

Sheldon T, Cullum N, Dawson D, Lankshear A, Lowson K, Watt I *et al.* (2004) What's the evidence that NICE guidance has been implemented? Results from a national evaluation using time series analysis, audit of patients' notes, and interviews. *British Medical Journal* **329**: 999.

Ubbink DT, Vermeulen H, Goossens A, Kelner RB, Schreuder SM, Lubbers MJ (2008) Occlusive vs gauze dressings for local wound care in surgical patients: a randomized clinical trial. *Archives of Surgery* **143**: 950–955.

Websites

www.cochrane.org/index0.htm – Cochrane Library: contains databases of systematic reviews and of trial reports (freely available via www to people in England, Wales, Scotland, Northern Ireland and Southern Ireland).

www.ethics-network.org.uk/educational-resources/mental-capacity-act-2005 – Resource on the Mental Capacity Act.

www.jameslindlibrary.org – James Lind Library: history of trials in medicine and why we need them.

www.phru.nhs.uk/Pages/PHD/resources.htm – Critical Appraisal Skills Programme: resources to help appraise clinical studies such as trials.

18 Surveys

Hugh McKenna, Felicity Hasson
and Sinead Keeney

Key points

- Descriptive surveys aim to describe what exists, whereas correlational and comparative surveys investigate and compare the relationship between variables.

- Surveys can capture the time dimension by being retrospective (past behaviour) and prospective (future propensities).

- Longitudinal surveys are conducted to monitor changes across a period of time.

- Data collection methods used in surveys include questionnaires, interviews, observation and analysis of secondary data.

- Epidemiology is a form of survey research that is concerned with how and why diseases and risk factors occur in populations.

- Epidemiological research has a long tradition in medicine, but is less commonly applied to nursing.

HISTORICAL DEVELOPMENT OF SURVEY RESEARCH IN HEALTH

It is impossible to determine when the first survey was conducted. Several accounts are given in the Bible, beginning with a census taken after Moses ascended Mount Sinai (Weisberg *et al.* 1996). Later the Romans carried out censuses to prepare for taxation. The social surveys that were at the heart of the early 20th-century survey movement were also total censuses of the cities studied, merging census data with special surveys of topics, such as housing conditions. In England, 19th-century surveys were conducted by independent individuals and government

agencies in attempts to study social conditions and the nature of poverty. For instance, in 1902 Charles Booth conducted his monumental inquiry into the *Labour and Life of the People of London'* (1889–1902). In 1912, Bowley undertook a study of working-class conditions. This was published as *Livelihood and Poverty* (Bowley & Burnett-Hurst 1915). Bowley's great methodological contribution was his use of statistical sampling, which came to act as a decisive stimulus to social surveys (Moser & Kalton 1971).

At the end of the World War I, a new approach was adopted that was different to censuses; it used psychophysical laboratories in which a small number of consumers were brought in for standardised product testing (Rossi *et al.* 1983). Market research psychologists introduced the techniques of questioning people on their preferences to a range of issues. The mid-1930s saw an expansion in the use of survey methods in public opinion polling. This was pioneered by George Gallup in America.

At the beginning of the 21st century, the survey is an established method of social inquiry. Since the time of Booth and Bowley, great changes have occurred in the amount of survey activity and in the interest by the public to this research approach. There have been considerable changes in methods of collecting and storing survey data due specifically to technological developments.

DESCRIPTIVE SURVEYS

The most common objective of survey research is to describe. In descriptive surveys, statistics are collected about a large group: for example, the proportion of men and women who view a television programme or who participated in a health-screening programme. They can be designed to measure events, behaviour and attitudes in a given population or sample of interest. So a descriptive survey is used to obtain information on the current status of phenomena so as to describe '*what exists*' with respect to variables or conditions (Sim & Wright 2000).

For example, a Gallup poll conducted during a political election campaign has the purpose of describing the voting intentions of the electorate. Descriptive surveys are based on the assumption that the answer to the research question may exist in the present so the objective is to collect this information in a systematic way. They are indispensable in the early stages of studying a phenomenon (Dublin 1978) because the information gained helps to develop concepts that can then be developed into theories.

Descriptive surveys are also carried out to describe populations, to study associations between variables, and to establish trends and possible links between variables. While this is valuable, they cannot provide robust evidence about the direction of cause-and-effect relationships. Research Example 18.1 provides an example of such a survey.

Descriptive surveys have several advantages over other types of survey, but perhaps the main one is that they are relatively easy to undertake as they involve only one contact with the study population. However, there is the potential problem that the respondents give the answers that they believe the researcher wants to hear, rather than their true views. Another, disadvantage is that they cannot measure change, so if things change rapidly, the survey information may

---

RESEARCH EXAMPLE

18.1 A Descriptive Survey

Zilembo M, Monterosso L (2008) Nursing students perceptions of desirable leadership qualities in nurse preceptors: a descriptive survey. *Contemporary Nurse* **27**(2): 194–206.

There is a paucity of literature examining the context of leadership within the clinical preceptor–undergraduate nursing student relationship and the relevance of this to the clinical learning environment. This study used a mixed methodological survey approach to explore the leadership qualities in nurse preceptors that are considered desirable and contribute to positive practicum experiences from the perspective of 23 undergraduate nurses. Findings showed students both want and need leadership from their preceptors in order to develop psychomotor skill competency and to experience orientation to the real world of nursing care. Gaining insight into the leadership qualities that students perceive as desirable to enhance the practical experience is vital since that practical experience is viewed as the making or breaking of many students and influences retention in undergraduate education and within the profession post registration.

easily become outdated. To measure change it is necessary to have at least two observations, that is at least two cross-sectional studies, at two points in time, on the same population. Furthermore, the results of surveys can be wrong. One of the most famous examples of this was the survey poll that predicted a landslide victory of Thomas E Dewey over Harry S Truman in the 1948 presidential elections. Truman won with a two million majority.

CORRELATIONAL AND COMPARATIVE SURVEYS

These types of survey are devoted to investigating and comparing the relationship between variables. For example, a questionnaire may be administered to a large number of patients to find out whether there is a difference in the self-reported levels of postoperative stress between those who received information and those who did not. In each case, the question is whether there is a relationship between variable X and variable Y. In correlational studies, a researcher can collect demographic details such as age, occupation, gender and educational background, and seek to establish links between these and other characteristics of participants such as their beliefs and behaviours (Parahoo 1997). The purpose is often to develop hypotheses and in turn contribute to theory development. It does so from theory-based expectations on how and why variables should be related. Hypotheses can be basic (i.e. relationships exist) or directional (i.e. the relationship is positive or negative). Such surveys only tell us that there is a relationship between the two variables; they do not tell us whether one variable 'caused' the other. Correlational studies have little control over the respondents' environment and thus have difficulty ruling out alternative explanations for causation.

In comparative surveys, data are collected that allow comparisons to be made according to demographic features such as age, gender or class. Therefore, the main purpose of such studies is to compare variables across people, places or time. If changes are surveyed over time we may need to compare data collected as a baseline with those collected some time later. If we want to know the effects of behaviour such as smoking or drinking, we can compare those who indulge in these practices with those who do not. Such studies can be quantitative, qualitative or both.

Comparative surveys encounter a number of potential limitations, including problems in ensuring comparable measures and samples. For example, over 65 countries participate in the World Values Survey (www.worldvaluessurvey.org). This involves comparing results across countries. Different sample designs in different countries, different methods of administering surveys, different acceptance of survey research and different levels of interviewer training and technique can cause problems. This can result in design-based measurement errors, in which the same methods of data collection and the same questions are used in very different cultural contexts.

Prospective and retrospective survey designs

Surveys can capture a snapshot of the attitudes, beliefs and behaviours of individuals and groups in the present, and they can also be applied retrospectively and prospectively.

A retrospective design is one in which researchers study a current phenomenon by seeking information from the past. Researchers have to work backwards and search for variables or factors to help shed light on issues. Such a design aims to describe or explain a phenomenon by examining factors with which it was associated. For example, patients' notes hold a considerable amount of information on the treatment and progress of their illness as well as demographic details. These can be used retrospectively to explain phenomena. Most cross-sectional studies are retrospective. This is a relatively inexpensive research method as large numbers of people can be surveyed quickly and data are easily coded (Bowling 1997).

One of the main drawbacks of retrospective designs is that the researcher relies on existing data that were, most probably, not collected for research purposes and therefore lack the required rigour. Furthermore, many archives that could be of interest to future researchers are being lost. For example, with the closure of many psychiatric hospitals, patients' notes and other materials are being destroyed. Also, descriptions of past behaviour may be highly subjective, and records may be incomplete and/or rely on respondents' memories. For instance, respondents may be asked questions about past diet and other lifestyle factors, and the potential for selectivity in recollection and recall bias is great. Despite these shortcomings, retrospective studies have been useful in, for example, studying the perspectives of older women regarding their experiences of living with ovarian cancer (Fitch *et al.* 2001).

The prospective survey is one that takes place over the forward passage of time with more than one period of data collection. Such studies attempt to establish the outcome of an event or explore what is likely to happen. For example, nurses may want to know the effects of new practices on patients' behaviour. Researchers using this design can have control over what they want to include in their study and how data are collected. Another example could be noting if and how the lifestyles of newly diagnosed cancer patients change over time. The researcher may compare this group of respondents with another group who do not have the illness (control group). With this design, data are collected at one or multiple points in the future. Such studies require careful definitions of the groups under study and careful selection of variables for measurement.

Prospective surveys can be expensive, take a long time, need a great amount of administration (e.g.

update and trace addresses) and can suffer from high sample attrition through natural loss, geographical mobility or refusals over time. Respondents can also become conditioned to the study and learn the responses that they believe are expected of them. In addition, there can be reactive effects of the research arrangements – the 'Hawthorne effect' – as people change simply as a result of being studied (Roethlisberger & Dickson 1939). Chapter 16 has a fuller discussion of this effect in experimental research. There needs to be a clear rationale to support the timing of repeated survey points, retaining the respondents' interests and participation and using sensitive instruments with relevant items that will detect change.

LONGITUDINAL SURVEYS AND COHORT STUDIES

Longitudinal surveys are normally conducted over a long period of time. Data collection takes place at regular intervals throughout the life of the study. The purpose of this is to monitor changes over time. Such surveys are sometimes referred to as panel studies. The British Household Panel Survey (Research Example 18.2) is a large-scale example of a longitudinal survey. The purpose of this survey is to monitor householders over a long period of time to analyse their responses to changes in the social and economic environment.

RESEARCH EXAMPLE

18.2 British Household Panel Survey

The British Household Panel survey began in 1991 and has followed the same group of respondents over the past 28 years. The main aim of the survey is to gain insight into social and economic change at the individual and household level. The survey is a resource for a wide range of social science disciplines and supports interdisciplinary research in many subject areas. It is a household-based study interviewing every adult member of a sampled household. It contains representation from different social groups, such as the elderly. The original panel consisted of 5,500 households from 250 areas of Great Britain. This equated to 10,300 individuals. In 1999, 1,500 households from Scotland and 1,500 households from Wales were added. In 2000, a further sample of 2,000 households from Northern Ireland were added.
www.statistics.gov.uk/STATBASE/Source.asp?vlnk=1308

The longitudinal survey may be of particular use in nursing research as certain phenomena from this field lend themselves to being studied over a long period of time. Parahoo (1997) used the example of people coming to terms with the loss of a spouse and the different phases that they may go through. It is obvious that in this case the collection of data on one isolated occasion would not be as beneficial as the collection of data at regular intervals over several years.

A cohort study is a form of longitudinal survey that uses a specific group of respondents for the entire study. Cohort studies chart the development of these groups from a particular time point, either prospectively or retrospectively. Such studies are concerned with life histories of sections of populations. They provide information on developmental changes across stages of life in any domain, including employment, education, housing, family and health.

Cohort studies have been used to study nurses. The most notable of these studies is the American Nurses Cohort Study (www.channing.harvard.edu/nhs/history/index.shtml). The original Nurses Cohort Study was established by Dr Frank Speizer in 1976 and was funded by the National Institutes of Health. The primary idea behind the survey was to investigate the potential long-term consequences of oral contraceptives, diet and lifestyle risk factors. Over 170,000 nurses completed baseline questionnaires for this study. Questionnaires are administered to the cohort every four years.

One of the main problems of longitudinal and cohort studies is that the respondents may drop out of the study. This is termed 'mortality' or 'attrition' (Parahoo 1997), and it can affect the success of a cohort study. Researchers can also move on to other roles or jobs and it is not uncommon to find that a succession of researchers have worked on the survey over the years.

Another difficulty with longitudinal studies is the effect of the research on the attitudes and behaviours of the respondents. By their very nature, longitudinal studies could serve to raise the awareness of the respondents and introduce bias. Time and cost are other inevitable consideration with longitudinal studies. In addition, it may be difficult to ensure continuity among respondents. In some cohort studies,

the researchers send Christmas cards and birthday cards to respondents to encourage continued participation.

SOURCES OF DATA IN SURVEY RESEARCH

Most people will have encountered a survey at some stage, either as a respondent to a postal survey or when approached by a market researcher in a supermarket, for example, or on the telephone. Organisations carry out surveys for a wide variety of reasons and results are used for different purposes, from changing policy to making decisions on a marketing strategy. Social researchers regard surveys as a valuable source of data about respondents' attitudes, beliefs, experience and behaviour.

Questionnaires and interviews

Chapters 28 and 30 describe the main data collection tools for surveys in more depth. Here we will discuss the relative merits of questionnaires and interviews for the purpose of a brief comparison of the two methods. There is no universal agreement among researchers about what should be called a questionnaire. It can mean a document containing a list of questions for respondents to complete on their own (the self-completion questionnaire) or it can mean a set of questions that a researcher reads out to a respondent. For the purpose of this chapter, a questionnaire will be considered to be a list of questions contained in a document that respondents complete themselves.

Questionnaires are usually distributed by post, although they can be distributed by hand, for example to patients or visitors in a hospital. More recently, researchers have been distributing questionnaires by email using a distribution list or simply by asking respondents to complete an online questionnaire (see Morris *et al.* 2004).

Generally, questionnaires follow a standardised format in which questions are pre-coded to provide a list of responses for selection by the respondent (tickbox questions). However, open-ended questions can be included with space to allow the respondent to provide a written answer. Questions should be easily comprehensible, as the respondent will not be able to seek clarification. For this reason, a questionnaire is often 'piloted' with a small subsection of the target population to ascertain if it is understandable, valid and acceptable. This may result in changes being made to question content or the length of the questionnaire. For a fuller discussion of questionnaires, turn to Chapter 30.

Face-to-face interviews use a list of questions sometimes called an interview guide. This guide may contain open or closed questions, or a combination of both. There is an important distinction between an interview schedule and an interview guide. An interview schedule uses a set of questions in a predetermined order that is adhered to during the interview. An interview guide is a list of areas to be covered, leaving the exact wording and order of the questions to be determined by the interviewer.

As the name implies, structured interviews tend to use an interview schedule with very explicit questions and leave no room for veering off the topic. Semi-structured interviews use the interview guides referred to above and there is room for exploration and for altering the questions based on a respondent's circumstances of replies. In contrast, unstructured interviews are totally open and the researcher has freedom to explore a range of issues around a general subject area. The internet also facilitates opportunities to conduct electronic interactive interviews via email or through the use of chat rooms. However, although electronic technologies are convenient and low cost for the researcher, they are still novel and raise many ethical questions.

Within face-to-face interviews, researchers may record responses by pen or directly on to a laptop computer. This approach is generally reserved for structured interviews that include many closed questions. For interviews using more open-ended questions, the interview is usually audio-recorded. This recording would subsequently be transcribed as an interview transcript. Generally data from questionnaires are analysed using computerised database and statistical analysis software such as the Statistical Package for Social Scientists (SPSS). Chapter 28 provides a more detailed consideration of interviewing.

Self-completion questionnaires and face-to-face interviews are long-established methods of data collection and each have their own strengths and weaknesses (see Table 18.1).

Table 18.1 Face-to-face interviews versus self-completion questionnaires

Face-to-face interviews	Self-completion questionnaires
Costly due to time-intensive nature	Less costly – slower data collection method
Longer and more complex questions are possible	Limited in length and complexity
High response rates	Often associated with poor response rates
Can adapt to include visual materials, e.g. show cards	Excludes the less literate and those who may have a disability, e.g. dyslexia, blind
Provides additional opportunities to clarify questions and responses	No opportunity to explain complex instructions, to answer questions or to probe for more detail on open-ended questions
Interviewee is not anonymous	Respondent cannot be connected to their response. As a result more honest responses may be provided
Can be subject to bias – acquiescence and social desirability bias – if not carefully recruited	Respondents have more time to weigh the issues carefully before responding – less prone to acquiescence
Enables interviewer to ensure data are being collected from the correct sample	Researcher cannot ensure the target person completes the questionnaire. For example, a questionnaire aimed at exploring the views of a patient may be completed by a carer

Interview schedules are also used for interviews carried out over the telephone. Telephone surveys have similar benefits to face-to-face interviews, but also facilitate reaching a much wider population at less cost. Telephone surveys are less popular with social researchers than they are with market and commercial researchers. While they may be less expensive to undertake than face-to-face interviews, telephone surveys do not take cognisance of non-verbal cues and surroundings, and certain groups may have to be excluded from the survey because they do not have a telephone. The issue of the growing ownership of mobile phones is also creating problems for researchers. Nicolaas (2004) has identified sampling problems in relation to mobile phone users who tend not to be listed in phone directories. Furthermore, mobile phone numbers cannot be linked to a geographical area and they tend to belong to one individual rather than a household. However, recently Ipsos MORI (2009) identified that as of August 2007, 87% of people in the UK owned a mobile phone. On average in the UK, 6.5 billion text messages are sent every month equating to 1.4 million text messages every day (Mobile Data Association 2008). Figures from the Mobile Data Association (2008) have also shown that more than 12.3 million people used their mobile phone to access the internet in the last quarter of 2006. This could be viewed as an interesting and important way to reach participants to complete surveys. Organisations such as Ipsos MORI have panels of mobile phone users, in this case 11,000 people willing to take part in surveys via mobile phone. Among the advantages of this method of data collection are wide geographical reach, fast response, wide demographic reach and immediacy.

Secondary data sources

Gilbert asserted that it is 'a truism of social research that almost all data are seriously under-analysed' (Gilbert 1993: 256). This may be one of the reasons why analysis of secondary data sources is continuing to grow in popularity with social researchers. Secondary analysis of data sources implies that the data are being subjected to further analysis than that for which it was originally collected. There are many

sources of data that can be used for secondary analysis. Examples include patient or public records, such as medical records, audit data, attendance records, nationally available statistics stored in data banks, government data, academic data and research data collected for other purposes. Hospitals retain patient medical records, attendance records, complaints records and other statistical data on both patients and staff.

Census data are also available for secondary analysis. The National Statistics Office is responsible for UK census data. It can provide access to the UK data bank and this can provide large amounts of data on many and varied topics across a lengthy period of time. In the UK, the National Data Archive is located at the University of Essex. It holds mainly UK data but has reciprocal arrangements with other countries for access to their national data. However, the secondary analysis of some of these data may raise ethical questions and may be difficult to access. After all, respondents provide the data for a specific purpose and to use it for another purpose without their consent is potentially problematic.

Observation

Moser and Kalton described observation as 'the classic method of scientific enquiry' (Moser & Kalton 1971: 245). Nonetheless, social researchers use observation relatively infrequently. One type of observation used in survey research is non-participant observation. Chapter 32 deals in more detail with this and other ways of using observation for research purposes.

In terms of practicality and validity, direct observation can have a number of advantages to using a questionnaire or an interview schedule. For example, studies of children may have to rely on observational techniques as children may not be able to verbalise or write down answers. Responses provided within questionnaires or interviews may also be inaccurate, whereas observation will provide a true picture of the situation. For instance, interview data on how nurses' practise may differ from data collected through observing them working.

Observation also has limitations. Non-participant observation does not allow the researcher to explore people's attitudes or perceptions. It is also difficult to ensure representativeness using observational techniques. Furthermore, there are obvious ethical issues relating to seeing unsafe practices while being a non-participant observer.

EPIDEMIOLOGY

Epidemiology is the study of how often diseases occur in different groups of people, why they occur (Coggon *et al.* 1997) and the risk factors for these diseases (Bowling 1997). Historically, the impact of epidemiology on the health of the nation has been far-reaching (Whitehead 2000). There has been a long-standing tradition of epidemiology within healthcare. This is due to the fact that epidemiological research is used to plan and evaluate strategies to prevent illness and as a guide to the management of patients who have already developed a disease (Coggon *et al.* 1997). Epidemiology is concerned with observing, measuring and analysing health-related occurrences in human populations (Trichopoulos 1996). As nursing roles become more involved in preventative care and public health, epi-

demiology will become increasingly appropriate as a research method. There are four main types of epidemiological survey.

Descriptive study

Descriptive epidemiology describes the health status of a population or characteristics of a number of patients and attempts to find correlations among such characteristics as diet, air quality and occupation. Research Example 18.3 gives an example of such a study. As alluded to earlier, descriptive studies may be considered weak because they make no attempt to link cause and effect and therefore no causal association can be determined.

Cross-sectional studies

A cross-sectional study measures the prevalence of health outcomes or determinants of health, or both, in a population at a point in time or over a short period (Coggon *et al.* 1997). For example, such designs have been used to explore insulin resistance and depression (Timonen *et al.* 2005). However, associations must be interpreted with caution as bias

RESEARCH EXAMPLE

18.3   Descriptive Epidemiological Survey

Morize V, Nguyen DT, Lorente C, Desfosses G (1999) Descriptive epidemiological survey on a given day in all palliative care patients hospitalized in a French university hospital. *Palliative Medicine* **13**: 105–117.

This descriptive study was undertaken in a French university hospital with all inpatients requiring palliative care on one particular day. A team made up of doctors and nurses identified patients and described their needs, treatment, social and family circumstances, and outcomes by completing a standardised questionnaire. Inclusion criteria stated that participants should be inpatients in the hospital with advanced or terminal-stage life-threatening conditions. Two hundred and forty-five patients were included in the study. Results show that 66% of subjects suffered from physical discomfort and 80% suffered psychologically. Patients received specific treatment for their condition in 45% of cases. Social problems were identified in medium- or long-term care inpatients who made up 36% of the total inpatient population. Findings also showed that 25% of participants had requested assistance from the Palliative Care Unit's support team, mainly to provide psychological support for the patient. The results have led to reconsideration of the general organisation of palliative care in the healthcare system in France.

18.4 Epidemiological Cohort Study

Morgan J, Scholtz S, Lacey H, Conway G (2008) The prevalence of eating disorders in women with facial hirsutism: an epidemiological cohort study. *International Journal of Eating Disorders* **41**(5): 427–431.

The prevalence of eating disorders was evaluated in a population of women with increased facial hair (facial hirsutism). The structured clinical interview and the eating disorder evaluation were administered to 80 hirsute women presenting routinely to an endocrine outpatient clinic. Objective phenotypic severity of hyperandrogenic (increased masculinity) symptoms, gender role, self-esteem and social adjustment were quantified using validated measures, and weight height, and fertility were assessed during the interview. The prevalence of eating disorders was 36.3% (22.5% eating disorder not otherwise specified, 12.6% bulimia nervosa, 1.3% anorexia nervosa). Depression, anxiety, low self-esteem and poor social adjustment were more common in participants suffering from an eating disorder, and co-morbidity was universal in eating-disordered cases. The study demonstrates that hirsute women are at high risk of developing an eating disorder. Factors associated with eating disorders are examined and explanatory hypotheses are suggested for the possible underlying mechanisms in these women.

may arise because of selection into or out of the study population.

Case-controlled studies

A case-controlled study is a retrospective comparison of exposures of persons with disease (cases) with those of persons without the disease (controls). In case-controlled studies, such individuals are selected with and without the particular disease and asked about past exposure. Exposure rates within the two groups are compared. Case-controlled studies offer several advantages in that they are quick and relatively inexpensive to conduct and are suitable for studying multiple exposures and rare diseases. However, they present possible biases, such as recall bias and interviewer bias.

Cohort studies

A cohort study is a study in which a group of healthy people are either followed over time to measure their exposure to certain conditions or receive a particular

treatment and are compared with another group who are not affected by the condition under investigation. As with general cohort studies, they are expensive, time-consuming and logistically difficult; however, the design is less subject to bias because it measures exposure before researchers learn the health outcome. Research Example 18.4 provides an example of an epidemiological cohort study.

CONCLUSIONS

This chapter has set the survey in its historical context and outlined the main types of survey used within nursing research. The sources of data are discussed and the pros and cons of self-completion questionnaires, face-to-face interviews and telephone interviews considered. Other methods used within survey research are also explored, including secondary data analysis and observations. Epidemiological research and its applicability to nursing research is also outlined. With the nursing body of knowledge still in the early stages of development there is every indication that survey research will continue to be popular for some time to come.

References

Booth C (ed) (1889–1902) *Labour and Life of the People of London* (17 volumes). London, Macmillan.

Bowley AL, Burnett-Hurst AR (1915) *Livelihood and Poverty: a study in the economic conditions of working-class households in Northampton, Warrington, Stanley and Reading.* London, Bell.

Bowling A (1997) *Research Methods in Health: investigating health and health services.* Buckingham, Open University Press.

Coggon D, Rose G, Barker DJP (1997) *Epidemiology for the Uninitiated*, 4th edition. London, BMJ Publishing.

Dublin R (1978) *Theory Building.* New York, The Free Press.

Fitch MI, Gray RE, Franssen E (2001) Perspectives on living with ovarian cancer: older women's views. *Oncology Nursing Forum* **28**(9): 1433–1442.

Gilbert N (1993) *Researching Social Life.* London, Sage.

Ipsos MORI (2009) *Research via Mobile Phones* (www.ipsos-mori.com/researchtechniques/techniques-methodologies/onlineresearch/research-via-mobile-phones.ashx; accessed 26 January 2009).

Mobile Data Association (2008) *The Q3 2008 UK Mobile Trends Report.* MDA, London.

Morgan J, Scholtz S, Lacey H, Conway G (2008) The prevalence of eating disorders in women with facial hirsutism: an epidemiological cohort study. *International Journal of Eating Disorders* **41**(5): 427–431.

Morize V, Nguyen DT, Lorente C, Desfosses G (1999) Descriptive epidemiological survey on a given day in all palliative care patients hospitalized in a French university hospital. *Palliative Medicine* **13**: 105–117.

Morris DL, Fenton MV, Mercer ZB (2004) Identification of national trends in nursing education through the use of an online survey. *Nursing Outlook* **52**: 248–254.

Moser C, Kalton G (1971) *Survey Methods in Social Investigation.* London, Heinemann.

Nicolaas G (2004) *Sampling Issues for Telephone Surveys in Scotland.* Survey Methods Unit, National Centre for Social Research (available online at www.bioss.ac.uk/rss/gerry_nicolaas.ppt).

Parahoo AK (1997) *Nursing Research Principles, Process and Issues.* London, Macmillan.

Roethlisberger EJ, Dickson WJ (1939) *Management and the Worker.* Cambridge, Harvard University Press.

Rossi P, Wright J, Anderson A (1983) *Handbook of Survey Research.* New York, Academic Press.

Sim J, Wright C (2000) *Research in Health Care. Concepts, designs and methods.* Cheltenham, Stanley Thornes.

Timonen M, Laakso M, Jokelainen J, Rajala U, Meyer-Rochow BV, Keinänen-Kiukaanniemi S (2005) Insulin resistance and depression: cross sectional study. *British Medical Journal* **330**: 17–18.

Trichopoulos D (1996) The future of epidemiology. *British Medical Journal* **313**: 436–437.

Weisberg H, Krosnick J, Bowen B (1996) *An Introduction to Survey Research, Polling and Data Analysis*, 3rd edition. Thousand Oaks, Sage.

Whitehead D (2000) Is there a place for epidemiology in nursing? *Nursing Standard* **14**(42): 35–38.

Zilembo M, Monterosso L (2008) Nursing students perceptions of desirable leadership qualities in nurse preceptors: a descriptive survey. *Contemporary Nurse* **27**(2): 194–206.

Further reading

Alreck PL, Settle RB (1995) *The Survey Research Handbook: guidelines and strategies for conducting a survey*, 2nd edition. New York, McGraw-Hill.

Bailey L, Vardulaki K, Langham J, Chandramohan D (2006) *Introduction to Epidemiology (Understanding Public Health).* New York, Open University Press.

Bruce N, Pope D, Stanistreet D (2008) *Quantitative Methods for Healthcare: a practical interactive guide to epidemiology and statistics.* London, John Wiley & Sons.

Bulmer M, Sturgis PJ, Allum N (2009) *The Secondary Analysis of Survey Data (Sage Benchmarks in Social Research Methods Series).* London, Sage.

Chang CL, Donaghy M, Poulter N (1999) Migraine and stroke in young women: case-control study. *British Medical Journal* **318**: 13–18.

De Vaus D (2002) *Surveys in Social Research*, 5th edition. New South Wales, Allen & Unwin.

Feldkamp ML, Reefhuis J, Kucik J, Krikov S, Wilson A, Moore CA *et al.* (2008) Case-control study of self reported genitourinary infections and risk of gastroschisis: findings from the national birth defects prevention study, 1997–2003. *British Medical Journal* **336**: 1420–1423.

French S, Peterson CB, Story M, Anderson N, Mussell MP, Mitchell JE (1998) Agreement between survey and interview measures of weight control practices in adolescents. *International Journal of Eating Disorders* **23**: 45–56.

Jinks MA, Lawson V, Daniela R (2003) A survey of the health needs of hospital staff: implications for health care managers. *Journal of Nursing Management* **11**: 343–350.

Mulhall A (1996) *Epidemiology, Nursing and Healthcare: a new perspective.* Houndsmill, Palgrave Macmillan.

Ray LM, Parker RA (2005) *Designing and Conducting Survey Research: a comprehensive guide.* San Francisco, Jossey Bass.

Websites

www.isworld.org/surveyinstruments/tutor.htm – a tutorial on survey instruments.

www.socialresearchmethods.net/kb/survey.php – Research Methods Knowledge Base: Survey Research.

www.worldvaluessurvey.org/ – World Values Survey are designed to provide a comprehensive measurement of all major areas of human concern, from religion to politics to economic and social life.

19 The Delphi Technique

Sinead Keeney

Key points

- The Delphi technique is an approach used to gain consensus on a certain issue or set of issues. It is based on the assumption that group opinion is more valid than individual opinion.

- The Delphi technique is a structured process that uses a series of questionnaires to gather information from a panel of experts and is continued until group consensus is reached. The number of rounds depends on how easily consensus is reached on a topic, the time available and the type of Delphi approach used.

- The Delphi technique has evolved into a number of modifications. Each type of Delphi has the same aim, to gain consensus on the issue at hand, but differs in the process used to reach this consensus.

- Consensus reached using the Delphi technique does not mean that the correct answer has been found, but rather that the experts have come to an agreement on the issue or issues under exploration.

INTRODUCTION

The Delphi technique is a research approach used to gain consensus on a certain issue or set of issues. It is a structured process that uses a series of questionnaires or rounds to gather information and is continued until group consensus is reached (Hasson *et al.* 2000). The name 'Delphi' is derived from the site of legendary Oracle of Delphi (the most important oracle in the classical Greek world) where anyone could visit the oracle to ask a question and receive an answer.

The main premise of the Delphi technique is based on the assumption that group opinion is more valid than individual opinion. A novel and contemporary way of illustrating this is through the use of 'ask the audience' in the popular television game show *Who Wants to be a Millionaire?*. The audience effectively acts as the 'expert panel' – as experts in general knowledge – and the contestant asks for their opinion on a certain question. The audience members give their opinion on the answer using a keypad and the results are displayed in a bar chart format showing where the consensus lies. Obviously the word 'expert' is used loosely here, but this demonstrates the main premise of the Delphi technique that group opinion is considered more 'valid' and 'reliable' than individual opinion.

The Delphi technique has been used by nurse researchers in a variety of studies over the past three decades. The purpose of these studies has been to identify research priorities for a particular area within nursing (Drennan *et al.* 2007; McCance *et al.* 2007; Bäck-Pettersson *et al.* 2008) to gain consensus on an issue or set of issues within nursing (Handler *et al.* 2008; Polivka *et al.* 2008; Jirwe *et al.* 2009); or to solve a particular problem (Wagenaar *et al.* 2003; McKeown & Gibson 2007). There have been numerous variations in application, design, administration and analysis of the Delphi technique within these studies, which demonstrates the flexibility and diversity of the technique. Research Example 19.1 illustrates the use of the Delphi within a nursing research study.

DEFINING THE DELPHI TECHNIQUE

The original advocates of the Delphi technique, Dalkey and Helmer (1963), defined it as a method used to obtain the most reliable consensus of opinion of a group of experts by a series of intensive questionnaires interspersed with controlled feedback. With increasing usage, other definitions have been put forward. For instance, Reid (1998) described the Delphi as a method for the systematic collection and aggregation of informed judgement from a group of experts on specific questions and issues, whereas Lynn *et al.* (1998) described it as an iterative process designed to combine expert opinion into group consensus. However, common among all definitions is the intention to achieve consensus among a group of experts on a certain issue through using a forecasting process to determine, predict and explore group attitudes, needs and priorities. Box 19.1 sets out the characteristics of the classical Delphi approach.

THE EXPERT PANEL

The popularity of the Delphi technique has centred on the fact that it allows the anonymous inclusion of a large number of individuals across diverse locations and expertise, and avoids the situation where a spe-

---

RESEARCH EXAMPLE

19.1   Delphi Study

Jirwe M, Gerrish K, Keeney S, Emami A (2009) Identifying the core components of cultural competence: findings from a Delphi study. *Journal of Clinical Nursing* **18**: 2622–2634.

The aim of this study was to identify the core components of cultural competence from a Swedish perspective. The methodology comprised a four-round modified Delphi technique. The initial round involved individual semi-structured interviews with a purposive sample of 24 experts (eight nurses, eight researchers, eight lecturers) who were knowledgeable in multicultural issues. The interviews explored the knowledge, skills and attitudes that formed the components of cultural competence. Content analysis of interview transcripts yielded statements that were developed into a questionnaire. Respondents scored questionnaire items in terms of perceived importance. The consensus level was set at 75%. Statements that reached consensus were removed from questionnaires used in subsequent rounds. Three rounds of questionnaires were distributed in total.

Consensus was reached on 118 of the 137 questionnaire items. These were grouped into five categories: cultural sensitivity; cultural understanding; cultural encounters; understanding of health, ill health and healthcare; and social and cultural contexts.

Acquisition of the knowledge, skills and attitudes identified should enable nurses to meet the needs of patients from different cultural backgrounds. The components of cultural competence can form the basis of nursing curricula.

Box 19.1 Characteristics of a classical Delphi

1 The use of a panel of 'experts' for obtaining data
2 Participants do not meet in face-to-face discussions
3 The use of sequential questionnaires and/or interviews
4 The systematic emergence of a concurrence of judgement or opinion
5 The guarantee of anonymity for participants' responses
6 The use of frequency distributions to identify patterns of agreement
7 The use of two or more rounds, between which a summary of the results of the previous round is communicated to and evaluated by panel members

(McKenna 1994a)

cific expert might be anticipated to dominate the consensus process (Jairarth & Weinstein 1994). It uses a purposive sample of 'experts' rather than a random sample that is representative of the target population. An expert has been defined as an informed individual (McKenna 1994a), a specialist in the field (Goodman 1987) or someone who has knowledge about a specific subject (Green *et al.* 1999).

Choosing an appropriate expert panel is critical for success (Hung *et al.* 2008). It is the first stage of the Delphi process and regarded as the 'lynchpin of the method' (Green *et al.* 1999). However, the selection of the expert sample raises some methodological concerns. The claim of the Delphi to represent valid expert opinion has been criticised as scientifically untenable and overstated (Strauss & Zeigler 1975). It is not surprising that Goodman (1987) warns about the 'pitfalls of illusory expertise' and the 'potentially misleading title of expert'.

Simply because individuals have knowledge of a particular topic does not necessarily mean that they are appropriate 'experts'. Those who are willing to engage in discussion are more likely to be affected directly by the outcome of the process and are also more likely to become and stay involved in the study. Hence, the commitment of participants is related to their interest and involvement with the issue being addressed. However, respondents must be relatively impartial so that the information obtained reflects current knowledge or perceptions (Goodman 1987). This balance is difficult to achieve and justify to the consumers of the finished research.

Size of the expert panel

There is little agreement about the size of the expert panel, the relationship of the panel to the larger population of experts and the sampling method used to select such experts (Williams & Webb 1994). Sample size and heterogeneity depend on the purpose of the project, design selected and time frame for data collection (McKenna 1994a; Green *et al.* 1999). For the conventional Delphi, a heterogeneous sample is used to ensure that the entire spectrum of opinion is determined (Moore 1987). Sampling different groups of experts such as nurse educators and nurse students may ensure heterogeneity.

There is no agreed optimum expert panel size. Dalkey and Hemler (1963) proposed a minimum number seven experts, Burns (1998) suggests an optimum number of 15, Alexander and Kroposki (1999) argued for 60, whereas Linstone (1978) reported on studies that had used several hundred panellists. However, panels of between 20 and 50 participants are most frequently recommended (Endacott *et al.* 1999).

It can be helpful to specify inclusion criteria to create boundaries around an expert panel (Keeney *et al.* 2006). These criteria may include, for example, specific qualifications, number of publications in the area of expertise, geographical location or years experience in a particular area. Consideration also needs to be given to the workload generated by the various rounds, which needs to be balanced with the time available to complete the study. A large panel of experts will require more time to administer the questionnaires and to follow up people who fail to respond than a smaller and more manageable sample.

DELPHI ROUNDS

The Delphi technique employs a number of rounds in which questionnaires are sent out until consensus is reached (Beretta 1996). In each round, a summary of the results of the previous round is included and evaluated by the panel members to facilitate the systematic emergence of a concurrence of opinion among the panel of experts (McKenna 1994a). The number of rounds depends on the time available and whether the first round is intended to generate items to be considered in subsequent rounds or whether the items are identified by the researcher in advance.

The process raises the question of how many rounds it takes to reach consensus. The classical original Delphi used four rounds (Young & Hogben 1978). However, this has been modified by many to suit individual research aims and in some cases it has been shortened to two or three rounds (Beech 1997). It can be difficult to retain a high response rate in a Delphi study that has many rounds. The topic needs to be of great interest to the panel members or they need to be rewarded in other ways.

Round one

Round one of the classical Delphi (see Box 19.1) starts with an open-ended set of questions, thus allowing panel members freedom in their responses. The number of items generated can be extremely large and can lead to a very lengthy second-round questionnaire if the researcher opts to include all panel members' round one views. This may put panel members off participating and it can become very difficult to sustain the experts' interest in the study (Green *et al.* 1999).

Traditionally, round one is used to generate ideas and the panel members are asked for their responses to or comments about an issue. There is now some support for revising the approach and providing pre-

existing information (for example from the literature) for ranking. However, it must be recognised that this approach could bias the responses or limit the available options. Nonetheless, a clear advantage to commencing the process in this way is that it is more time efficient (Jenkins & Smith 1994).

Subsequent rounds

Subsequent rounds generally take the form of structured questionnaires incorporating feedback to each panel member. The data from each round are analysed and circulated to panel members. In this way, the Delphi allows efficient and rapid collection of expert opinions, while the feedback is controlled (Buck *et al.* 1993). This process encourages panel members to become more involved and motivated to participate (Walker & Selfe 1996) and can lead to perceptions of ownership and acceptance of the findings (McKenna 1994a).

The Delphi study might encounter problems due to a decline in response rate because, in order to achieve consensus, it is important that those panel members who have agreed to participate stay involved until the process is completed (Buck *et al.* 1993). However, poor response rates are often a characterisation of the fourth and final round of the Delphi. This could be why many researchers are now stopping at two or three rounds rather than the originally recommended four rounds.

Number of rounds

One of the basic principles underpinning the Delphi technique is to have as many rounds as are required to achieve consensus or until the law of diminishing returns occurs (McKenna 1994a). Provision for feedback and opportunity to revise earlier responses obviously requires that the Delphi has at least two rounds. However, the number of rounds can be a matter of dispute. There are no strict guidelines on the correct number of rounds, and the number in a particular study can depend on the time available and whether the researcher ignited the Delphi sequence with one broad question or with a list of questions or events.

RESPONSE RATES

In general, questionnaire research is notorious for its low response rates. Researchers often have to send out two or three reminder letters to non-responders. With anything up to four rounds of questionnaires, a Delphi study asks much more of respondents than a simple survey and the potential for low response rates increases dramatically.

To enhance response rates in Delphi rounds it is critical that participants are interested in the topic and feel that they are partners in the study. The researcher should take every opportunity to remind participants that each round is constructed entirely on their responses to previous rounds, encouraging ownership and active participation. This attempt to encourage participants psychologically to sign up to a study is common in longitudinal cohort studies where researchers send regular update newsletters to participants as well as sometimes birthday or Christmas cards.

McKenna (1994b) suggested that the personal touch could help enhance return rates. Using face-to-face interviews as his first round, he achieved a 100% response rate, which is rare in a Delphi study. Such a relationship is necessary to increase the likelihood of ongoing commitment from the participant. It starts at initial contact where the researcher gains informed consent and explains either in writing or verbally the nature of the research, what the participant's role is and what is required of them. Recruiting letters should include an explanation of the study, anticipated number of rounds, outline of time commitment and a consent form or confirmation of acceptance to take part in the study. The idea behind this is to get the expert panel to sign up to take part in the study before it begins.

The follow-up of non-respondents is essential. Researchers may do this in different ways, including sending follow-up letters, a further copy of the questionnaire or a follow-up phone call or email (McKenna & Keeney 2004). Prompt and appropriate feedback can also facilitate a high response rate as it keeps the members of the expert panel on board. If weeks or even months pass before panel members receive feedback on the previous round they are likely to lose interest.

MODIFICATIONS OF THE DELPHI TECHNIQUE

Since its inception, the Delphi technique has evolved into a number of modified versions. Each type of Delphi has the same aim – to gain consensus on the issue at hand – but differs in the process used to reach this consensus. There are numerous accounts in the literature reporting Delphi studies using these different manifestations and this is tribute to the flexibility of the method.

At present there are no formal, universally agreed guidelines on the use of the Delphi, nor does any standardisation of methodology exist (Evans 1997). Consequently, there is flexibility in the design and format of the Delphi and it often depends on the study's aims and objectives. The most popular formats include:

- the modified Delphi (McKenna 1994b)
- the policy Delphi (Turoff 1970; Crisp *et al.* 1997)
- the decision Delphi (Couper 1984)
- the real-time Delphi (Beretta 1996)
- the e-Delphi (Sheikh *et al.* 2008).

Box 19.2 shows the different forms and main characteristics of these types of Delphi.

The approaches used with a Delphi study may differ. For example, in the traditional design (Linstone 1978), the content for the first round is normally obtained from the literature rather than the qualitative views of participants or from other secondary data. Other variations to the Delphi exist, for example Procter and Hunt (1994) sent participant nurses three patient profiles with the remit to identify the care needs of each patient, while Jones *et al.* (1992) involved the use of face-to-face meetings of participants after two initial Delphi rounds.

The lesson here is to acknowledge that if modification of the technique is not systematic and rigorous it may be problematic. For example, using literature sources as the basis for round one can cause premature closure of ideas and bias the results. Without care, this could result in a self-fulfilling prophecy where participants could be steered to agree on a highly visible issue in the literature. The researcher

Box 19.2   Types of Delphi and main characteristics

Classical Delphi	uses factual based information to elicit opinion and gain consensus (e.g. first round based in literature in the area); uses three or more postal rounds
Modified Delphi	modification usually takes the form of replacing the first postal round with face-to-face interviews or focus group; may use fewer than three postal rounds
Decision Delphi	same process usually adopted as a classical Delphi; focuses on making decisions rather than coming to consensus
Policy Delphi	uses the opinions of experts to come to consensus and agree future policy on a given topic
Real-time Delphi	similar process to classical Delphi except that experts may be in the same room and consensus reached in real time rather than by post; sometimes referred to as a consensus conference
e-Delphi	similar process to the classical Delphi but administered by email or online web survey
Technological Delphi	similar to the real-time Delphi but using technology such as hand-held keypads allowing experts to respond to questions immediately while the technology works out the mean/median and allows instant feedback allowing experts the change to re-vote moving towards consensus in the light of group opinion

should allow participants freedom to bring their views to the first round.

TIME FRAME

The time it takes to administer a Delphi study varies considerably and depends on several factors, not least of which the type of Delphi used. Obviously a real-time Delphi study will be completed in one day, whereas a classical Delphi study could take over six months to complete. The size of expert panel will be a major determining factor in the time frame of the study. The more participants there are in an expert panel, the more views and opinions will be elicited in the first place and the wider the spread of opinion is likely to be. This in turn can lead to a greater number of rounds being needed to reach consensus.

ANONYMITY

The intention in a Delphi study is to seek to ensure anonymity whereby panel members are not known to each other. Anonymity provides an equal chance for each panel member to present and react to ideas without being influenced by the identities of other participants (Goodman 1987). Reactions are given independently, so each opinion carries the same weight and is given equal importance in the analysis. In this way subject bias is eliminated (Jeffery *et al.* 1995).

This promise of anonymity facilitates respondents' openness about their views on certain issues, which in turn provides insightful data for the researcher. Furthermore, it gives each participant the opportunity to express an opinion to others without feeling pressured by more influential panel members (Couper 1984). It is unclear at present whether respondents in a Delphi process change their opinions on the basis of new information or, despite the protection of anonymity, feel pressurised to conform to the group's view.

However, complete anonymity cannot be guaranteed when using the Delphi technique. First, the researcher knows the panel members and their responses, and second, it is often the case that panel members know each other. However, they cannot attribute responses to any one member. McKenna (1994b) coined the term 'quasi-anonymity' for when the respondents may be known to one another, but their judgements and opinions remain anonymous.

GAINING CONSENSUS

The reason for using the Delphi technique is to gain consensus or a judgement among a group of perceived experts on a topic. However, expert opinions can differ and it would be difficult to gain 100% agreement on all issues. Therefore, a key question in any Delphi study is what percentage agreement a researcher would accept as synonymous with consensus. As with most aspects of the Delphi, the literature provides few clear guidelines on what consensus level to set. Loughlin and Moore (1979) suggested that consensus should be equated with 51% agreement among respondents. Any views that receive less than this percentage cut-off point are rejected and not used in subsequent rounds. By contrast, Green *et al.* (1999) used an 80% consensus level. Establishing the standard is crucial, since the level chosen determines what items are discarded or retained as the rounds unfold. It is good practice to establish the consensus level before data collection.

INTERPRETING RESULTS

According to Evans (1997) the terms 'agreement' and 'consensus' are essentially two different ideologies. Is there a difference between the extent to which each participant agrees with the *issue* under consideration and the extent to which participants agree with *each other*? When reporting findings, few studies do so in the context of these different principles. Most researchers report findings on participants' agreement with *each other*. However, the extent to which participants agree with each other does not mean that consensus exists, nor does it mean that the 'correct' answer has been found. This is especially the case when the issues have ethical implications.

Advocates of the Delphi approach would argue that panel members change their minds and move towards consensus because they see that someone else has identified a more relevant issue that they had not thought of. Delphi cynics would assert that panel members are cajoled to change their minds because of a possible mistaken belief that the views expressed by the majority of the panel must be right. The obvious conclusion of this assertion is that strong-willed panel members hold rigidly to their views across rounds and weak-willed panel members alter theirs. If true, this challenges seriously the validity and reliability of Delphi findings.

Therefore, there is a danger of placing too much reliance on the results without acknowledging the influence of bias and other factors of validity and reliability. Ultimately, there is the possibility of obtaining the 'wrong' answer from the participants. A number of strategies can be used to enhance authenticity. For instance, pilot testing, the integration of an additional methodological technique such as focus groups, or the comparison with secondary validated data.

SKILLS OF THE RESEARCHER

The success of a Delphi study relies on the skills of the researcher. These include establishing an administration system and analysing and presenting both qualitative and quantitative data. While these skills are not paid much attention in the literature, their presence is vital for an effective and efficient Delphi study.

Researchers must design their own administrative system to allow for tracking of individual responses for each round, which will enable non-respondents to be traced and targeted. Using self-administrative questionnaires requires the establishment of a mail base and the allocation of physical and financial resources to cover costs of postage, printing, telephone bills and photocopying. Like most research studies, the Delphi study will fail if administrative systems are not in place to ensure that proper processes are followed. Due to the multiple rounds that make up a Delphi study, high-quality administrative systems are crucial for success.

CRITIQUE OF THE TECHNIQUE

There are many advantages to using the Delphi technique but also some limitations, and these should be considered before beginning a study using the Delphi. Box 19.3 summarises the advantages and limitations of the technique.

It should be noted that the existence of consensus from a Delphi study does not mean that the correct answer has been found. There is a danger that the Delphi can lead the researcher to place greater reliance on the results than might otherwise be warranted. In addition, the Delphi has been criticised as a method that forces consensus and is weakened by not allowing participants to discuss issues, providing no opportunity for respondents to elaborate on their views (Walker & Selfe 1996).

ETHICAL CONSIDERATIONS

A Delphi study is subject to the same ethical considerations as any postal survey (see Chapter 18). However, there are some particular ethical issues that merit consideration. The issue of anonymity has been discussed earlier in this chapter and it has been noted that despite the researcher's best endeavours, participants may be known to each other, especially when the field from which the experts can be drawn is small. Nevertheless, it is important that the researcher does not disclose the responses from individual respondents to other panel members

Beretta (1996) has drawn attention to a study by Hitch and Murgatroyd (1983), who maintained telephone contact with respondents while waiting for their questionnaire to be returned. Beretta (1996) suggested that this could cause respondents to feel coerced into returning the questionnaire, even though they may wish to withdraw from the study. Care should therefore be taken in following up panel members.

Box 19.3 Advantages and criticisms of the Delphi technique

Advantages	Criticisms
• Versatile technique	• No universally agreed guidelines
• Relatively inexpensive	• Potential for lack of methodological rigour
• Simple technique to use	• True anonymity?
• Confidentiality of responses	• Lack of evidence of reliability and validity
• No geographic restrictions	• No pilot testing reported in literature
• Protects participants' anonymity	• Lack of consideration of ethical implications
• Avoids 'group think'	• Time commitment from participants
• Cost-effective	• Potential for low response rate
• 'Two heads are better than one'	

CONCLUSIONS

The Delphi technique is a valuable method for achieving consensus on issues where none previously existed. The versatility of the technique lends itself to a wide range of applications and topics within nursing. The benefits are many, including simplicity of use, inexpensive nature, wide geographical reach, confidentiality and quasi-anonymity for expert panel members, and ultimately gaining consensus on important issues while avoiding 'group-think'. However, researchers considering using the technique should contemplate its complexity before use to ensure that they get the best from the technique in attempting to address the research objectives of their study.

References

Alexander J, Kroposki M (1999) Outcomes for community health practice. *Journal of Nursing Administration* **29**: 49–56.

Bäck-Pettersson S, Hermansson E, Sernert N, Björkelund C (2008) Research priorities in nursing – a Delphi study among Swedish nurses. *Journal of Clinical Nursing* **17**(16): 2221–2231.

Beech BF (1997) Studying the future: a Delphi survey of how multi-disciplinary clinical staff views the likely development of two community mental health centres over the course of the next two years. *Journal of Advanced Nursing* **25**: 331–338.

Beretta R (1996) A critical review of the Delphi technique. *Nurse Researcher* **3**(4): 79–89.

Buck AJ, Gross M, Hakim S, Weinblatt J (1993) Using the Delphi process to analyse social policy implementation – a post hoc case from vocational rehabilitation. *Policy Sciences* **26**(4): 271–288.

Burns FM (1998) Essential components of schizophrenia care: a Delphi approach. *Acta Psychiatrica Scandinavica* **98**: 400–405.

Couper MR (1984) The Delphi technique: characteristics and sequence model. *Advances in Nursing Science* **71**: 72–77.

Crisp J, Pelletier D, Duffield C, Adams A, Nagy S (1997) The Delphi method. *Nursing Research* **46**(2): 116–118.

Dalkey N, Helmer O (1963) Delphi technique: characteristics and sequence model to the use of experts. *Management Science* **9**(3): 458–467.

Drennan J, Meehan T, Kemple M, Johnson M, Treacy M, Butler M (2007) Nursing research priorities for Ireland. *Journal of Nursing Scholarship* **39**(4): 298–305.

Endacott R, Clifford CM, Tripp JH (1999) Can the needs of the critically ill child be identified using scenarios? Experiences of a modified Delphi study. *Journal of Advanced Nursing* **30**: 665–676.

Evans C (1997) The use of consensus methods and expert panels in pharmacoeconomic studies – practical applications and methodological shortcomings. *Pharmacoeconomics* **12**(2): 121–129.

Goodman CM (1987) The Delphi technique: a critique. *Journal of Advanced Nursing* **12**: 729–734.

Green B, Jones M, Hughes D (1999) Applying the Delphi technique in a study of GPs information requirement. *Health and Social Care in the Community* **7**(3): 198–205.

Handler SM, Hanlon JT, Perera S, Roumani YF, Nace DA, Fridsma DB *et al.* (2008) Consensus list of signals to detect potential adverse drug reactions in nursing homes. *Journal of the American Geriatrics Society* **56**(5): 808–815.

Hasson F, Keeney S, McKenna HP (2000) Research guidelines for the Delphi technique. *Journal of Advanced Nursing* **32**(4): 1008–1015.

Hitch PJ, Murgatroyd JD (1983) Professional communications in cancer care: a Delphi survey of hospital nurses. *Journal of Advanced Nursing* **8**: 413–422.

Hung HL, Altschuld JW, Lee YF (2008) Methodological and conceptual issues confronting a cross-county Delphi study of educational program evaluation. *Evaluation and Program Planning* **31**: 191–198.

Jairath N, Weinstein J (1994) The Delphi methodology (part one): a useful administrative approach. *Canadian Journal of Nursing Administration* **7**(3): 29–40.

Jeffery G, Hache G, Lehr R (1995) A group based Delphi application: defining rural career counselling needs. *Measurement and Evaluation in Counselling and Development* **28**: 45–60.

Jenkins D, Smith T (1994) Applying Delphi methodology in family therapy research. *Contemporary Family Therapy* **16**(5): 411–430.

Jirwe M, Gerrish K, Keeney S, Emami A (2009) Identifying the core components of cultural competence: findings from a Delphi study. *Journal of Clinical Nursing* **18**: 2622–2634.

Jones J, Sanderson C, Black N (1992) What will happen to the quality of care with fewer junior doctors? A Delphi study of consultant physician's views. *Journal of the Royal College of Physicians* **26**(1): 36–40.

Keeney S, Hasson F, McKenna HP (2006) Consulting the oracle: ten lessons from using the Delphi technique in nursing research. *Journal of Advanced Nursing* **53**(2): 1–8.

Linstone HA (1978) The Delphi technique. In: Fowles RB (ed) *Handbook of Futures Research*. Westport CT, Greenwood, pp 271–300.

Loughlin KG, Moore LF (1979) Using Delphi to achieve congruent objectives and activities in a paediatrics department. *Journal of Medical Education* **54**(2): 101–106.

Lynn MR, Layman EL, Englebardt SP (1998) Nursing administration research priorities: a national Delphi study. *Journal of Nursing Administration* **28**(5): 7–11.

McCance TV, Fitzsimons D, Keeney S, Hasson F, McKenna HP (2007) Capacity building in nursing and midwifery research and development: an old priority with a new perspective. *Journal of Advanced Nursing* **59**(1): 57–67.

McKeown C, Gibson F (2007) Determining the political influence of nurses who work in the field of hepatitis C: a Delphi survey. *Journal of Clinical Nursing* **16**(7): 1210–1221.

McKenna HP (1994a) The Delphi technique: a worthwhile approach for nursing? *Journal of Advanced Nursing* **19**: 1221–1225.

McKenna HP (1994b) The essential elements of a practitioners' nursing model: a survey of clinical psychiatric nurse managers. *Journal of Advanced Nursing* **19**: 870–877.

McKenna HP, Keeney S (2004) Leadership within community nursing in Ireland north and south: the perceptions of community nurses, GPs, policy makers and members of the public. *Journal of Nursing Management* **12**: 69–76.

Moore CM (1987) Delphi technique and the mail questionnaire. *Group Techniques for Idea Building: applied social research methods*. Newbury Park, Sage.

Procter S, Hunt M (1994) Using the Delphi survey technique to develop a professional definition of nursing for analysing nursing workload. *Journal of Advanced Nursing* **19**: 1003–1014.

Polivka BJ, Stanley SA, Gordon D, Taulbee K, Kieffer G, McCorkle SM (2008) Public health nursing competencies for public health surge experts. *Public Health Nursing* **25**: 159–165.

Reid N (1998) The Delphi technique: its contribution to the evaluation of professional practice. In: Ellis R (ed) *Professional Competence and Quality Assurance in the Caring Profession*. London, Croom Helm, pp 223–262.

Sheikh A, Major P, Holgate ST (2008) Developing consensus on national respiratory research priorities: key findings from the UK Respiratory Research Collaborative's e-Delphi exercise. *Respiratory Medicine* **102**(8): 1089–1092.

Strauss HJ, Ziegler LH (1975) The Delphi technique: an adaptive research tool. *British Journal of Occupational Therapy* **61**: 4153–4156.

Turoff M (1970) The policy Delphi. *Journal of Technological Forecasting and Social Change* **2**: 2.

Wagenaar D, Colenda CC, Kreft M, Sawade J, Gardiner J, Poverejan E (2003) Treating depression in nursing homes: practice guidelines in the real world. *Journal of the American Osteopath Association* **103**(10): 465–469.

Walker AM, Selfe J (1996) The Delphi method: a useful tool for the allied health researcher. *British Journal of Therapy and Rehabilitation* **3**(12): 677–681.

Williams PL, Webb C (1994) The Delphi technique: An adaptive research tool. *British Journal of Occupational Therapy* **61**(4): 153–156.

Young WH, Hogben D (1978) An experimental study of the Delphi technique. *Education Research Perspective* **5**: 57–62.

Further reading

Keeney S, Hasson F, McKenna HP (2001) A critical review of the Delphi technique as a research methodology for nursing. *International Journal of Nursing Studies* **38**: 195–200.

Linstone HA, Turoff M (2002) *The Delphi Method: techniques and applications*. Reading, MA, Addison-Wesley.

Mullen PM (2000) *When is Delphi not Delphi?* Birmingham, Health Services Management Centre, School of Public Policy, University of Birmingham.

Websites

http://is.njit.edu/pubs/delphibook – The Delphi Method: techniques and applications. Free digital version of Linstone and Turoff's 2002 book on the technique.

www.iit.edu/~it/delphi.html – the Delphi technique: definition and historical background. Website hosted by the Illinois Institute of Technology giving comprehensive background to the technique and detailed overview of using the method.

20 Case Study Research

Charlotte L Clarke and Jan Reed

Key points

- Case study research explores a phenomenon in its context and assumes that this context is of significance to the phenomenon.

- It is a flexible and holistic approach to research design in which data collection is shaped by the boundaries of the case being studied.

- A critical step is to define the case, making sure that it illustrates the issue under investigation.

- Insider knowledge of the context, or at least the ability to access it, is important in shaping the sampling and data collection methods.

- The ability to transfer knowledge beyond the case is important in developing high-quality case study research.

INTRODUCTION

For many practitioners the idea of case study methodology strikes several chords. As practitioners have become more aware of the importance of taking an holistic and individualised approach to care, a research method that is in tune with these ideas seems a natural fit. Case study methodology has a connection with the ways in which nurses and other healthcare practitioners think about practice, in terms of 'cases' or individual service users. This connection between research and practice is perhaps most clearly demonstrated by the use of the 'case study' in healthcare practice. The medical profession, for example, has a long tradition of using 'cases' as a method of exploring practice, from the case conference where people gather to assess and plan care, to the case study publication in professional journals, where an example of a patient's history and treatment is presented.

As such, case study research offers a valuable means of exploring a phenomenon in its context and assumes that the context is of significance to understanding the phenomenon. Phenomena may be conceptual (e.g. vulnerability), as in instrumental case studies (Stake 1995), about people or organisations, depending on the focus of the research being undertaken. This emphasis on knowing the phenomenon in its context and as it occurs in practice characterises case study research, and even those forms of case study that are single-case clinical trials (e.g. testing in a single individual whether a new medication improves their health) assume the need to understand the impact of the context on the establishment, processes and outcomes of the phenomenon.

Using case studies in research, then, has a resonance with professional practice. It offers the opportunity of learning in a way that pays attention to and respects the individuality and unique nature of service users and services.

In addition, it is a way of exploring the dimensions of each case in an holistic way, where key factors or variables can be investigated as their relevance becomes evident in each case, rather than to a pre-set research design.

This flexibility and individuality, however, leads to the main difficulties of case study research. First, there is the problem of relevance to other cases, sometimes expressed in other research traditions as 'generalisability'. In other words, there is a question about how the phenomenon observed in one case can have any relevance to other cases – after all, if it has no relevance then the effort to learn has very little benefit for wider practice. As Kozma and Anderson (2002) argue:

'In instrumental case studies, the focus of the analysis is on underlying issues, relationships, and causes that may generalise beyond the case. With this type of case study, the focus is not on the uniqueness of a special case but on what can be taken away from it and cases are selected for this purpose. Analysis of instrumental case studies goes beyond the specific case to examine an underlying issue or research question' (Kozma & Anderson 2002: 387)

The second difficulty is one of structure and design, that is if case studies are too flexible and data can be collected in an ad-hoc way as and when they look interesting or become available, then there is a danger of the original questions being lost in a sea of data, producing findings which do not go very far towards addressing the issues which gave rise to the study.

Both of these points have been raised in the literature discussing case study research (see for example Meyer 2003; Corcoran *et al.* 2004; Yin 2009). Writers have either dismissed case studies as a useful approach because of perceived methodological limitations, or argued that their potential has not been realised because researchers have had only a superficial

understanding of the methodology, seeing it simply as a convenient label to describe their small-scale studies. Writers have exhorted case study researchers to pay more attention to the theoretical and methodological aspects of case studies in order to move beyond these limitations. As Corcoran *et al.* (2004) have argued:

'case-study research … falls short of its promise due to a lack of theorising about the research methodology or an understanding about the methodology' (Corcoran *et al.* 2004: 7)

It is useful to outline some of the measures that allow case study research to confidently challenge these criticisms and ensure high-quality research. In principle, the measures are no different from those needed in high-quality research of any design, namely that the researcher should:

- have an effective conceptualisation of the issue under study and the research questions. For case study research this means knowing how to define 'the case', something that is somewhat harder to achieve than may at first appear
- have a good understanding of the research philosophy that is being used. This will ensure that the data collected 'fits' together, it all contributes to addressing the question and helps to avoid the risk of collecting whatever data is to hand (the magpie effect)
- think through carefully what is being learnt from the case study and how this can contribute to learning that is beyond the specific case. For example, case study methods may be best at answering questions about processes and the notion of a population from which a sample is drawn may be very different to that of other research approaches.

It is important to emphasise that case study research is complex and tackles real-life issues in their full glory in practice. The scale and scope of case studies is extremely variable and they can be very substantial multi-site studies. It is certainly not a way of adding gloss to a poor-quality and poorly developed research design, whether small or large scale. This chapter includes illustrations from several studies that we have been involved with which use case study approaches, either as part of a larger study or as the primary research design.

DEFINITIONS OF CASE STUDY METHODOLOGY

One of the most commonly quoted definitions of case study methodology is that of Yin (2009), who described the case study as an approach to empirical enquiry that:

> 'investigates a contemporary phenomenon within its real-life context, when the boundaries between phenomenon and context are not clearly evident' (Yin 2009: 13)

There are, of course, other definitions, but this one is used frequently, perhaps because it comes from one of the key writers on case studies, whose book, first published in 1984, has become an important resource for researchers. It also points to some of the features of a research question that would make case study methodology appropriate. First there is the emphasis on the contemporary nature of the phenomenon, second there is the importance placed on its 'real-life' nature and finally, and most importantly, there is the idea that a division between setting and phenomenon is difficult to draw: the phenomenon is intimately connected to the context, and to research one without the other would be to produce only a partial account of what is happening. A similar definition is offered by Robson (2002) who defines case study as 'a strategy for doing research which involves an empirical investigation of a particular contemporary phenomenon within its real life context using multiple sources of evidence'. This points to another dimension, the complexity of real life and the need for multiple sources of data to capture this.

Case study research then, is about treating the phenomenon being researched as a distinct entity or case, and exploring it in the context in which it occurs. This, however, does not explain what a case is, or how this can be demarcated, so further clarification is needed. This is quite a difficult move to make, paradoxically, because the links between phenomena and context that are so integral to the justification of using a case study approach make it difficult to put boundaries around a case for the purposes of definition.

One way to approach this is to eschew an overall definition of a case, which could be applied across studies, and to see this definitional process as one that each researcher needs to engage with: in other words that the definition of a case needs to be thought through carefully in the light of the research goals of the study. For example, if the goal is to understand the experiences of an individual service user, then the case can be defined around that service user, their experiences and thoughts. If the study is about how an organisation responds to change, then the case can be defined as an organisation.

This is not to say that the case needs to be defined as an inviolable unit that cannot be thought of in different ways; there may be a utility in breaking down a case into subunits for the purpose of data collection and analysis. A case study of a family, for example, may be broken down at some point into parents and children as subunits, depending on the questions being asked. Matching the boundaries of the case study to the research questions being asked enables the data collection and analysis to be focused and relevant. Defining the case, then, can be seen as a process not reliant on textbook terminology but on the specific aims and focus of the research.

Defining the case depends much on the 'pre-understanding' of the researcher (Gummesson 1998). Meyer (2003) has described this pre-understanding as potentially arising from 'general knowledge such as theories, models and concepts or from specific knowledge of institutional conditions and social patterns' (Meyer 2003: 331). Researchers come to projects from a range of different experiences and debates about the researched topic. Building on 'pre-understanding' leads to the definition of the case and its boundaries, the processes of data collection and the process of data analysis. As Gummesson (1998) has argued, the challenge for researchers is not to split their pre-understanding from their research, but to be 'able to balance on a razor's edge using their pre-understanding without being its slave' (Gummesson 1998: 58). Pre-understandings lead to research aims and questions, which then lead to specific definitions of what a case is for a particular study.

Nurses and other healthcare practitioners have a particular advantage in pre-understanding the issues and contexts they seek to research as they possess considerable 'insider' knowledge from their practice experiences (Reed *et al.* 1996). The challenge lies in using this insider knowledge effectively to shape research questions and design. An example is Lovell (2006), who used his work with people with learning difficulties to identify and explore the issues arising in one specific case.

Much like grounded theory, case study approaches to research may integrate sampling with data collection and with data analysis, each informing the other. For example, the analysis of one piece of data may suggest that the study could be informed by data collected from a different part of an organisation. This allows for structured and defensible flexibility in the research and maximises the ability of the study to respond to the theoretical sensitivity of the researcher.

RESEARCH QUESTIONS

A fundamental part of carrying out a case study is to identify the research questions. This is pertinent, of course, in any study, but because of the individual nature of the case study, the research questions and the ways of answering them are correspondingly individual, and need careful thinking through. Methodology cannot be simply 'off the peg', i.e. standardised and pre-determined. Bergen and While (2000) describe how case study method has derived from a wide variety of disciplines, each with their own methodological orientation (e.g. pure science through to sociology) and implications for the research questions asked. Case study methodology can be either quantitative or qualitative, that is the research questions can be about exploring the case either in words or numbers. In addition, case studies may have goals or questions that are about describing phenomena or making links (often causal between aspects of phenomena). These different aims give rise to questions as follows.

■ How does this family deal with and manage the implications of this family member's health problem?

■ How are services for people with this health problem organised?
■ How do staff manage appointments in this clinic?
■ Has the reorganisation of the system for making appointments reduced non-contact time for the staff?

These questions are a mix of the descriptive, 'what is happening here', and the inferential, 'how are these things linked here?' They will vary according to the research aims and how it is hoped they will inform and contribute to debates about practice, policy or theory. There should be a logical flow from the research question to the selection of the case and the process of data collection and analysis.

SELECTION OF CASES

Discussions of sampling in case study methodology are somewhat different from those of other research approaches. They go back to the pre-understanding of the researcher and what they want to do with their research, and are therefore about how a case can be defined, its constituents and its boundaries. Some approaches, for example Soft Systems Methodology (SSM) (Checkland & Scholes 1999), can work well with case study methodology because they have a theoretical framework that is specific about the dimensions of the phenomena being studied. SSM focuses on the communication patterns within and between organisations, and provides a framework for identifying what the constituents of a system might be. It is based on the idea that the way to understand organisational activity is to think of it as being part of a communication system, and that exploration should focus on the way that communication happens across the system. SSM has an inherent set of research goals and a way of defining a case as the system of communications between and within organisations. Starting off with one point in the system, the boundaries of the case can be mapped out by asking who communicates with whom at this point. The identification of the sample is shaped by the theory underpinning the study. An example of SSM in a case study design is given in Research Example 20.1.

20.1 Using Soft Systems Methodology in Practice Development Research

Clarke CL, Wilcockson J (2001) Professional and organisational learning: analysing the relationship with the development of practice. *Journal of Advanced Nursing* **34**: 264–272.

Clarke CL, Wilcockson J (2002) Seeing need and developing care: exploring knowledge for and from practice. *International Journal of Nursing Studies* **39**: 397–406.

The study aimed to understand how developments in practice spread and were sustained within an organisation. Three case study sites were identified as NHS organisations with a good level of practice development. Approximately 15 people in each organisation were interviewed about the ways in which they develop practice and why. The Soft Systems Methodology guided questions about the social and political aspects of practice development as well as organisational structures and allowed theory to be developed and explored with the participants.

Table 20.1 Sampling criteria for case study sites for specialist services and older people survey

Sampling criteria	Rank
Roles of specialised staff (i.e. whether they are used as advisors to other staff or have a direct role in care provision)	1
How does the service utilise user opinion/feedback/advocacy groups (e.g. in service development or service audit)?	2
Integration and partnership of healthcare organisation activity across the whole system of service provision (i.e. whether the role is restricted to the healthcare organisation or has the potential to impact on other agencies)	3
How the client group has been demarcated (i.e. whether older people are explicitly identified as a group or whether this is subsumed under other headings, such as medical speciality or type of provision)	4
How the service/post has been developed	5
How does the service offer services for older people of diverse ethnic backgrounds/or cater for older people of all ethnic backgrounds?	6
Which National Service Framework – Older Person themes and/or standards does this service contribute to?	7

Where a theoretical framework is not so clear, however, researchers need to think through their definition of the phenomenon under study very carefully in order to map out its dimensions. It may be necessary for some preliminary work to be done to make sure that the cases chosen will help to answer the research questions. This issue arose in a study that examined specialist services for older people (Reed *et al.* 2005a, 2006, 2007). It began with a national survey to identify the scope and range of specialist services, and then explored the processes of development in more detail, focusing on the development of specialist nursing roles. The sampling matrix shown in Table 20.1 was circulated to the research steering group so that the variables identified by the project team could be ranked by steering group members in order of importance to the project aims (the final ranking is given in the right-hand column).

The ranking of the variables was based on the research objectives and was translated into a sampling matrix (Reed *et al.* 1996). Matrix sampling is a process where the key variables of interest in a study are laid out in matrix form. Possible cases for inclusion in a study are entered into the matrix so that the characteristics are set out in a way that makes selection processes visible to researchers and readers. In this case it allowed the team to match up case study sites with the research priorities and ensure that there was a range of cases that would explore key issues and reflect the range of models of specialist services that had been developed.

A further concern is whether a sample should be homogenous or heterogeneous, in other words whether the case study should include similar or dissimilar phenomena. Again this is a product of the study aims: it may be that a case study will seek out a range of phenomena in order to broaden the understanding of difference, or it may be that a study would select similar examples to increase the amount of data available over a narrower range.

This discussion of sampling echoes the earlier discussions about the definitions of a case. Case study approaches can involve 'subunits' where a case may have different components, so a case study of an organisation may involve a number of different departments or partners or clients, which may be chosen because of their similarities or differences. Moving up a level of unit of analysis, the sampling strategy for the study as a whole may involve multiple case study sites, which may, as with case subunits, be selected to provide contrasting examples or similar ones.

The context dependency of case study research leads to the need for local knowledge to ensure that sampling reflects this context. As a result, sampling in case study research for researchers who are unfamiliar with the area can be particularly complex. One approach that we have developed and used in a number of studies takes a multi-stage approach to sampling. For example, Box 20.1 illustrates the sampling flow from issue to unit of data collection within a case. Research Examples 20.2 and 20.3 describe studies that illustrate this process in practice.

RESEARCH DESIGN

The idea of flexible sampling is linked to the idea of a flexible research design. The design, for example, can have a built-in facility for inductive sampling (where subsequent samples are based on previous analysis of data and intended to allow deeper analysis of the phenomenon), as an initial case study leads to

---

Box 20.1 Sampling in case study research

Phenomenon under investigation
↓

Identification of characteristics of the phenomenon to create case criteria
↓

Data collection to inform matrix sampling to identify illustrative case(s)
↓

Identification of those with local context knowledge as 'informants'
↓

Identification of sample inclusion / exclusion criteria
↓

Matrix sampling to identify data collection sample

20.2 Case Study Sampling in a Leadership Course Evaluation

Clarke C, Reynolds J, McClelland S, Reed J (2004a) *Evaluation of the NHS Leading Modernisation Programme*. Final Report. Northumbria University, Newcastle.

In an evaluation of a leadership course for modernisation leads in Strategic Health Authorities (SHAs) that was commissioned by the NHS Modernisation Agency:

- the phenomenon was defined as the processes of modernisation activity in SHAs
- the case criteria (identified after various forms of data collection and analysis) were:
  - gender of SHA modernisation lead
  - geographical location
  - doctoral level registration status of SHA modernisation lead as part of the leadership course
  - whether posts had been held outside the NHS
  - level of academic qualification
  - pre-course profile of individual in relation to leadership and modernisation activity
  - general management and/or clinical background
- five SHAs were selected as case study sites following matrix mapping of all 28 SHAs against the case criteria
- the informants were identified as the SHA modernisation leads who were participants in the leadership course
- the sampling criteria within each SHA sought to identify a sample of stratified maximum variation, which is designed to maximise the generation of information rather than seeking generalisation
- using the sampling criteria the informants each identified 24 people in their SHA (e.g. 'people who have most influenced the way that I modernise', 'people who I think have implemented modernisation activities across boundaries and/or agencies') and mapped them on a further sampling matrix against various criteria (e.g. 'this person has been particularly involved with leadership/care delivery systems/improvement science', 'this person is employed by NHS/ other organisation'). From this pool of nominated people, the research team selected 15 for interview in each site, ensuring diversity and breadth in the sample.

a need to explore the research question with further cases chosen for their utility in exploring key issues. Alternatively, the design can be planned from the outset. Yin (2009) has talked about multiple case studies, where parallel investigations can be carried out, again either to explore differences or similarities as indicated in the research question.

There are, though, challenges to achieving consistency across multiple case study sites. Research Example 20.4 describes a multinational study into the strategies that older people use to maintain wellbeing. Appreciative Inquiry gave the research a coherence, which could have been missing given the diversity of the study sites and the differences in background and

experience of the researchers. Appreciative Inquiry is an approach to organisational evaluation and learning that begins by identifying and examining examples of successful working and further explores ways of building on these (Reed *et al.* 2002, Reed 2006). This allowed the analysis to identify the unique developments in the study sites and the lessons to be learned across sites.

DATA ANALYSIS

This chapter began by pointing out the criticism levied at case studies about the failure of the meth-

RESEARCH EXAMPLE

20.3   Case Study Sampling in Dementia Care Research

Clarke CL (1999) Family caregiving for people with dementia: some implications for policy and professional practice. *Journal of Advanced Nursing* **29**: 712–720.

In this case study, the issue concerned the experiences of someone with dementia, and so the case was that of an individual who had dementia and their family and non-family carers. Each of the nine cases was identified through services to which they were known, and these people with dementia in turn nominated a family member and identified non-family carers who could be approached for interview. In this way, each case involved data collection with the person with dementia, one family member and up to three non-family carers.

Clarke C, Luce A, Gibb C, Williams L, Keady J, Cook A, Wilkinson H (2004b) Contemporary risk management in dementia: an organisational survey of practices and inclusion of people with dementia. *Signpost* **9**(1): 27–31.
   Clarke CL, Gibb C, Keady J, Luce A, Wilkinson H, Williams L, Cook A (2009) Risk management dilemmas in dementia care: An organisational survey in three UK countries. *International Journal of Older People Nursing* **4**: 89–96.

In a study exploring how people with dementia construct and manage risk, the 56 people with dementia (who were interviewed twice over 2 months) each nominated a family member and a non-family carer for interview. In this way many case studies were created and this high number of cases to explore the issue under investigation poses particular challenges at the point of analysis.

odology to reach its potential because of the lack of rigour in analysis. As case studies are so embedded in particular contexts, it is tempting to produce an analysis with only local relevance. There is a huge difference between simply saying 'this is what happened in this case' and extending this to discuss the relevance of the case to broader issues.

There are three approaches that can be taken to consider the way in which case study research can contribute to broader issues. First, this needs to be built into the research questions and study design from the outset. Appropriate modelling and theorising of the phenomenon from its conception will ensure that the study is set up to produce data amenable to analysis that can make a wider contribution. For example, the project described in Research Example 20.2 was commissioned as an evaluation of a leadership course, but was also designed to contribute to a knowledge base about the processes of practice and service development. As much was learned about the ways in which people and services modernise as was learned about the leadership course. To

achieve this, the research team needed to know how to access local, on-the-ground knowledge to ensure context sensitivity. They also had to be sufficiently aware of the contemporary knowledge base and philosophical options to allow theoretical sensitivity to inform the project development.

Second, having collected the data there is a need to analyse it in two ways. Initially, the internal patterns in the data must be carefully teased out and confirmed, whether through qualitative or quantitative data analysis methods. This is the level of analysis that is most often described and concerns getting to grips with the detail of the data itself and organising it in a way that allows those patterns to be described. In the second part of the analysis, which may be concurrent with the first or most often will follow it, the results of the data analysis need to be analysed in relation to the external knowledge base generated by other research and the practice and policy environment. This can be best described as external patterning. In this way, the contribution of the internal data analysis can be explored in relation

RESEARCH EXAMPLE

20.4   Using Appreciative Inquiry to Guide Data Collection

Reed J, Richardson E, Marais S, Moyle W (2008) Older people maintaining well-being: an International Appreciative Inquiry study. *International Journal of Older People Nursing* **3**: 168–176.

The study used Appreciative Inquiry as the methodological basis for the case studies. Appreciative Inquiry is a 'strengths-based' approach, which begins from an exploration and appreciation of the ways in which participants have acted positively in their lives. These issues play out in different ways across different cultures and countries, as service development has taken place against the background of different policy frameworks. To explore these processes, this study has identified a number of different international settings, or cases, as follows:

- UK – welfare state structure and services
- Germany – voluntary sector/Church sector and services
- Australia – private sector and services
- South Africa – limited service development.

Appreciative Inquiry focus groups/individual interviews have been held in each of these countries, and the initial questions were as follows.

- What strategies have you developed to respond to physical challenges? What sort of challenges were these, and did your strategies involve any of the following examples – thinking through strategies, using aids or assistance, changing or reflecting on lifestyles, or any other responses?
- What strategies have you developed to respond to psychological challenges? What sort of challenges were these, and did your strategies involve any of the following examples – thinking through strategies, using aids or assistance, changing or reflecting on lifestyles, or any other responses?
- What strategies have you developed to respond to social challenges? What sort of challenges were these, and did your strategies involve any of the following examples – thinking through strategies, using aids or assistance, changing or reflecting on lifestyles, or any other responses?

The data from each focus group in each case study country will be pooled and used to explore different theoretical dimensions, but prior to this the context in each case will be described using the Community Capitals Framework (Flora *et al.* 2004). In this way the diversity of cases and their common themes are identified. The data analysis will contribute towards a framework for international service and practice development.

to the external knowledge environment and the study's contribution to that knowledge base carefully articulated.

Third, there needs to be careful consideration of the transferability of the results of the study from one context to another. This has some similarities to the process of generalising from a sample to a wider population in that the researcher needs to know what characteristics of the sample must be present in the wider population to legitimately claim that the results can be generalised from one to the other.

In case study research, with dependence on context, there needs to be an examination of the factors that reside in the context that can be found in other contexts to which claims of transferability may be made with some credibility. The classic example is a case study of some innovative development that is perceived to have happened 'only because Mary is here' and that if others had a Mary then they would achieve the same development. It is important to move beyond the 'Mary factor' and analyse just what it is about the way in which Mary works and has been able to work within the organisation that has allowed an innovation to occur. In this way, having examined and analysed data within its context, the next step required is that of de-contextualising the issue, transferring it to another context and re-contextualising it there. In other words, the analysis needs to identify the critical aspects of context that would allow something to be used elsewhere, so long as those certain critical aspects of context were (or were not) present.

One important consideration in the analysis of data in multiple case study research is the extent to which data are analysed within or across cases. It may be that the cases have been purposefully selected to reflect different dimensions of the phenomenon. In this situation, analysis across cases is necessary to ensure that all dimensions are taken into account in developing the findings from the data. Cross-case analysis can be used to emphasise commonality or difference between cases. Within case analysis each case is taken in turn and analysed as an interdependent set of data. This will maximise identification of the context-dependent aspects of the phenomenon. For example, Stake (1995) refers to seeking to refine an understanding of an issue by searching for patterns across a number of cases. For most studies, some analysis at both 'within-' and 'across-case' level is appropriate. In the study of care management conducted by Bergen and While (2000), Yin's (2009) ideas of designating a unit smaller than the case for the purposes of analysis was adopted; the case was care management and the unit of analysis was individual community nurse's practice.

Data analysis in case study research requires attention to the analytical demands of the very wide range of data sources that may be involved. Yin (2009) refers to documentation, archival records, direct observation, participant observation, interviews and physical artefacts as of equal relevance to case study research. Many of these, such as documentary analysis are a way of using pre-existing materials as data sources (Reed 1992). While such data has the advantage of being relatively 'untouched' by the research process, as it was written for other reasons, it has

been produced for particular audiences, and these need to be borne in mind when analysing these data.

PRESENTATION AND REPORTING

The presentation and reporting of any research study requires consideration of the audience. In case study research this is coloured by issues such as maintaining confidentiality and the plurality of audiences in particular. As case study research is context dependent it is necessary to describe organisations and people in considerable detail, and even if anonymity of names is maintained this level of context description may make it quite easy for people and places to be identified. This should be acknowledged with participants at the start of the research and it may be necessary for some forms of reporting to obscure the association between place/person and reported detail. This may be most easily achieved through cross-case reporting which does not seek to portray each case individually.

On the other hand, people and organisations can become very involved in case study research and naturally wish to see their role profiled appropriately. They may also wish to learn what they can from the work, and in this instance they may find it most helpful to receive the research presented in a way that is very explicit about each case. For example, in one study (Reed *et al.* 2005b), additional brief reports of each case study site were written that did not appear in the overall (and more public) report of the research in which only the cross-case analysis was presented.

In addition, reporting to people and organisations in a way that is accessible for their practice needs to be complemented by making the findings of the research accessible to the wider academic and practice communities through publication and presentations. To achieve this effectively will require the work to have relevance beyond the local case study sites, as described above. There also needs to be a level of theoretical analysis in presenting and disseminating the work so it can be transferred to other settings and can have the catalytic ability to make people think about their current knowledge and practice.

CONCLUSIONS

Case study research is unique in the emphases it places on the importance of the context and the impact of the context on the phenomenon under investigation. The design, sampling and data collection methods reflect this emphasis on context dependency. There is, however, a need to analyse the data and articulate the findings in a way that is both respectful of this context and that allows the research to be transferred to other environments. It is a form of research that is attractive to researchers and practitioners alike, and draws on the knowledge base of both.

References

Bergen A, While A (2000) A case for case study studies: exploring the use of case study design in community nursing research. *Journal of Advanced Nursing* **31**: 926–934.

Checkland P, Scholes J (1999) *Soft Systems Methodology in Action*. Chichester, Wiley.

Clarke CL (1999) Family caregiving for people with dementia: some implications for policy and professional practice. *Journal of Advanced Nursing* **29**: 712–720.

Clarke CL, Gibb C, Keady J, Luce A, Wilkinson H, Williams L, Cook A (2009) Risk management dilemmas in dementia care: an organisational survey in three UK countries. *International Journal of Older People Nursing* **4**: 89–96.

Clarke C, Luce A, Gibb C, Williams L, Keady J, Cook A, Wilkinson H (2004b) Contemporary risk management in dementia: an organisational survey of practices and inclusion of people with dementia. *Signpost* **9**(1): 27–31.

Clarke CL, Reynolds J, McClelland S, Reed J (2004a) *Evaluation of the NHS Leading Modernisation Programme*. Final Report. Northumbria University, Newcastle.

Clarke CL, Wilcockson J (2002) Seeing need and developing care: exploring knowledge for and from practice. *International Journal of Nursing Studies* **39**: 397–406.

Clarke CL, Wilcockson J (2001) Professional and organisational learning: analysing the relationship with the development of practice. *Journal of Advanced Nursing* **34**: 264–272.

Corcoran PB, Walker KE, Wals AEJ (2004) Case-studies, make-your-case studies, and case stories: a critique of case-study methodology in sustainability in higher education. *Environmental Education Research* **10**(1): 7–21.

Flora, CB, Flora JL, Fey S (2004) *The Community Capitals Framework. Rural Communities: legacy and change*, 2nd edition. Boulder, CO, Westview Press.

Gummesson E (1998) *Qualitative Methods in Management Research*. Lund, Studentlitteratur, Chartwell-Bratt.

Kozma RB, Anderson RE (2002) Qualitative case studies of innovative pedagogical practices using ICT. *Journal of Computer Assisted Learning* **18**: 387–394.

Lovell A (2006) Daniel's story: self-injury and the case study as method. *British Journal of Nursing* **15**(3): 167–170.

Meyer CB (2003) A case in case study methodology. *Field Methods* **13**: 329–352.

Reed J (2006) *Appreciative Inquiry: research for change*. London, Sage.

Reed J (1992) Secondary data in nursing research. *Journal of Advanced Nursing* **7**: 877–883.

Reed J, Cook M, Cook G, Inglis P, Clarke C (2006) Specialist services for older people: issues of negative and positive ageism. *Ageing & Society* **26**: 849–865.

Reed J, Inglis P, Cook G, Clarke C, Cook M (2007) Specialist nurses for older people: implications from UK development sites. *Journal of Advanced Nursing* **58**(4): 368–376.

Reed J, Jones A, Irvine J (2005b) Appreciating impact: evaluating small voluntary organisations in the United Kingdom. *Voluntas: International Journal of Voluntary and Non-profit Organisations* **16**: 123–141.

Reed J, Pearson P, Douglas B, Swinburne S, Wilding H (2002) Going home from hospital – an Appreciative Inquiry study. *Health and Social Care and the Community* **10**: 36–45.

Reed J, Procter S, Murray S (1996) A sampling strategy for qualitative research. *Nurse Researcher* **3**(4): 52–68.

Reed J, Richardson E, Marais S, Moyle W (2008) Older people maintaining well-being: an International Appreciative Inquiry study. *International Journal of Older People Nursing* **3**(1): 68–76.

Reed J, Watson B, Cook M, Clarke C, Cook G, Inglis P (2005a) Developing specialist practice for older people in England: responses to policy initiatives. *Practice Development in Health Care* **4**(4): 192–202.

Robson C (2002) *Real World Research*, 2nd edition. Oxford, Blackwell.

Stake RE (1995) *The Art of Case Study Research*. Thousand Oaks, Sage.

Yin RK (2009) *Case Study Research: design and methods*, 4th edition. Thousand Oaks, Sage.

21 Evaluation Research

Colin Robson

Key points

- Evaluation is an inescapable feature of modern life in general, and nursing in particular.

- Evaluation research is different from other forms of research in terms of purpose rather than the methods used.

- There is a range of models of evaluation research available, and selection of the model and type of data collection are largely dependent on the type of question to which answers are sought.

- Evaluations affect people and their interests; they are inevitably sensitive.

- An objective in all evaluations should be to improve the service or practice evaluated.

WHAT IS EVALUATION?

An evaluation seeks to assess the worth or value of something. Newspapers, magazines, television and other media are awash with evaluations of cars, household goods, restaurants, films, theatre productions, concerts, investments and sports performances, to name but a few. Those working in hospitals and other health-related settings and services are not immune to evaluation pressures, as many nurses are only too aware. Such pressures are part of a drive to make both public and private services accountable, to seek reassurance that the resources devoted are achieving the results hoped for and that there is value for money.

On balance, I regard this as a good thing. Resources are not limitless, and we need to make the best use of them. There is considerable satisfaction in finding out that you are providing a valued and effective service, or if things are not working well to know this and to have suggestions about how improvements might be made. However, evaluations are not necessarily benign. They may be carried out for questionable motives, for example to give spurious authenticity to a decision made to close a service or to cut costs. They can be carried out incompetently or insensitively. They can engender a climate of fear and suspicion, even in situations where the evaluation is being carried out in good faith.

WHY EVALUATION RESEARCH?

Evaluation research is a type of research. It is distinguishable from other types or forms of research because of its purpose, which, as indicated above, is to assess the worth or value of whatever is evaluated. In nursing, and other health-related areas, this is typically a service, programme, innovation or intervention, but it can be any aspect of what nurses and other health professionals get involved in. Bringing it under the umbrella of research provides certain safeguards. As discussed in Chapter 1, for a study to qualify as research, not only are certain competencies in the researcher called for, but there is also a commitment to the study being carried out in accordance with stringent ethical guidelines (see Chapter 3).

The position taken here is that, while evaluation research has a distinctive purpose, it is not restricted in any way as to the type or style of research that can be used. Evaluation research can use an experimental design and can rely on methods producing quantitative data. But it can in appropriate circumstances be purely qualitative; indeed any of the approaches in Section 3 of this book may be used, including action research or case study.

How do you decide which is appropriate? The choice is largely determined, as in other forms of research, by the questions to which you are seeking answers. The rest of this chapter is mainly concerned with introducing a range of possible approaches. Let us start by considering the type of evaluation which seems to spring to many people's mind when first asked to evaluate.

THE SATISFACTION QUESTIONNAIRE

In its simplest form this tries to find out what people who have been involved with a service, or whatever, thought about it. It is typically a short, self-completion questionnaire concentrating on areas such as usefulness and relevance, mainly consisting of questions with a fixed set of possible answers, and one or two open questions where the response is up to them. As with all methods of data collection this can be done well or poorly. Careful attention needs to be given to the wording of questions, as discussed in Chapter 30. It is crucially important that a high response rate is achieved as, logically, you do not know what non-respondents would have said. When questionnaires are completed in your presence, you should be able to set up the situation so that non-

response is rare. However, with postal questionnaires this can be a real problem, calling for sustained efforts to achieve acceptable response rates.

This type of simple evaluation has its value, and continues to be both used and published (e.g. Sutherland *et al.* 2008 who used questionnaires to elicit the views of people with cancer, their family and friends, about a cancer education programme). Somewhat more complex designs can be used, as in Allinson (2004), who incorporated a control group (see Research Example 21.1). Satisfaction questionnaires can also be incorporated into a range of designs, including randomised controlled trials (e.g. Giallo & Gavidia-Payne 2008).

Satisfaction studies are not necessarily small-scale. For example, Beecroft *et al.* (2006) present results from a six-year study of cohorts of new graduate nurses focusing on their perception of the mentoring they received. Aspects studied through survey questionnaires included the extent to which they were satisfactorily matched with mentors, received guidance and support, attained socialisation into the nursing profession, benefited from having a role model for acquisition of professional behaviours and maintained contact with mentors, as well as their general satisfaction with the mentorship.

Beech and Leather (2003) castigate reliance on subjective responses to satisfaction questions, which they refer to as 'happy sheets'. In evaluating a management of aggression course unit for student nurses they, among other things, use aggression scenarios; these are presented to students, who have to identify risk factors within the scenario. Their demonstration of increases in factors identified from before, to during, to after the course, provides one route to assessing more objectively the effects of the course on those involved.

It will, I hope, be clear from these examples that evaluations can focus on a variety of things in addition to, or instead of, the satisfaction of those involved. The next section discusses some possible foci.

MODELS OF EVALUATION

Evaluations can focus on many different things, including the following.

RESEARCH EXAMPLE

21.1 An Evaluation of Satisfaction

Allinson V (2004) Breast cancer: evaluation of a nurse-led family history clinic. *Journal of Clinical Nursing* **13**: 765–766.

A study based on a convenience sample of 46 women who were to attend the clinic within a 3-month period. A two-part questionnaire was used. The first part, given to the patients before their consultation, asked about the service they had received in the symptomatic clinic the previous year. It was anticipated that this might cause problems with recall; therefore, a control group of 15 women who had yet to be allocated to the nurse-led clinic was also recruited. This group saw the doctor alone and completed the first part of the questionnaire the same day. The second part of the questionnaire was given after the consultation with the nurse. The response rate was very high (44 out of 46; and all 15 in the control group) 'as women were asked to complete the questionnaires before leaving the department'. Very similar responses were received from the two groups on the first part, suggesting that the time delay was not affecting responses. Very high satisfaction rates for the nurse-led clinics were obtained and key elements (particularly discussion of family history) isolated. It was acknowledged that 'positive skew is a recognised flaw in patient satisfaction surveys' and possibly that 'patients may have been unwilling to complain about this new service thinking it might be withdrawn'.

- Finding out if needs are being met, answering questions such as: 'Are clients' needs being met?' or 'Are we reaching the target group?'
- Assessing the outcomes: 'Is the service effective?' or 'What happens to clients using the service?'
- How the service is operating: 'What is actually happening?' or 'Is it operating as planned?'
- Assessing efficiency: 'How do costs compare with benefits?' or 'How does its efficiency compare with possible alternatives?'

Note that, for 'service' you can also read 'procedure', or 'programme', or 'intervention', or 'innovation', depending on the situation.

The different approaches are sometimes referred to as '*models of evaluation*'.

Needs-based evaluation

When the focus is on client needs, it is necessary to establish what these needs are. While the needs that many nursing services seek to meet may appear self-evident to those providing the service, a strong principle behind this approach is that, because it is the client or recipient of the service who has the needs, they should have a strong voice in saying what they are. For example, Chien *et al.* (2006) sought to establish the needs of family members who had a relative admitted to an intensive care unit of a Hong Kong regional hospital, through the use of a version of the Critical Care Family Needs Inventory (Lee *et al.* 2000). The evaluation produced evidence that sessions based on the assessed needs did in fact meet these needs. Note that this study was also outcomes based (see below). A quasi-experimental design showed that, when compared with a control following a standard introduction to the ICU environment, an experimental group that had the needs-based programme had reduced anxiety and an increase in satisfaction of family needs (Chiu *et al.* 2004).

A needs assessment can provide the means of determining needs. It is not an evaluation of an existing service, but a way of finding out in advance what type of service would be found valuable. Carrying out an initial needs assessment before developing the service helps to tailor the service to these needs. It makes it less likely that resources are wasted on a service, and also provides a useful agenda to focus an evaluation when the service is up and running.

Houston and Cowley (2002) show a way of using needs assessment in the context of health visiting to provide a means of empowering clients. Horne and Costello (2003) describe how a health needs assessment of a community was conducted using action research. The study involved local people and a multi-agency steering group, within a primary healthcare setting. Six focus groups, with varying sections of the community, were used to elicit community perceptions of their health needs.

Outcome-based evaluation

This is a traditional form of evaluation that many, including administrators and service-providers, assume (mistakenly) to be the only valid approach. Undoubtedly, assessing the outcomes of a service, intervention or whatever, is often the main priority. However, outcomes can mean many things. If the service has specified goals or objectives then an obvious outcome is to assess whether they have been achieved. A serious shortcoming of this tight, objectives-linked approach is that services and interventions involving people are notorious for having unintended and unanticipated consequences (either in addition to, or instead of, the planned ones). Hence there is advan-

tage in spreading the net wide when considering the possible outcomes of involvement with a service.

The simple satisfaction questionnaire is one form of outcome evaluation. As discussed above, it has serious limitations. However, if the patients find something an unsatisfactory experience, this outcome is likely to have an adverse effect on other aspects.

Edwards *et al.* (2007) evaluated the effectiveness of a peer education programme in developing paediatric nurses' evidence-based knowledge and attitudes towards fever management and the sustainability of these changes. They carried out a quasi-experimental outcome design using an experimental group that received the peer education programme (peer support and education were provided for those unable to attend the sessions). A control group continued its normal practices. Statistically, the experimental group nurses demonstrated significantly more knowledge of general fever management principles four months after the intervention than control group nurses, and compared with their own knowledge before the intervention.

Wilkinson *et al.* (2007) provide an example of a randomised controlled design for an evaluation (Research Example 21.2). The randomised controlled trial is considered in some influential quarters as the

---

RESEARCH EXAMPLE

21.2 Evaluation Using a Randomised Controlled Trial

Wilkinson SM, Love SB, Westcombe AM, Gambles MA, Burgess CC, Cargill A *et al.* (2007) Effectiveness of aromatherapy massage in the management of anxiety and depression in patients with cancer: a multicenter randomized controlled trial. *Journal of Clinical Oncology* **25**: 532–539.

Two hundred and eighty-eight cancer patients referred to complementary therapy services with clinical anxiety and/or depression were allocated randomly to a course of aromatherapy massage or usual supportive care alone. The authors found that one session of aromatherapy massage each week for four weeks resulted in a statistically significant decrease in clinical anxiety and/or depression experienced by cancer patients up to two weeks after the end of the intervention, compared to the control group. However, this benefit was not sustained at six weeks post intervention. Although improvement in self-reported anxiety was evident up to six weeks post intervention, they found no evidence of benefit for aromatherapy massage on pain, insomnia, nausea and vomiting, or global quality of life at either assessment point. The authors claim that this is the first large, multicentre, randomised controlled trial of a complementary therapy in a healthcare setting.

'gold standard' for evaluation (and other) research, but it is not without its critics (see the discussion in Robson 2002: 116–123). Lindsay (2004) analyses 47 published randomised controlled trials in the field of nursing research that were published in 2000 or 2001. He identifies bias and unreliability in all of the studies, suggesting that inadequate study design is widespread in such trials of nursing interventions.

Process evaluation

This style of evaluation seeks to find out how the programme or service works in practice. What is the experience of those involved? What actually happens on the hospital ward or wherever? Outcome evaluation is typically (though not necessarily) based on methods of data collection that yield quantitative data. Process evaluations typically rely on methods such as observation and interviews, where the data are commonly qualitative. If it has been planned that the service should be delivered in a particular way, one concern for a process evaluation is possible discrepancies between the planned and the actual.

Heaman *et al.* (2006) used a descriptive, qualitative evaluation of an early childhood home visiting programme to establish the factors that appeared to be important for its success. In-depth interviewing was carried out with public health nurses, home visitors and parents. Important components included voluntary enrolment of parents, regularly scheduled home visits and a curriculum to structure the home visitor's interventions. Evaluations such as this, which include the views of several different groups (or 'stakeholders'), are sometimes referred to as a 'pluralistic evaluation' (Hall 2004). Carr *et al.* (2008) provides a further example (Research Example 21.3).

Cost-benefit evaluation

Assessment of the costs expended in running a service in relation to the benefits accruing is of obvious interest and importance. In cost-benefit analysis the costs measured in monetary terms (pounds, euros, dollars or whatever) are compared with the benefits, also in monetary terms. This is not an easy task in practice, as difficult decisions have to be made, both about what to include and how to reach the monetary values. Yates (1997) considers problems with the common assumption that outpatient care is far less expensive than inpatient care. For example, the fact that families who play a part in home care will typically have reduced opportunities for employment in addition to restrictions on their private and social life, could reasonably be entered into the 'costs' side of

---

Q RESEARCH EXAMPLE

21.3   A Pluralistic Evaluation

Carr SM, Lhussier M, Wilcockson J (2008) Transferring palliative care knowledge: evaluating the use of a telephone advice line. *International Journal of Palliative Nursing* **14**: 303–308.

The evaluation design combined methodology using action research and pluralistic evaluation of a Palliative Care Advice Line (PCAL) providing 24-hour telephone advice to local health and social care professionals. This allowed formative, ongoing feedback into the advice line service during the evaluation, with a strong emphasis on learning and an iterative relationship between theory and practice. It also acknowledged a potential diversity of views on what 'success' is, and consequently on what a 'successful service' might achieve. Six different data collection methods were employed, including collaborative learning groups, interviews, use of routinely collected data, a survey of doctors and a focus group. The authors claim that the PCAL was a successful service development that achieved multiple positive outcomes. They discuss issues worthy of discussion to inform future practice innovations seeking to provide a mechanism to transfer knowledge between expert and generalist health and social care professionals.

the equation. In general, however, the relative costing of two or more services or variants of services is somewhat more straightforward and conclusions about the 'best buy' are easier to make. Robson (2000) provides an introduction to carrying out these analyses. Recently published examples include Ipsen *et al.* (2006) on a health promotion programme for individuals with mobility impairments, and Allsup *et al.* (2005), who carried out a cost–benefit evaluation of routine influenza immunisation in older people.

In cost-effectiveness analysis, benefits are assessed in non-monetary terms. Gift *et al.* (2006), who describe a cost-effectiveness evaluation of a jail-based chlamydia screening programme for men, and Williams *et al.* (2005), who studied the cost-effectiveness of a new nurse-led continence service, provide examples. Jester and Hicks (2003a,b) use cost-effectiveness analysis to compare 'hospital at home' and inpatient interventions. The first paper showed hospital at home to be significantly more effective in terms of patient satisfaction and reduced joint stiffness, and at least as effective as inpatient care on a range of other indicators. The second paper is essentially a worked example of how a variety of approaches, including cost-benefit and cost-effectiveness analyses, can be used. It is practical and lucid, and is strongly recommended to nurses and others interested in carrying out these types of analyses. Glick *et al.* (2007) provide a practical handbook on carrying out cost-effectiveness analyses as part of randomised trials.

Formative and summative evaluations

A formative evaluation seeks to promote the development of the service or intervention evaluated. A summative evaluation seeks to describe what effect a service or intervention has had on those involved. Outcome evaluations are sometimes characterised as summative, and process evaluations as formative. However, the distinction is not clear-cut.

A process evaluation provides information about one aspect of the effects that the intervention is having, i.e. it is in that sense summative. The outcomes of a service or intervention can have a formative influence. Positive outcomes can lead to its continuation and possible extension. Equivocal ones may hasten closure.

A common aphorism is that 'the purpose of evaluation is to improve rather than prove'. Indeed, it could be argued that all evaluations should have a concern for the improvement of whatever is being evaluated. Outcome evaluations are deficient in this respect. Whatever the outcomes, they give little or no direct guidance about what could or should be changed to lead to improvement. Put another way, few evaluations (and in particular outcome evaluations) ask, or seek answers to, the 'why' question. Why does the service or intervention have the effects that it does?

An approach called 'realistic evaluation' (Pawson & Tilley 1997) follows this route. They argue in favour of adopting a realist philosophy, where the task is to identify the mechanisms operating in a situation that lead to the observed effects. Building on the finding that most social interventions produce weak overall group effects, they set the task as 'finding what works, for whom, in what situations'. Their highly polemical text, which includes a swingeing critique of the utility of randomised control group methodology in evaluation research, has been influential. McEvoy and Richards (2003) make a strong case for a particular form of realism, known as critical realism, providing a basis for a way forward for evaluation research in nursing (see also Angus *et al.* 2006). They stress the importance of nursing interventions being properly understood if they are to be used effectively in the context of clinical practice. Examples of evaluations following this approach in the nursing context include Clark *et al.* (2007), who discuss a programme of research into secondary prevention programmes for heart disease drawing on critical realism, and Wilson *et al.* (2005), who employ the approach to evaluate emancipatory practice development processes and outcomes in a special care nursery.

QUANTITATIVE OR QUALITATIVE?

The examples discussed above incorporate both quantitative and qualitative data collection methods. It is worth reiterating the point made previously, that the choice of quantitative or qualitative methods should be largely dependent on the questions to which you seek answers when doing evaluation research. Pragmatically, it is the case that some audiences find numbers and statistical analysis persuasive. These audiences, including many administrators and managers, typically call for outcome evaluations that almost inevitably incorporate the collection of quantitative data. Conversely, some audiences, including practitioners and client groups, often more readily empathise with vivid accounts and other forms of qualitative data analysis.

This does not have to be an either/or decision. There can be advantages in asking a range of evaluation questions and using a corresponding range of both quantitative and qualitative data collection methods. Such designs are sometimes referred to as mixed method. The benefits of such an approach are illustrated in a study by Morgan and Stewart (2002). They describe how the use of quantitative (quasi-experimental) and qualitative (grounded theory) methods in an evaluation of new dementia special care units led to a better understanding of how the nursing home environment affects residents with dementia. This study also emphasises the valuable point that evaluation research cannot be perfectly pre-planned. It is a process that involves ongoing decisions and management of unexpected events. They describe the sequence of key methodological decisions made during the planning, implementation and integration phases of the study, conducted over a 21-month period. Happ *et al.* (2006) describe a range of techniques for mixed methods data combination and analyses using different design approaches. Chapter 27 discusses mixed methods research in more detail.

THE POLITICAL NATURE OF EVALUATION

Evaluations inevitably impinge in various ways on those involved. They can affect people's lives, primarily through the ways in which the findings and recommendations are acted upon. But the mere fact that an evaluation is taking place increases the sensitivity of all involved. As a researcher you can try to make it clear that it is the service, innovation or whatever, that is the focus of the evaluation. Staff will still suspect it is their performance that is being assessed.

In other words, evaluations always take place in a political context. The various interest groups, including politicians, administrators, medical staff, nurses, patients, etc., are likely to be influenced or affected by policy decisions arising from the research. Each of these groups may seek to influence the evaluation to best serve their interests.

This poses problems for an evaluator. Are you the 'hired hand' in the pay of those in powerful positions? Or are you representing the interests of the relatively powerless? The former is ethically dubious, particularly if the choice of evaluation questions is limited to those that the sponsor is comfortable with. The latter is advocated by some and, in seeking to redress inequalities, has its attractions. However, an evaluation that has a concern for all stakeholders, as well as being ethically sound, is likely to be most useful and most likely to be used.

EVALUATION RESEARCH AND EVIDENCE-BASED PRACTICE

Evaluation research and evidence-based practice (as discussed in Chapter 38) have similar concerns. They are both in the business of assessing value, and both fall within an accountability, value-for-money agenda. As currently conceived, evaluation research would seem to have the wider remit; anything and everything is grist to the evaluation mill, whereas evidence-based practice is self-evidently restricted to practice.

Early evaluation research was firmly within the experimental, comparison groups paradigm. Later developments have a much more broad church view, which this chapter has sought to reflect. To a relative outsider, evidence-based practice shows signs of moving on a similar journey. A quantitative and statistical view where the best, to some the only, evidence comes from randomised controlled trials appears to be now under question, with wider views of what is meant by 'evidence'.

CONCLUSIONS

A central aim of this chapter is to make it clear that evaluation research can come in many forms and styles. It can vary from a one-off, small-scale study by someone evaluating a situation or practice with which they are directly involved, to a multi-site extended evaluation of national initiatives by a large research team.

Finally, do remember that evaluation research is inevitably political (in that it is likely to affect the interests of one or more groups) and, partly because of this, is always sensitive. Make sure that you have given serious attention to the ethical issues involved.

References

Allinson V (2004) Breast cancer: evaluation of a nurse-led family history clinic. *Journal of Clinical Nursing* **13**: 765–766.

Allsup S, Gosney M, Haycox A, Regan M (2005) Cost–benefit evaluation of routine influenza immunization in people 65–74 years of age. *International Journal of Technology Assessment in Health Care* **21**: 144–150.

Angus J, Miller KL, Pulfer T, McKeever P (2006) Studying delays in breast cancer diagnosis and treatment: critical realism as a new foundation for inquiry. *Oncology Nursing Forum* **33**: 64–70.

Beech B, Leather P (2003) Evaluating a management of aggression unit for student nurses. *Journal of Advanced Nursing* **44**: 603–612.

Beecroft PC, Santner S, Lacy ML, Kunzman L, Dorey F (2006) New graduate nurses' perceptions of mentoring: six-year programme evaluation. *Journal of Advanced Nursing* **55**: 736–747.

Carr SM, Lhussier M, Wilcockson J (2008) Transferring palliative care knowledge: evaluating the use of a telephone advice line. *International Journal of Palliative Nursing* **14**: 303–308.

Chien WT, Chiu YL, Lam LW, Ip WY (2006) Effects of a needs-based education programme for family carers with a relative in an intensive care unit: a quasi-experimental study. *International Journal of Nursing Studies* **43**: 39–50.

Chiu YL, Chien WT, Lam LW (2004) Effectiveness of a needs-based education programme for families with a critically ill relative in an intensive care unit. *Journal of Clinical Nursing* **13**: 655–656.

Clark AM, MacIntyre PD, Cruickshank J (2007) A critical realist approach to understanding and evaluating heart health programmes. *Health: An Interdisciplinary Journal for the Social Study of Health, Illness and Medicine* **11**: 513–539.

Edwards H, Walsh A, Courtney M, Monaghan S, Wilson J, Young J (2007) Improving paediatric nurses' knowledge and attitudes in childhood fever management. *Journal of Advanced Nursing* **57**: 257–269.

Giallo R, Gavidia-Payne S (2008) Evaluation of a family-based intervention for siblings of children with a disability or chronic illness. *Australian e-Journal for the Advancement of Mental Health* **7**(2); www.auseinet.com/journal/vol7iss2/giallo.pdf (accessed 9 September 2008).

Gift TL, Lincoln, T, Tuthill R, Whelan M, Briggs P, Conklin T, Irwin KL (2006) A cost-effectiveness evaluation of a jail-based chlamydia screening program for men and its impact on their partners in the community. *Sexually Transmitted Diseases* **33**(October Suppl): S103–S110.

Glick HA, Doshi JA, Sonnad SS, Polsky D (2007) *Economic Evaluation in Clinical Trials*. Oxford, Oxford University Press.

Hall JE (2004) Pluralistic evaluation: a situational approach to service evaluation. *Journal of Nursing Management* **12**: 22–27.

Happ MB, Dabbs AD, Tate J, Hricik A, Erlen J (2006) Exemplars of mixed methods data combination and analysis. *Nursing Research* **55**(Suppl 1): S43–S49.

Heaman M, Chalmers K, Woodgate R, Brown J (2006) Early childhood home visiting programme: factors contributing to success. *Journal of Advanced Nursing* **55**: 291–300.

Horne M, Costello J (2003) A public health approach to health needs assessment at the interface of primary care and community development: findings from an action research study. *Primary Health Care Research & Development* **4**: 340–352.

Houston AM, Cowley S (2002) An empowerment approach to needs assessment in health visiting practice. *Journal of Clinical Nursing* **11**: 640–650.

Ipsen, C, Ravesloot C, Seekins T, Seninger S (2006) A financial cost–benefit analysis of a health promotion program for individuals with mobility impairments. *Journal of Disability Policy Studies* **16**: 220–228.

Jester R, Hicks C (2003a) Using cost-effectiveness analysis to compare hospital at home and in-patient interventions. Part 1. *Journal of Clinical Nursing* **12**: 13–19.

Jester R, Hicks C (2003b) Using cost-effectiveness analysis to compare hospital at home and in-patient interventions. Part 2. *Journal of Clinical Nursing* **12**: 20–27

Lee IYM, Chien WT, Mackenzie AE (2000) Needs of families with a relative in a critical care unit in Hong Kong. *Journal of Clinical Nursing* **9**: 46–54.

Lindsay B (2004) Randomized controlled trials of socially complex nursing interventions: creating bias and unreliability? *Journal of Advanced Nursing* **45**: 84–94.

McEvoy P, Richards D (2003) Critical realism: a way forward for evaluation research in nursing? *Journal of Advanced Nursing* **43**: 411–420.

Morgan DG, Stewart NJ (2002) Theory building through mixed-method evaluation of a dementia special care unit. *Research in Nursing & Health* **25**: 479–488.

Pawson R, Tilley N (1997) *Realistic Evaluation*. London, Sage.

Robson C (2000) *Small-scale Evaluation: principles and practice*. London, Sage.

Robson C (2002) *Real World Research: a resource for social scientists and practitioner-researchers*, 2nd edition. Oxford, Blackwell.

Sutherland G, Hoey L, White V, Jefford M, Hegarty S (2008) How does a cancer education program impact on people with cancer and their family and friends? *Journal of Cancer Education* **23**: 126–132.

Wilkinson SM, Love SB, Westcombe AM, Gambles MA, Burgess, CC, Cargill A *et al.* (2007) Effectiveness of aromatherapy massage in the management of anxiety and depression in patients with cancer: a multicenter randomized controlled trial. *Journal of Clinical Oncology* **25**: 532–539.

Williams KS, Assassa RP, Cooper NJ, Turner DA, Shaw C, Abrams KR *et al.*, The Leicestershire MRC Incontinence Study Team (2005) Clinical and cost-effectiveness of a new nurse-led continence service: a randomised controlled trial. *British Journal of General Practice* **55**: 696–703.

Wilson VJ, McCormack BG, Ives G (2005) Understanding the workplace culture of a special care nursery. *Journal of Advanced Nursing* **50**: 27–38.

Yates BT (1997) Formative evaluation of costs, cost-effectiveness, and cost-benefit: toward cost–procedure–process–outcome analysis. In: Bickman L, Rog DJ (eds) *Handbook of Applied Social Research Methods*. Thousand Oaks, Sage, pp 285–314.

Further reading

Bamberger MJ, Rugh J, Mabry L (2006) *RealWorld Evaluation: working under budget, time, data and political constraints*. Thousand Oaks, Sage.

Brophy S, Snooks, H, Griffiths L (2008) *Small-Scale Evaluation in Health: a practical guide*. Thousand Oaks, Sage.

Robson C (2000) *Small-scale Evaluation: principles and practice*. London, Sage.

Websites

http://gsociology.icaap.org/methods/ provides valuable free resources for anyone carrying out evaluation research (particularly those without easy access to academic libraries). The focus is on 'how to do' evaluation research, and the methods used; covering, for example, surveys, focus groups, sampling and interviews. Most of these links are to resources that can be read over the web. It is a site provided for the general good by an American academic.

www.intute.ac.uk/healthandlifesciences/nursing/ – the Intute: health and life sciences site is a major UK gateway to internet research in nursing, midwifery and allied health areas (formerly known as NMAP); when searched on 'evaluation research' it provides a wide range of useful links to relevant sites. They include full evaluation reports not available as journal articles, all of which have been quality assessed.

www.jameslindlibrary.org/ – to give a broader, historical, perspective on evaluation research, I recommend the James Lind library website marking the 250th anniversary of James Lind's evaluation of different treatments for scurvy, which details the evolution of tests of treatment effects, ranging from an Old Testament (Daniel, chapter 1:16) description of a controlled test of diets, through an 11th-century Chinese evaluation of the effects of ginseng, to the present day. The text of *Testing Treatments: better research for better healthcare*, a 100-page book published by the British Library in 2006 is available as a free download.

www.policy-evaluation.org/ – the WWW Virtual Library has a site devoted to evaluation with extensive links to resource guides and databases. There are also links to mailing lists, including EVALTALK (a general and lively discussion group on issues involved with doing evaluation research) and GOVTEVAL (which focuses on public sector evaluations) among many others. It can be fascinating to 'lurk' on these lists (i.e. to join but not make contributions yourself), and members are typically very helpful to new evaluators with queries.

www.york.ac.uk/inst/crd/ – the website of the Centre for Reviews and Dissemination includes databases on NHS Economic Evaluations (NHS EED) and of abstracts of reviews of effects (DARE).

22 Action Research

Julienne Meyer

Key points

- Action research is a research approach that involves interpreting and explaining social situations while implementing a change intervention.

- Action researchers adopt a participatory approach, involving participants in both the change and the research process.

- Both qualitative and quantitative methods of data collection may be employed during the three phases of action research: exploration, intervention and evaluation.

- Action researchers act as agents of change and need skills not only in research, but also in change management.

- Although sometimes criticised as unscientific, action research has a real-world focus and directly seeks to improve practice.

PRINCIPLES OF ACTION RESEARCH

Action research is an approach to research, rather than a specific method of data collection. The approach involves doing research *with* and *for* people (users and providers of service), in the context of its application, rather than undertaking research *on* them. The action researcher is seen as a facilitator and evaluator of change, whether the focus is on their own practice or the practice of others. Typically in health and social care settings, action researchers begin by exploring and reflecting on patient and/or client experience and, through a process of feeding back findings to providers of services (formal and informal), go on to identify gaps in care that those

engaged in the research would like to improve. Through an ongoing process of consultation and negotiation that gives democratic voice to all participants about the best way forward, the action researcher then works to support and systematically monitor the process and outcomes of change. An eclectic approach to data collection is taken, using whatever methods best address the problem being researched, although often action research is written up in its rich contextual detail as a case study.

From case studies of action research, two types of knowledge can be generated – theoretical and practical. In contrast to other forms of research, the action researcher cannot predetermine the nature of the study, as it is dependent on the views and wishes of those with whom they are collaborating. Action researchers thus have to work in a flexible and responsive way to deal with issues as they naturally occur in practice. In so doing, they have to rely as much on their interpersonal skills as their research skills. This requires special thought to be given to how those involved in the research can be protected from harm. Gaining formal ethical approval for the study is not enough. It is important to agree a code of ethical practice at the start of the study that allows participants control over what change happens, how it is researched and how the findings are shared with others.

As a nurse, I am particularly attracted to the underlying characteristics of action research (see Figure 22.1), namely its emergent developmental form, its focus on practical issues, the creation of knowledge in action, its links to participation and democracy, and its interest in human flourishing (Reason & Bradbury 2001). Action research typically blurs the boundaries between education, practice and research. If nothing else is gained as a result of the research, at least participants in the study should learn and develop from the process of being actively involved with it. Too much research is built around the researcher as expert, with a 'hit and run' approach to data collection; at least this approach aims to give something back (social change) at the same time as contributing to social knowledge.

COMMON MODELS OF WORKING WITH ACTION RESEARCH IN NURSING

Action research is not easily defined, as there are many different models, largely influenced by the level of focus (own practice, collective practice of others, wider political events), degree of participation and vision of knowledge (Whitelaw *et al.* 2003). A recent systematic review of the uptake and design of action research in published nursing research by Munn-Giddings *et al.* (2008) found that 24 different terms were used to define the action research approach, including, for example, *collaborative action research, emancipatory and enhancement action research, participatory research* and *evaluative action research*.

Reason and Bradbury (2008) view action research as a 'family of practices of inquiry' and offer the following broad definition:

'Action research is a participatory process concerned with developing practical knowing in the pursuit of worthwhile human purposes. It seeks to bring together action and reflection, theory and practice, in participation with others, in the pursuit of practical solutions to issues of pressing concern to people, and more generally the flourishing of individual persons and their communities' (Reason & Bradbury 2008: 4)

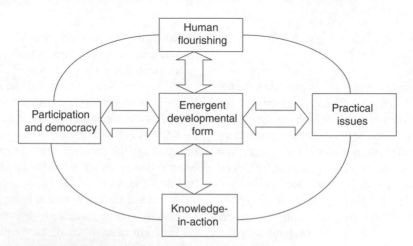

Figure 22.1 Characteristics of action research
Reproduced by permission of Sage Publishing from Reason P, Bradbury H (2008) *The Sage Handbook of Action Research Participative Inquiry and Practice*, 2nd edition. London, Sage.

They suggest that for some, action research is primarily an individual affair concerned with how practice might be improved. For others, it is more concerned with organisational development; whereas for a third group, it is more about how imbalances of power in society can be restored so that ordinary people can better manage their everyday lives. They argue that there can never be one 'right way' of doing action research and urge readers to value and embrace its many varied forms (Reason & Bradbury 2008). Whitelaw *et al.* (2003) have argued that the majority of literature on action research advocates critical and emancipatory approaches and suggest that exponents have paradoxically therefore been uncritical in their portrayal of action research by ignoring the potential of other models to influence practice.

Action research is complex and it is not easy to categorise any specific study neatly into a particular type. However, typologies of action research can help us appreciate and articulate the complexity of action research, even if we would be unwise to label and categorise individual studies using these typologies.

In my view, Hart and Bond (1995) provide one of the most accomplished typologies of action research. They suggest that there are seven criteria, which not only distinguish action research from other methodologies, but also determine the range of approaches used in action research. They present a typology of action research identifying four basic types (see Table 22.1):

- experimental
- organisational
- professionalising
- empowering.

They suggest that each type embodies a different theoretical perspective on society.

Hart and Bond's (1995) typology provides a useful framework for critiquing individual studies and, in particular, for thinking about how concepts are operationalised, the features of particular settings and the contribution of the people within those settings to solutions.

It is worth noting that, over time, health-related action research appears to have moved away from 'experimental' to more 'empowering' models of research. However, empowering models have to be used with care. Within an emancipatory action research project, practitioners, as co-researchers, need to make a commitment to the project in terms of reflecting on their practice and working towards changing the way they work. This can be very challenging and researchers should not make the assumption that practitioners will be willing or able to engage at this level. Dewing (2005) found that the emancipatory approach originally used in the Admiral Nursing Competency Project did not suit the context or existing culture and a more participatory approach needed to evolve. Somekh (1994) reiterates this point, arguing that different occupational cultures can affect action research methodology. For this reason, she suggests that action research should be grounded in the values and discourse of the individual or group rather than rigidly adhering to a particular methodological perspective.

ACTION RESEARCH IN HEALTHCARE PRACTICE

Action research is particularly useful when:

- no evidence exists to support or refute current practice
- knowledge, skills and attitudes are too poor to carry out evidence-based practice
- gaps have been identified in service provision
- services are under-utilised or deemed inappropriate
- new roles are being developed and implemented
- working across traditional conflicting boundaries.

More recently, it has been suggested that action research could help nurses better articulate the nature of their practice to address the invisibility of nursing work and to illuminate the significance of their contributions to healthcare and society (Canam 2008). It has also been suggested that it could have a more significant role in knowledge transfer science (Kitson 2009).

Table 22.1 Action research typology

Action research type: distinguishing criteria	Consensus model of society / Rational social management		Conflict model of society / Structural change	
	Experimental	Organisational	Professionalising	Empowering
1 Educative base	Re-education	Re-education/training	Reflective practice	Consciousness-raising
	Enhancing social science/administrative control and social change towards consensus	Enhancing managerial control and organisational change towards consensus	Enhancing professional control and individual's ability to control work situation	Enhancing user-control and shifting balance of power; structural change towards pluralism
	Inferring relationship between behaviour and output; identifying causal factors in group dynamics	Overcoming resistance to change/restructuring balance of power between managers and workers	Empowering professional groups; advocacy on behalf of patients/clients	Empowering oppressed groups
	Social scientific bias/researcher focused	Managerial bias/client focused	Practitioner focused	User/practitioner focused
2 Individuals in groups	Closed group, controlled, selection made by researcher for purposes of measurement/inferring relationship between cause and effect	Work groups and/or mixed groups of managers and workers	Professional(s) and/or (interdisciplinary) professional group/negotiated team boundaries	Fluid groupings, self-selecting or natural boundary or open/closed by negotiation
	Fixed membership	Selected membership	Shifting membership	Fluid membership
3 Problem focus	Problem emerges from the interaction of social science theory and social problems	Problem defined by most powerful group; some negotiation with workers	Problem defined by professional group; some negotiation with users	Emerging and negotiated definition of problem by less powerful group(s)
	Problem relevant for social science/management interests	Problem relevant for management/social science interests	Problem emerges from professional practice/experience	Problem emerges from members' practice/experience
	Success defined in terms of social sciences	Success defined by sponsors	Contested, professionally determined definitions of success	Competing definitions of success accepted and expected

4 Change intervention	Social science, experimental intervention to test theory and/or generate theory	Top-down, directed change towards predetermined aims	Professionally led, predefined, process led	Bottom-up, undetermined, process led
	Problem to be solved in terms of research aims	Problem to be solved in terms of management aims	Problem to be resolved in the interests of research-based practice and professionalisation	Problem to be explored as part of process of change, developing an understanding of meaning of issues in terms of problem and solution
5 Improvement and involvement	Towards controlled outcome and consensual definition of improvement	Towards tangible outcome and consensual definition of improvement	Towards improvement in practice defined by professionals and on behalf of users	Towards negotiated outcomes and pluralist definitions of improvement: account taken of vested interests
6 Cyclic processes	Research components dominant	Action and research components in tension; action dominated	Research and act on components in tension; research dominated	Action components dominant
	Identifies causal processes that can be generalised	Identifies causal processes that are specific to problem context and/or can be generalised	Identifies causal processes that are specific to problem and/or can be generalised	Changes course of events; recognition of multiple influences on change
	Time limited, task focused	Discrete cycle, rationalist, sequential	Spiral of cycles, opportunistic, dynamic	Open-ended, process driven
7 Research relationship, degree of collaboration	Experimenter/respondents	Consultant/researcher, respondent/participants	Practitioner or researcher/ collaborators	Practitioner researcher/ co-researchers/co-change agents
	Outside researcher as expert/research funding	Client pays an outside consultant – 'they who pay the piper call the tune'	Outside resources and/or internally generated	Outside resources and/or internally generated
	Differentiated roles	Differentiated roles	Merged roles	Shared roles

Reproduced by permission of the Open University Press from Hart E, Bond M (1995) *Action Research for Health and Social Care: a guide to practice.* Buckingham, Open University Press, pp 40–43.

Action research has much to offer healthcare practice. Munn-Giddings *et al.* (2008) found that action research has a strong presence within nursing research, but is mainly focused on organisational/professional development/education settings. Participation of practitioners within the research process is very strong, though few studies involved service users and/or carers. While many action research studies highlight the difficulties of changing practice (Meyer *et al.* 2000), there have been some more notable successes (for instance, Kilbride 2007).

Exemplar study 1: Local level

This two-year study, 'Inside the Black Box: creating excellence in stroke care through a community of practice' (Kilbride 2007), looked at the lessons learnt from setting up a new inpatient stroke service in a London teaching hospital. The aim of the study was to use a collaborative action research approach to achieve an interventional change, while generating new knowledge from practice by studying the process and outcomes of change. Key participants included members of the multiprofessional stroke team and support staff, the hospital management team and representatives drawn from patients and informal carers. Mixed methods were used to generate data. These included focus groups, in-depth interviews, documentary analysis, audits and participant observation. Prior to the study there was no specialist stroke service for the approximately 325 patients who were admitted to the trust each year; stroke care was fragmented, uncoordinated and spread over 18 wards. Local and national stroke audits showed there was much room for improvement in the care provided, with the hospital being placed in the bottom 5% in the country. Over the course of the study and beyond, a culture of sustained service improvement emerged, demonstrated by consistent placement in the top 5% in the National Sentinel Stroke Audits (Clinical Effectiveness & Evaluation Unit 2002, 2004, 2006). This remarkable success of moving from bottom to the top resulted in the unit receiving a national award for clinical service redesign in 2005 (*Health Service Journal* 2005). Overall stroke care improved markedly within the hospital, with death rates falling, higher results achieved on the national sentinel stroke audit and the

establishment of a hospital-based stroke prevention service. However, it should be noted that the success of action research does not depend on whether the intended goals are achieved or the change sustained. It is unrealistic to assume that change will be sustained in ever-changing healthcare contexts. It can take a long time for new ideas to become embedded in practice. However, intended goals are often linked to policy initiatives and much can be learned from trying to put policy into practice. The success of Kilbride's (2007) action research can be best seen in the learning from the systematic monitoring of the emergent processes in the study. Four main themes emerged from the process which had contributed to the local success:

- building a team
- developing practice-based knowledge and skills in stroke
- valuing the central role of the nurse in stroke care
- creating an organisational climate for supporting change.

While the previous body of knowledge had shown stroke units to be linked to better patient outcomes, these findings address a gap in the body of knowledge on how to set up an effective stroke unit. In addition to providing useful practical knowledge, it also adds to theoretical knowledge by showing how the emergent findings linked to the development of a community of practice. Recent literature suggests that communities of practice have a key role to play in implementing evidence-based practice (Fitzgerald *et al.* 2006), and this study provides some supporting evidence to this fact and reveals for the first time the practical knowledge and skills required to develop this style of working.

While action research predominately focuses on a local level, as in the above study, it has also been used to develop national guidance. Interestingly, this also took a community of practice approach.

Exemplar study 2: National level

This five-year project sought to provide evidence of the impact of the Caledonian practice development model on processes and outcomes of nursing practice with older people (Tolson *et al.* 2006). The model involved practitioners in a transformational learning experience supporting local practice development actions designed to promote the implementation of evidence-based practice. Learning was enabled through membership of a community of practice that collaborates and shares knowledge through an internet-based practice development college.

Twenty-four nurses from 18 sites representing three different care environments were recruited to form three communities of practice, covering both the NHS and independent sector. The study intervention focused on facilitating the nurses' practice development skills and the enablement of evidence-based practice through the implementation of an NHSQIS Best Practice Statement chosen by each community.

The impact of the model was assessed in two ways.

1 The impact on the practice area, using baseline and outcome audits of individual patient care and unit-level facilities.
2 The impact on the nurses, using three standardised questionnaires and focus group interviews recorded at the study's completion.

At follow-up eight months later, the practice evaluations demonstrated improvements in the quality of care of individual patients and in the practitioner questionnaires the nurses reported experiencing significantly greater autonomy and feelings of organisational support in their roles. The study provides encouraging evidence of the positive impact of the Caledonian practice development model, although a cautionary note is made with regard to the readiness of the practice environment to embrace internet-enabled approaches to learning and the availability of resources to enrich the learning environment. This study reaffirms the importance of communities of practice in implementing evidence-based guidance. It also demonstrates how a community of practice can be achieved nationally through an internet-based practice development college.

THE ROLE OF THE RESEARCHER IN ACTION RESEARCH

Critics suggest that action research is no different to what goes on in everyday practice, for example prac-

tice development, medical audit, clinical governance and good management. However, as stated before, the essential difference is the focus on systematically evaluating the process and outcomes of change and reflecting on, and disseminating, findings in relation to what is already known about the topic under study. If, as Stringer (1999) suggests, research is:

'systematic and rigorous inquiry or investigation that enables people to understand the nature of problematic events or phenomena' (Stringer 1999: 5)

then the role of the researcher in action research is to make this happen. Modifying ideas from Mills (2003) in relation to teaching, I would argue it involves a process of working with participants to:

- describe the problem and area of focus
- define the factors involved (e.g. community and agencies involved, healthcare setting within its historical and sociopolitical context, current practice, patient, practitioner and practice outcomes)
- develop research questions
- describe the intervention or innovation to be implemented
- develop a timeline for implementation
- describe the membership of the action research group
- develop a list of resources to implement the plan
- describe the data to be collected (qualitative and quantitative)
- develop a data collection and analysis plan
- gain ethical approval and permission to undertake the study
- select appropriate tools of inquiry
- carry out the plan (implementation, data collection, data analysis)
- reflect on and report the results (e.g. final report, professional and academic journals, local newsletters).

Not all practitioners have the skills to undertake research and it is important that they seek adequate levels of support. Action research is often undertaken as part of academic study and supervised by colleagues in higher education. Given its emphasis on learning, action research provides an ideal opportunity for the different agencies involved to personally benefit from the process, for example submitting work in relation to the study to contribute to academic qualifications. However, academic study is not for everyone and other types of support might be more appropriate. There are a number of commercially available toolkits for action research (see Hart & Bond 1995 for a good example).

ETHICAL ISSUES

An important role of the researcher in action research is to ensure the wellbeing of participants. This is normally achieved by going through a process of formal ethical approval. However, the non-predictive nature of action research means that it is also important to mutually agree an ethical code of practice at the start of the study. Winter and Munn-Giddings (2001) highlight a number of ethical issues and principles of procedure. First they emphasise the importance of maintaining a professional relationship, guided by a duty of care and respect for the individual regardless of gender, age, ethnicity, etc., along with a respect for cultural diversity and individual dignity,

as well as protection from harm. This last principle is part of any social researcher's role, in addition to the need for informed consent and honesty. However, Winter and Munn-Giddings (2001) suggest that there are other principles of procedure that should be followed in action research (see Box. 22.1).

Having an ethical code of practice does not negate the additional need for research governance and formal ethical approval for action research. However, these quality processes are made all the more complex by the action researcher not being able to say in advance what the research will do. Action research proposals need to be written in collaboration with participants, often as co-applicants, with an inbuilt degree of flexibility. The action researcher should indicate the likely course of the study, specify the need for flexibility and enter into open and ongoing dialogue with funders and ethical committees to seek approval for emergent changes in design.

METHODS OF DATA COLLECTION

While action research is often written up as a case study and tends to draw on qualitative methods

---

Box 22.1   Ensuring ethical practice – principles of procedure for action research

- Make sure discussions are fully documented
- Establish procedures for taking joint decisions
- Ensure the work of the project remains 'visible' to all participants
- Check back and get any interpretations authorised before wider circulation
- Enable participants to amend their contribution before its circulation
- Ensure progress reports and invite suggestions on future developments
- Differentiate between what is confidential to participants and intended for wider publication
- Negotiate acceptable rules of confidentiality
- Give participants the right to withdraw material containing any reference that may identify them
- Negotiate in advance how disagreements will be resolved
- Ensure participants seek the group's permission to use material for academic study
- Draw up clear statement of principles of procedure, early in the work

Adapted from Winter R, Munn-Giddings C (2001) *A Handbook for Action Research in Health and Social Care.* London, Routledge, pp 220–224.

(Meyer 2000), an eclectic approach to data collection is taken. Usually data collection focuses on three stages of the inquiry (exploration, intervention and evaluation) and, where possible, involves participants as co-researchers in the design and execution of the study.

Exploration phase

In the exploratory phase of the study, action researchers gather data to explore the nature of the problem and focus of the study. Data are typically generated through questionnaires, interviews and focus groups in order to seek participant opinion as to what needs to change. If the action researcher is an outsider, this phase often includes some participant observation so that the researcher can familiarise themselves with the context and establish good working relationships with participants. It helps if the action researcher has some familiarity with the setting, as the clinical credibility of the action researcher can aid entry into the field. Through a process of feeding back findings to participants, the focus of the study (action) is negotiated. The end of the exploration phase usually involves gathering data in relation to the focus of the study in order to establish a baseline from which to measure change over time. Typically this involves data being generated from audits of practice.

Intervention phase

During this phase, a number of action research cycles usually emerge, as spirals of activity. Each action research cycle comprises a period of planning, acting, observing, reflecting and re-planning. Action research should offer the capacity to deal with a number of problems at the same time and often spirals of activity lead to other spin-off spirals of further work. It would be wrong to give the impression of order and linearity, although action research is often written up in this way so as not to confuse the reader. During this period of intense activity it is important to monitor the process of change and reflect on learning being gained.

Data are thus usually generated through participant observation methods, reflective journals, diaries, fieldnotes and narratives of practice. During the intervention phase, interim findings are fed back to participants to guide their action. Meanwhile, the action researcher should keep self-reflective fieldnotes throughout the study to acknowledge their own subjectivity and demonstrate freedom from bias. It is important that they not only represent the views of all participants, including their own, but that they are also clear about whose voice they are representing and when.

Evaluation phase

There is no neat end to an action research project, as often participants wish to continue with the change processes. However, action researchers need to withdraw from the field to analyse and reflect on what has been learnt in the context of the wider body of knowledge. Before leaving the field, they typically repeat baseline measures to see if change has occurred over time and invite participants to reflect on what has been achieved (or not) and their explanations for this. In the evaluation phase, it is possible to analyse existing documents and protocols to enhance findings and further set the study in context. Most importantly, all findings should be shared with participants to allow them to comment critically on whether they feel their views have been represented adequately and for them to check that they are happy for the material to be shared with a wider audience.

In the Central and East London Education Consortium (CELEC) Action Research Project (Meyer *et al.* 2003, 2004) a variety of data collection methods were used to evaluate the process and outcomes of change. The exploration phase involved establishing a baseline from which to measure change over time in each of the seven organisations. This was done using the audit instruments Monitor 2000, a tool to measure quality of nursing care (Fearon & Goldstone 1995); and SQUIS, a tool to measure quality of social interaction between nursing staff and patients (Dean *et al.* 1993). Stakeholders (lead R&D nurses, trust and university staff, and representatives of the funder) were also interviewed to explore potential areas in need of development and to determine how to take the project forward. During the intervention phase, a large volume of documentary evidence was collected, including minutes of meetings and internal reports (e.g. annual reports) and, with their agreement, data were also gathered about the issues and concerns that the lead R&D nurses presented in monthly action learning sets.

At the end of each year, the lead R&D nurses were invited to design their own evaluation of the project and to report findings in whatever way they chose. In addition, the project co-ordinator and each of the seven lead R&D nurses kept reflective fieldnotes to capture achievements and lessons learnt. Finally, in the evaluation phase, the baseline measures (Monitor and SQUIS) were repeated and stakeholders re-interviewed to ascertain their views on what had been achieved, problems they had encountered and what had been learnt from the experience. Using these data collection methods, it was possible to:

- demonstrate concrete evidence of improvement over time (improved scores in Monitor and SQUIS)
- draw attention to other tangible outcomes (e.g. additional funding awarded to extend the way of working into the independent care home sector)
- describe perceived benefits (e.g. seen as effective way of commissioning nurse education)
- describe the lessons learnt (e.g. support needs for change agents).

For further details of the project see Meyer *et al.* (2004).

ASSESSING QUALITY

What makes action research data trustworthy? Waterman *et al.* (2001) provide 20 questions for assessing action research proposals and projects (see Box 22.2).

These criteria were later modified by Greenhalgh *et al.* (2004), but others would question the value of even having such standards or criteria (Lyotard 1979). Bradbury and Reason (2002) engage in this debate and conclude with the need to consider five overlapping issues of quality.

- Was the action research group set up for maximal involvement?
- Was the action research useful?
- Did the action research study acknowledge different ways of viewing the world?
  - ensure conceptual-theoretical integrity?
  - embrace ways of knowing beyond the intellect?
  - intentionally choose appropriate research methods?
- Was the action research perceived to be worthwhile?
- Did the action research lead to significant change in understanding or practice?

Bradbury and Reason (2002) suggest that while these issues deserve our attention, they should only be seen as checkpoints to engage in further dialogue about our work. They recognise that different people will wish to place different emphasis on each issue and, rather than aiming to judge action research as being 'good' or 'bad', these five issues of quality should be used to assess whether action researchers have been explicit about their work.

In addition to addressing trustworthiness of data, it is also important to consider their transferability. Action research is often written up as a case study. As such, the findings are reported in their rich contextual detail so that the reader can judge the relevance to their own practice situation. Sharp (1998) suggests that case studies also lend themselves well to theoretical generalisation, but acknowledges that this is not always attempted. This opens up debates about whether there is any general learning to be gained from specific cases. Bassey (1999) advocates that case study researchers should have more confidence in making fuzzy generalisations about their work. By clearly stating from single cases what researchers consider to be 'possible', 'likely' or 'unlikely' in similar contexts, they protect themselves from the charge of being engaged in trivial pursuit. Meyer *et al.* (2000), drawing on findings that compared a single case of action research with those generated by a systematic review of action research, caution against ignoring the findings from the single case. They argue that the findings from a single case of action research more closely reflect reality and are

Box 22.2   Questions for assessing action research proposals and projects

1   Is there a clear statement of the aims and objectives of each stage of the research?
2   Was the action research relevant to practitioners and/or users?
3   Were the phases of the project clearly outlined?
4   Were the participants and stakeholders clearly described and justified?
5   Was consideration given to the local context while implementing change?
6   Was the relationship between researchers and participants adequately considered?
7   Was the project managed appropriately?
8   Were ethical issues encountered and how were they dealt with?
9   Was the study adequately funded/supported?
10 Was the length and timetable of the project realistic?
11 Were data collected in a way that addressed the research issue?
12 Were steps taken to promote the rigour of the findings?
13 Were data analyses sufficiently rigorous?
14 Was the study design flexible and responsive?
15 Are there clear statements of the findings and outcomes of each phase of the study?
16 Do the researchers link the data that are presented to their own commentary and interpretation?
17 Is the connection with an existing body of knowledge made clear?
18 Is there discussion of the extent to which aims and objectives were achieved at each stage?
19 Are the findings of the study transferable?
20 Have the authors articulated the criteria upon which their own work is to be read/judged?

Reproduced with permission of Department of Health from Waterman H, Tillen D, Dickson R, de Koning K (2001) Action research: a systematic review and guidance for assessment. *Health Technology Assessment Monograph* **5**: 23. London, Department of Health, pp 48–50.

potentially more valid and meaningful to others. These issues relating to case study research are examined in more detail in Chapter 20.

RESEARCH AS AN AGENT OF CHANGE

It could be argued that the ultimate aim of all research is to improve practice. However, most research relies on practitioners to implement findings. Slowly the limitations to this segregated approach of research and development are being recognised. A recent report describing a systematic review of the literature on the spread and sustainability of innovations in health service delivery and organisation (Greenhalgh *et al.* 2004) recommended 'participatory action research' along with 'realistic evaluation' as the way forward. They saw these approaches as being based on a 'whole-systems' approach, in as much as they are:

- theory-driven
- process rather than 'package-oriented'
- participatory
- collaborative and co-ordinated
- addressed using common definitions, measures and tools
- multidisciplinary and multimethod
- meticulously detailed
- ecological (relational to people and context).

Whole-systems approaches to change management are now favoured, as they recognise the complexity and inevitability of change.

Clearly in action research, research is being used as an agent of change. This implies that the action researcher not only needs research skills, but also an understanding of change and skills in change management. The literature about change management is large and not easy to access. Sometimes change is deliberate, a product of conscious reasoning and actions. This type of change is called 'planned change'. In contrast, change sometimes unfolds in an apparently spontaneous and unplanned way. This type of change is known as 'emergent change'.

According to Isles and Sutherland (2001) change can be emergent in two ways: first, managers can make decisions based on unspoken, and sometimes unconscious, assumptions about the organisation, its environment and the future; and second, external factors (such as the economy, competitors' behaviour and political climate) or internal features (such as the relative power of different interest groups, distribution of knowledge and uncertainty) can influence the change in directions outside the control of managers.

This highlights the need to identify, explore and, if necessary, challenge the assumptions that underlie decisions. Further, it is important to understand that organisational change is a process that can be facilitated. Isles and Sutherland (2001) conclude that it is vital to recognise that organisation-level change is not fixed or linear in nature but contains an important emergent element. Gibbons *et al.* (1994) suggest that there is a need to break away from linear thinking to more flexible and creative systems that allow true expertise to flourish. As can be seen from what is written above, action researchers take account of these issues in both the design and execution of their studies. Indeed, it has been argued that nurses are leading these developments in the field of health services research (Meyer 1997).

ADVANTAGES AND DISADVANTAGES OF ACTION RESEARCH

Waterman *et al.* (2001) identify eight categories of pivotal factor that can be used to demonstrate the strengths and limitations of action research:

Box 22.3 Advantages and disadvantages of action research

Advantages	Disadvantages
In situations where: – no evidence exists to support or refute current practice – poor knowledge, skills and attitudes to carry out evidence-based practice – gaps have been identified in service in service provision – services are underused or deemed inappropriate – new roles are being developed and implemented – work is across traditional conflicting boundaries	– not viewed as science – findings not generalisable – vulnerability of participants – depends on collaboration – difficult to achieve and sustain change – feedback can be threatening – change hard to measure – poor development of theory

- participation
- key persons
- action researcher–participant relationship
- real-world focus
- resources
- research methods
- project process and management
- knowledge.

They argue that for each of these factors there are opposing aspects that help to provide possible avenues for reconceptualising understanding of the process of action research in healthcare and offer ideas for its further development. These issues can be summarised into a number of advantages and disadvantages, which are presented in Box 22.3.

CONCLUSIONS

This chapter has explored the nature of action research and demonstrated its value at the 'D' end of the 'research and development' spectrum. It has identified common models of working with action research in nursing and suggests caution in adopting any one particular model. It has reflected on the role of the researcher in action research, highlighting the need for a mutually agreed ethical code of practice. In addition it has described the methods of data collection in relation to three phases of action research (exploration, intervention and evaluation) and given some consideration to the idea of research being an agent of change. Finally, consideration has been given to the advantages and disadvantages of action research. In conclusion, it would appear that action research has much to offer health services research, and it is suggested that nurses are leading the way.

References

Bassey M (1999) *Case Study Research in Educational Settings*. Buckingham, Open University Press.

Bradbury H, Reason P (2002) Conclusion: broadening the bandwidth of validity: issues and choice-points for improving the quality of action research. In: Reason P, Bradbury H (eds) *Handbook of Action Research: partici-patory inquiry and practice*. London, Sage, pp 447–455.

Canam C J (2008) The link between nursing discourses and nurses' silence: implications for a knowledge-based discourse for nursing practice. *Advances in Nursing Science* **31**(4): 296–307.

Clinical Effectiveness and Evaluation Unit (2002) *National Sentinel Audit of Stroke 2001/2*. Report for site code 175. Prepared on behalf of the Intercollegiate Stroke Group by Clinical Effectiveness and Evaluation Unit. London, Royal College of Physicians.

Clinical Effectiveness and Evaluation Unit (2004) *National Sentinel Audit of Stroke 2004*. Report for site code 230. Prepared on behalf of the Intercollegiate Stroke Group by Clinical Effectiveness and Evaluation Unit. London, Royal College of Physicians.

Clinical Effectiveness and Evaluation Unit (2006) *National Sentinel Audit of Stroke 2006*. Report for site code 230. Prepared on behalf of the Intercollegiate Stroke Group by Clinical Effectiveness and Evaluation Unit. London, Royal College of Physicians.

Dean R, Proudfoot R, Lindesay J (1993) The quality of interaction schedule (QUIS): development, reliability and use in the evaluation of two domus units. *International Journal of Geriatric Psychiatry* **8**: 819–826.

Dewing J (2005) Admiral nursing competency project: practice development and action research. *Journal of Clinical Nursing* **14**: 695–703.

Fearon MM, Goldstone LA (1995) *Monitor 2000. An audit of the quality of nursing care for medical and surgical wards*. Newcastle upon Tyne, Unique Business Services Ltd.

Fitzgerald L, Dopson S, Ferlie E, Locock L (2006) Knowledge in action. In: Dopson S, Fitzgerald L (eds) *Knowledge to Action? Evidence-based Healthcare in Context*. Oxford, Oxford University Press, pp 155–181.

Gibbons M, Limoges C, Nowotny H, Schwartzman S, Scott P, Trow M (1994) *The New Production of Knowledge: the dynamics of science and research in contemporary societies*. London, Sage.

Greenhalgh T, Robert G, Bate P, Kyriakidou O, Macfarlane F, Peacock R (2004) *How to Spread Good Ideas: a systematic review of the literature on diffusion, dissemination and sustainability of innovations in health service delivery and organization*. Report for the National Co-ordinating Centre for NHS Service Delivery and Organisation R & D (NCCSDO). London, London School of Hygiene and Tropical Medicine.

Hart E, Bond M (1995) *Action Research for Health and Social Care: a guide to practice*. Buckingham, Open University Press.

Isles V, Sutherland K (2001) *Managing Change in the NHS. Organisational Change: a review for health care managers, professionals and researchers*. Report for the National Co-ordinating Centre for NHS Service Delivery and Organisation R & D (NCCSDO). London, London School of Hygiene and Tropical Medicine.

Kilbride, C (2007) Inside the Black Box: creating excellence in stroke care through a community of practice. Unpublished PhD thesis. London, City University.

Kitson AL (2009) The need for systems change: reflections on knowledge translation and organizational change. *Journal of Advanced Nursing* **65**(1): 217–228.

Lyotard JF (1979) *The Postmodern Condition: a report on knowledge* (trans. Bennington G, Massimi B). Manchester, Manchester University Press.

Meyer J (2000) Using qualitative methods in health related action research. *British Medical Journal* **320**: 178–181.

Meyer J (1997) Action research in health-care practice: nature, present concerns and future possibilities. *NT Research* **2**: 175–184.

Meyer J, Johnson B, Bryar R (2004) CELEC Action Research Project: care for older people. Unpublished report. London, City University.

Meyer J, Johnson B, Bryar R, Procter S (2003) Practitioner research: exploring issues in relation to research-capacity building. *NT Research* **8**: 407–417.

Meyer J, Spilsbury K, Prieto J (2000) Comparison of findings from a single case in relation to those from a systematic review of action research. *Nurse Researcher* **7**(2): 37–53.

Mills GE (2003) *Action Research: a guide for the teacher researcher*. Upper Saddle River, Merrill/Prentice Hall.

Munn-Giddings C, McVicar A, Smith L (2008) Systematic review of the uptake and design of action research in published nursing research, 2000–2005. *Journal of Research in Nursing* **13**(6): 465–477.

Reason P, Bradbury H (2001) Inquiry and participation in search of a world worthy of human aspiration. In: Reason P, Bradbury H (eds) (2001) *Handbook of Action Research*. London, Sage, pp 1–14.

Reason P, Bradbury H (2008) Introduction. In: Reason P, Bradbury H (eds) *The Sage Handbook of Action Research Participative Inquiry and Practice*, 2nd edition. London, Sage.

Sharp K (1998) The case for case studies in nursing research: the problem of generalisation. *Journal of Advanced Nursing* **27**: 785–789.

Somekh B (1994) Inhabiting each other's castles: towards knowledge and mutual growth though collaboration. *Educational Action Research Journal* **2**(3): 357–381.

Stringer E (1999) *Action Research*, 2nd edition. London, Sage.

Tolson D, Booth J, Lowndes A, Baxter S, Smith J, Hoy D, Schofield I (2006) *The Gerontological Nursing Demonstration Project. Caledonian Practice Development Model Practice Impact Study*. Final Report, Centre for Gerontological Practice, Glasgow Caledonian University.

Waterman H, Tillen D, Dickson R, de Koning K (2001) Action research: a systematic review and guidance for assessment. *Health Technology Assessment Monograph* **5**: 23.

Whitelaw S, Beattie A, Balogh R, Watson J (2003) *A Review of the Nature of Action Research*. Welsh Assembly Government, Sustainable Health Action Research Programme.

Winter R, Munn-Giddings C (2001) *A Handbook for Action Research in Health and Social Care*. London, Routledge.

Further reading

Reason P, Bradbury H (eds) (2008) *The Sage Handbook of Action Research Participative Inquiry and Practice*, 2nd edition. London, Sage.

Susman GI, Evered RD (1978) An assessment of the scientific merits of action research. *Administrative Science Quarterly* **December**: 582–603.

Websites

www.bath.ac.uk/carpp/ – Centre for Action Research in Professional Practice (CARP).

www.did.stu.mmu.ac.uk/carnnew/ – Collaborative Action Research Network, based at Manchester Metropolitan University, provides a network of action researchers linked to the international journal *Educational Action Research*.

www.parnet.org/ – Participative Action Research Network (PARnet), an action research site in North America offering valuable resources and links to other sites.

www.scu.edu.au/schools/gcm/ar/arr/links.html – action research resources at Southern Cross University, Australia, provides a list of sites offering links and resources to action research, and related topics.

www.uea.ac.uk/care/ – Centre for Applied Research in Education (CARE), a UK action research site at the University of East Anglia offering resources and links to other websites.

23 Practitioner Research

Jan Reed

Key points

- Every researcher with experience of contributing to practice provision is a practitioner researcher.

- This approach shapes research decisions in ways that may be different to traditional research.

- Practitioner research involves a number of issues relating to integration with research participants.

- Transparency is needed to make the rationale for these decisions clear and open to evaluation.

- A practitioner research culture is needed to support practitioner research development.

INTRODUCTION

Many of us are practitioner researchers, that is we have been trained as practitioners and are also doing research. We may be nurses investigating our own practice or researchers investigating someone else's, but we are likely to share a language, values and outlook. As such, these issues shape the way we engage with research, the way we generate it, plan it, do it, use it and disseminate it. Not surprisingly, the balancing of practice experience with the traditional 'distance' or objectivity of research is challenging and complex, particularly if we are hoping to carry out studies that meet the criteria for research quality set by various external bodies, such as publishers and

funders. We do not always want to keep research to ourselves, and we may want to share it or develop it further, but the channels we can use may not seem welcoming – publishers or funders may not seem supportive.

Rolfe (1998) has outlined these criteria and ideas of valid evidence pointing to a hierarchical structure, where evidence is ranked according to perceived strength. At the top of this is the traditional randomised controlled trial – as the name suggests, this is research that selects participants randomly, and controls interventions and evaluations; neither aspect is compatible with engaged practitioner person-centred care. As this hierarchy implies, any other form of research, such as qualitative research, is ranked lower. This ranking prioritises what is very similar to the model of research use named by Schön (1983) as 'technical rationality', which is the development of a highly specialised form of statistically valid knowledge and application to practice, not necessarily with the understanding of practitioners. In contrast, Schön has also pointed to the 'messiness' of practice, and the way that it is often embroiled in dilemmas and debates. Rolfe attributes the lack of practitioner confidence and the 'theory–practice gap' to this 'technical rationality' way of applying knowledge, and the consequent devaluing of the messiness of practitioner experience and knowledge.

If we want to address this, we have two options. We can either try to comply with traditional research criteria or we can develop and apply our own. The first option runs the risk of us becoming so compliant with traditional research criteria that we lose integration with practice. The second option, however, runs the risk of losing integration with resources – if we set our own practice-relevant criteria, then we may not have access to funding or effective means of dissemination.

So what do we do? One response could be to examine and reflect on the issues of practitioner research and the potential that it has for developing nursing, and in this way to develop and strengthen it. The term 'practitioner research' is one that encapsulates two key ideas. First, it emphasises the salience of interactions with those providing and using nursing services. Second, there is the inclusion of the word 'researcher', which indicates an exploration and investigation of nursing practice. This is what this chapter is about, a way of combining these two activities, that is to say, developing knowledge that informs and reflects practice engagement.

Of course, this combination has been visited before, and discussions have had a variety of goals and focused around a number of different processes. The section on the background to practitioner research lays out some of this context, but as the chapter progresses, more detailed debate is offered and the stages of research are explored with their attendant concerns and questions. This chapter then offers a process for researchers exploring these stages and checking that they meet requirements for practice validity.

BACKGROUND TO PRACTITIONER RESEARCH

There has been a long development in nursing calling for practice to be founded on evidence rather than tradition. This movement has been attributed to many drivers and motives. One driver may simply be the realisation that much of what nurses do has little justification and we may not only be not helping patients, but we may also be doing them harm. Another, perhaps more cynical, line of thinking is that much of this search for justification can be traced back to competition with other disciplines, particularly medicine, which has a history of applying research-based evidence to practice. The place of custom in determining practice can, of course, be discerned, and there are likely to be gaps in studies exploring the myriad dimensions of care, but the principle of using research to inform practice is a constant theme.

Evidence-based practice

One development has been the movement to encourage evidence-based practice (EBP) (see Chapter 38 for more discussion of this concept). This has involved practitioners or their managers finding studies that answer questions about practice (or the questions that researchers pose, which may be different), and applying this evidence. The skills required are seen as the ability to understand and apply the research findings. Examples of this are given by Rolfe (1998), who refers to both the UK Department of Health and the International Council of Nurses directives on using research in practice, and comments that:

> 'research is therefore seen ... as a specialist, even elitist activity carried out by a select group comprised mainly of academics. These researchers then pass down their findings to practitioners to implement in what has been referred to as research-based or evidence-based practice' (Rolfe 1998: 673)

These directives may seem dated, but there is some indication that this model of evidence-based practice, where the evidence is developed by researchers and then applied to practice, is still a matter of current debate. French (2002), for example, has argued that for much evidence-based practice there is little evidence. Many of the papers on evidence-based practice that French analysed were diverse and shared little conceptual foundation.

Moreover, Baumbusch *et al.* (2008) have argued that:

> 'With regards to the definition of best evidence, theoretical and methodological approaches that are used in nursing research, such as qualitative research, participatory action research, research underpinned by critical inquiry, are often not included or fall at the bottom of EBP hierarchies (Baumbusch *et al.* 2008: 133)

This makes the hierarchy of EBP incongruent with many of the sources of knowledge that nurses use, such as philosophic, aesthetic, theoretical, personal and practice knowledge, as Reimer-Kirkham *et al.* (2007) have argued.

This is reflected in many discussions of how EBP can be achieved. Profetto-McGrath *et al.* (2005), for example, argue that EBP must be accompanied by critical thinking in order to apply evidence to practice, and talk about a two-stage process. The first stage is generating knowledge from research, and the second is examining this evidence to see how it could inform practice, which is where critical thinking comes in. The EBP debate, then, has moved on here, with there being no automatic process of evidence application. There is still, however, an idea that evidence should be developed by scientists outside practice, and then applied to it. There is still a separation between the generators and the users of knowledge.

The place of critical thinking is emphasised in this discussion, and a similar stance is taken by Baumbusch *et al.* (2008) in their discussion of 'knowledge translation' (see Chapter 39 for a more in-depth discussion of knowledge translation). This discussion moves from the unidirectional 'transfer' of knowledge to a more interactive and collaborative process, where practitioners are not simply passive recipients of information, but play an active part in the synthesis and use of evidence. This reflects the importance of practice experience, a point also made by McCracken and Marsh (2008) when they argue that:

> 'far from being a mechanistic process that ignores practitioner expertise, reflection and critical thinking

are essential to implementing EBP in real-world clinical practice (McCracken & Marsh 2008: 301)

Nonetheless, the EBP movement is accompanied by calls for practitioners to use research generated by others, rather than generate their own.

Practice development

A step towards practitioners generating their own knowledge is demonstrated by debates on practice development initiatives. Here, practice development is seen as a continual process, as practice responds to changing environments. Garbett and McCormack (2002), for example, have defined practice development as 'built-in' continuous action to change practice:

> 'a continuous process of improvement designed to promote increased effectiveness in patient-centred care. It is brought about by enabling health care teams to develop their knowledge and skills and in doing so, transform the culture and context of care. It is enabled and supported by facilitators who are committed to systematic, rigorous and continuous processes of change that will free practitioners to act in new ways that better reflect the perspectives of both service users and service providers' (Garbett & McCormack 2002: 87)

The process of practice development uses research from a variety of methodological schools, and therefore looks at relevance rather than methodological ranking. It also draws on practitioner knowledge and motivation to effect change and development (McCormack 2003).

The localised nature of practice development means that learning and sharing outside these localities may be limited. This limited generalisation comes partly from methodological complexities, in that the forms of knowledge that practice development draws on are difficult to use to inform other practices. The application of formal research depends on translating research that has usually been developed elsewhere by non-practitioners who act according to research criteria. The use of practitioner knowledge, on the other hand, is usually an informal process and as such is not easily shared with other practitioners working in other places – we do not know how this knowledge was generated, articulated or evaluated, and it is this lack of discussion that makes sharing more difficult.

Bringing practice and research together

These brief discussions of moves towards evidence-based practice (EBP) and practice development have pointed to some of the strengths of these approaches, that they make us think carefully about what we do. They also point towards some of the issues that arise from this, that research and practice are separated, and the development of practice knowledge is not articulated clearly.

These two issues make a case for bringing research and practice together. This is not necessarily a matter of reconciling opposing activities, as we can identify a range of ideas shared between the two. Larsen *et al.* (2002), for example, have argued that there is no gap 'per se' between research and practice as both develop in different contexts and 'theory and practice have different logics; they are not on a continuum nor are they hierarchically ordered'. This argument criticises the 'barrier paradigm', which postulates the existence of gaps between activities and suggests that this is not necessarily the case – research and practice are just different. Perhaps the key to this argument lies in the statement that research and practice are not differently ranked, but the statement that they are different does suggest that the nature of practice knowledge needs to be explored more openly. Research knowledge is often scrutinised and critiqued in the process of funding and publication, and indeed, if this public scrutiny were not possible, then the research would lose credibility.

Larsen *et al.* (2002), despite their claims, do distinguish between research and practice, but their argument also points to a way forward, and that is the process of opening up practitioner research to this process of open scrutiny. Baumbusch *et al.* (2008) in their discussion of knowledge transfer and translation also see differences as insignificant due to shared agendas and concerns, most clearly a concern with transparency, rigour and questioning.

The concern shared by both research and practice is that practice is informed and shaped by knowledge that is open to challenge and debate. In the case of traditional research this might be through the application of traditional research criteria of validity and reliability. For practitioner research these criteria might be different. Dadds (2008), for example, has suggested that 'empathetic validity' may be a key element of research. 'Empathetic validity' can be defined as the potential of practitioner research in its processes and outcomes to transform the emotional dispositions of people towards each other, such that greater empathy and regard are created. Practitioner research that is high in empathetic validity contributes to positive human relationships and, as such, is an important form of research in an age of increasing violence, as well as stress and tension in the workplace. The paper makes a distinction between internal empathetic validity (that which changes the practitioner researcher and research beneficiaries) and external empathetic validity (that which influences audiences with whom the practitioner research is shared). This idea of validity comes closer to identifying what sort of criteria practitioner research may employ – if we have regard for our colleagues and patients, in accordance with our professional values of individual needs and development, then empathetic validity fits with these values.

McCormack (2003) has also pointed to the resonance of practice development with practitioner research as a way of bridging the divide between the 'knowledge generators' and the 'knowledge users'. He goes on to describe the development of practitioner research as a way of developing a research culture in practice. In other words, practitioner research is not simply a single study but a continuous process of exploration and reflection. He uses the definition of practitioner research offered by Brooker and McPherson (1999):

> 'Practitioner research is a formal and systematic attempt made by practitioners alone or in collaboration with others to understand practitioners' work with the intended purpose of transforming self, colleagues and work contexts and the development of new understandings of practitioners' work' (McCormack 2003: 207)

In this definition the notion of collegiality and engagement with practice are clear, indicating the importance of developing a culture of inquiry, a point that we return to in the conclusion.

To explore these issues and identify potential frameworks for evaluating practitioner research we need to work through the process of carrying out practitioner research and identify the way in which we can do this, the issues that can arise and the way we might reflect on the way that we do this. This moves away from ideas of technical rationality to ideas of reflective research (Reed & Procter 1995) and provides a starting point for development. In the interests of reflective research, then, this is offered as a starting point for debate rather than a set of procedures, and as Reimer-Kirkham *et al.* (2007) have argued:

'autonomy is eroded if nurses use evidence as recipes, without drawing on their professional knowledge and clinical judgment to interpret evidence, and make decisions about best evidence in context – this is the core of professional practice' (Reimer-Kirkham 2007: 29)

INSIDER AND OUTSIDER POSITIONS

One of the first activities to engage in is the review and reflection of your position as researcher. The term 'position' sounds very fixed, and it is more likely that you will move in and out of positions at different times and in different contexts, or even occupy several positions at the same time. Nonetheless, thinking about your position can be a helpful activity that can alert you to ways in which your research can be shaped by, and can itself shape, different discussions.

Reed and Procter (1995) presented a 'position continuum', which suggests the range of positions that can be taken (see Box 23.1).

Looking at this continuum, it is possible to reflect on where you can place yourself at different points in the research process. As an 'insider' you may be directly engaged with practice, perhaps involved in service delivery or development. As an 'outsider' you may be able to step away from this and be more

---

Box 23.1   Position Continuum

POSITION	'OUTSIDER'– primarily a researcher with no or little engagement with practice	'INSIDER'– primarily engaged with practice and carrying out research into this practice
AIMS	To explore a social phenomenon (nursing) in order to contribute to the body of social science knowledge	To solve a critical problem, thereby contributing to the body of nursing knowledge
ACCESS	Choice of research setting wide, but contact transient and superficial	Setting limited by practice contacts, but this is sustained and intimate
ROLE	Researcher is a guest	Researcher is a member
DESIGN AND PLANNING	Informed by knowledge of research methods	Informed by knowledge of practice
ANALYSIS	Does not share taken-for-granted assumptions, and adopts a naive stance towards the data	Shares taken-for-granted assumptions, and needs to reflectively adopt a naive stance towards the data
CONTRIBUTION	To academic community and the development of theory	To colleagues and the academic community and the development of practice

Adapted from Reed J, Proctor S (1995) *Practitioner Research in Health Care*. Chapman and Hall, London.

directly involved in external worlds, such as the academic world of examination and awards.

Reflecting on this general placing, it then becomes more possible to examine and explore some of the assumptions that are brought to the study. As Nagel (1986) asserted, there is no 'view from nowhere'. In other words, we all approach situations with some assumptions and preconceptions, or as Lykkeslet-Molde and Gjengedal (2007) argue:

> 'A researcher never enters the field, be it a foreign or familiar one, fresh and without preconceptions. All she observes will be influenced by her previous experiences and her pre-understanding. It takes time and effort to develop a way of distinguishing between the field as viewed by a fieldworker and the same field viewed by the practitioner' (Lykkeslet-Molde & Gjengedal 2007: 700)

Following this advice, the following section explores these pre-understandings throughout the process of research. This idea of process suggests that this can be clearly identified and defined, but it may not be the case. As anyone who has thought about doing research will know, the neat and tidy description of a 'research process' belies the chaos, confusion and weaving backwards and forwards that research can involve. It is more astute then to regard what follows and the stages of research that are discussed as tools for working through practitioner research issues rather than a definitive description.

At each of these stages of research we echo the comments of Lykkeslet-Molde and Gjengedal (2007: 699) when they flag up two key debates in what they term 'practice-close' research. These debates are:

- the researcher's ability to explicate their preconceptions
- the researcher's interaction with the participants in the study.

There are, of course, other issues at play here, and some of these have already been debated in this chapter, namely the issue of 'approved' or 'legitimate' knowledge in the context of traditions of hierarchies of knowledge. Another issue, which we return to at the end of this discussion of the research process, is the issue of ethics and values, and the relationship between research and practice views of these.

REFLECTING ON THE PRACTITIONER RESEARCH PROCESS

Research questions

One of the first steps in a research study is to think about the focus of the study, the issues it will explore and the questions it will ask. An overview of the positions of 'outsider' and 'insider' is given below.

OUTSIDER
Is the question determined by gaps in academic knowledge and formulation?

INSIDER
Is the question determined by gaps in practical knowledge and understanding?

As an 'outsider', for our purposes a traditional academic researcher, questions can be directed by an awareness of gaps or deficits in existing knowledge. These gaps can be identified through a trawl of existing studies (published in journals that adhere to traditional criteria for validity), which will indicate where previous studies have identified confusions, gaps or overlaps. The task of any proposed study, then, is to address these. As such, the logic of a study focus is straightforward, as the goals of a study are to contribute to this academic body of knowledge.

As an 'insider', the questions can be very different, and may well be about the ways in which practice could be developed in the context of the practice environment. This context, and the resources and systems that shape it, will determine what services are offered, and to whom. While these factors may be minimised or controlled in outsider research, they are simply part of the environment in most practitioner research studies. If the environment needs to be adapted for the study, the practitioner researcher's colleagues will be the people who can do this. Colleagues can also stimulate ideas for research, and conversations about possibilities can be fruitful in making concerns and priorities clear.

There are, however, some disadvantages in being an insider. As Whitehead has said, being an insider can make it difficult to see the obvious:

> 'Familiar things happen and people don't take notice of them. It takes an unusual mind to discover the obvious' (cited in Lykkeslet-Molde & Gjengedal 2007: 701)

23.1 Identifying Questions

Reed J, Bond S (1991) Nurses' assessment of elderly patients in hospital. *International Journal of Nursing Studies* **28**(1): 55–64.

In a study about older person care, I undertook some unstructured observation of early morning practice, in order to find a focus to my questioning. I spent several mornings observing staff, and each time I came away with a blank sheet of paper, with no notes, comments or observations on it.

Following this I discussed my experiences with academic colleagues. They were intrigued by the possibilities of using observation of everyday practice to explore concepts such as institutionalisation, autonomy or depersonalisation.

I also discussed my experiences with practice colleagues, who were amazed at my lack of insight, commenting on how hard the staff were working and how they responded to the diverse needs of patients.

I had seen 24 patients helped out of bed, taken to the toilet, given breakfast and medicines, but as an insider had taken it all for granted. My academic colleagues had raised some interesting conceptual points, and practice colleagues had raised some practical points, but I had not raised any questions.

This 'taking for granted' makes identifying questions difficult for insider researchers. As the example in Research Example 23.1 suggests, this can be an issue that researchers have to consider carefully.

Sample

A next stage may be to decide who will be the participants in the study, sometimes referred to as a 'sample.'

OUTSIDER	INSIDER
Is the sample determined by academic concerns about generalisation?	Is the sample determined by accessibility contingent on practice roles and practice goals?

For an outsider, samples and settings are selected according to their meeting of criteria for inclusion, and these criteria are, in turn, determined partly by the research question(s). This directs the population to be studied, and the sample is taken from this population, often using random methods of selection. This random generation does not take into account any characteristics of the population other than the features being studied. If a sample is generated which does take the characteristic of accessibility or avail-ability into account, then this can be called a 'convenience sample' and it is not regarded as statistically worthy as a random sample, as the data it produces cannot be generalised (see Chapter 12 for further discussion of sampling techniques).

For an insider, accessibility may be a key characteristic of a sample. That is, an insider researcher may want to study the environment and actors engaged in practice. This may mean that the population is whatever or whoever is, in the researcher's professional judgement, significant in increasing understanding of practice. The sample may be the population, i.e. there may be no selection, and if there is any selection, accessibility may be the basis for this. If, for example, a practitioner is working with a client group in a particular area, the population may be that client group.

This suggests that the criterion of random sampling may not apply – the criterion may be practice relevance rather than statistical relevance. Statistical processes allow for generalisability, i.e. the findings can be generalised to the whole population. With a practice sample, the process may be different, and the use of study findings in other areas may be more a matter of professional judgement. If a study was done in a particular setting, then a researcher may need to note the similarities and differences between that setting and their practice, to decide which findings are useful and which are not.

This does not mean that sampling is straightforward in practitioner research – accessing chosen samples may be fraught with difficulties in negotiation. Sometimes gatekeepers might block access or they might encourage it – and both responses can create difficulties. Apart from an overenthusiastic coercion to take part in a study, there are some theoretical issues to be aware of. As Lykkeslet-Molde and Gjengedal (2007) argue 'having a good relationship with the people being studied is … potentially a double-edged sword'. They then go on to refer to Hammersley and Atkinson who argued that those who participate in studies are exploited, because 'they give information that is used by the researcher and receive little or nothing in return' (Lykkeslet-Molde & Gjengedal 2007: 702).

Research Example 23.2 gives an example of someone working with people living in the country who wanted to explore how rurality affected their lives. This meant that the people she was researching were often her own clients, and the temptation was to involve them in the study on the basis of professional knowledge. As part of her response to this she involved a colleague in what could have been a coercive or not transparent process.

Methods

When we identify methods to use in any research there are two basic forms – watch people or talk to them. Most usually we will do both, whether by accident or design. If you are watching people you will be talking (or not talking) to them. As Watzlawick *et al.* (1967) put it:

> 'there is no such thing as non-behavior or, to put it even more simply: one cannot not behave. Now, if it is accepted that all behaviour, in an interactional situation has message value, i.e. is communication, it follows that no matter how one may try, one cannot not communicate' (Watzlawick *et al.* 1967: 48–49)

Similarly, if you are talking to people then these conversations will be accompanied by some watching of the setting and the interviewees.

The position of the researcher becomes important in this debate, as it reflects the goals and messages of data collection. As an outsider, methods may be driven by methodological concerns – the focus is on finding the right way to explore a theoretical issue and maintain methodological integrity. As an insider, any data collection will happen in the context of current relationships with colleagues and clients. This is summarised below.

RESEARCH EXAMPLE

23.2 Sampling Strategy

Bell A (2008) An exploration of 'choice' in relation to social care for older people in a rural area. Unpublished PhD proposal, University of Northumbria.

This study sought to explore the experiences of older people living in a rural area where the researcher was a member of the community team.

The sampling strategy was purposive sampling, with the objective of identifying information rich cases for in-depth analysis. A small group of service users was selected from two rural district social care offices. The researcher relied on care managers' professional judgement to ascertain whether service users were physically and psychologically well enough to consent and participate in the study. If they were willing the researcher would then make telephone contact to discuss the project again and confirm their agreement prior to visiting. The care manager would identify if there were any service users for whom telephone contact would not be appropriate, in which case a pre-interview visit was carried out.

OUTSIDER	INSIDER
Are methods determined by concerns about academic integrity and theoretical frameworks?	Do methods reflect and respond to practice relationships and processes?

The idea that the outsider position is more distant and the methods chosen would be unencumbered by insider assumptions can certainly be challenged. We have already seen arguments about the impossibility of 'non-behaviour', where messages are sent or received regardless of researcher intentions (Watzlawick *et al.* 1967). Kvale and Brinkmann (2008) also have something to say about the idea of the egalitarian interview where researchers hope to carry out conversations with no imbalance of power, but can find that assumptions of status permeate interviews. Lykkeslet-Molde and Gjengedal (2007) summarise this as follows.

'The difference between the interviewer and the interviewee with respect to power and resources might seem to disappear. A dialogue engaged in for purposes such as these might also have an aspect of control, as the situation tends to conceal the power and the freedom the researcher possesses to use the information as he or she sees fit. It is therefore important to see the interview as an asymmetrical relationship. The conversation is the means by which the researcher attains his or her goal; the conversation is not an end in itself (Lykkeslet-Molde & Gjengedal 2007: 703)

The suggestion that the relationship between researcher and researched is unequal indicates that some examination of this relationship is needed in the analysis and presentation of studies. Moreover, it suggests that efforts should be made to address this imbalance, particularly as this may conflict with practice values. Research Example 23.3 gives an example of this, as a researcher found an interview methodology that allowed research to go some way towards respecting practice values. Research Example 23.4 gives an example of how practitioner research can lead to innovations in methodology, in this case developing drama as a data source, a process that relied on practitioner support in the process. Research Example 23.5 shows how the skills of a practitioner are closely related to the skills required by researchers.

Analysis

As data are collected, researchers engage in a process of meaning making, and that meaning is shaped by the goals and questions that the study began with. We

---

RESEARCH EXAMPLE

23.3 Selecting Methods

Hibberd P (2008) Family-centred admiral nursing: re-conceptualising practice values. Unpublished PhD report, University of Northumbria.

The revisiting or 'unearthing' of problems did not sit comfortably with my approach to working with carers and people with dementia. In the clinical area I prefer to approach a therapeutic intervention/relationship using a solution-focused approach (De Shazer 1988). My experiences as a practitioner in the NHS have heightened my awareness of how colleagues feel and are treated when being asked to participate in research and organisational change. In my experience this has always been from a problem-based approach leaving participants feeling weary, overworked and undervalued. The suggestion and then study of an Appreciative Inquiry approach (Reed 2007) started to appear to relate to my positive and relational approach to working. Initial 'testing' of the approach first at home (instigating positive change of teenage behaviour) and then in class with continuing professional development students in dementia care were promising. Students became noticeably engaged and empowered when asked to cite positive experiences and build on them.

23.4   Developing Innovative Methodology with Practitioner Research

Keady J, Williams S (2007) Co-constructed inquiry: a new approach to generating, disseminating and discovering knowledge in qualitative research. *Quality in Ageing* **8**: 27–37.

John Keady and Sion Williams developed co-constructed inquiry in partnership with specialist nurse practitioners, university-based researchers (with a clinical background in stroke and dementia care) and people living with long-term conditions. This introduces the language of drama and theatre into the theory building and reporting process and consists of three stages: building the set; performing the production; and bringing down the curtain. People with long-term conditions explored their experiences through the production of a life story script, a personal theory and, eventually, a collective theory. This exploration involved collaboration with practitioners and researchers, who shared insights and goals. The outcomes informed practice and care, and the study explored methods of articulation and collaboration in drama, an activity that is not often used as a research methodology.

23.5   Using Practice Skills in Research

Way R (2008) Discovery Interviews with older people: reflections from a practitioner. *International Journal of Older People Nursing* **3**: 211–216.

Discovery Interview technique was originally developed for use in service improvement programmes run by the National Health Service (NHS) Heart Improvement Programme. It involves practitioners conducting one-to-one, face-to-face, semi-structured interviews with service users, which focus on the interviewee describing their experiences in their own words. Stories are then shared more widely with local teams with a view to stimulating service improvements.

In this paper a practitioner reflects on his use of the method, and the outcomes of the interviews. He found that the method was useful, but that he needed to adapt it to the context of the unit. He also found that Discovery Interviews led to ideas for service development, including improving communication and delivering care adapted to the environment. In carrying out the interviews, he was using practitioner skills in communicating with patients.

can summarise this with reference to possible researcher positions.

OUTSIDER	INSIDER
Is meaning principally shaped by the context of academic discourses on theory and methodology?	Is meaning principally shaped by the challenges of practice?

The range of potential ways of meaning making, and the different interests and questions, is illustrated in Research Example 23.6. A study was carried out where four research groups from four different countries interviewed local groups of older people to explore their strategies for developing wellbeing. Each research team was working in a different service system and had different academic and practice interests. To address this wide range of potential meanings, four strands of analysis were identified, as shown in Research Example 23.6. In this framework, there were strands of analysis from theoretical ideas, service configuration, service use and individ-

RESEARCH EXAMPLE

23.6   Analysis

Reed J, Richardson E, Marais S, Moyle W (2008) Older people maintaining well-being: an International Appreciative Inquiry study. *International Journal of Older People Nursing* **3**(1): 68–76.

This study on the strategies older people use to maintain their well being involved four teams of researchers from four countries. In order to include the cultural and national differences and similarities between the countries, and to explore practitioner concerns, the following levels of analysis were used.

Meta-level –   the presentation of data in reports and papers might use some of these meta-level theories, and we noted down our ideas about theories as they occurred to us throughout the study.
Macro-level –   we summarised 'society' as a whole, including national parties, political systems, service organisation, health and social care systems.
Mezzo level –   we examined responses to institutions and organisations (families, business, civil service, associations) in the data we collected.
Micro-level –   we examined our interview data to explore face-to-face, social interaction and personal experiences.

RESEARCH EXAMPLE

23.7   Outcomes of Practitioner Research

Shur R, Simons N (2008) Quality issues in health care research and practice. *Nursing Economics* **26**(4): 258–263.

The authors describe a programme of quality improvement, and argue that 'This work was performed by practitioner-researchers and efficiency consultants from many disciplines. The resulting recommendations are striking in their straightforward practicality and in their insistence that process factors determine output' (Shur & Simons 2008: 258).

This points to a potential outcome of practitioner research that findings can be used in practice. Moreover, practitioner research can challenge orthodox thinking from its basis in practice.

ual experiences. This clarified the analysis process and made it possible to identify routes of meaning making.

Research Example 23.7 summarises a paper which argues that the outcomes of practitioner research are very practical and challenging. Practitioner research, then, can be pragmatic and also lead to theoretical developments.

ETHICAL ISSUES

Throughout the process of carrying out research, the relationships with colleagues, service providers and service users have been indicated as a fundamental dimension of research. The outsider position, with traditional research mores, can adopt a disengaged and distant stance, whereas an insider researcher practises

RESEARCH EXAMPLE

23.8 Setting Up Resources for Practitioner Research

Darbyshire P, Downes M, Collins C, Dyer S, Day B (2005) Moving from institutional dependence to entrepreneurialism. Creating and funding a collaborative research and practice development position. *Journal of Clinical Nursing* **14**: 926–934.

This paper describes the development of the rationale behind and the external funding of a collaborative research-clinical practice development position, and discusses the issues of funding such an enterprise. The paper argues that nurses should look to a range of funders, and also that a practitioner research project, with a focus on developing interventions, is well placed to attract this support.

This is one way in which practitioner research can be resourced and supported, and a culture of research and collaboration can be developed.

with research participants, and the relationships that have arisen there will permeate any study that is done. Participation does not stop because a study has begun.

Perhaps this point is best made in the following quote:

> 'As practitioner researchers, our ontological position is one of democratic participation and inclusion; our epistemological stance is associated with socially critical constructions of knowledge; and our methodological approach is "working with" rather than "working on" people. For us, people are research participants and research colleagues, and not research subjects' (Macpherson *et al.* 2004: 95)

If we think of practitioner research as being an extension of practice, then the values of autonomy and independence that inform practice will inform research too. However, the issue may be that if we think this merging is 'unscientific' then we may hide theses values rather than explore them.

CONCLUSIONS

This chapter has argued that one of the ways to develop practitioner research is to identify and explore the issues that can arise. In doing this, we can work towards developing a set of criteria that we can use to evaluate studies, criteria that may be different from those of traditional science, and reflective of

practice engagement. To do this is a tall order and, like practitioner research itself, is something that needs wide support. This points towards developing a culture of enquiry, where reflection and thought are encouraged. Practitioner research, then, can be a starting point for wider development.

Research Example 23.8 gives an example of how this may be resourced, and how funding may be attracted by practitioner research, which is driven by practice concerns. This focus may be one that is the foundation of bids for support: research that integrates practice with research.

References

Baumbusch JL, Reimer-Kirkham S, Basu Khan K, McDonald H, Semeniuk P, Tan E, Anderson JM (2008) Pursuing common agendas: collaborative model for knowledge translation between research and practice in clinical settings. *Research in Nursing & Health* **31**: 130–140.

Bell A (2008) An exploration of 'choice' in relation to social care for older people in a rural area. Unpublished PhD proposal, University of Northumbria.

Brooker R, MacPherson I (1999) The processes and outcomes of practitioner research: an opportunity for self-indulgence or serious professional responsibility? *Educational Action Research* **7**(2): 207–220.

Dadds M (2008) Empathetic validity in practitioner research. *Educational Action Research* **16**(2): 279–290.

Darbyshire P, Downes M, Collins C, Dyer S, Day B (2005) Moving from institutional dependence to entrepreneurialism. Creating and funding a collaborative research and practice development position. *Journal of Clinical Nursing* **14**: 926–934.

De Shazer S (1988) *Clues: investigating solutions in brief therapy*. New York, Norton.

French P (2002) What is the evidence on evidence-based nursing? An epistemological concern. *Journal of Advanced Nursing* **37**(3): 250–257.

Garbett R, McCormack B (2002) A concept analysis of practice development. *Nursing Times Research* **7**: 87.

Hibberd P (2008) Family-centred admiral nursing: reconceptualising practice values. Unpublished PhD report, University of Northumbria.

Keady J, Williams S (2007) Co-constructed inquiry: a new approach to generating, disseminating and discovering knowledge in qualitative research. *Quality in Ageing* **8**(2): 27–37.

Kvale S, Brinkmann S (2008) *InterViews. Learning the Craft of Qualitative Research Interviewing*, 2nd edition. Thousand Oaks, Sage.

Larsen K, Adamsen L, Bjerregaard L, Madsen JK (2002) There is no gap 'per se' between theory and practice: research knowledge and clinical knowledge are developed in different contexts and follow their own logic. *Nursing Outlook* **50**(5): 202–212.

Lykkeslet-Molde E, Gjengedal E (2007) Methodological problems associated with practice-close research. *Qualitative Health Research* **17**(5): 699–704.

McCormack B (2003) Knowing and acting – a strategic practitioner-focused approach to nursing research and practice development. *Nursing Times Research* **8**: 86–100.

McCracken SG, Marsh JC (2008) Practitioner expertise in evidence-based practice decision making. *Research on Social Work Practice* **18**: 301–310.

Macpherson I, Brooker R, Aspland T, Cuskelly E (2004) Constructing a territory for professional practice research Some introductory considerations. *Action Research* **2**(1): 89–106.

Nagel T (1986) *The View from Nowhere*. New York, Oxford University Press.

Profetto-McGrath J (2005) Critical thinking and evidence-based practice. *Journal of Professional Nursing* **21**(6): 364–371.

Reed J (2007) *Appreciative Inquiry Research for Change*. London, Sage.

Reed J, Bond S (1991) Nurses' assessment of elderly patients in hospital. *International Journal of Nursing Studies* **28**(1): 55–64.

Reed J, Procter S (1995) *Practitioner Research in Health Care*. London, Chapman and Hall

Reed J, Richardson E, Marais S, Moyle W (2008) Older people maintaining well-being: an International Appreciative Inquiry study. *International Journal of Older People Nursing* **3**(1): 68–76.

Reimer-Kirkham S, Baumbusch J, Schultz A, Anderson J (2007) Enhancing professional nursing practice through evidence-based practice: insights and opportunities from a post colonial feminist perspective. *Advances in Nursing Science* **30**: 25–40.

Rolfe G (1998) The theory-practice gap in nursing. *Journal of Advanced Nursing* **28**(3): 672–679.

Schön DA (1983) *The Reflective Practitioner*. London, Temple Smith.

Shur R, Simons N (2008) Quality issues in health care research and practice. *Nursing Economics* **26**(4): 258–263.

Watzlawick P, Beavin AB, Jackson MD (1967) *Pragmatics of Human Communication*. New York, Norton.

Way R (2008) Discovery Interviews with older people: reflections from a practitioner. *International Journal of Older People Nursing* **3**: 211–216.

24 Systematic Reviews and Evidence Syntheses

Andrew Booth, Angie Rees and Claire Beecroft

Key points

- Evidence syntheses, in particular systematic reviews, contribute to evidence-based practice by using explicit methods to identify, select, critically appraise and summarise large quantities of information to aid the decision-making process.

- The three main types of evidence syntheses are systematic reviews, practice guidelines and economic evaluations.

- Regardless of the type of evidence synthesis, several discrete, but interconnected, stages are followed: writing a research protocol, systematically searching the literature, selecting relevant studies, assessing the quality of the literature, extracting key information from the selected studies, summarising, interpreting and presenting the findings, and writing up the research in a structured manner.

INTRODUCTION

This chapter builds on Chapters 7 and 8 to provide a practical introduction to conducting evidence synthesis (i.e. reanalysing existing research), with specific reference to systematic reviews. Readers are advised to refer to these two earlier chapters for more detailed information about the skills required to access and appraise research literature. A worked example relating to antibiotics and antiseptics for venous leg ulcers (taken from a completed Cochrane review from the Cochrane Library) is used throughout (see Research Example 24.1).

BACKGROUND TO EVIDENCE SYNTHESIS

The knowledge base for any evidence-based profession is founded on evidence syntheses. By reanalysing previously collected data from original (primary) studies within research syntheses, it is possible to summarise large volumes of information in a succinct manner. This not only increases the precision of the overall result, but also assists in establishing generalisability of findings and examining conflicting results. It also provides an opportunity to identify gaps in the current knowledge base and hence suggest future primary research areas.

RESEARCH EXAMPLE

24.1   A Cochrane Plain Language Summary and Review Abstract

Summary

Antibiotics and antiseptics to help healing venous leg ulcers

Venous leg ulcers are a type of wound that can take a long time to heal. These ulcers can become infected and this might cause further delay to healing. Two types of treatment are available to treat infection: systemic antibiotics (i.e. antibiotic tablets or injections) and topical preparations (i.e. applied directly to the wound). Whether systemic or topical preparations are used, patients will also usually have a wound dressing to cover the wound and maybe a bandage too. This review was undertaken to find out whether using antibiotics and antiseptics works better than usual care for healing venous leg ulcers, and if so, to find out which antibiotic and antiseptic preparations are better than others. In terms of topical preparations, there is some evidence to support the use of cadexomer iodine. Further good quality research is required before definitive conclusions can be made about the effectiveness of systemic antibiotics and topical agents such as povidone iodine, peroxide-based preparations, ethacridine lactate and mupirocin in healing venous leg ulceration.

This record should be cited as: O'Meara S, Al-Kurdi D, Ovington LG (2008) Antibiotics and antiseptics for venous leg ulcers. Cochrane Database of Systematic Reviews Issue 1. Art. No.: CD003557. DOI: 10.1002/14651858.CD003557.pub2. This version was first published online 23 January 2008.

Abstract

Background

Venous leg ulcers are a type of chronic wound affecting up to 1% of adults in developed countries at some point during their life. Many of these wounds are colonised by bacteria or show signs of clinical infection. The presence of infection may delay ulcer healing. There are two main strategies used to prevent and treat clinical infection in venous leg ulcers: systemic antibiotics and topical antibiotics or antiseptics.

Objectives

The objective of the review is to determine the effects of systemic antibiotics and topical antibiotics and antiseptics on the healing of venous ulcers.

Search strategy

The following databases were searched up to October 2007: the Cochrane Wounds Group Specialised Register; the Cochrane Central Register of Controlled Trials; MEDLINE; EMBASE; and CINAHL. In addition, the reference lists of included studies and relevant review articles were examined.

Continued

Selection criteria

Randomised controlled trials recruiting people with venous leg ulceration that evaluated at least one systemic antibiotic, topical antibiotic or topical antiseptic and reported an objective assessment of wound healing (e.g. time to complete healing, frequency of complete healing, change in ulcer surface area) were eligible for inclusion. Selection decisions were made by three authors working independently.

Data collection and analysis

Information on the characteristics of participants, interventions and outcomes were recorded on a standardised data extraction form. In addition, aspects of trial methods were extracted, including methods of randomisation and allocation concealment, use of blinded outcome assessment, intention-to-treat analysis, reporting of patient follow-up and study group comparability at baseline. Data extraction and validity assessment were conducted by one author and checked by a second.

Main results

Twenty-two trials were identified of different antibiotics and antiseptics, including systemic antibiotics (five trials). The remainder were topical preparations. For the systemic antibiotics, the only comparison where a statistically significant between-group difference was detected was that in favour of the antihelminthic levamisole when compared with placebo. This trial, in common with the other evaluations of systemic antibiotics, was small and so the observed effect could have occurred by chance. In terms of topical preparations, there is some evidence to suggest that cadexomer iodine generates higher healing rates than standard care. One study showed a statistically significant result in favour of cadexomer iodine when compared with standard care (not involving compression) in terms of frequency of complete healing at six weeks (RR 2.29, 95% CI 1.10 to 4.74). The intervention regimen used was intensive, involving daily dressing changes, and so these findings may not be generalisable to most everyday clinical settings. When cadexomer iodine was compared with standard care with all patients receiving compression, the pooled estimate from two trials for frequency of complete healing at 4 to 6 weeks indicated significantly higher healing rates for cadexomer iodine (RR 6.72, 95% CI 1.56 to 28.95). Surrogate healing outcomes such as change in ulcer surface area and daily or weekly healing rate showed favourable results for cadexomer iodine, peroxide-based preparations and ethacridine lactate in some studies. These surrogate outcomes may not be valid proxies for complete healing of the wound. Most of the trials were small and many had methodological problems such as poor baseline comparability between groups, failure to use (or report) true randomisation, adequate allocation concealment, blinded outcome assessment and analysis by intention-to-treat.

Authors' conclusions

At present, there is no existing evidence to support the routine use of systemic antibiotics to promote healing in venous leg ulcers. However, the lack of reliable evidence means that it is not possible to recommend the discontinuation of any of the agents reviewed. In terms of topical preparations, there is some evidence to support the use of cadexomer iodine. Further good-quality research is required before definitive conclusions can be made about the effectiveness of systemic antibiotics and topical preparations such as povidone iodine, peroxide-based preparations, ethacridine lactate and mupirocin in healing venous leg ulceration. In light of the increasing problem of bacterial resistance to antibiotics, current prescribing guidelines recommend that antibacterial preparations should only be used in cases of defined infection and not for bacterial colonisation.

Systematic reviews

A '*systematic review*' (or '*overview*') is:

'a review of the evidence on a clearly formulated question that uses systematic and explicit methods to identify, select and critically appraise relevant primary research, and to extract and analyse data from the studies that are included in the review' (Khan *et al.* 2001: 4)

Whereas 'review' (sometimes referred to as a narrative or traditional review) is a general term used to describe a synthesis of the results and conclusions of two or more publications on a given topic, a systematic review strives for comprehensive identification and synthesis of all literature on a given topic. A systematic review, aims to be:

- systematic (e.g. in its identification of literature)
- explicit (e.g. in its statement of objectives, materials and methods)
- reproducible (e.g. in its methodology and conclusions) (Greenhalgh 2000).

The term '*meta-analysis*' is often used interchangeably with 'systematic review'. However, it describes a statistical technique used to combine the results of several studies into a single estimate (Khan *et al.* 2001).

Examples of systematic reviews in nursing include reviews on infection control strategies for methicillin-resistant *Staphylococcus aureus* (MRSA) in nursing homes for older people (Hughes *et al.* 2008), nursing interventions for smoking cessation (Rice & Stead 2008) and specialist breast care nurses for supportive care of women with breast cancer (Cruickshank *et al.* 2008). All these examples can be found on The Cochrane Library (www.cochrane.org).

Practice guidelines and economic evaluations

Other examples of evidence synthesis are practice guidelines and economic evaluations. Practice guidelines are:

'Directions or principles presenting current or future rules of policy for the health care practitioner to assist him in patient care decisions regarding diagnosis, therapy, or related clinical circumstances … The guidelines form a basis for the evaluation of all aspects of health care and delivery' (Clinical Practice Guidelines, National Library of Medicine, MeSH Browser)

Many evidence-based guidelines, such as those produced in the UK by the National Institute for Health and Clinical Excellence (NICE), have implications for nursing. Examples include 'Antenatal care – routine care for healthy pregnant women' (2008), 'Prevention and treatment of surgical site infection' (2008) and 'Diabetes in pregnancy' (2008). These can be accessed on the NICE website (www.nice.org. uk).

An '*economic evaluation*' entails drawing up a balance sheet of the advantages (benefits) and disadvantages (costs) associated with different healthcare options so that choices can be made (Robinson 1993). Published examples include an economic evaluation of in-reach specialist nursing teams for residential care homes (Szczepura *et al.* 2008) and cost and clinical outcomes of a back injury clinic (New & Winecoff 2007).

Advantages of evidence synthesis

Well-conducted evidence syntheses offer several advantages over single primary research studies (Mulrow 1995; Greenhalgh 2000). For example:

- large amounts of information can be assimilated quickly and efficiently, thereby assisting in the decision-making process
- the use of explicit methods helps to limit bias in identifying and excluding studies
- the results of different studies can be formally compared to establish generalisability of findings and consistency of results
- reasons for inconsistency in results across studies can be identified and new hypotheses generated
- quantitative techniques, such as meta-analysis, increase the precision of the overall result
- Conclusions are thus considered to be more reliable and accurate.

Stages in conducting evidence synthesis

For each of the above types of evidence synthesis, the researcher typically follows discrete, but interconnected, stages:

- writing a research protocol, outlining the purpose and methods of the research
- systematically searching the literature
- selecting relevant studies
- assessing the quality of the literature
- extracting key information from the selected studies
- summarising, interpreting and presenting the findings
- writing up the research in a structured manner.

This chapter focuses on systematic reviews, the most common of research syntheses, but the described methods apply, to varying degrees, to other types of evidence synthesis.

WRITING A SYSTEMATIC REVIEW PROTOCOL

The first step in undertaking a systematic review is to establish whether there is sufficient need for a review. This starts with a comprehensive search for existing reviews addressing the same (or similar) research question(s) and critical appraisal of the quality of any potentially relevant reviews. Existing and ongoing systematic reviews can be identified by searching:

- the Cochrane Database of Systematic Reviews (CDSR) – www.cochrane.org/reviews
- the Database of Reviews of Effects (DARE) – www.crd.york.ac.uk/crdweb
- major health-related databases, such as MEDLINE, using methodological search filters designed to retrieve systematic reviews (e.g. www.ncbi.nlm.nih.gov/entrez/query/static/clinical.shtml#reviews). Box 24.1 provides an example of such a filter. Local healthcare librarians can provide advice and support in identifying and using search filters.

If existing reviews are outdated, or of poor quality, it may be necessary to update them or to conduct a new review from scratch. The key to a successful systematic review lies in the reviewer's ability to be precise and specific when stating the problems to be addressed. A structured approach to framing questions should be used. To the four components of PICO (**P**atients (or population), **I**nterventions (or

---

Box 24.1 Methodological search filter designed to retrieve systematic reviews in MEDLINE (Dialog)

The following search filter, originally designed by Ann McKibbon at McMaster University in Canada, can be added to any subject search in MEDLINE (Dialog interface).

1 review-academic.pt.
(pt means publication type)
2 review-tutorial.pt.
3 systematic NEAR review.ti,ab,de.
(NEAR means the two words must be within 5 words of each other)
(ti,ab,de looks for the words in the title, abstract and MeSH heading (descriptor) field)
4 systematic NEAR overview.ti.ab.de.
5 (metaanaly$ OR meta analy$ OR meta-analy$).ti,ab,de.
($ is the truncation symbol)
6 meta-analysis.pt.
7 1 or 2 or 3 or 4 or 5 or 6.

exposures) **C**omparison and **O**utcomes) that apply to all types of question (see Chapter 6) you will find it helpful to add a further component specifically for the purpose of a systematic review, namely the **S**tudy design(s) that are suitable for addressing the review question (Khan *et al.* 2004). This stage in the systematic review process is perhaps the most difficult, yet most important to get right. A review protocol is drawn up specifying the plan that the review will subsequently follow. It is a key reference document throughout the review process. Modifications should only be made to the protocol if there is a genuine reason (for example, if an additional outcome measure is identified on closer examination of the literature).

A review protocol typically includes the following.

- *Background and rationale to the review.* This includes a justification for the review being undertaken, as well as a preliminary assessment of potentially relevant literature and its size.
- *Review question(s).* The review question(s) should be well focused in terms of the population, intervention and outcome(s).
- *Inclusion criteria.* These should follow on logically from the review question(s), and cover any restrictions regarding study design or publication type, language or year of publication. Any exclusion criteria should be stated explicitly and reasons given. Where feasible, these criteria should be applied to the studies by two independent reviewers.
- *Literature search strategy.* This should outline details of the sources to be searched and a sample search strategy.
- *Quality assessment strategy.* This should provide details of the critical appraisal checklist or scale (preferably validated) used to assess the quality of the included studies.
- *Data extraction strategy.* Where possible, a sample data extraction form should be included, indicating the information to be collected from each study (e.g. details about the participants, methods, interventions, results, etc.).
- *Proposed analysis.* This should document the type of data most likely to be found (e.g.

quantitative or qualitative), and the proposed data synthesis and presentation strategy (e.g. meta-analysis).
- *Plans for reporting and dissemination.* This should describe the strategy for reporting and disseminating the findings to relevant audiences.
- *Members of the review team.* Ideally a systematic review should be undertaken by a review 'team', although many smaller reviews are written by lone researchers. Members of a review team should include an information specialist to identify, locate and store relevant references; someone to review the literature; a methodologist (such as a statistician); and content experts, possibly in the form of an advisory group.
- *Project timetable.* Include a draft timetable outlining each stage in the systematic review.
- *Proposed costings.* Even small-scale reviews entail costs (e.g. staff time, obtaining articles, etc.). It is important to be aware of these costs at the outset and, if necessary, apply for additional funding.

SYSTEMATICALLY SEARCHING THE LITERATURE

The aim of a systematic literature search is 'to provide a list as comprehensive as possible of primary studies, both published and unpublished' (Khan *et al.* 2001: 21).

Refining the review question

The search starts by refining the review question and translating it into a search strategy that can be used to interrogate electronic bibliographic databases. As well as searching the literature to identify existing systematic reviews, 'scoping' searches will ensure that the final strategy reflects all components of the review question(s). Research Example 24.2 applies the PICOS approach to the review of antibiotics and antiseptics for venous leg ulcers.

24.2 A Refined Review Question: Antibiotics and Antiseptics for Venous Leg Ulcers (O'Meara *et al.* 2008)

	Components	Keywords	Synonyms (i.e. alternative search terms)
P	Patient/Problem/Population	venous leg ulcers	varicose ulcer (MeSH) leg ulcer (MeSH) venous ulcers
I	Intervention	antibiotics	exp antibacterial-agents (MeSH) antibiotics penicillin cephalosporin aminoglycosides gentamicin quinolones ciprofloxacin clindamycin metronidazole trimethoprim
C	Comparison	antiseptics	exp anti-infective agents, local (MeSH) antiseptics disinfectants
O	Outcomes	wound healing	wound healing (MeSH) ulcer healing wound size wound duration
S	Study design	randomised controlled trials	randomised controlled trial [publication type] clinical trial [publication type] randomised controlled trials (MeSH) Random* control* trial*

Selecting relevant sources to search for a systematic review

A review team should search a wide variety of sources for published, as well as unpublished, literature including:

- large electronic bibliographic databases, such as MEDLINE, CINAHL, EMBASE and the Web of Knowledge[1]

[1]While some database names originated as meaningful acronyms it is common practice to identify and to refer to these resources by their abbreviated forms.

- subject-specific electronic bibliographic databases, such as AMED (for allied health literature and complementary and alternative medicine), PsycINFO (for psychological and psychiatric literature), AgeINFO (for literature relating to older people), etc.
- research and trials registers, such as CCTR (formerly the Cochrane Controlled Trials Register), Current Controlled Trials, National Research Register, Index to Theses and Dissertation Abstracts
- grey literature databases, such as the Health Management Information Consortium (HMIC)

database, a compilation of data from the library and information services of the Department of Health and the King's Fund

- the Internet, including generic search engines (e.g. Google Scholar) and subject-specific search engines (e.g. Intute, a free online service providing a database of hand selected web resources for education and research)
- hand searching the table of contents of key journals
- checking the reference lists of selected articles
- contacting experts and key organisations
- conducting citation searches on key articles and authors using the Web of Knowledge or Google Scholar.

Developing sensitive search strategies

Systematic literature searches use highly sensitive search strategies to ensure that no relevant studies are overlooked. This means a reviewer will look through a larger set of references (usually hundreds, or even thousands) to minimise the chance of missing relevant items. Using 'specific' search strategies means that the search retrieves fewer, but more highly relevant references, but the reviewer runs the risk of missing relevant studies. The reviewer, therefore, aims to achieve the right balance between 'sensitivity' and 'specificity' when designing search strategies.

The sensitivity of a search strategy can be increased by:

- including more search terms and thesaurus terms (identified from previously retrieved references)
- using truncation ('*' or '$') or wildcards ('?' or '#') in free text searches
- using 'OR' to combine terms within the same concept
- using 'NEAR' to retrieve terms within the same sentence
- using a combination of free text and thesaurus search terms
- 'exploding' thesaurus search terms
- selecting 'all subheadings' for thesaurus search terms

- searching only on the 'population' and 'intervention', i.e. not introducing 'outcomes' or 'comparisons' into the strategy
- not applying date, language, or study design limits to the search strategy
- using 'sensitive' methodological search filters (see below).

Methodological search filters

Methodological search filters are strategies that are added to the subject search and are designed to retrieve different types of evidence from the search. Filters have been developed for the major types of question (i.e. therapy, prognosis, diagnosis and aetiology) and the major types of study (i.e. qualitative research, economic evaluations and clinical guidelines). Sample filters can be found at the InterTASC Information Specialists' Sub-Group Search Filter Resource (www.york.ac.uk/inst/crd/intertasc).

Most of the major databases (for example Ovid MEDLINE, PubMed and the National Library for Health's Search 2.0 function) now include a pre-stored facility to enable use of methodological filters. Although these should be used with caution when conducting a *sensitive* search, for systematic review purposes they do provide a useful and *specific* way of scoping the quantity and quality of the literature prior to developing a review protocol.

Addressing publication bias

Publication bias means that studies with significant results are more likely to be published (Khan *et al.* 2004). Debate centres on whether systematic reviews should identify and include non-English language or unpublished research (Egger *et al.* 2003; Easterbrook *et al.* 1991). For example, McAuley *et al.* (2000) have shown that if unpublished studies are not included in meta-analyses the effectiveness of an intervention may be overestimated. However, even the most comprehensive literature search cannot eliminate the possibility of publication bias. For example, studies are published two or more years after the research was conducted; other studies are never published; there is a tendency towards 'selective reporting', i.e. where only studies that show statistically significant results are published; and multiple publication of the same results from a single study in several different journals is common. Techniques to address 'publication bias' are given under 'Summarising, interpreting and presenting the findings' below.

Managing large sets of references

It is essential to use a reference management system to manage the large numbers of references. Chapter 7 introduced electronic reference management software packages such as Reference Manager, EndNote and Procite. These packages allow the reviewer to:

- store and maintain references (journals, books, reports, websites, theses, etc.)
- import references directly from major electronic bibliographic databases, such as MEDLINE
- keep track of references ordered from libraries
- assign keywords to references (e.g. the keyword 'RCT' can be applied to references retrieved from a clinical trials search)
- retrieve sets of references by author, publication year, title, keywords, etc.
- insert personal notes and comments relating to individual references
- automatically create reference lists in the reviewer's preferred journal style
- insert references directly into word-processed reports.

Documenting a systematic literature search

The review team should keep an accurate record of the search strategy used. This helps to avoid duplicated effort and provides a basis for updating the review in the future. Information to be recorded includes the date of the search, the sources searched, the search terms used and the number of references retrieved.

Selecting relevant studies

When selecting studies for inclusion the aim is to identify those articles that address the question(s) being posed. It is important to screen all the references retrieved and obtain the full text of studies that potentially meet the inclusion criteria. These criteria should stem directly from the review question(s) and relate to the core components of the question, i.e. participants, interventions, outcomes and study design. Research Example 24.3 lists criteria for considering studies for inclusion in the antibiotics and antiseptics for venous leg ulcers review.

Criteria should be set in advance and piloted to check that they can be applied consistently. Final decisions about inclusion and exclusion are made after reading the full-text of articles. Reasons for exclusion are recorded. Errors of judgement in study selection can be reduced by using two independent reviewers. However, this is not always feasible and it may be acceptable to assess a sample of studies independently.

ASSESSING THE QUALITY OF THE LITERATURE

Study quality refers to the degree to which a study takes steps to minimise bias and error in its design, conduct and analysis (Khan *et al.* 2004). Once studies of a minimum acceptable quality (based on the study design) have been selected, an in-depth critical appraisal is required. It is important to determine whether there is a quality (or study design) threshold that defines the weakest acceptable study to be included. For example, many Cochrane reviews only include randomised controlled trials (RCTs).

Detailed quality assessment of studies within a systematic review (Khan *et al.* 2004) aims to:

- describe the quality of studies included in the review
- explore whether different effects in different studies can be explained by variations in their quality
- decide whether to pool the effects observed in included studies

24.3   Criteria for Considering Studies for Review: Antibiotics and Antiseptics for Venous Leg Ulcers (O'Meara *et al.* 2008)

Types of participant

Trials recruiting people described in the primary studies as having venous leg ulcers were eligible for inclusion. Trials recruiting people with different types of wound (e.g. arterial ulcers, diabetic foot ulcers) were included if the results for patients with venous ulcers were presented separately or if the majority of participants (at least 75%) had leg ulcers of venous aetiology. Selection of trials was not restricted to those with a certain wound status at baseline (i.e. those with colonised or infected wounds); where information was given about these variables it was recorded (see data extraction).

Types of intervention

The primary intervention is antibiotics (topical or systemic) or antiseptics (topical) prescribed for venous leg ulceration. Systemic preparations could be given orally or parenterally (for example by intravenous administration), and administered singly or in combination. Control regimens could include placebo, an alternative antibiotic or antiseptic, any other therapy, standard care or no treatment. Both intervention and control regimens could consist of combinations of antibiotics and antiseptics. Interventions could be delivered in any setting (inpatient, outpatient, nursing home, plus any others). Trials evaluating topical silver-based preparations or the use of honey in wound healing were excluded as these interventions have been, or will be, covered in other Cochrane reviews).

Types of outcome measure

Primary outcomes

Trials reporting any of the following outcomes at any endpoint were eligible.

1   Time to complete ulcer healing
2   Proportion of ulcers completely healing during the trial period (frequency of complete healing)
3   Objective measurements of change in ulcer size
4   Healing rate (e.g. mm^2 ulcer surface area reduction per week)

Secondary outcomes

Where reported, the following outcomes were also recorded.

1   Changes in signs and/or symptoms of clinical infection
2   Changes in bacterial flora
3   Development of bacterial resistance
4   Ulcer recurrence rates
5   Adverse effects of treatment
6   Patient satisfaction
7   Quality of life
8   Costs

Continued

Studies were only eligible for inclusion if they reported a primary outcome, since those reporting solely secondary outcomes could introduce reporting bias. Findings from methodological research suggest that failure to report the full range of available outcomes assessed within a trial is associated with statistically non-significant results. This can result in the presentation of a selective and biased subset of study outcomes.

Types of study

Prospective randomised controlled trials (RCTs) evaluating topical or systemic antibiotics or antiseptics in the treatment of venous ulcers were included.

- determine the strength of inferences from the data
- recommend how future studies should be conducted.

When conducting a systematic review, it is essential to identify suitable checklists for each study design that meets the inclusion criteria. If a checklist does not exist, then adapting existing tools that reflect generic issues relating to validity, reliability and applicability is preferable to developing an unvalidated checklist.

EXTRACTING KEY INFORMATION FROM THE SELECTED STUDIES

'*Data extraction*' involves identifying and recording important items (such as details of the author, the setting, the participants, the interventions, the outcomes and the main results) from each study. Data extraction forms are used to facilitate this; these should be piloted so as to reduce errors and minimise bias. For example, the data extraction form must accommodate all eligible study designs and ensure that the researcher consistently collects the same type of data from each study. Sample data extraction forms are provided in the second edition of CRD Report Number 4 (Khan *et al.* 2001; www.york.ac.uk/inst/crd/CRD_Reports/crdreport4_app3.pdf). Research Example 24.4 documents the proposed data extraction strategy for the antibiotics and antiseptics for venous leg ulcers example.

SUMMARISING, INTERPRETING AND PRESENTING THE FINDINGS

Having extracted all relevant data, this information must then be synthesised. In many cases this entails providing a descriptive summary ('*narrative commentary*'), possibly supported by a tabular presentation ('*summary tables*'). Where possible, quantitative data are combined in a '*meta-analysis*' to quantify the benefits (or harms) of an intervention. Before undertaking such an analysis it is important to establish whether it is appropriate to do so. For example, there is no value in pooling results if:

- only one study has estimated the effect of an intervention
- significant differences in participants, interventions and/or setting could substantially affect the outcomes ('*clinical heterogeneity*')
- there is excessive variation in the results of the studies ('*statistical heterogeneity*')
- outcome(s) have been measured in different ways in each study
- studies do not contain the required information.

In simple terms, a meta-analysis involves taking individual results for the same outcome from several studies and calculating a 'single summary statistic' (sometimes referred to as an '*effect measure*'). Standard effect measures include 'odds ratio', 'relative risk', 'risk difference', 'number needed to treat', 'standardised mean difference' and 'weighted mean

RESEARCH EXAMPLE

24.4 Data Extraction and Management: Antibiotics and Antiseptics for Venous Leg Ulcers (O'Meara *et al.* 2008)

Details of the studies were extracted and summarised using a standardised data extraction sheet. If data were missing from reports, study authors were contacted and asked to provide missing information. Studies that had been published in duplicate were included only once, ensuring that all relevant data from all publications were included. Data extraction was undertaken by one author (DAK) and checked for accuracy by a second author (SO).

Types of data extracted included the following.

1 Study authors
2 Year of publication
3 Country where study performed
4 Study design (RCT)
5 Method of randomisation
6 Unit of randomisation
7 Overall sample size and methods used to estimate statistical power (relates to the target number of participants to be recruited, the clinical difference to be detected and the ability of the trial to detect this difference)
8 Outcomes measured
9 Setting of treatment
10 Duration of treatment
11 Participant selection criteria
12 Details of interventions (including specific antibiotics and antiseptics used) per study group, including concurrent interventions such as compression
13 Numbers per study group
14 Baseline characteristics of participants per treatment group (gender, age, ethnicity, baseline ulcer area, ulcer duration, prevalence of co-morbidities such as diabetes, prevalence of clinically infected wounds with definition as used in the trial, prevalence of colonised wounds with definition as used in the trial, identity of microorganisms isolated)
15 Methods used for identifying microorganisms
16 Statistical methods used for data analysis
17 Results per group for each outcome
18 Withdrawals (per group with numbers and reasons)

difference'. 'Relative risk' (RR) and 'odds ratio' (OR) are the most common measures. Both measures relate the proportion of participants who are observed to experience an event in the intervention group to the proportion of participants who experience the same event in the control group. Although the way the statistics are calculated is slightly different, it is easy to remember that for both measures an RR/OR of 1 indicates no difference between the groups being compared (Khan *et al.* 2001).

Where studies examine 'similar' groups, effect sizes across studies should be compared and an overall effect calculated by taking a weighted average of the individual study effects. However, not all readers are comfortable with interpreting the statistical measures involved. Results of a meta-analysis can be presented graphically as a '*forest plot*', sometimes referred to as a 'blobbogram' or 'odds ratio diagram'. This represents the individual study results within the review, together with the combined result of the meta-analysis. An example is provided in Figure 24.1.

The vertical line represents the line of no effect, i.e. where the group receiving the intervention are no

Review: Home care by outreach nursing for chronic obstructive pulmonary disease
Comparison: 01 Respiratory outreach nurse vs control
Outcome: 05 Mortality

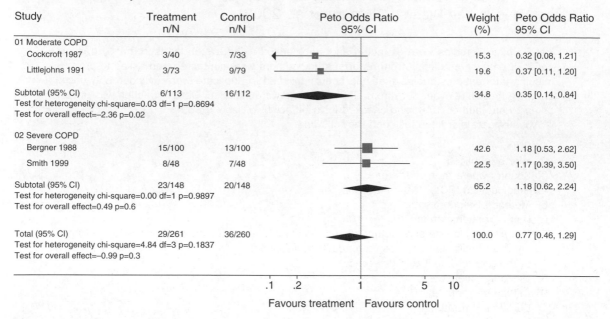

Figure 24.1 An example of a Forest plot
From: Smith B, Appleton S, Adams R, Southcott A, Ruffin R (2003) Home care by outreach nursing for chronic obstructive pulmonary disease (protocol for a Cochrane Review). *The Cochrane Library*, Issue 3.) Reproduced with permission from John Wiley and Sons.

better or worse off than the control group or, in other words, where the odds ratio (OR) is equal to 1. The small 'blobs' represent the results of individual trials. The area of each 'blob' represents the weight given to each study in the meta-analysis. Larger, higher-quality studies receive more weight than smaller, lower-quality ones. The larger diamond-shaped 'blob' next to the 'Total' row represents the overall meta-analysis result when all the studies are pooled together. The horizontal lines associated with each 'blob' represent the confidence interval (in this case, 95%) for each result. The confidence interval tells us how much uncertainty is associated with each result. Narrow confidence intervals indicate that the same result is likely to occur were the study to be repeated many times. Wider confidence intervals mean that different results are more likely to occur. In the example in Figure 24.1, comparing respiratory outreach nurses with a control, the overall pooled result indicated by the diamond lies to the left of the line of

no effect. This indicates less of the outcome (mortality) in the treatment (respiratory outreach nurse) group. However, the horizontal points of the diamond, indicating the confidence interval when all the studies are pooled together, cross the line of no effect, which means that the result is not significant. Closer examination of the plot and the text of the review reveals that the authors have pooled studies including people with both moderate and severe chronic obstructive pulmonary disease, and the overall effect 'mixes up' people most likely to benefit from the treatment with those who are less likely to benefit.

A meta-analysis is a complex mathematical calculation often requiring input from a statistician. Fortunately several software packages (such as Review Manager; www.cc-ims.net/RevMan) are available to facilitate this process.

Even rigorously conducted systematic reviews cannot eliminate the risk of 'publication and related biases'. Therefore every review should incorporate a formal assessment of such risks. Statistical and modelling techniques, such as '*funnel plots*', exist to assist in highlighting these biases. These plot individual effects from studies against some measure of study information (e.g. study size). If the resulting inverted funnel is asymmetrical this may indicate the presence of bias, although the possibility of chance cannot be excluded.

WRITING UP THE REVIEW

A succinct report of the review allows readers to judge its validity and the implications of its findings (Khan *et al.* 2001). All Cochrane reviews are reported in a consistent manner that includes a structured abstract, background, objectives, criteria for considering studies, search strategy, methods of the review, description of studies, methodological quality, results, summary of analyses, discussion, reviewers' conclusions (including implications for practice and research) and references. A similar structure should be adopted when writing up any systematic review. The QUOROM (QUality Of Reporting Of Meta-analyses) statement outlined a standard for the quality of reporting of systematic reviews of RCTs (Moher *et al.* 1999). It is currently being updated under the more memorable acronym PRISMA (Preferred Reporting Items for Systematic Reviews and Meta-Analyses).

SYSTEMATIC REVIEWS OF QUALITATIVE RESEARCH

Techniques for identifying and synthesising qualitative research have been at the forefront of recent methodological developments, although there remains little consensus as to which methods should be used for searching, appraising and synthesising good-quality studies (Booth 2001). Part of this complexity stems from the diversity of qualitative research. Some argue that a particular method of appraisal or analysis may privilege specific types of qualitative research. Evans and Pearson (2001) provide a good overview of the main issues for qualitative systematic reviews for nurses. They characterise these under six stages of the review process:

- defining the focus
- locating studies
- selecting studies for inclusion in review
- critical appraisal
- data extraction
- data synthesis.

The stages of the systematic review process are thus common to both quantitative and qualitative research. However, similarities and differences between methods used and their underlying principles exist for quantitative and qualitative syntheses at each stage of the review process.

Approaches to syntheses of qualitative research tend to divide into those that regard syntheses of qualitative research as broadly equivalent to those for quantitative research and those that state that qualitative evidence synthesis is, in fact, conceptually aligned to primary qualitative research. Both approaches work from the premise that systematic reviews of qualitative research should be systematic, explicit and reproducible, but other concepts strongly associated with quantitative systematic reviews, such as the requirement to be 'comprehensive', mark the battle lines.

Aside from such conceptual differences the review community is at least starting to identify some broad operating principles. For example, if an established conceptual framework already exists for a topic under exploration, then some type of framework analysis approach may be appropriate; if, however, the topic is still fluid and being defined, then a grounded theory approach may be chosen. Similarly, if the main intent of the review is descriptive, then an aggregative approach, such as employed by the Joanna Briggs Institute (Pearson 2004), may be most suitable. If, however, the primary intent is analytical, requiring some degree of conceptual innovation, then an interpretative approach, such as meta-ethnography or critical interpretive synthesis, may be considered. Such principles cannot be prescriptive, however, and those planning a qualitative evidence synthesis may find it helpful to look at compilations of methodological alternatives, such as the book by Pope *et al.* (2007), the report by Dixon-Woods *et al.* (2004) or guidance from the Cochrane Collaboration's Qualitative Research Methods Group (www.joannabriggs.edu.au/cqrmg).

RESEARCH EXAMPLE

24.5   A Qualitative Meta-synthesis of Directly Observed Therapy for Tuberculosis (Noyes & Popay 2007)

Background

DOT is part of a World Health Organization (WHO)-branded package of interventions to improve the management of TB and adherence with treatment (Maher et al. 2003). DOT involves asking people with TB to visit a health worker, or other appointed person, to receive and be observed taking a dose of medication. To supplement a Cochrane Intervention review of trials of DOT, we conducted a synthesis of qualitative evidence concerning people with, or at risk of, TB, service providers and policy makers, to explore their experience and perceptions of TB and treatment. Findings were used to help explain and interpret the Cochrane Intervention review and to consider implications for research, policy and practice.

Review questions

Two broad research questions were addressed.

1   What are the facilitators and barriers to accessing and complying with tuberculosis treatment?
2   Can exploration of qualitative studies and/or qualitative components of the studies included in the intervention review explain the heterogeneity of findings?

Method

Search methods: a systematic search of the wider English-language literature was undertaken. The following terms were used: DOT; DOTS; directly observed therapy; directly observed treatment; supervised swallowing; self-supervis*; in combination with TB and tuberculosis. We experimented with using methodological filters by including terms such as 'qualitative', but found this approach unhelpful as the Medline MeSH heading 'Qualitative Research' was only introduced in 2003, and even after 2003 many papers were not identified appropriately as qualitative. We searched MEDLINE, CINAHL, HMIC, Embase, British Nursing Index, International Bibliography of the Social Sciences, Sociological Abstracts, SIGLE, ASSIA, Psych Info, Econ lit, Ovid, Pubmed, the London School of Hygiene and Tropical Medicine database of TB studies (courtesy of Dr Simon Lewin), and Google Scholar. Reference lists contained within published papers were also scrutinised. A network of personal contacts was also used to identify papers. All principal researchers involved in the six randomised trials included in the Cochrane Intervention review were contacted and relevant qualitative studies obtained.

Selection and appraisal of studies: the following definition was used to select studies: 'papers whose primary focus was the experiences and/or perceptions of TB and its treatment among people with, or at risk of, TB and service providers'. The study had to use qualitative methods of data collection and analysis, as either a stand-alone study or a discrete part of a larger mixed-method study. To appraise methodological and theoretical dimensions of study quality, two contrasting frameworks were used independently by JN and JP (Popay 1998; Critical Appraisal Skills Programme 2006). Studies were not excluded on quality grounds, but lower-quality studies were reviewed to see if they altered the outcome of the synthesis – which they did not.

Analysis: thematic analysis techniques were used to synthesise data from 1990–2002, and an update of literature to December 2005. Themes were identified by bringing together components of ideas, experiences and views embedded in the data – themes were constructed to form a comprehensive picture of participants' collective experiences. A narrative summary technique was used to aid interpretation of trial results.

Findings: 58 papers derived from 53 studies were included. Five themes emerged from the 1990–2002 synthesis, including: socioeconomic circumstances, material resources and individual agency; explanatory models and knowledge systems in relation to tuberculosis and its treatment; the experience of stigma and public discourses around tuberculosis; sanctions, incentives and support; and the social organisation and social relationships of care. Two additional themes emerged from the 2005 update: the barriers created by programme implementation, and the challenge to the model that culturally determined factors are the central cause of treatment failure.

Conclusions: the Cochrane Intervention review did not show statistically significant differences between DOT and self-supervision, suggesting that it was not DOT per se that led to an improvement in treatment outcomes. Variants of DOT differed in important ways in terms of who was being observed, where the observation took place and how often observation occurred. The synthesis of qualitative research suggests that these elements of DOT will be crucial in determining how effective a particular type of DOT will be in terms of increased cure rates. The qualitative review also highlighted the key role of social and economic factors and physical side effects of medication in shaping behaviour in relation to seeking diagnosis and adhering to treatment. More specifically, a predominantly inspectorial approach to observation is not likely to increase uptake of service or adherence with medication. Inspectorial elements may be needed in treatment packages, but when the primary focus of direct observation was inspectorial rather than supportive in nature, observation was least effective. Direct observation of an inspectorial nature had the most negative impact on those who had the most to fear from disclosure, such as disadvantaged women who experienced gender-related discrimination. In contrast, treatment packages in which the emphasis is on person-centred support are more likely to increase uptake and adherence. Qualitative evidence also provided insights into the type of support that people with TB find most helpful. Primarily, the ability of the observer to add value depended on the observer and the service being able to adapt to the widely varying individual circumstances of the person being observed (age, gender, agency, location, income, etc.). Given the heterogeneity among those with TB, findings support the need for locally tailored, patient-centred programmes rather than a single worldwide intervention.

Recent methodological developments in qualitative evidence synthesis have challenged the idea of singularly unidirectional migration of approaches from quantitative syntheses to qualitative syntheses. It is clear that methods from primary qualitative research can not only inform the conduct of qualitative reviews but can also benefit systematic reviews in general. For example, iterative approaches typically used to develop and refine interpretation of qualitative data challenge the prescriptively sequential model of reviews perpetuated by the quantitative model. Furthermore, there is increasing acknowledgement that *comprehensiveness of a search strategy* is not in itself a defining characteristic of a systematic review. Instead the *appropriateness of the sampling strategy* for identifying the literature, be it comprehensive, purposive, theoretical or random, is a much more tenable principle focusing, as it does, on 'fitness for purpose'. Liberation from this unforgiving principle of comprehensiveness not only benefits qualitative evidence synthesis but also time-limited quantitative approaches such as health technology assessments.

Syntheses of qualitative research include a meta-synthesis of directly observed therapy in tuberculosis (Research Example 24.5) (Noyes & Popay 2007) and a systematic review of qualitative reports of support for breastfeeding mothers (McInnes & Chambers 2008). Although it is helpful to recognise that the intent of evidence syntheses, whether quantitative or qualitative, may be primarily aggregative (in bringing the evidence together in an additive way) or interpretative (in broadening our understanding of a specific phenomenon) (Noblit & Hare 1988), it must be acknowledged that this is a continuum. Approaches that can integrate both quantitative and qualitative data, and that can fulfil aggregative and interpretive functions, will become increasingly important especially as mixed-method approaches continue to grow in popularity.

CONCLUSIONS

Evidence syntheses, in the form of systematic reviews, practice guidelines and economic evaluations, provide the opportunity to generate a synthesis of research evidence to inform practice. Explicit methods are used to identify, select, critically appraise and summarise large quantities of information. Irrespective of the type of evidence synthesis, several discrete, but interconnected, stages are followed. These include:

- writing a research protocol
- systematically searching the literature
- selecting relevant studies
- assessing the quality of the literature
- extracting key information from the selected studies

- summarising, interpreting and presenting the findings
- writing up the research in a structured manner.

References

Booth A (2001) Cochrane or cock-eyed? how should we conduct systematic reviews of qualitative research? Presented at the Qualitative Evidence-based Practice Conference, Taking a Critical Stance. Coventry University, May 14–16 (www.leeds.ac.uk/educol/documents/00001724.htm).

Critical Appraisal Skills Programme (2006) Public Health Resource Unit, Oxford (www.phru.nhs.uk/pages/PHD/CASP.htm).

Cruickshank S, Kennedy C, Lockhart K, Dosser I, Dallas L (2008) Specialist breast care nurses for supportive care of women with breast cancer. *Cochrane Database of Systematic Reviews* 2008, Issue 1. Art. No.: CD005634. DOI: 10.1002/14651858.CD005634.pub2.

Dixon-Woods M, Agarwal S, Young B, Jones D, Sutton A (2004) *Integrative Approaches to Qualitative and Quantitative Evidence*. London, Health Development Agency.

Easterbrook PJ, Berlin JA, Goplan R, Matthews DR (1991) Publication bias in clinical trials. *Lancet* **337**: 867–872.

Egger M, Juni P, Barlett C, Holenstein F, Sterne J (2003) How important are comprehensive literature searches and the assessment of trial quality in systematic reviews? *Health Technology Assessment* **7**: 1–76 (available at www.ncchta.org/execsumm/summ701.htm).

Evans D, Pearson A (2001) Systematic reviews of qualitative research. *Clinical Effectiveness in Nursing* **5**: 111–119.

Greenhalgh T (2000) *How to Read a Paper: the basics of evidence based practice*, 2nd edition. London, BMJ Books.

Hughes C, Smith M, Tunney M (2008) Infection control strategies for preventing the transmission of methicillin-resistant *Staphylococcus Aureus* (MRSA) in nursing homes for older people. *Cochrane Database of Systematic Reviews*, Issue 1. Art. No.: CD006354. DOI: 10.1002/14651858.CD006354.pub2.

Khan KS, Kuna R, Kleijnen J, Antes G (2004) *Systematic Reviews to Support Evidence-based Medicine*. London, Royal Society of Medicine.

Khan KS, ter Riet G, Glanville J, Sowden AJ, Kleijnen J (eds) (2001) *Undertaking Systematic Reviews of Research on Effectiveness. CRD's guidance for carrying out or commissioning reviews*, 2nd edition. CRD Report No. 4. York, NHS Centre for Reviews and Dissemination, University of York.

McAuley A, Pharm B, Tugwell P, Moher D (2000) Does the inclusion of grey literature influence estimates of intervention effectiveness reported in meta-analyses? *Lancet* **356**: 1228–1231.

McInnes RJ, Chambers JA (2008) Supporting breastfeeding mothers: qualitative synthesis. *Journal of Advanced Nursing* **62**(4): 407–427.

Maher D, Uplekar M, Raviglione M (2003) Treatment of tuberculosis. *British Medical Journal* **327**: 822–823.

Moher D, Cook DJ, Eastwood S, Olkin I, Rennie D, Stroup DF (1999) Improving the quality of reports of meta-analyses of randomised controlled trials: the QUOROM statement. Quality of Reporting of Meta-analyses. *Lancet* **354**: 1896–1900.

Mulrow C (1995) Rationale for systematic reviews. In: Chalmers I, Altman DG (eds) *Systematic Reviews.* London, BMJ Publishing, pp 1–8.

National Library of Medicine. Medical Subject Headings (MeSH) from PubMed, MeSH browser. Available at: www.ncbi.nlm.nih.gov/entrez/query.fcgi?db=mesh

New FR, Winecoff A (2007) Cost and clinical outcomes of a back injury clinic. *Nursing Economics* **25**(2): 127–129.

Noblit GW, Hare RD (1988) *Meta-ethnography: synthesizing qualitative studies.* Paper series on Qualitative Research Methods, Volume **11**. Newbury Park, Sage.

Noyes J, Popay J (2007) Directly observed therapy and tuberculosis: how can a systematic review of qualitative research contribute to improving services? A qualitative meta-synthesis. *Journal of Advanced Nursing* **57**(3): 227–243.

O'Meara S, Al-Kurdi D, Ovington LG (2008) Antibiotics and antiseptics for venous leg ulcers. *Cochrane Database of Systematic Reviews* Issue 1. Art. No.: CD003557. DOI: 10.1002/14651858.CD003557.pub2.

Pearson A (2004) Balancing the evidence: incorporating the synthesis of qualitative data into systematic reviews. *JBI Reports* **2**(2): 45–64.

Popay J, Rogers A, Williams G (1998) Rationale and standards for the systematic review of qualitative literature in health services research. *Qualitative Health Research* **8**: 314–351.

Pope C, Mays N, Popay J (2007) *Synthesising Qualitative and Quantitative Health Evidence. A guide to methods.* Milton Keynes, Open University Press.

Rice VH, Stead LF (2008) Nursing interventions for smoking cessation. *Cochrane Database of Systematic Reviews* Issue 1. Art. No.: CD001188. DOI: 10.1002/14651858.CD001188.pub3.

Robinson R (1993). Economic evaluation and health care. What does it mean? *British Medical Journal* **307**: 670–673.

Smith B, Appleton S, Adams R, Southcott A, Ruffin R (2003) Home care by outreach nursing for chronic obstructive pulmonary disease (protocol for a Cochrane Review). *The Cochrane Library.* Issue 3. Chichester, John Wiley.

Szczepura A, Nelson S, Wild D (2008) In-reach specialist nursing teams for residential care homes: uptake of services, impact on care provision and cost-effectiveness. *BMC Health Services Research* **8**(1): 269.

Further reading

Aveyard H (2007) *Doing a Literature Review in Health and Social Care: a practical guide*. Milton Keynes, Open University Press.

Bero LA, Grilli R, Grimshaw JM, Harvey E, Oxman AD, Thompson MA (1998) Closing the gap between research and practice: an overview of systematic reviews of interventions to promote the implementation of research findings. The Cochrane Effective Practice and Organization of Care Review Group. *British Medical Journal* **317**: 465–468.

Chalmers I, Altman DG (eds) (1995) *Systematic Reviews.* London, BMJ Publishing Group.

Egger M, Davey-Smith G, Altman DG (Eds) (2001) *Systematic Reviews in Health Care. Meta-analysis in context.* London, BMJ Publishing Group (see www. systematicreviews.com).

Glasziou P, Irwig L, Bain C, Colditz G (2001) *Systematic Reviews in Health Care. A practical guide.* Cambridge, Cambridge University Press.

Mulrow CD, Cook D (eds) (1998) *Systematic Reviews. Synthesis of best evidence for health care decisions.* Philadelphia, American College of Physicians.

NHS Centre for Reviews and Dissemination (2009) *Systematic Reviews: CRD's guidance for undertaking reviews in health care.* York, University of York.

Pope C, Mays N, Popay J (2007) *Synthesising Qualitative and Quantitative Health Evidence. A guide to methods.* Milton Keynes, Open University Press.

Torgerson C (2003) *Systematic Reviews.* London, Continuum International Publishing Group.

Websites

www.campbellcollaboration.org – The Campbell Collaboration.

www.cochrane.org – The Cochrane Collaboration.

www.thecochranelibrary.com – The Cochrane Library.

www.york.ac.uk/inst/crd/intertasc/ – InterTASC Information Specialists' Sub-Group Search Filter Resource.

25 Realist Synthesis

Jo Rycroft-Malone, Brendan McCormack, Kara DeCorby and Alison Hutchinson

Key points

- Realist synthesis is a new and emerging approach to evidence review. It is particularly appropriate for unpacking the impact of complex interventions because it works on the premise that one needs to understand how interventions work in different contexts, and why.

- Realist synthesis is premised on a set of principles rather than a formula. Stages of review include theory formulation, bespoke data extraction form development, finding and appraising evidence, data synthesis and narrative construction. Fundamentally, realist synthesis is concerned with developing and refining theory through this process.

- The demands on a realist synthesiser are different to those expected in a Cochrane-type review. Quality assurance within realist synthesis is dependent on the reviewers' explicitness and reflexivity. In turn, this requires a high level of expertise in reasoning, research methods and quality appraisal.

INTRODUCTION

The research evidence base for healthcare policy and practice is huge, and most of us would not have the time to search, appraise and interpret this volume of available information. Evidence reviews, specifically systematic reviews, have become a popular mechanism for the identification, appraisal and synthesis of research-based evidence about the effectiveness of a particular intervention (Green *et al.* 2008). Traditional systematic reviews, which tend to include research evidence according to specific eligibility criteria that favour the hierarchy of evidence, and which answer focused questions, have been criticised for being too specific and inflexible (Pawson *et al.* 2004, 2005;

McCormack *et al.* 2007a). This critique becomes particularly relevant when considering the complexity of implementing healthcare interventions. The context of healthcare is complex, multifaceted and dynamic, which means that rarely, if ever, would the same intervention work in the same way in different contexts. As such, conventional systematic review approaches to evaluating the evidence of whether they work (or not) will result in limited answers such as 'to some extent' and 'sometimes' (Pawson *et al.* 2004; Pawson 2006). Realist synthesis has emerged as a new strategy for synthesising evidence that focuses on providing explanations for why interventions may or may not work, in what contexts, how and in what circumstances.

REALIST SYNTHESIS: PHILOSOPHY AND PRINCIPLES

Traditional systematic reviews are rooted in positivism. In contrast, a realist synthesis has its roots in realism. Realism as a philosophy of science is situated between the extremes of positivism and relativism (Delanty 1997). Realism involves identifying underlying causal mechanisms and how they work under what conditions (Pawson & Tilley 1997; Pawson 2002; McEvoy & Richards 2003). Because causal mechanisms always occur in a particular social context, there is a need to understand the complex relationship between these mechanisms and the effect the context has on their effectiveness. Complex interventions, according to Pawson *et al.* (2004), are comprised of theories, involve the actions of people, consist of a chain of steps or processes that interact and are rarely linear, are embedded in social systems, are prone to modification and exist in open systems that change through learning. Pawson and Tilley (1997) within their approach to realistic evaluation sum this up as: context + mechanism = outcome.

Realist synthesis draws on the principles of realistic evaluation and is underpinned by the philosophy of realism to evaluate and synthesise multiple sources of evidence. For Pawson (2006), any synthesis of evidence needs to investigate why and how interventions might work, in what contexts. The aim then is:

> '... to articulate underlying programme theories and then to interrogate the existing evidence to find out whether and where these theories are pertinent and productive' (Pawson 2006: 74)

In this case 'theory' is construed and defined differently from positivistic interpretations. For realist synthesis a theory is framed in terms of a proposition about how interventions work, e.g. if you implement an intervention in this way, in this context, you may get x result (Pawson *et al.* 2004, 2005; Pawson 2006).

REALIST SYNTHESIS: EXAMPLES

As a relatively new approach to evidence review, published examples of realist synthesis, particularly

in the nursing literature, are rare. Examples from the health-related literature more broadly include a review by Greenhalgh *et al.* (2007) that sought to understand the efficacy of school feeding programmes. In this example the authors set out to examine studies from a Cochrane review, using realist synthesis. Through this process, in contrast to simply finding out whether feeding programmes worked, they were able to determine what it was about school feeding programmes that made them work. Greenhalgh *et al.* (2004) also used some principles of realist synthesis in a meta-narrative review of the diffusions of innovation literature. This resulted in a theoretical framework that represents the multiple factors and interactions that might arise in particular contexts and settings, which may determine the success or failure of innovation adoption. Similarly, within a realistic evaluation of protocol-based care within the UK National Health Service, Rycroft-Malone and colleagues (2008a,b) used the principles of realist synthesis to review relevant literature in order to develop a number of propositions that were then tested through the evaluation study. McCormack and colleagues (McCormack *et al.* 2006, 2007a,b,c,d) conducted an extensive realist synthesis, which critically evaluated the evidence base underpinning approaches to practice development.

STAGES IN CONDUCTING A REALIST SYNTHESIS

We draw on two examples within this chapter to illustrate the stages in conducting a realist synthesis; first a published example McCormack *et al.* (2006), and second a realist synthesis currently being undertaken by an international team (the ReS-IS Project; Realist Synthesis of Implementation Strategies), which is answering the question 'what are the interventions and strategies that are effective in enabling evidence-informed healthcare?'

A realist synthesis follows similar stages to a traditional systematic review, with some notable differences (see Table 25.1). However, as realist methodologies are predicated on the existence of mechanisms in contexts, then realist synthesis

Table 25.1 Approach to realist synthesis (adapted from Pawson *et al.* 2004)

Define the scope of the review	Identify the question	What is the nature and content of the intervention?
		What are the circumstances or context of its use?
		What are the policy intentions or objectives?
		What are the nature and form of its outcomes or impacts?
		Undertake exploratory searches to inform discussion with review commissioners/decision makers
	Clarify the purpose(s) of the review	Theory integrity – does the intervention work as predicted?
		Theory adjudication – which theories around the intervention seem to fit best?
		Comparison – how does the intervention work in different settings, for different groups?
		Reality testing – how does the policy intent of the intervention translate into practice?
	Find and articulate the programme theories	Search for relevant 'theories' in the literature
		Draw up list of programme theories
		Group, categorise or synthesise theories
		Design a theoretically based evaluative framework to be 'populated' with evidence
Search for and appraise the evidence	Search for the evidence	Decide and define purposive sampling strategy
		Define search sources, terms and methods to be used (including cited reference searching)
		Set the thresholds for stopping searching at saturation
	Appraise the evidence	Test relevance – does the research address the theory under test?
		Test rigour – does the research support the conclusions drawn from it by the researchers or the reviewers?
Extract and synthesise findings	Extract the results	Develop data extraction forms or templates
		Extract data to populate the evaluative framework with evidence
	Synthesise findings	Compare and contrast findings from different studies
		Use findings from studies to address purposes(s) of review
		Seek both confirmatory and contradictory findings
		Refine programme theories in the light of evidence including findings from analysis of study data
Draw conclusions and make recommendations		Involve commissioners/decision makers in review of findings
		Draft and test out recommendations and conclusions based on findings with key stakeholders
		Disseminate review with findings, conclusions and recommendations

methodology is framed around a number of key principles.

- The review focus is derived from a negotiation between commissioners (of the review) and the researchers. Therefore the extent of stakeholder involvement throughout the process is high.
- The search and appraisal of evidence is purposive and theoretically driven with the aim of refining theory.
- Multiple types of information and evidence are included.
- The process is iterative.
- The outcome is always 'explanatory', i.e. the findings focus on explaining to the reader why (or not) the intervention works and in what ways, to enable informed choices about further use and/or research.

Pawson *et al.* (2004) set out the following steps for a realist synthesis approach.

Phase 1: Concept mining and theory formulation

Developing the focus of the study and the theories to be examined is an important aspect of a realist synthesis study as it provides the structure for examining a diverse body of evidence (Pawson *et al.* 2004). Phase 1 is therefore concerned with concept mining and theory formulation: digging through the literature for key terms, ideas, middle range theories and hypotheses that begin to provide some explanations to your subject of interest (Pawson *et al.* 2006). The challenge of developing the framework for a realist synthesis is to find the level of abstraction that allows the reviewers to both stand back from the mass of detail and variation in the data set and also meet the purpose of the review. Additionally, as a realist synthesis focuses on determining 'what works' within differing contextual configurations, a theoretical model must be outcome focused.

McCormack *et al.* (2006) developed a theoretical model derived from the project steering group's ideas and questions, the project team's constructions and conceptualisations of practice development found in the literature. These ideas and conceptual connec-

tions were referred to by McCormack *et al.* as *theoretical fragments* as they are the basis for constructing the theoretical model. Following discussion of these theoretical fragments among the project team and the project steering group, a theoretical model was developed around the 'who, what/why, how and by whom' of practice development (Figure 25.1).

The model has four theoretical areas containing 13 areas of focus with themes for exploration as follows.

Theory area 1 – Properties of the people and context in practice development

- What impact does the extent of involvement of different stakeholders have on the outcomes of practice development?
- What impact does the scale of a study have on the outcomes of practice development?
- How do contextual factors in the study setting have an impact on the outcomes of practice development?
- How do cultural factors in the study setting have an impact on the outcomes of practice development?
- How do styles of leadership in the study setting have an impact on the outcomes of practice development?

Theory area 2 – Properties of the people involved in developing practice

- How does the location of a practice developer have an impact on the outcomes of practice development?
- How do the means by which the practice developer gains access to the practice environment have an impact on the outcomes of practice development?
- How do the methodological positions taken by practice developers have an impact on the outcomes of practice development?

Theory area 3 – Issues surrounding the initiation and carrying out of practice development

- How do factors involved in the initiation of practice development have an impact on its outcomes?

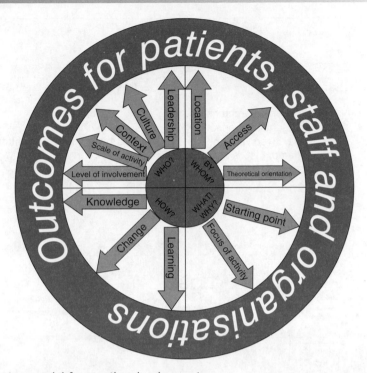

Figure 25.1 Explanatory model for practice development
Reproduced from McCormack B, Wright J, Dewer B, Harvey G, Ballintine K (2007a) A realist synthesis of evidence relating to practice development: methodology and methods. *Practice Development in Health Care* 6(1) 5–24 (page 15) with permission from John Wiley and Sons.

- What are the foci of practice development activity and how do they have an impact on its outcomes?

Theory area 4 – Approaches to the use of knowledge, bringing about change and supporting learning in practice development

- How do approaches taken to support learning within practice development have an impact on outcomes?
- How do approaches taken to bringing about change within practice development have an impact on outcomes?
- What forms of knowledge use and knowledge generation are used in practice development and what are the consequences for the outcomes?

In the ReS-IS project 'theory formulation' occurred through an iterative process of workshops, telephone conferences and 'blog discussions'. All project team members were immersed in knowledge utilisation research. Discussion at the first workshop centred on the purpose of the synthesis being to establish 'what works for whom, in what circumstances, in what respects, and how?' (Pawson *et al.* 2004). Following a brainstorming exercise, five key concepts for examination emerged:

- change agency (person, roles)
- levels (target of intervention)
- technology (mechanisms)
- education and learning strategies
- systems change (group or social processes).

These concepts were then framed to construct a theoretical model with *dose* (what quantity of an intervention is needed), *theory* and *contextual factors* (evidence of particular theory and context issues shaping the mechanism) as central factors and *outcomes* as the encompassing factor (Figure 25.2).

The ReS-IS model had four theoretical areas and 13 theoretical foci.

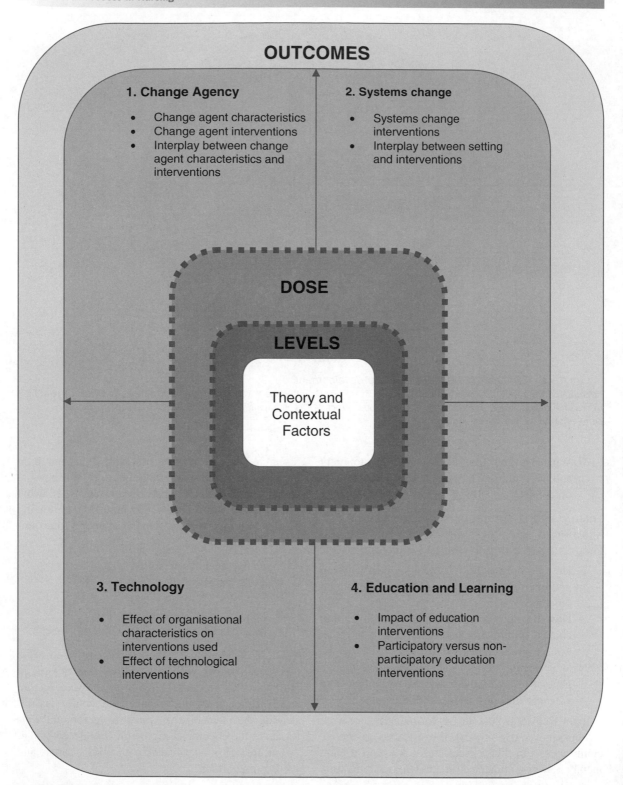

Figure 25.2 A theoretical model to explain knowledge utilisation in the context of evidence-informed healthcare (the ReS-IS model)

Theory area 1 – Properties of change agency in evidence-informed healthcare (E-IHC)

- What impact do the characteristics of the change agent have on E-IHC?
- What is the overall impact of the change agent intervention on E-IHC?
- What impact does the interaction between the change agent and the setting have on E-IHC?

Theory area 2 – System change in E-IHC

- What impact do characteristics of the systems change intervention(s) have on E-IHC?
- What is the overall impact of the system change intervention(s) used?
- What impact does the interaction between the system change and the setting have on E-IHC?
- What impact do senior leadership roles have in creating practice environments that integrate daily use of evidence at the point of care delivery?

Theory area 3 – Properties of technologies (paper and electronic) used in E-IHC

- What impact do the characteristics of the technological intervention(s) have on E-IHC?
- What is the overall impact of the technological intervention(s) used?
- What impact does the interaction between the technological intervention and the setting have on E-IHC?

Theory area 4 – Education interventions in E-IHC

- What impact do the characteristics of the education intervention(s) have in enabling E-IHC?
- What is the overall impact of the education intervention(s) used?
- What impact does the interaction between the education intervention and the setting have on E-IHC?

The breadth of the theoretical areas outlined in both these examples clearly suggests a considerable scope and degree of work. Pawson *et al.* (2004) caution that totally comprehensive reviews are impossible and that the task is to prioritise and agree on which theories are to be inspected. For example, McCormack and colleagues used the concerns of the project steering group to focus the work. In addition, the steering group identified their desired use of the review outcomes (e.g. information to inform commissioning, funding and dissemination of practice development approaches) that helped provide a direction for key areas of work to target.

The ReS-IS team engaged in discussion with the wider knowledge utilisation community through workshops, presentations and discussions, and as a result adopted a pragmatic approach that resulted in the prioritisation of one theory area for a first review.

Data extraction forms

The theoretical model is made visible in a realist synthesis through the 'data extraction forms'. This is a unique feature of realist synthesis in that unlike traditional systematic reviews, a *bespoke* set of data extraction forms are developed. Figure 25.3 provides examples of data extraction forms developed by McCormack *et al.* (2006).

Phase 2: Evidence synthesis

Finding and appraising the evidence

In a realist synthesis, a systematic approach is adopted to the finding, analysis and synthesis of evidence. The approach needs to reflect the concerns of the research methodology being used; in realist synthesis the literature needs to be scrutinised to identify 'programme theories' (Pawson *et al.* 2004). It is worth reiterating that from a realist perspective a 'theory' is an intervention *and* it is a theory because it is always based on a hypothesis (evidence of y requires x intervention) and if the intervention is used in a particular context it will bring about a particular outcome (if I do x then y will/might happen).

The searching for evidence is guided by the theoretical model developed in phase 1. A number of approaches can be applied to literature searching, including:

THEORY AREA 1 – PROPERTIES OF THE PEOPLE AND CONTEXT IN PRACTICE DEVELOPMENT
What impact does the extent of involvement of different stakeholders have on the outcomes of practice development?
What impact does the scale of a study have on the outcomes of practice development?
How do contextual factors in the study setting have an impact on the outcomes of practice development?
How do cultural factors in the study setting have an impact on the outcomes of practice development?
How do styles of leadership in the study setting have an impact on the outcomes of practice development?
THEORY AREA 2 – PROPERTIES OF THE PEOPLE INVOLVED IN DEVELOPING PRACTICE
How does the location of a practice developer have an impact on the outcomes of practice development?
How do the means by which the practice developer gains access to the practice environment have an impact on the outcomes of practice development?
How do the methodological positions taken by practice developers have an impact on the outcomes of practice development?

Figure 25.3 Example of data extraction form

Reproduced from McCormack B, Wright J, Dewer B, Harvey G, Ballintine K (2007a) A realist synthesis of evidence relating to practice development: methodology and methods. *Practice Development in Health Care* **6**(1): 5–24 (page 22) with permission from John Wiley and Sons.

THEORY AREA 3 – ISSUES SURROUNDING THE INITIATION AND CARRYING OUT OF PRACTICE DEVELOPMENT

How do factors involved in the initiation of practice development have an impact on its outcomes?

What are the foci of practice development activity and how do they have an impact on its outcomes?

THEORY AREA 4 – APPROACHES USED TO THE USE OF KNOWLEDGE, BRINGING ABOUT CHANGE AND SUPPORTING LEARNING IN PRACTICE DEVELOPMENT

How do approaches taken to support learning within practice development have an impact on outcomes?

How do approaches taken to bringing about change within practice development have an impact on outcomes?

What forms of knowledge use and knowledge generation are used in practice development and what are the consequences for the outcomes?

CRITIQUE

(from CASP 2002)

Was there a clear statement of the aims of the research?

Was the research design appropriate to address the aims of the research?

Figure 25.3 *Continued*

Was the recruitment strategy appropriate to the aims of the research?
Were the data collected in a way that addressed the research issue?
Has the relationship between researcher and participants been adequately considered?
Was the data analysis sufficiently rigorous?
Is there a clear statement of findings?
Additional comments   Would it be useful to get hold of the full report for this study: Yes: No:
REFERENCES TO FOLLOW UP:

Figure 25.3 *Continued*

- searching using key words
- mapping of commonly used subject headings onto concepts (theoretical fragments) of the theoretical model
- mapping key words on to concepts of the theoretical model.

McCormack and colleagues (2006) experimented with all three approaches and found that the approach of mapping key words on to concepts of the theoretical model was the most efficient and yielded the best results. They believe this was the case because the term 'practice development' is not a search term available on most databases and thus does not stand alone as a key word or as a subject heading. McCormack *et al.* negotiated with a university librarian to use the concepts from the theoretical model as a checklist to guide the selection of papers found using the terms 'practice' and 'development' across a range of databases. While use of these terms was not specific, it had the advantage of at least identifying those papers that used the terms in the specific way that distinguishes practice development from other forms of managed change. Using the concepts helped to increase the rigour and specificity of the selection of papers for in-depth scrutiny. The possible drawback of this approach is that it assumed the quality of the previous studies and ran the risk of 'closing down' the possible range of programme theories that would be identified. Nonetheless, McCormack and colleagues argued the need to look for instances of the term 'practice development' being used as a descriptor for specific ways of working as a precursor to looking in greater depth at the programme theories that are described in the practice development literature. The search included the databases listed in Table 25.2.

Table 25.2 Databases searched

Databases	References identified
British Nursing Index	63
CINAHL	203
First Search	52
MEDLINE	33
National Electronic Library for Health (NeLH)	0
PsycINFO	10
Social Science Citation Index	11
AMED	0
HMIC	0
Bandolier (www.jr2.ox.ac.uk/bandolier/)	4

Reproduced from McCormack B, Wright J, Dewer B, Harvey G, Ballintine K (2007a) A realist synthesis of evidence relating to practice development: methodology and methods. *Practice Development in Health Care* 6(1): 5–24 (p 19), with permission from John Wiley and Sons.

Table 25.3 Classification of papers

Category	Number of papers
1 Explicitly use practice development as a study methodology or study the experience of involvement in practice development	71
2 Scholarly reviews of practice development literature	30
3 Concept analyses	6
4 Studies in which practice development approaches are implicit (for example using facilitative approaches to change)	29
5 Papers based on empirical research but did not contain evidence about practice development processes or outcomes	33

Reproduced from McCormack B, Wright J, Dewer B, Harvey G, Ballintine K (2007a) A realist synthesis of evidence relating to practice development: methodology and methods. *Practice Development in Health Care* 6(1): 5–24 (p 19), with permission from John Wiley and Sons.

A list of 376 references was developed, to which were added 14 papers that the researchers were aware of but that were not found in the searches. However, examination of the list showed that entries in different databases may use different conventions, resulting in duplication. In this case, 38 papers were entered twice and a further 183 papers were excluded because they were descriptive papers, editorials, news stories or despite previous searches did not meet criteria as practice development papers. The remaining 169 papers formed the basis of the first phase review. The 169 papers remaining after removing the duplicates were classified as shown in Table 25.3.

To ensure reliability, papers were read in parallel by two members of the research team using the bespoke data extraction form. In addition the papers were critiqued by the whole research team to ensure congruity with the conceptual framework.

In the ReS-IS study, two members of the research team developed a directory of terms to accompany and provide context for the theoretical model. They circulated an initial list of terms and invited the whole group to add to the list. The final list of terms, in conjunction with relevant indexing terms, was used to guide the searches. The first search focused on literature relevant to the change agency theory area. Two team members conducted the searches of six online databases: MEDLINE, CINAHL, EMBASE, PsycINFO, Sociological Abstracts and Web of Science. Health sciences librarians were consulted in the process of constructing the search. Consistent with the purpose of the review to examine the effectiveness of interventions and strategies to enable evidence-informed *healthcare* (in general), the search strategies were deliberately broad and did not include discipline-related terms, with one exception. In CINAHL, the indexing term 'nursing knowledge' was combined, using the Boolean operator 'OR', with the term 'knowledge' in order to capture all papers indexed using either 'knowledge' or 'nursing knowledge'.

A 10-year publication period was searched. As a quality measure, one group member reviewed the indexes of 14 journals that publish articles about knowledge utilisation issues. A second group member determined that relevant papers from these journals were adequately indexed in the databases selected. Additionally, using their knowledge of the literature, all team members reviewed the final reference list to ensure that potential relevant papers were not missed by the search strategy.

Over 15,000 electronic references were returned from the *change agency* search strategies. Preliminary screening of the article titles retrieved in the search reduced the list of potentially relevant papers to 196. The preliminary screen was intentionally inclusive to capture all articles potentially relevant to the review's purpose of addressing what change agency interventions worked, for whom, in what circumstances, in what respects and how. At this stage, all seemingly relevant papers were retrieved in full text for a more detailed relevance test. Second-level screening resulted in the exclusion of further papers, bringing the final tally of papers relevant to the theory area to 52.

The group divided into five subgroups and the references were divided evenly across the subgroups. Within each subgroup, articles were initially screened for relevance to the theory area and study purpose. If a reviewer considered that an article did not meet the relevancy requirement, a second subgroup member reviewed it. Discrepancies in opinions about relevancy of articles were resolved through discussion. The rationale for exclusion of any articles was documented. If considered relevant, data were extracted from the article and this extraction was then peer reviewed/validated by a second member of the subgroup.

Once all subgroups had completed data extraction for the articles they deemed relevant to the project, the respective data extraction tables were amalgamated to form a single data extraction table for all articles addressing *change agency*. Data pertaining to the target population and discipline for each study were when extracted within the subgroups.

Pawson *et al*. (2004) argue that a thorough realist synthesis should not rely on published papers alone, but that all forms of evidence should be taken into account. In addition, the non-linear nature of realist synthesis methodology and its focus on meeting the needs of key stakeholders means that an iterative approach needs to be adopted in the appraising of evidence. In their study, McCormack *et al*. (2006) included an analysis of grey literature sourced from national and international practice development networks and contacts.

DATA SYNTHESIS

In the published works of Pawson and colleagues little, if any, guidance on data synthesis is offered. They suggest that synthesis focus on four dimensions:

- questioning the integrity of a theory
- adjudicating between competing theories
- considering the same theory in comparative settings
- comparing the 'official' theory with actual practice.

However, detail about how to undertake the actual synthesis of evidence is not provided.

In their study, McCormack *et al*. (2006) adopted an eight-step process to data synthesis, drawing on classical approaches to thematic analysis in qualitative research. The data from the individual data extraction forms for the published literature were extracted and copied on to 'theory synthesis forms' for each of the four theory areas. The data consisted of direct quotes, researchers' commentaries and impressions. These data were grouped according to the particular emphasis in the data and researchers' impressions of the specific meanings. Each theory synthesis form was read and re-read to gain overall impressions of the data, and rough notes were made. Data from each theory synthesis form were then themed. In some cases, the original papers were revisited to clarify meanings and finalise themes. A draft report was formulated and presented to the project steering group for discussion, clarification and challenge.

The grey literature data were then fed into the 'theory synthesis forms' for each of the theory areas to form a complete data set. The data were re-read and the initial themes reconsidered based on the evidence from the grey literature. Few themes changed significantly, but instead the grey literature either strengthened or weakened initial themes. The themes were constructed into a narrative and these narratives formed the structure of the findings section of the report.

The final stage consisted of an analysis of the telephone interviews, which were themed under the questions on the interview schedule. Key quotes and comments were highlighted and these were fed into the discussion of the data to highlight particular issues, confirm themes from the literature, verify or contradict the strength of claims made in the literature analysis, and identify novel issues and themes. This final stage resulted in the identification of four overarching themes and nine subthemes, and these formed the structure for the data synthesis (Box 25.1).

Figure 25.4 shows the iterative approach adopted by McCormack *et al.* (2006).

The ReS-IS research team adopted an alternative approach to data synthesis, derived from the principles underpinning realistic evaluation. Thematic analysis was first conducted by three subgroups who themed the extracted data according to one of three questions.

1 What impact do the characteristics of the change agent have on knowledge use?
2 What is the overall impact of the change agent intervention on knowledge use?
3 What impact does the interaction between the change agent and the setting have on knowledge use?

Subgroup members independently themed the data extracted from each article using the question assigned to their subgroup. The subgroup then collated the themes identified by each of the members. From here the subgroup members identified overarching themes or 'chains of inference'. A chain of inference is a connection that can be made across articles based on the themes identified. The connection may not be explicit, but a possible relationship between the theme and the outcome under consideration may have been highlighted. Subgroup members each shared the

---

Box 25.1 Data analysis themes and subthemes

Theme	Subtheme
1. Unidisciplinary versus multidisciplinary approaches	• None
2. Stakeholders	• Managers • Service users • Practice development roles and relationships • HEI relationships • Learning
3. Methodologies and methods	• Methodological perspectives • Methodologies in use • Methods • The cost/funding of practice development
4. Outcomes arising from practice development	• None

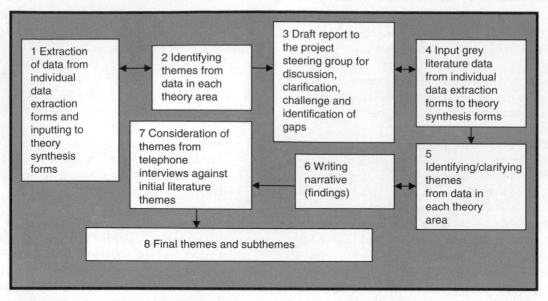

Figure 25.4   Data extraction, analysis and synthesis

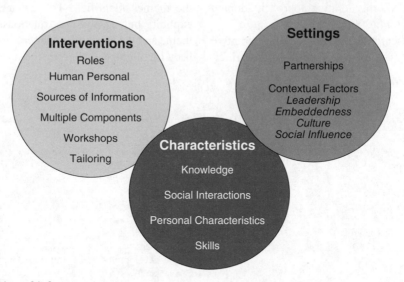

Figure 25.5   Chains of inference

chains of inference they had identified. Figure 25.5 shows the chains of inference identified by the group.

Discussion, amendment and/or confirmation of the chains of inference that had been proposed happened via teleconference. For each chain of inference, articles linking themes and chains of inference were recorded to create an audit trail. Table 25.4 shows an example of some chains of inference linked to themes and original articles.

In a face-to-face meeting, the team identified connections between the chains of inference and their impact on evidence-informed practice. Having articulated the connections, the group formulated hypotheses regarding the chains of inference. A chain of

Table 25.4 Chains of inference linked to themes and original articles

Chains of inference	Derived from the following themes	Articles
Knowledge	Professional qualifications Expert knowledge Knowledgeable Local knowledge Research knowledge Practice knowledge	1, 3, 6, 7, 10, 11, 13, 14, 15, 16, 18, 19, 20, 21, 22, 23, 25, 29, 35, 36, 37, 39
Skills	Communication skills Leadership skills Thinking skills Clinical skills Cognitive skills Evaluation skills Political skills Facilitation skills Reflective skills	2, 4, 5, 6, 7, 8, 9, 10, 11, 12, 13, 14, 15, 16, 17, 18, 19, 20, 21, 22, 24, 25, 27, 28, 32, 33, 34, 36, 38, 39, 40
Personal characteristics	Role model Positive attitude Responsibility/accountability Respected Information seeking Positive attitude Accessible Age Teacher Culturally compatible Objectivity Years of experience	1, 2, 4, 6, 7, 8, 13, 14, 15, 16, 17, 18, 22, 28, 29, 30, 31, 32, 33, 35, 36, 37, 38, 39
Social interaction	Social influence Networking Shared ownership	5, 8, 12, 15, 18, 31, 39, 40

inference is, therefore, linked to each hypothesis and for each chain of inference themes from the literature are also linked. Further, all papers from which the themes related to the respective chains of inference were drawn are clearly identified. Table 25.5 provides an illustration of this process.

NARRATIVE CONSTRUCTION

Adopting a systematic approach to the writing up of the review is an important consideration. Essential to the decision is the format of the report. Like all systematic reviews, the reader needs to be able to clearly see each stage of the review process and the decisions made in each stage. This is important in order to:

- make a judgement about the overall quality of the review processes
- build on the review (e.g. conduct a repeat review using literature not included in the published review)
- make a judgement about the conclusions made by the authors and the implications of the conclusions for practice
- undertake further research drawing on the review conclusions.

317

Table 25.5 Hypotheses linked to chains of inference

Hypotheses	Chain of onference (theory level)	Chain of inference (sub-theory level)	Themes from the literature	Papers addressing the theme
An opinion leader and their personal characteristics are dependent on contextual factors in order to have an impact on E-IHC A facilitator and their personal characteristics are dependent on contextual factors in order to have an impact on E-IHC	The nature of the relationship between the change agent's personal characteristics, the role adopted, and contextual influences and the impact of E-IHC	Roles Personal characteristics Contextual factors	Opinion leader (OL) Facilitator (FAC) Change agent (CA)	*Papers with mixed and positive effects, only:* 6 OL (Wright, Chaillet, Curran, Moore, Davies, Majumdar) 6 FAC (internal/ external and external facilitators included), (Stetler, Cranney, Gerrish, Milner, Thomas, Hutt) Total 18 CA papers, 12 OL and FAC

Typically the writing of the review follows the theoretical model developed. McCormack *et al.* (2006) adopted a two-stage approach to the reporting of findings. First, the literature analysis relating to each of the subtheory areas (13) was presented in detail. Each subtheory area was concluded with a data summary to show the relationships between data themes in the final synthesis (see Box 25.1 above) and the theory areas. The synthesised findings were then presented using these data themes. Pawson *et al.* (2004) do not recommend the making of 'recommendations' in realist synthesis as the purpose of a realist synthesis is not to determine 'best' practice but instead describes the relationships between interventions and the contexts in which those interventions occur. However, because of the iterative approach adopted, McCormack *et al.* did make recommendations. These were derived from a discussion of the findings with the project steering group and their interpretation of actions that should be recommended arising from the synthesised findings. However, recommendations were made concerning the development of a practice development (theoretical) model rather than a list of recommendations for 'doing practice development'.

In the ReS-IS project the narrative was constructed around the identified hypotheses for the theory area. In collaboration with the whole research team, the structure of the report and the approach to its construction were agreed. Four members (the authors of this chapter) worked together to write the narrative. Unlike McCormack *et al.*, the analysis and synthesis was written as one account. This was possible because of the use of hypotheses, which acted as synthesised statements of findings against which the previous stages of analysis could be presented.

STRENGTHS AND LIMITATIONS OF REALIST SYNTHESIS

As Pawson and colleagues have noted, unlike some other review processes one of the strengths of a realist approach to review is that it has firm roots in philosophy and social sciences (Pawson *et al.* 2004, 2005). Rather than being a method or formula, it is a 'logic of enquiry' (2004: 37), which enables a flexible, all-embracing approach to explanation (what works for whom in what circumstances and in what respects) rather than judgement. Rather than controlling for real-life events, realist synthesis has the capacity to work with, and untangle, complexities. This allows for an equal focus on what works and what does not work in an attempt to learn from failures and maximise learning across policy, disciplinary and organisational boundaries. Furthermore, realist synthesis is inherently stakeholder driven, which facilitates engagement and the inclusion of multiple perspectives.

The strengths of realist synthesis underpin its limitations. Realist synthesis is premised on a set of principles rather than a formula and while this allows for flexibility and inclusivity, it means that the review is not reproducible. The two examples used in this chapter are good examples of how taking a set of principles and developing a particularised approach result in similar, but not identical processes. For example, it follows that if the appraisal and data extraction needs to be bespoke to the particular review questions that arise from the theoretical framework, these will be different for each review. Furthermore, given that the fundamental interest in realist synthesis is about finding out what works in what contexts, the recommendations one can make will not be generalisable. However, findings are theoretically transferable; ideas ('theories') that can be tested in different contexts, with different stakeholders. Pawson *et al.* (2004) suggest that realist syntheses are not for novices. Unlike a Cochrane review, for example, which relies on standardised protocols and tools, the demands on a realist synthesiser are different. For example, quality assurance within realist synthesis is dependent on the reviewers' explicitness and reflexivity. In turn, this requires a high level of expertise in reasoning, research methods and quality appraisal.

CONCLUSIONS

Realist synthesis is a new but emerging approach to evidence review. It is particularly appropriate for unpacking the impact of complex interventions because it works on the premise that one needs to understand how interventions work in different contexts, and why. It is not an easy option, and the fact that as yet there are not many published reviews available is unhelpful. As the two examples used in this chapter show, there is no one prescribed approach to doing a realist synthesis; there is a set of principles that the reviewer must particularise to the issue being explored while being sympathetic to the philosophy of realism. This presents unique challenges, but with it, the opportunity to develop more pragmatic conclusions than some other approaches to systematic reviewing.

ACKNOWLEDGEMENTS

The authors would like to acknowledge the work of the ReS-IS Project team who have collectively contributed to the design and management of the ReS-IS study. The ReS-IS co-investigators are Tracey Bucknall (Australia), Kara DeCorby (Canada), Alison Hutchinson (Australia/Canada), Bridie Kent (Australia), Brendan McCormack (UK), Jo Rycroft-Malone (UK), Alyce Schultz (USA), Erna Snelgrove-Clarke (Canada), Cheryl Stetler (USA), Lars Wallin (Sweden), Marita Titler (USA) AND Val Wilson (Australia).

References

Critical Appraisal Skills Programme (CASP) (2002) *Evidence-based Health Care: an open learning resource for health care practitioners*. Oxford, CASP.

Delanty G (1997) *Social Science: beyond constructivism and realism*. Buckingham, Open University Press.

Green S, Higgins JPT, Alderson P, Clarke M, Mulrow CD, Oxman AD (2008) 'Part 1: Cochrane Reviews – Introduction. In: Higgins JPT, Green S (eds) *Cochrane Handbook for Systematic Reviews of Interventions* Version 5.0.1 [updated September 2008]. The Cochrane Collaboration 2008 (available from www.cochrane-handbook.org).

Greenhalgh T, Kristjansson E, Robinson V (2007) Realist review to understand the efficacy of school feeding programmes. *British Medical Journal* **335**: 858–861.

Greenhalgh T, Robert G, Bate P, Kyriakidou O, MacFarlane F, Peacock R (2004) *How to Spread Good Ideas: a systematic review of the literature on diffusion, dissemination and sustainability of innovation in health service delivery and organisation*. Report for the National Co-ordinating Centre for NHS Service Delivery and Organisation R&D (NCCSDO), University College London.

McEvoy P, Richards D (2003) Critical realism: a way forward for evaluation research in nursing? *Journal of Advanced Nursing* **43**: 411–420.

McCormack B, Dewar B, Wright J, Garbett R, Harvey G, Ballantine K (2006) *A Realist Synthesis of Evidence Relating to Practice Development*. Final Report To NHS Education For Scotland and NHS Quality Improvement Scotland (www.nhshealthquality.org/nhsqis/3134.html; accessed 5 January 2009).

McCormack B, Wright J, Dewer B, Harvey G, Ballintine K (2007a) A realist synthesis of evidence relating to practice development: methodology and methods. *Practice Development in Health Care* **6**(1): 5–24.

McCormack B, Wright J, Dewer B, Harvey G, Ballintine K (2007b) A realist synthesis of evidence relating to practice development: findings from the literature review. *Practice Development in Health Care* **6**(1): 25–55.

McCormack B, Wright J, Dewer B, Harvey G, Ballintine K (2007c) A realist synthesis of evidence relating to practice development: interviews and synthesis of data. *Practice Development in Health Care* **6**(1): 56–75.

McCormack B, Wright J, Dewer B, Harvey G, Ballintine K (2007d) A realist synthesis of evidence relating to practice development: recommendations. *Practice Development in Health Care* **6**(1): 76–80.

Pawson R (2006) *Evidence-based Policy: a realist perspective*. London, Sage.

Pawson R (2002) Evidence-based policy: the promise of realist synthesis. *Evaluation* **8**: 340–358.

Pawson R, Greenhalgh T, Harvey G, Walshe K (2005) Realist review – a new method of systematic review designed for complex policy interventions. *Journal of Health Service Research & Policy* **10**(3): 21–34.

Pawson R, Greenhalgh T, Harvey G, Walshe K (2004) *Realist Synthesis: an introduction. RMP Methods Paper 2/2004*. Manchester, Centre for Census and Survey Research, University of Manchester.

Pawson R, Tilley N (1997) *Realistic Evaluation*. London, Sage.

Rycroft-Malone J, Fontenla M, Bick D, Seers K (2008a) Protocol-based care evaluation project. Final Report for the National Institute for Health Research Service Delivery and Organisation Programme (available at www.sdo.nihr.ac.uk/sdo782004.html; accessed 5 January 2009).

Rycroft-Malone J, Fontenla M, Bick D, Seers K (2008b) Protocol-based care: impact on roles and service delivery. *Journal of Evaluation in Clinical Practice* **14**: 867–873.

26 Historical Research

Anne Marie Rafferty and Rosemary Wall

Key points

- Historical research is valuable for health policy making and implementation of innovations as we learn from the past.

- Undertaking historical research is a complex and time-consuming experience, but can bring rich rewards in understanding our past.

- There are various methodologies and methods of interpretation used in historical research.

- This chapter gives some practical guidelines to researching the history of nursing.

INTRODUCTION

People study history for a variety of reasons: for pleasure, as a form of intellectual training, for the light it sheds on contemporary problems and as a contextual guide to decision making. Marwick (1970: 17) and Evans (1997) argue that the study of the past contributes greatly to our understanding of contemporary problems, human behaviour and the forces driving social change. In Britain, the use of historical evidence in justifying the case for change was prominent in the United Kingdom Central Council for Nursing, Midwifery and Health Visiting *Project 2000* document, which owed much to the inspiration of Celia Davies as project officer and her research experience in historical sociology (UKCC 1986).

As researchers we are attracted to different subject areas, methodologies and research environments for different reasons. Some people love laboratory work, others libraries; some thrive on social and collabora-

tive contact, others on solving problems solo; some rejoice in large-scale data sets and statistical modelling, while others prefer the participant observation of ethnography. But the key ingredient that unites many researchers is passion – emotional and often political commitment to their field. This can apply as much to scientists as historians, and the history of science provides ample evidence of faith and political beliefs driving innovation as much as reason (Pickering 1992).

Historical research was not included in the previous volume of this book. There are several reasons why historical research might not feature. The first is the size of the field. History is very much a minority interest within the profession. It does not fit readily into the traditional R&D model of impact and outcomes-driven outputs or funding regimes. Moreover, it is rare for nurses to have a background in history so those who choose historical research usually do so against the grain. Many nurses who embark on historical research do so mid-career, so there is usually some catching up to do. The purpose of this chapter is to identify what historical research has to offer the would-be nurse researcher, and to provide an overview of where we have been and where we are heading in the field.

First, we must define our terms. Although history is a field of inquiry, the term historiography is often used to describe not only the study of history, the academic tools, methods and approaches that are deployed, but the different ways in which that history is interpreted. However, the notion that students would be trained in historical methodology is relatively recent. As with nursing, you became a historian by doing, serving an apprenticeship, being socialised into the discipline. History is often regarded by its practitioners as a craft that you learn by reading, writing, excavating the evidence, weighing up and interpreting its significance for the argument. Like nursing then, history is a broad church embracing both qualitative and quantitative methods and multi-method approaches where warranted. Analytical methods also expand as new sources and methods are added to the repertoire. Oral history, film studies, visual and material culture have become more prominent features of nursing historiography in recent years (Lewenson & Herrmann 2008).

The scholarly and innovative merit of an historical work may hinge on the extent to which it is based on primary sources or reinterprets secondary sources in a novel way. Primary sources are the raw, unedited data (the minutes, papers and correspondence of individuals or organisations such as the now defunct General Nursing Council for England and Wales) on which historical interpretation is based. They can also include sources such as newspapers and published papers written at the time of the topic being studied, in addition to the non-textual sources already mentioned, such as films, photographs and objects. Secondary sources refer to the digested, interpreted or reported data of primary historical material. Generally, the secondary literature is mastered before the primary data are mined to provide the necessary contextual material for the account, but this order may not be strictly adhered to as new lines of inquiry emerge. Arguments will usually be suggested by the data, and are subject to change as different types of

source emerge and are explored and re-read at different stages in the research. Interpretation is a dynamic and interactive process.

Until the early 1960s, the writing of nursing history was dominated by nurses and nurse leaders who used history as a vehicle to promulgate a professional agenda. This largely self-congratulatory and at times hagiographic approach has given way to a more critical, astringent form of analysis. The entry of researchers from fields outside of nursing has brought fresh, and at times critical, perspectives to bear on nursing history, opening up not only new avenues for analysis but introducing new methodologies in the process. Sociologists, historians of medicine, feminist, labour and social historians introduced a revisionism that changed the field forever, for which the publication of *Rewriting Nursing History* marked the watershed (Davies 1981a).

Some may argue, though, that we lose something by removing the cosy reassurance that nursing history has traditionally provided by painting a positive portrait of the past. Nursing is not alone in looking to history to boost morale. It is common for professions to use history to prop up their ego, but this 'insider' history is increasingly giving way to a historiography that reflects the combined expertise of nurses and historians (Godden *et al.* 1993).

WHY STUDY HISTORY?

Let us explore the value that history might hold for the would-be nurse researcher and what might motivate nurses to choose historical research as the method for research. Within nursing research, history helps us to understand what gets researched by whom, when and how. An analysis of nursing research characterised it as having certain features called 'endogenous'; endogenous research being conducted by nurses about nurses, often self-funded and undertaken as a lone activity. This contrasted with exogenous research, which fitted more readily with the medical model; it addressed patient problems, often in teams, and tended to be funded by external sources. The argument was that nursing research needed to move from the endogenous to the exogenous model to secure its legitimacy and sustainability in investment terms (Traynor *et al.* 2001). History helps us to understand why research in nursing has been shaped the way it has, its success and impacts on the profession, policy makers and patients. What appear to be novel ideas and innovations often turn out to have a pedigree in the past, or represent recurrent problems which are never fully resolved but which wax and wane over time. The nursing shortage is cyclical but each time the context and strategies for solution differ. Another current example of this is the revival of polyclinics, which have been presented as a new idea in the 2008 NHS Next Stage Review, and yet were first discussed and trialled in the 1920s and 1930s (Carrier & Kendall 2008; Berridge 2008a). Questions need to be asked regarding recurrences like this – why did the practical implementation fail in the medium term previously and why might it be the same or different this time?

Virginia Berridge (2008b) has examined the use of history in health policy making. Although her clear message is that history and the knowledge of historians are not used enough, there are cases where history has been used regularly in 21st-century debates. History has been used in discussing legacy and traditions; to examine precedents in legal styles of argument; and perhaps most importantly has been referred to in order to learn from the past. However, Berridge writes that health policy specialists have considered that a main reason for organisational problems is the failure to learn from experience.

One powerful example of the use of history in policy is the Committee on Nursing chaired by Lord Asa Briggs and published as the Briggs report in 1972. The fact that Briggs was a historian is in itself significant, and his historical sensibility permeated the report that bears his name (DHSS 1972). The report was also an historical landmark in its own right as one of the most influential in the history of nursing policy. Commissioned by a Labour government and implemented by a Conservative government it bears re-reading for its prescience and relevance to the challenges we face today; the image of the profession, educational preparation of the profession and the research base on which key decisions can be made. Its findings had far-reaching effects on the profession. The Nurses, Midwives and Health Visitors

Act of 1979 replaced the General Nursing Council, established in 1919, with the UKCC. The apprenticeship system of paid nurse training on the wards was replaced by college-based higher education and the move towards the much prized supernumerary status for students, as a step towards aligning such experience with that of other students within the higher education sector. It advocated the basic curricular structure that we have today of an 18-month common curriculum followed by modular courses leading to registration. It also famously advocated that research should be part of the 'mental equipment' of every nurse and midwife and that the professions should be more research based. The recruitment base should target more A-level, undergraduate and graduate students. Nursing was contextualised within a system reform model that strove to integrate hospital and community with social services and move towards more community-based care.

History also helps us to understand the process of change, be it in methods used to treat pressure sores or the introduction of new ways of organising care. One of the first evaluation studies of team nursing, for example, was published in the late 1950s by a Canadian nurse (Jenkinson 1953). Where did the idea and method originate? Was it significant that this innovation was promoted by a nurse from North America? What was it about the organisational climate at the hospital in question (St George's, London) that favoured the implementation of new ideas? Was the then matron, Muriel Powell, a crucial influence in supporting the change? In relation to nursing research, historical research can help us to understand more fully the factors that transform a 'good idea' into standard practice and help to explain why some research findings are implemented and not others.

SHIFTING SANDS

The study of nursing history appears to be more embedded within the research base of nursing itself, although its star has risen and fallen. Once regarded as an essential of the Diploma in Nursing curriculum, history is now regarded as an expendable luxury propagated only where local enthusiasm or expertise allows. Historical research in nursing has developed significantly since Celia Davies (1981a) led us into the new and exciting terrain of her innovative edited collection of feminist and labour history interpretations of nursing history in the early 1980s.

Early commentators such as Lynaugh and Reverby (1987) in the US and Davies (1981b) and Maggs (1978) in the UK advocated a move from the hero-centred view of history to a more critical form of research which located nursing within its wider social and political context as women's history, labour history and imperial history, subsequently evolving into questions of race, class and gender, and the manner in which these intersect with each other (Carnegie 1991; Marks 1994). Patricia D'Antonio's review essay summarises these trends and more in the 1980s and 1990s, such as their role in political movements and the extent of autonomy in the nursing profession, providing an extensive bibliography (D'Antonio 1999). She challenges us to draw connections with the wider historical community and set up a dialogue, the two-way street of cross-disciplinary reciprocity.

Historical research is not just practised by nurses who delve into history and develop their skills as historians, but also by historians who focus on nursing. The more this dialogue occurs the more enriched the field will become. It is significant that both Patricia D'Antonio and Sioban Nelson have dual training as historians and nurses. Nelson (2002) advocates a reappraisal of the professional agenda in nursing history and asks the question not only 'What is nursing history for?' but 'Who is the audience?' She urges us to locate nursing history within the wider historiographical shifts in the field, to absorb those shifts within our own thinking and stimulate historians to ask new questions of their own data and inject a nursing presence into the historical debates.

The historian Anne Borsay (2009) argues for the relevance of history to nursing in terms of the way in which history challenges orthodoxies of the past and renders power relations more nuanced. Moreover, history can recover clinical practices of the past as well as parts of the patient experience which otherwise condense into crude categories and stereotypes if left unchallenged. History can blow away assumptions and demonstrate the negotiated nature of practice. History can be liberating, as new methods as well as new sources and analytical techniques challenge assumptions.

VOYAGE OF DISCOVERY OR JOURNEY WITHOUT MAPS?

Joan Lynaugh (1998) has argued that 'history is like real life; it is contingent'. Just as history itself is contingent so too is the historical record and the research process allied with it. Although undoubtedly historical research may be motivated by the politics and values of the researcher as much as the intellectual challenge that lies within, there is also a large emotional component that makes it quite magical. Historians rarely talk about the experience of doing research in this way, but research not only has to engage the intellect but the passions. The archives draw you into another world and in doing so bring you into direct and intimate contact with your subject. The bond may be especially intense where that research is biographical in nature. So the archive can be a place of enchantment, where the voice of your subject is heard sometimes for the first time since records were written. For those of us who love the archives there is nowhere quite like it. As such it is also a place of privilege and responsibility but one that is necessarily governed by ethical standards in research more generally, particularly where records are not publicly available. In particular, oral history can throw up surprises taking participants into uncharted waters emotionally.

Archival research can be frustrating as well as rewarding. Hours spent searching for a particular source of evidence may yield nothing, but it is also possible to stumble on a goldmine of information: a personal diary, an album of photographs, a clutch of newspaper cuttings. The records of the past were not written with the needs of the historian in mind, although public bodies do have preservation policies implemented by officials trained to evaluate the historical importance of documents. As nurses and historians, we should take an active role in trying to influence preservation policies to maximise their utility for future generations of historians, nurses and researchers.

It is best to try and identify sources well in advance where possible, as this can help to refine the research question prior to embarking on the research project or submitting a funding application. By the same token try not to rely on a single source of data, and diversify where possible. Cross-fertilisation will pay dividends not only in the richness and range of perspectives that can be brought into play, but also by triangulating sources, testing and corroborating evidence, and refining conclusions based on different sources. The direction and outcome of the research will be dependent on the use that can be made of the sources and, consequently, the question asked may change dramatically in the course of investigation. For this reason there is no recipe to order the inquiry or orderly progression of steps or stages to follow and one is likely to come and go between primary and secondary material as the data demands. Make friends with the archivist as their role can be crucial in guiding you, greatly enhancing the relevance and efficiency of retrievals.

Generally speaking, however, the problem of 19th- and 20th-century historical research is not one of finding sufficient material, but of containing the huge volumes of paper generated by organisations. Documents, journals and personal papers should be systematically screened for relevant material and this can mean hours of laborious scrutiny and scanning. All research has its routine tasks, but this is labour that may be crucial to how the account will be organised and presented. In determining the division of labour, it may be advisable to tackle the records of one organisation at a time. If events are particularly current, it is desirable to interview the participants themselves.

Oral history requires specific methodological and ethical considerations and has acquired the status of a subdiscipline within history itself (Thompson 1978; Boschma *et al.* 2008). It may serve a variety of purposes: to fill gaps in the documentation, uncover details of decisions, generate evidence missing from the records or allow the clarification of factual points. Oral history may be invaluable as an insight into an individual's thought processes, the discovery of new and important information and, more generally, in enriching the quality of data. In some cases it may be the only evidence available. There are many pitfalls, as well as great potential in the use of oral testimony, some of which have to do with the power relations and social characteristics of the interviewer and interviewee (see Chapter 28 on interviewing).

The Royal College of Nursing (RCN) sponsored a project concerned with collecting the career histories of a cohort of retired nurse leaders. This top-down history has been supplemented more recently by a bottom-up approach to the oral history of nurses who were trained in and practised in the 1930s and is logged with the RCN archives in Edinburgh. The Florence Nightingale Museum researched and exhibited a project entitled 'Hospital Voices' from 2007–2008, recording patients', nurses' and politicians' memories of Guy's, St Thomas' and Evelina Children's hospitals. Julie Fairman (2008) has shown the value of interweaving the insights from oral history with traditional text-based research in her history of nurse practitioners.

PILGRIMS OF PROGRESS?

The writing of history through the story of progress and great men, biased to one side of events, was recognised and derided by Herbert Butterfield as *The Whig Interpretation of History* in 1931. The term whiggism was drawn from histories of the Whig political party in the UK, which picked out of the past a story of progress, highlighting events and institutions leading to constitutional liberty. Whiggish history is a term applied more widely to presentist and biased history in general (Butterfield 1931; Carr 1964). While it is tempting to view the changes of the past as the fulfilment of progress, this assumes that the past is governed by law-like mechanisms, and tends to underplay the conflict and complexities of rival forces competing for power.

Much of the recent research in the history of nursing rejects this view as failing to account for the tensions between historical agencies and the intricacies of power differentials, which favour one set of conditions rather than another. The past as representing progress, while psychologically gratifying, prejudges it and forces it into a false mould, which empirical research may contradict. For example, although increases in nurses' pay in the UK have occurred since the introduction of the National Health Service, the fluctuating pattern of relativities suggests that the story of nurses' pay has not been one of onward and upward (Gray 1989). It is notable that Brian Abel-Smith's (1960: xi) contention, that nursing 'as an activity or skill, what it was like ... to nurse ... or receive nursing care' remained largely absent from history, remains relevant today.

For a profession that often declares itself a practice profession this omission is at odds with the professional ideology it espouses. Interestingly, D'Antonio (2006) argues that the very presence of the clinical psyche and training intrudes inadvertently into the historical process and shapes the kinds of question we as historians ask in ways we may be unaware of. D'Antonio raises the legitimate point that while we complain about the absence of nursing from histories of hospitals and other venues, we have likewise excluded other actors, aides and doctors from our histories. There are notable exceptions, especially where clinical specialisation has been involved as case studies of intensive and coronary care illustrate (Fairman & Lynaugh 1998; Keeling 2004).

However we conceptualise the challenge, there is still relatively little application of historical research as a means of recouping and recovering everyday practice. Where such studies have been undertaken they have often challenged stereotypes and received wisdom. In examining the development of the nurse practitioner movement in the US, Julie Fairman (2002) demonstrates how much of the advancement of practice has relied on relationships of trust, subtle and sophisticated processes of negotiation and risk taking by physicians and nurses alike. Oral history provided a key ingredient in unravelling the experiences of doctor and nurse pioneers in ways that would not be possible from using written records alone. Film can also provide vivid portraits of practice. In a study of US recruitment and training films held at the National Library of Medicine in Washington DC, we have uncovered films of nurses involved in a range of roles and practices that have become redundant, notably massage and diagnostics work hitherto the province of the nurse. Textbooks of the period also provide valuable guides to pedagogical theory as well as traces of practice. Fairman and D'Antonio (2008) take their lead from Charles Rosenberg (1992), reminding us that practice is contingent, with no fixed boundaries and liable to change over time. The negotiated order of the clinic is one in which nursing makes medicine possible and has been and become a symbiotic, pragmatic relationship, resulting from the rise of the hospital and biomedicine in the 19th century, rather than one of inevitable and straight forward subordination (Rafferty 1996).

INTRICACIES OF INTERPRETATION

Although presentism and bias should be avoided, interpretation lies at the heart of the historiographical endeavour. Historians will attach greater or lesser significance to the influence of particular variables on events and outcomes. Under the influence of postmodernism, history has been convulsed by culture wars. Such debates revolve around the proposition that a text is a text is a text. Thus, the border between fact and fiction, authorship and authority, breaks down. The historian is merely an author like any other, having no apparatus of authority to which to appeal in the case of competing interpretations of events except their own. Evans (1997) rejects this view and has mounted a stirring defence of the discipline from what he implies are its academic assailants. His defence of a more liberal approach to history is far more pragmatic; we can know something about the past, although there are no hard and fast rules about its interpretation.

Berridge considers that few people in the health field have reached the understanding that history is interpretation rather than 'incontrovertible' facts. Therefore although policy makers use history, usually stories of 'great men', they do not see 'historians or historical interpretation as a necessary part of the frame' (Berridge 2008b: 318). Carr (1964) has defined history as 'the continuous interaction between the historian and his facts, an unending dialogue between the present and the past' (Carr 1964: 24). Although it may seem on the surface that historians are at the mercy of their sources, all researchers are in fact dependent on their evidence and subject to economic and ethical constraints. Historical research is particularly sensitive to chronology of the question(s) being asked. In attempting to identify the 'causes' of wound healing, for example, a historical survey of past treatments may cast light on the mechanisms underlying changes in the theory and practice of wound care. The Hippocratic and Galenic medical theory of the fifth century BC to the second century AD, for example, maintained that suppuration and the production of so-called 'laudable pus' was an essential part of wound healing (Cartwright 1977).

This reasoning contrasts vividly with current theory of wound care, the object of which is to prevent infection. What the historian attempts to understand is how such theory was shaped and the factors that brought about change at any given point in time. Studying the history of nursing research helps us to understand that knowledge is provisional and apt to alter with the generation of fresh findings. While more sophisticated analyses of the theory–practice gap and implementation process in nursing research are beginning to emerge, historical studies of specified nursing 'inventions' can enhance our understanding of the politics of innovation and research utilisation.

CALCULATING CHANGE

History does not lend itself easily to estimating the precise effect of confounding variables, those that produce an interactive effect and therefore require correction to ascertain the effect of each individually. History is not, however, devoid of or divorced from the world of statistics. Indeed, there is a subdiscipline of history called *cliometrics*, which deals precisely with this. History and computing are growing areas of interest for researchers skilled in the management of large data sets, working at the interface between demography and history. The advent of information technology penetrated every sphere of life, including history. Quantitative methods in the history of medicine were the subject of a book by Porter and Wear (1987). Examples from the history of medicine of the collection and use of large data sets, analysed quantitatively and qualitatively, are John Harley Warner's *The Therapeutic Perspective* (1997), which analyses case notes for interventions and for language, and Anne Crowther and Marguerite Dupree's *Medical Lives in the Age of Surgical Revolution* (2007), which examines cohorts of medical students through prosopography, meaning collective biography. These approaches could be applied to nursing practice and cohorts.

Historians also talk about the strength of their evidence in terms of causation. Stone (1972), in his discussion of the causes of the English Civil War, divides the causal factors into three chronological groups: long-term preconditions, medium-term precipitants and short-term triggers. For example, if studying the origins of *Project 2000* in the UK and the 'causes' of its success, one of the major questions the historian would ask is 'Why has *Project 2000* apparently succeeded as a reform strategy where others seem to have failed?' (UKCC 1986). What factors have promoted its implementation: the merits of the case; demographic pressures; the social, political and economic environment; the fit with government policy; administration of the health, educational and social services; or all of these? If so, were all of equal importance? Immediately, we are confronted with the problems of historical evaluation.

- What in historical terms counts as success or failure?
- How can we measure historical change?
- Which outcome variables should we consider?
- Whose view(s) should we take into account – practising nurses, nurse leaders, the project team, government officials?
- Which sources should we use and how should we prioritize them?

Successful state-sponsored change in nursing can often be explained as the product of three overlapping forces: context, convergence and contingency – these were all present in *Project 2000* (Traynor & Rafferty 1998). The context and backdrop was the so-called demographic time bomb that threatened to explode in the employment market for nurses. Convergence consisted in the fit that the mobility and multipurpose employment ethos of *Project 2000* had with Thatcher's policy on flexible workforces, casualisation of the labour force and deregulation of the public sector. Finally, contingency resulted from the fortuitous timing that coincided with wider policy changes within higher education.

A similar set of forces can be seen at work in the entry of nursing into higher education itself. Although as far back as 1948 it was recognised that 10–15% of the nursing workforce qualified for university entrance, the seismic shift in policy only occurred when the context of the government objectives for higher education changed in the late 1980s. For once, the female dominance of the workforce converged with government's agenda as canny vice chancellors and policy makers cashed in on nursing's generous dowry of gender. Together, contingency ensured that nursing and health sciences made a significant contribution to the growth of higher education by broadening access, especially to women.

REPERTOIRE OF RESOURCES

In theory, one can study nursing history wherever there are resources to do so. While both historians and scientists may have to negotiate access to the research site through gatekeepers such as ethics committees, health service managers and keepers of manuscripts, the historian may have their work predetermined by virtue of the preservation or destruction of records. The historian traversing unknown territory may have little idea of what, if anything, primary sources, once located, will reveal.

Public records may be stored at the National Archives, Kew, the Scottish equivalent, the National Archives of Scotland, or regional records offices such as the London Metropolitan Archive and County Records Offices, or other local repositories such as (in Scotland) the Lothian Health Trust Medical Archives Centre housed in Special Collections at Edinburgh University Library. Some hospitals store their own records, but the stage of preservation varies enormously. The Hospital Records Database, an online resource created by the National Archive and the Wellcome Library, provides an excellent tool for discovering the location of and a brief guide to holdings for hospitals in the UK. The RCN employs a full-time archivist, based at the Scottish headquarters

in Edinburgh. The Wellcome Library's Archives and Manuscript Collection contains a number of different sources that are relevant to nursing, including the Queen's Institute of District Nursing and the records of the Community Practitioners and Health Visitors Association. In the UK, help and advice can be offered by members of the RCN History of Nursing Society and also through an increasing number of university centres of the history of medicine and related disciplines, especially those where academics with expertise in the history of nursing reside, such as those at King's College London, Manchester, Glasgow, Birmingham, Exeter and Oxford.

Historical sources are also subject to a particular set of regulations concerning access and closure, which may be crucial in determining the research that can be undertaken. The '30-year rule' in the UK closes access to public records for 30 years after the date of the last item in the file. 'Public' may be defined as those records deriving from organisations that are accountable to public bodies such as Parliament, with all records of the NHS authorities falling into this category. Medical records of patients in the UK are only usually open to the public after 100 years. In exceptional cases, organisations may decide to waive the rules normally governing access to material under their jurisdiction, usually through applications to ethics committees, and open files earlier than the statutory period to *bona fide* researchers, provided precautions to safeguard anonymity and the conditions of the Data Protection Act in publications are adhered to. Since the Freedom of Information Act 2000 (FOI) and the review of the 30-year rule, these rules are subject to change. The public can now request access to information, but in practice, it is often difficult for historians to know exactly what material to request under FOI if documents are not yet catalogued, and in any case access can still be denied. The independent review recommended that public records should in the future be available after 15 years rather than after 30.

CONCLUSIONS

The above discussion represents only the briefest outline of some signposts to historical research in nursing. In many ways, historical research may be compared to mining; extensive exploratory work may be necessary to refine an area for further investigation. Diligent excavation may reveal a wealth of resources. For this reason, and the fact that only in exceptional cases will records be susceptible to computer analysis, the process of extracting and analysing the data and formulating interpretations is time-consuming and labour intensive. It can be expensive in time and resources, and there are no immediate practical spin-offs in terms of a product to justify research investment. It also tends to be an individualistic enterprise and less frequently undertaken as part of a multidisciplinary project. Teamwork is rarer in historical research than health services research, although the history of the International Council of Nurses was very much a team effort (Brush & Stuart 1994). However, historical research has helped to shed important light on the multiple meanings of nursing and has provided a vehicle for setting a challenging political agenda for nurses. It provides an important vehicle to give expression to the different voices of nurses and nursing through documentary, oral or visual sources, such as film and photography. It enriches our experience, and our sense of identity. History anchors us in who we are, and provides role models for who we just might want to be.

References

Abel-Smith B (1960) *History of the Nursing Profession.* London, Heinemann.

Berridge V (2008a) Polyclinics: haven't we been there before? *British Medical Journal* **336**: 1161–1162.

Berridge V (2008b) History matters? History's role in health policy making. *Medical History* **52**(3): 311–326.

Borsay A (2009) Nursing history: an irrelevance for nursing practice? *Nursing History Review* **17**: 14–27.

Boschma G, Scaia M, Bonifacio N, Roberts E (2008) Oral history research. In: Lewenson SB, Herrmann EK (eds) *Capturing Nursing History: a guide to historical methods in research*. New York, Springer, pp 79–98.

Brush B, Stuart M (1994) Unity amidst difference: the ICN project and writing international nursing history. *Nursing History Review* **2**: 191–204.

Butterfield H (1931) *The Whig Interpretation of History.* London, Bell.

Carnegie ME (1991) *The Path We Tread: blacks in nursing 1854–1990*, 2nd edition. New York, National League for Nursing.

Carr EH (1964) *What is History?* 2nd edition. London, Penguin.

Carrier J, Kendall I (2008) 'Twas ever thus: why Darzi is 90 years too late. *Health Service Journal* **28 February**: 16–17.

Cartwright FF (1977) *A Social History of Medicine.* London, Longman.

Crowther MA, Dupree MW (2007) *Medical Lives in the Age of Surgical Revolution*. Cambridge, Cambridge University Press.

D'Antonio P (2006) History for a practice profession. *Nursing Inquiry* **13**(4): 242–248.

D'Antonio P (1999) Revisiting and rethinking the rewriting of nursing's history. *Bulletin of the History of Medicine* **73**(2): 268–290.

Davies C (ed) (1981a) *Rewriting Nursing History*. London, Croom Helm.

Davies C (1981b) Introduction: the contemporary challenge in nursing history. In: Davies C (ed) *Rewriting Nursing History*. London, Croom Helm, pp 1–17.

DHSS (1972) *Briggs Report: Report of the Committee on Nursing*. Cmnd. 5115 London, HMSO.

Evans RJ (1997) *In Defence of History*. London, Granta.

Fairman JA (2002) The roots of collaborative practice: nurse practitioner pioneer stories. *Nursing History Review* **10**: 159–174.

Fairman JA (2008) *Making Room in the Clinic: nurse practitioners and the evolution of modern health care*. New Brunswick, NJ, Rutgers University Press.

Fairman JA, D'Antonio P (2008) Reimagining nursing's place in the history of clinical practice. *Journal of the History of Medicine and Allied Sciences* **63**(4): 435–446.

Fairman JA, Lynaugh J (1998) *Critical Care Nursing: a history*. Philadelphia, University of Pennsylvania Press.

Godden J, Curry G, Delacour S (1993) The decline of myths and myopia? The use and abuse of nursing history. *Australian Journal of Advanced Nursing* **10**(2): 27–34.

Gray AM (1989) The NHS and the history of nurses' pay. *Bulletin of the History of Nursing Group at the Royal College of Nursing* **2**(8): 15–29.

Jenkinson V (1953) Case assignment method of nursing. *Nursing Mirror* **116**: i–iv.

Keeling AW (2004) Blurring the boundaries between medicine and nursing: coronary care nursing, circa the 1960s. *Nursing History Review* **12**: 139–164.

Lewenson SB, Herrmann EK (eds) (2008) *Capturing Nursing History: a guide to historical methods in research*. Springer, New York.

Lynaugh J (1998) Editorial. *Nursing History Review* **1**: 1.

Lynaugh J, Reverby S (1987) Thoughts on the nature of history. *Nursing Research* **36**: 1, 4 & 69.

Maggs CJ (1978) Towards a social history of nursing, parts 1 and 2. *Nursing Times* **74**(20–21) (Occasional papers): 53–58.

Marks S (1994) *Divided Sisterhood: race, class and gender in the South African nursing profession*. London, MacMillan.

Marwick A (1970) *The Nature of History*. London, Macmillan.

Nelson S (2002) The fork in the road: nursing history versus the history of nursing. *Nursing History Review* **10**: 175–188.

Pickering A (1992) *Science As Practice and Culture*. Chicago, University of Chicago Press.

Porter R, Wear A (eds) (1987) *Problems and Methods in the History Medicine*. London, Croom Helm.

Rafferty AM (1996) *The Politics of Nursing Knowledge*. London, Routledge.

Rosenberg CE (1992) Framing disease: illness, society and history. In: Rosenberg CE, Golden J (eds) *Framing Disease: studies in cultural history*. New Brunswick, NJ, Rutgers University Press, pp xiii–xxvi.

Stone L (1972) *The Causes of the English Revolution*. London, Routledge.

Thompson P (1978) *The Voice of the Past*. Oxford, Oxford University Press.

Traynor M, Rafferty AM (1998) Context, convergence and contingency. *Journal of Health Services Research and Policy* **3**(4): 195–196.

Traynor M, Rafferty AM, Lewison G (2001) Endogenous and exogenous research? Findings from a bibliometric study of UK nursing research. *Journal of Advanced Nursing* **34**(2): 212–222.

United Kingdom Central Council for Nursing, Midwifery and Health Visiting (1986) *Project 2000: a new preparation for practice*. London, UKCC.

Warner JH (1997) *The Therapeutic Perspective: medical practice, knowledge and identity in America, 1820–1885*, 2nd edition. Princeton, NJ, Princeton University Press.

Websites

http://library.wellcome.ac.uk – Wellcome Library for the History of Medicine, London.

http://rcnarchive.rcn.org.uk – The Royal College of Nursing Archive, Edinburgh

www.30yearrulereview.org.uk – 'An independent review of the 30-year rule' (UK).

www.direct.gov.uk/en/Governmentcitizensandrights/Yourrightsandresponsibilities/DG_4003239 – Freedom of Information (UK).

www.florence-nightingale.co.uk/cms/index.php/whats-on/exhibitions/hospital-voices – Hospital Voices.

www.nationalarchives.gov.uk/hospitalrecords – Hospital Records Database.

www.nursing.manchester.ac.uk/ukchnm – UK Centre for the History of Nursing and Midwifery, University of Manchester.

www.nursing.upenn.edu/history – Barbara Bates Centre for the Study of Nursing in History, University of Pennsylvania.

www.nursing.virginia.edu/Research/cnhi – The Center for Nursing Historical Inquiry, University of Virginia.

www.rcn.org.uk/development/communities/specialisms/history_of_nursing – Royal College of Nursing, History of Nursing Society.

27 Mixed Methods

Lucy Simons and Judith Lathlean

Key points

- Mixed methods research refers to research where quantitative and qualitative methods are integrated within one project.

- Mixed methods are needed to reflect and account for complexity in contemporary healthcare.

- The nature and robustness of the integration contributes to the whole being more than the sum of the parts.

- This kind of research is challenging to undertake but rewarding for the additional insights gained.

DEFINING MIXED METHODS

Mixed methods research is that which combines the methods that cross the two primary research approaches or paradigms in the same study. Methods include the full range of techniques or strategies used, for example, to sample participants and collect and analyse data. Paradigm refers to the overarching perspective or worldview guiding an investigation. The two main perspectives, often placed in opposition to each other, are the interpretivist/constructivist (qualitative) paradigm and the positivist (quantitative) paradigm.

However, it is the process of blending or bringing together the methods within one study that makes a study mixed methods. It is not about employing qualitative or quantitative methods in tandem *without* some interaction between the components. Similarly,

some may use the term 'mixed methods' inappropriately to refer to research in which two or more methods from the same paradigm are involved, for example routinely collected statistics on health outcomes and a survey conducted on the relevant population. Arguably, it is also not helpful to label a situation as 'mixed methods' when findings from two different studies are brought together after the event. For it to truly count as a mixed methods approach, the data within one study, derived from the two methods, should be mutually illuminating (Bryman 2008a), resulting in an enhanced end product.

Other terms used to describe this approach are combined methods research, multi-method, multiple methods, multidisciplinary research and blended research (see Bryman 2008b for a discussion of the different language used), but the term 'mixed methods' is becoming increasingly accepted as standard for this type of research especially in health, social and behavioural sciences (O'Cathain *et al.* 2007a; Teddlie & Tashakkori 2003).

WHY MIXED METHODS?

Twinn (2003) reports on the increasing use of mixed methods designs in the nursing literature from 1985. In health services research, the proportion of studies commissioned by the English Department of Health Research and Development programmes increased from 17% in the early 1990s to 30% by 2004 (O'Cathain *et al.* 2007a). Indeed, many bodies funding health research are increasingly receptive to, and often demand, mixed method designs. This renewed interest in combining methods has led to a surge in research texts on mixed methods and the launch of journals and conferences specific to it. Two studies into the use of mixed methods, one focusing on health services research (O'Cathain *et al.* 2007a,b) and another on the social sciences (Bryman 2006) have helped map out the landscape in relation to

mixed methods research and are contributing to developing ideas about its quality.

One of the main reasons for seeing this increase in the use of mixed methods is the view that research methods need to account for, and reflect, the increasing complexity of contemporary understandings of health and healthcare. Added to this is the recognition by many that this complexity is best explored by tapping a multiplicity of sources of knowledge, and this is where mixed methods research can excel (Forthofer 2003). This is particularly so in nursing research, which requires a better understanding of the context and process of care and the influence this has on health outcomes in order to advance nursing and healthcare knowledge (Twinn 2003). For example, a researcher might be interested in both how many and the type of people that attend a primary care out-of-hours service and also their experiences of and views about the use of these services (see Research Example 27.1). Generating the knowledge to answer these questions will require more than one research approach.

It is also apparent that particular disciplines in the health arena have been closely associated with par-

---

RESEARCH EXAMPLE

27.1   The Complementarity of Mixed Methods

Turnbull J *et al.* (2008) Does distance matter? Geographical variation in GP out-of-hours service use: an observational study. *British Journal of General Practice* **58**: 471–477.

This study focused on the role of place (geographical distance) on access to general practitioner services outside normal surgery hours ('out of hours'). The mixed method design included a quantitative geographical analysis of the rates of service use and call outcome (home visit, primary care centre attendance or GP telephone advice), followed by a qualitative study designed to understand the experience of access from the patient point of view. The geographical study found that patients in rural areas and those who live at greater distances from primary care centres make fewer contacts with out-of-hours services. Also those at a greater distance were more likely to receive GP telephone advice. The greatest variation was seen for children aged 0–4, and therefore the qualitative study focused on the parents of young children. The integration of the key findings demonstrated how place may affect parents help-seeking behaviour in relation to out-of-hours services.

NB This paper reports on the geographical quantitative analysis only. Further detail of the qualitative study can be found in Turnbull J (2008) Out-of-hours general practice: an investigation of patients' use and experiences of access to services. Unpublished PhD thesis, University of Southampton.

ticular types of research approach. For example, medicine and public health research has largely been distinguished by quantitative methods, whereas nursing research often takes a qualitative approach. This simplistic characterisation of disciplines is becoming less relevant as more researchers recognise the legitimacy and value of different forms of knowledge and methods required to generate new understandings. As healthcare is increasingly delivered by multidisciplinary teams and high-quality care requires multiple perspectives, it is apparent that single method or single perspective research restricts understanding. Just as there is now greater recognition that no one method is superior to another, and that different research approaches are equally good at answering different types of research questions, there is increasing understanding that combining methods can bring added value to healthcare research.

CAN METHODS BE MIXED?

There are long-standing arguments in some research fields that mixing methods is not feasible because the two paradigms are incommensurate – that the underpinning view on the nature of reality and truth is different in each paradigm. The qualitative paradigm sees reality as constructed by the complex set of meanings people attribute to their experiences, and there can be multiple truths, whereas the quantitative paradigm holds that reality is a known fixed point that can be objectively measured (see Chapter 11 for more discussion of these issues).

Other researchers believe that while mixing methods across the paradigms is feasible and can broaden the dimensions of the research, one approach should always be dominant in each study, meaning the philosophical underpinnings or 'theoretical drive' are drawn from this paradigm (Morse 2003). In this way, the second method is viewed as supplementary to the main or primary method. For example, a qualitative component may be added to a quantitative survey, but both methods would still be driven by the deductive assumptions of the quantitative paradigm. Morgan (1998) takes this approach when writing about mixed methods and using the term priority instead of dominance, calling it the 'Priority-Sequence Model'. He presents a two-by-two table to present the way in which methods can be combined in this model (see Figure 27.1).

However, other researchers have taken a different stance where one method is not prioritised over another and there is the belief that mixing methods, to some extent, overcomes the paradigm arguments. First, there are those who consider methods as 'techniques' (Bryman 2008a) at the 'shop floor' level of research (Sandelowski 2000). Such methods are not necessarily tied to a particular philosophical position,

		Priority decision	
		Principal method: *Quantitative*	Principal method: *Qualitative*
Sequence decision	Complementary method: *Preliminary*	Design 1 qual → QUANT e.g. to generate hypotheses, develop questionnaires	Design 2 quant → QUAL e.g. to guide purposive sampling, identify areas to pursue in depth
	Complementary method: *Follow-up*	Design 3 QUANT → qual e.g. help to interpret poorly understood results, help explain divergent findings	Design 4 QUAL → quant e.g. to generalise results to other settings, test elements of emergent theories

Figure 27.1 Mixed methods – adapted from Morgan's (1998) Priority-Sequence Model

and so can be fused, *transcending* the paradigm wars. Second, by taking a pragmatic approach, it is argued mixed methods can *supersede* the paradigm wars. With such an approach the driver of research design, and thus method, is the research question. Rather than being tied to a particular research approach, researchers should choose the appropriate method for answering the research questions – it should be the research question that dictates the methods, not a particular paradigm (Tashakkori & Teddlie 1998). However, this remains a controversial area for some, in that they believe pragmatism and other associated positions gloss over, rather than tackle head on, the paradigm debates (Twinn 2003).

THE PURPOSE OF USING MIXED METHODS RESEARCH

Given the greater focus on the practice of mixed methods, a number of typologies have been developed to summarise the reasons for mixing methods. Some of these run into many items, creating an exhaustive catalogue of reasons and attempting to list every possible combination of methods that could occur. However, most of these reasons can be organised under three key concepts in relation to mixed methods – triangulation, facilitation (or development) and complementarity (Hammersley 1996; Sandelowski 2000).

Triangulation

The derivation of the term triangulation stems from navigation and geography, where it refers to a process of taking bearings from more than one landmark to locate a precise position – the point where the bearing lines converge. This notion of convergence underpins the meaning of triangulation in the research context in that it refers to a process of adopting two or more methods in order to corroborate the findings from one method with the other. With this process of cross-checking, it is intended that the confidence in the entire study will be enhanced.

Denzin (1970) identified four types of triangulation.

1 *Data* triangulation involves using a range of data sources, from different settings or across space and time.
2 *Investigator* triangulation is where more than one person investigates the phenomena to seek to reduce personal bias on the data.
3 *Theoretical* triangulation applies when researchers approach data from different theoretical perspectives to test the fit with the data.
4 *Methodological* triangulation is when methods either from within the same paradigm or across paradigms are used to study the same phenomena.

It is this final type of triangulation that has most relevance to mixed methods research.

An example of this type of triangulation featured in a study exploring a new type of mental health worker – the Mental Health Practitioner (MHP) (see Research Example 27.2). People involved in the training programme to become an MHP were invited to take part in a survey and a smaller number was sampled for individual interviews. In the interviews, trainee MHPs described how they found it difficult to distinguish their role from that of the mental health nurse. The survey revealed that most of the people acting as mentors, line managers and supervisors for the trainees were mental health nurses. In this case, the findings from each method were found to corroborate and explain each other – confirming the high presence of mental health nurses in the training of MHPs, which led to tensions over role identity for the new types of worker.

However, in other cases the findings from two parts of a mixed method study may not converge on the same point. In such situations the mix of methods often reveals a more complex picture where one set of methods uncovers further data, which may diverge from the findings of the other method. In fact, some authors describe triangulation as a way of gaining deeper or greater understandings of a phenomenon by investigating it from different perspectives. For example, Morse (2003) defined triangulation as:

'the combination of the results of two or more rigorous studies conducted to provide a more comprehensive picture of the results than either study could do alone' (Morse 2003: 190)

RESEARCH EXAMPLE

27.2   Methodological Triangulation

Brown J *et al.* (2008) New ways of working: how mental health practitioners' perceive their training and role. *Journal of Psychiatric and Mental Health Nursing* **15**: 823–832.

In this study the experiences of trainees taking part in a two-year training programme for the mental health workforce were of interest. Mixed methods were adopted as the study aimed to provide a snapshot of current trainees' experiences and explore in-depth perceptions of role development over time. Therefore, a postal questionnaire was administered to the whole population (first and second year trainees) while the first year cohort only was sampled for the interview phase. The ordering of the methods of data collection (interviews followed by the survey) was designed to ensure the exploratory semi-structured interviews were not influenced by the topics introduced in the questionnaire. In the analysis of the data, an iterative process, which entailed moving backwards and forwards between the two datasets, was developed. In this way the data were checked against each other and the research team was able to critically question emergent findings. In the presentation of the findings, the survey data were used to substantiate the themes derived from the qualitative data. The mixed methods revealed and corroborated the key finding of poor role clarity for trainees.

While this purpose of combining methods to achieve a broader, more comprehensive picture is not disputed, the use of the term triangulation in this context is. The etymology of the term suggests very clearly the idea of convergence and coming together at a particular point, whereas the idea of a more comprehensive picture suggests a widening out, a divergence away from the initial ideas. When this happens the researcher must carefully consider these divergences and reflect on the complexity revealed by mixed methods.

Using the same term to signify both processes serves to confuse. However, this dual meaning of the term may stem from the issue that it is almost impossible to know at the outset of a mixed method study whether the findings will converge or diverge. If this were known at the outset there would seem little reason to do the research. The term *complementarity* better describes the process in which mixed methods results in a more comprehensive understanding of the phenomena under study. Designating which term will be appropriate for describing a mixed method study may need to be postponed until the outcome of the study is known.

Although the term triangulation can be used to describe the process of corroborating findings by drawing attention to a single point, this suggests alignment with the quantitative paradigm, where there is belief in a single fixed reality (i.e. one truth) that can be objectively known through the use of multiple methods. However, as suggested earlier, many researchers operate from a stance which holds that multiple realities (i.e. many truths) are *de rigeur*. Indeed, many of the arguments used earlier in the chapter to justify the use of mixed methods recognise the multiple ways of knowing and the need for a range of ways of understanding the world to advance knowledge.

A further caution needed with triangulation is that while a greater air of validity or confidence in the findings might be suggested by the corroboration process, it is important to examine the way in which the methods have been applied in every study. Flawed methods might lead to a single point, but this does not mean additional confidence should be taken from the resultant findings.

Facilitation

The acceptance that there are alternative modes of knowing or understanding about a health problem can substantiate the use of mixed methods for the development or facilitation of research. Here, one method is used to facilitate the next stage of the research, for example in relation to the sampling strategy, for instrument development, as a process evaluation within a randomised controlled trial, or to develop or improve health interventions.

Research Example 27.3 provides an example of a facilitative mix of methods in relation to sampling. Here, the researcher adopted the sequential use of quantitative then qualitative phases. A survey was implemented, the results of which were used to purposively sample participants who held a range of views about the topic under investigation. Interestingly, this study is not identified as a mixed method study. However, the sampling strategy adopted would not have been possible without the initial survey. This study is also an example of the theoretical drive coming from one method, as in the reporting of the study the qualitative element is dominant and the theoretical justifications for the methods adopted are underpinned by an interpretive approach.

Another important way in which methods are combined to facilitate the research is to design, develop and test a research instrument. Most often this would take the form of qualitative methods, for example individual interviews or group discussions being used to understand the context, detail and language associated with an issue to enable the design of a survey instrument or questionnaire. In this way, the questionnaire should be more relevant to the issue being investigated and appropriate for the population under study than if the preliminary work had not been undertaken. This might be most useful for researching populations that have different characteristics from the research team, for example young people or populations from different cultural backgrounds. By undertaking preliminary work to better understand their perspectives and, importantly, their preferred way of talking about the issues being investigated, a research instrument such as a questionnaire is more likely to be relevant to those being asked to complete it.

Complementarity

The notion of complementarity in mixed methods research is grounded in the argument that the weaknesses of one method can be offset by combining them with an alternative method which offers different strengths – that is, methods are combined to complement one another. This broad concept covers a whole range of different rationales for why two or more methods would be better than a single method approach.

RESEARCH EXAMPLE

27.3   Mixed Methods to Facilitate Sampling

Summers A (2003) Involving users in the development of mental health services: a study of psychiatrists' views. *Journal of Mental Health* **12**(2): 161–174.

This study explored the views and attitudes of psychiatrists towards service user involvement in the development of mental health services. This mixed method study included a survey followed by qualitative interviews. The survey was sent to the total population of consultant and specialist registrar grades of psychiatrists in the study area. Sampling for the qualitative interviews was based on the survey results to achieve variation across a range of characteristics which were assumed to potentially influence attitudes. These were age, gender, employing trust, non-clinical roles, clinical experience and, finally, experience of and stated enthusiasm for user involvement. The findings indicated that in general the participants used a scientific, utilitarian frame of reference to talk about user involvement and could be clustered into three groups according to how much support they expressed for involvement (optimists, rationalists and sceptics).

First, there is the issue of *completeness* or *comprehensiveness*. As discussed above, not everything can be known or discovered through one way of looking at the social world; therefore by combining methods, knowledge that is not accessible through one route can be included in a study by the employment of alternative methods. A questionnaire can collect data on what people report they do or intend to do in a certain situation, for example how a clinician provides information to a patient during a consultation. However, by observing the clinic setting, data can be collected on how they actually do communicate with the patient.

Another way in which different methods complement each other is where qualitative methods are used to provide a detailed examination of the *context* for understanding the information gleaned with broad brush quantitative methods. In the presentation of findings from the research, qualitative data can then be used to *illustrate* some of the themes arising from the quantitative data. Alternatively, as in the example in Research Example 27.2, quantitative data can be used to *substantiate* the findings emerging from the interpretative analysis of qualitative data.

Third, qualitative methods might be combined with quantitative methods to help *explain* any association found between the factors (or variables) being studied. For example, quantitative methods can provide a snapshot of a particular issue and explore whether associations between various factors (or variables) are apparent. However, these methods would not shed light on why these associations have been found. Complementing the quantitative work with qualitative work would enable explanatory factors to be explored with the population under study. This was the rationale for using mixed methods undertaken by Turnbull and colleagues in the study presented in Research Example 27.1. The study was designed to explore the role of place (that is, urban or rural locations and geographical distance) in people's use and experiences of access to general practitioner services outside usual surgery hours (out of hours). By using a sequential design, the associations and patterns identified in the quantitative phase were further explored in the follow-on qualitative phase. In this way the qualitative work was able to develop further the insights gained from the initial results and at the same time offer some explanations as to why the associations between place and access to out-of-hours services had been found in the quantitative analysis.

Another example of where qualitative work can help explain quantitative work is within randomised controlled trials. This is most useful when complex interventions are being evaluated, such as psychological therapy or the organisation of specialist services (Medical Research Council 2000). Here, the quantitative method will be able to answer the question of whether one approach is more effective than another. Complementing a randomised controlled trial (RCT) study with qualitative methods will help to explain why this effect has been observed. In other words, where the trial methodology focuses on the *outcome* of the intervention, the qualitative methods will focus on the *process* of the intervention, which, as suggested earlier in the chapter, can have a significant effect on health outcomes (an example of combining qualitative methods with an RCT is given in Research Example 27.4).

THE IMPORTANCE OF INTEGRATION IN MIXED METHODS RESEARCH

Increasingly, an indicator of quality in mixed methods studies is the way in which the methods interact with each other. As argued earlier, it is the fact that mixed methods can bring something extra to the research process that distinguishes this approach from single method research or two methods used in tandem. It is this *integration* that brings the added value to the research. Integration may occur at one or many stages of the research process, from devising the research questions, through to writing up, including the stages of research design, sampling, analysis and interpretation of the results (O'Cathain *et al.* 2007b).

Research question

This is a key stage in the integration of mixed methods in any study, because it is the research question that is the driver over choice of research design. In the study presented in Research Example 27.1, it was the

27.4 Mixed Methods in the Design of a Randomised Controlled Trial

Donovan J *et al.* (2002) Improving design and conduct of randomised trials by embedding them in qualitative research: ProtecT (prostate testing for cancer and treatment) study. *British Medical Journal* **325**: 766–770.

The ProtecT study was designed to test the feasibility of screening and evaluating different treatments for prostate cancer in men aged 50–69. This health area, and thus the study, was controversial because of the variable complication rates across different treatment options. Low rates of recruitment and randomisation to the different treatment arms of the trial was found. Qualitative research methods were used to investigate the process of recruitment into the study. The findings from the qualitative work were communicated to those recruiting men into the study and had a direct impact on the conduct of the trial in four ways: organisation of study information; the terminology used in study information; specification and presentation of the non-radical treatment arm; and presentation of randomisation and clinical equipoise. Recruitment rates into the trial rose from 30–40% to 70% over the course of one year.

interest in both the use and experience of out-of-hours services that set the direction of the mixed method study. The quantitative part was designed to provide information about the use of out-of-hours services and the qualitative part designed to consider people's experiences of out-of-hours services.

Research design

Integration in the design stage has been highlighted above where mixed methods are used for facilitation and complementarity. An often cited good example of integrated research design is summarised in Research Example 27.4, where an RCT was embedded within qualitative research. This resulted in important changes being made to the trial design, which significantly increased the recruitment and randomisation rates to the trial.

Sampling

Methods are integrated where the sampling for one phase of a mixed method study is informed by the analysis of an earlier phase. It might be appropriate to sample case studies from the results of a survey, as in the study described in Research Example 27.3. In this study, the whole population of interest was surveyed about their experience and attitudes towards

service user involvement in mental health service development. Following this, a purposive sample of respondents holding a range of views towards involvement was invited to take part in an in-depth interview.

To maximise the potential of mixed methods, it is important to ensure that the analysis takes account of the sampling information (O'Cathain *et al.* 2007b). In a study that explored community mental health nurses' experiences of delivering brief interventions for anxiety and depression in the context of an RCT (Simons *et al.* 2008), nurses were sampled on the basis of the different interventions they had been delivering. In the analysis of the interviews, the commonalities and differences between the nurses' experiences were sought, depending on the type of intervention they had provided. It would not have been appropriate in this instance, to only look for themes that were common across the whole data set, because the participants had been sampled for this part of the study specifically because they had experience of the different interventions in the trial.

Analysis

In some cases it may be appropriate to analyse the two linked datasets separately, using techniques appropriate to each form of data. In this situation integration should take place at the interpretation stage (see below). However, at the analysis stage there are ways in which data sets can be combined or transformed into a single data set. The process of transforming qualitative data into quantitative data has been referred to as *quantitising*, while the process of converting quantitative data into qualitative data has been referred to as *qualitising* (Sandelowski 2000).

One way of quantitising qualitative data is transforming responses from a qualitative interview into variables for numerical analysis. This was the approach taken in a study in which 173 people were interviewed after discharge from an acute psychiatric hospital admission (Simons *et al.* 2002). Each person took part in a semi-structured interview consisting primarily of open-ended questions about their experience of the discharge procedure. After the interview the researcher completed a pro-forma in which the person's experience was converted into a number of broad categorical variables, for example the length of notice the person received about discharge from hospital and whether or not the person was involved in the decision to discharge. These data were then analysed statistically, while the full interview data were analysed using qualitative analysis techniques. This type of transformation should be approached cautiously because the sample size for many qualitative components would not yield sufficient data for a meaningful statistical analysis.

Interpretation

A key stage in mixed method research is bringing together the insights gained from both methods. This often takes place in the latter stages of the study once the main analysis has been completed. This further stage is referred to by some as 'crystallisation' (O'Cathain *et al.* 2007b), where there is a purposeful search for convergence, divergence and discrepancy between the findings from the different methods. It is important to ensure that this additional process in mixed method research is deliberately planned into the time and resources for the study at the outset. It is disappointing when reading a mixed method study to find that in the presentation of the results and sub-

sequent discussion both parts of the study are presented separately with no attempt made to bring the insights from the parts together.

Although specific examples have been used to illustrate integration at different stages of the research, integration does not need to take place at only one stage of the research. High-quality mixed method studies may have integrated elements throughout. To ensure that integration is apparent to readers of mixed methods studies it may be appropriate when presenting such studies to devise a diagram to demonstrate where integration takes place. For the study described in Research Example 27.1, a diagram was used in the written presentation of the research to clearly demonstrate the way in which the two components of the study were integrated. This is shown in Figure 27.2.

CHALLENGES WITH MIXED METHOD STUDIES

Although mixed methods research can bring many advantages to the research endeavour, careful consideration should be taken before embarking on a mixed methods study. Simply because many researchers are taking this approach and it seems fashionable at the present time is not sufficient justification. As with all research, the design should be driven by the research question and good rationale is required for any design adopted. Some of the challenges brought about by the rise in popularity and conduct of mixed method research are summarised below.

The strategic use of mixed methods

Researchers might propose a mixed method design as they believe it is favoured by funding bodies and that using this design will increase their chance of gaining funding. This is not sufficient justification to attempt a mixed method study, since a diverse range of skills and additional time and resources may be required to ensure an effective design (Forthofer 2003).

Mixed methods requires a range of expertise and skill

There are limited training programmes that specifically focus on how to conduct good-quality mixed

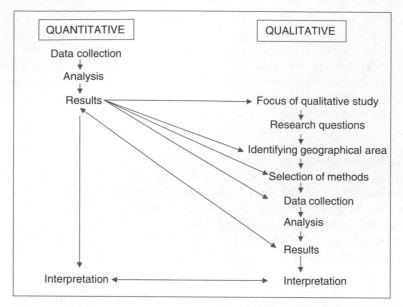

Figure 27.2 An example of how to represent mixed method integration in a diagram
Reproduced from Turnbull J (2008) Out-of-hours general practice: an investigation of patients' use and experiences of access to services. Unpublished PhD thesis, University of Southampton, with permission from Joanne Turnbull.

method studies. It is therefore unlikely that one researcher will have the range of necessary skills to ensure the quality of both methods within a mixed methods study. This means mixed methods studies are usually conducted by teams of researchers with complementary skills.

Multidisciplinary or interdisciplinary team working

The argument for working in teams when conducting mixed method research is strong. However, while this can often be a rich and rewarding experience, it also has the potential to give rise to tensions and difficulties. It is important to adopt respectful and collaborative practice to guard against 'silos' developing where a series of separate mini-projects are conducted rather than integrated mixed methods. This is particularly pertinent where one method has been the dominant approach in a particular discipline and there may be limited understanding of the other approach. It has been argued that rather than multidisciplinary

working, where each person brings their skills to the team but operates in isolation, interdisciplinary working is sought, with all members of a team contributing to and learning from each other (Simons 2007). In such cases it important for the team to pay attention to the process of doing the research as much as the outcome of the research. However, others have argued that this may be hard to achieve without creating overly burdensome research management processes (Tritter 2007).

Maintaining quality in mixed method research

If both qualitative and quantitative methods are being applied, there is a danger that neither approach will be conducted well. The overall quality of a mixed method study will always be constrained by the individual components. While there are as yet no established criteria or checklists for assessing the quality of mixed methods studies, this issue is being debated. For example, researchers in the field are asking whether it is appropriate to apply both sets of criteria to a mixed methods study. However, as the discussion about integration indicated, it may be the aspects of the research that are *distinctive* to mixed methods that should be assessed, rather than applying criteria developed for a different purpose.

CONCLUSIONS

Mixed methods research has gained greatly in popularity in recent years, but therein lies a danger. While it has the potential to provide positive and enriching experiences for researchers, as well as answers to complex healthcare questions, the term has been used as a 'catch-all' to lend credence to research that is not truly adopting the underpinning philosophy and principles. To ensure that the value, robustness and integrity of mixed methods approaches are maintained, attention must be paid to the integration of qualitative and quantitative date in a way that produces outcomes that are greater than the sum of the parts.

References

Brown J, Simons L, Zeeman L (2008) New ways of working: how mental health practitioners' perceive their training and role. *Journal of Psychiatric and Mental Health Nursing* **15**: 823–832.

Bryman A (2008a) Mixed methods research: combining quantitative and qualitative research. In: Bryman A. *Social Research Methods*, 3rd edition. Oxford, Oxford University Press, pp 603–625.

Bryman A (2008b) Why do researchers integrate/combine/mesh/blend/mix/merge/fuse quantitative and qualitative research? In: Bergman M (ed) *Advances in Mixed Methods Research*. Thousand Oaks, Sage, pp 87–100.

Bryman A (2006) Integrating quantitative and qualitative research: how is it done? *Qualitative Research* **6**: 97–113.

Denzin NK (1970) *The Research Act in Sociology: a theoretical introduction to sociological methods*. London, Butterworth.

Donovan J, Mills N, Smith M, Brindle L, Jacoby A, Peters T *et al.* for the Protect Study Group (2002) Improving design and conduct of randomised trials by embedding them in qualitative research: ProtecT (prostate testing for cancer and treatment) study. *British Medical Journal* **325**: 766–770.

Forthofer MS (2003) Status of mixed methods in the health sciences. In: Tashakkori A, Teddlie C (eds) *Handbook of Mixed Methods in Social and Behavioral Research*. Thousand Oaks, Sage, pp 527–540.

Hammersley M (1996) The relationship between qualitative and quantitative research: paradigm loyalty versus methodological eclecticism. In: Richardson JTE (ed) *Handbook of Qualitative Research Methods for Psychology and the Social Sciences*. Leicester, BPS Books, pp 159–174.

Medical Research Council (2000) *A Framework for Development and Evaluation of RCTs for Complex Interventions to Improve Health*. London, Medical Research Council

Morgan D (1998) Practical strategies for combining qualitative and quantitative methods: applications in health research. *Qualitative Health Research* **8**: 362–367.

Morse JM (2003) Principles of mixed methods and multi-method research design. In: Tashakkori A, Teddlie C (eds) *Handbook of Mixed Methods in Social and Behavioral Research*. Thousand Oaks, Sage, pp 189–208.

O'Cathain A, Murphy E, Nicholl J (2007a) Why, and how, mixed methods research is undertaken in health services research in England: a mixed methods study. *BMC Health Services Research* **7**: 85.

O'Cathain A, Murphy E, Nicholl J (2007b) Integration and publications as indicators of 'yield' from mixed method studies. *Journal of Mixed Method Research* **1**(2): 147–163.

Sandelowski M (2000) Combining qualitative and quantitative sampling, data collection and analysis techniques in mixed-method studies. *Research in Nursing and Health* **23**: 246–255.

Simons L (2007) Moving from collision to integration: reflecting on the experience of mixed methods. *Journal of Research in Nursing* **12**(1): 73–83.

Simons L, Lathlean J, Squire C (2008) Shifting the focus: sequential methods of analysis with qualitative data. *Qualitative Health Research* **18**(1): 120–132.

Simons L, Petch A, Caplan R (2002) *'Don't They Call It Seamless Care?': a study of acute psychiatric discharge*. Edinburgh, Scottish Executive Social Research.

Summers A (2003) Involving users in the development of mental health services: a study of psychiatrists' views. *Journal of Mental Health* **12**(2): 161–174.

Tashakkori A, Teddlie C (1998) *Mixed Methodology: combining qualitative and quantitative approaches*. Thousand Oaks, Sage.

Teddlie C, Tashakkori A (2003) Major issues and controversies in the use of mixed methods in the social and behavioral sciences. In: Tashakkori A, Teddlie C (eds) *Handbook of Mixed Methods in Social and Behavioral Research*. Thousand Oaks, Sage, pp 3–50.

Tritter J (2007) Mixed methods and multidisciplinary research in health care. In: Saks M, Allsop J (eds) *Researching Health: qualitative, quantitative and mixed methods*. Los Angeles, Sage, pp 301–318.

Turnbull J (2008) Out-of-hours general practice: an investigation of patients' use and experiences of access to services. Unpublished PhD thesis, University of Southampton.

Turnbull J, Martin D, Lattimer V, Pope C, Culliford D (2008) Does distance matter? Geographical variation in GP out-of-hours service use: an observational study. *British Journal of General Practice* **58**: 471–477.

Twinn S (2003) Status of mixed methods research in nursing. In: Tashakkori A, Teddlie C (eds) *Handbook of Mixed Methods in Social and Behavioral Research*. Thousand Oaks, Sage, pp 541–556.

Further reading

Andrew S, Halcomb E (2009) *Mixed Methods Research for Nursing and the Health Sciences*. Oxford, Wiley-Blackwell.

Bergman M (ed) (2008) *Advances in Mixed Methods Research*. Thousand Oaks, Sage.

Bryman A (ed) (2006) *Mixed Methods* (4 volumes). Thousand Oaks, Sage.

Creswell JW, Plano Clark VL (2007) *Designing and Conducting Mixed Methods Research*. Thousand Oaks, Sage.

O'Cathain A, Thomas K (2006) Combining qualitative and quantitative methods. In: Pope C, Mays N (eds) *Qualitative Research in Health Care*, 3rd edition. Oxford, Blackwell, pp 102–111.

Tashakkori A, Teddlie C (eds) (2003) *Handbook of Mixed Methods in Social and Behavioral Research*. Thousand Oaks, Sage.

Websites

http://mmr.sagepub.com/ – *Journal of Mixed Method Research*. Information about the journal, table of contents for each edition and request free sample copy.

www.mixedmethods.leeds.ac.uk/ – International Mixed Methods Conference. This site provides the information for the forthcoming conference plus an archive of the previous four conferences.

www.ncrm.ac.uk/ – ESRC National Centre for Research Methods training centre for innovations in methods. Hosted workshops on mixed methods are detailed on the site, plus a discussion paper about mixed methods written by Julia Brannen. Also seminars within the individual research programmes relevant to mixed methods.

Collecting Data

This section contains six practical chapters dealing with the common methods used in nursing research to collect data. A generic approach has been maintained, with several of the methods such as interviewing and observation being used in both qualitative and quantitative research.

Chapter 28 begins by tackling interviews, a versatile data collection method widely used in nursing research. This is followed by a chapter describing focus groups, increasingly popular as an adjunct to individual interviews or as a stand-alone tool. Both these chapters deal with the purposes to which the methods are best suited, the essential preparation for, and conduct of, the interview or focus group, and the practical and ethical issues raised.

Chapter 30 then deals with questionnaires, perhaps the most widely used method of data collection in healthcare research. This chapter has been completely rewritten for the 6th edition of the book by new authors, and discusses in detail some of the ways of testing validity and reliability of existing questionnaires, as well as giving advice to nurse researchers who are developing their own measure.

Observation, structured or unstructured, participant or not, is a powerful tool for data collection that is used less often than it might be, perhaps because of the demands made on the researcher. Observation is used differently in qualitative and quantitative research, and this chapter discusses each approach carefully. Ethical issues raised are considered, as are the problems of ensuring validity, reliability and trustworthiness of the data collected.

The final two chapters in this section have been newly written for this edition. Think aloud is a less well-known technique for data collection than many discussed in this section, but one that has unique ability to increase our understanding of clinical decision making. It can be combined with other data collection tools to increase the richness and validity of data gathered. Finally, Chapter 33 deals with outcome measures. Evaluation of clinical treatments is increasingly measured by patient-based outcomes, as well as scientifically observable physiological measures, although the latter are still, of course, important. This chapter, therefore, considers the range of measures that can be used to assess the effects of nursing care, and which are also vitally important in many research studies.

28 Interviewing

Angela Tod

Key points

- Interviews can be used to collect qualitative and quantitative data, and can vary in their degree of structure. The degree of structure is dictated by the research design and purpose.

- Key skills in conducting rigorous interviews include developing a well-designed data collection tool, selecting a suitable environment, establishing rapport, and balancing the direction and flexibility of questioning.

- Interviews can generate rich data reflecting the perspective of participants. Interviews can be of particular value when the research focus is a sensitive area.

- Interviews are labour intensive, expensive and can introduce bias.

- Interviews provide a unique opportunity to gain insight into a range of subjects and experiences related to nursing and health services.

INTRODUCTION

This chapter considers some of the key issues confronting the researcher in conducting a research interview. Brief attention is paid to the purpose and nature of the research interview. This is followed by an overview of different types of interview and some of the advantages and disadvantages of the different forms. The main issues to reflect on when undertaking research interviews are reviewed, followed by an outline of some factors relating to validity, reliability and ethics.

THE PURPOSE OF THE RESEARCH INTERVIEW

Conducting a research interview is one of the most exciting and fascinating methods of data collection in nursing and healthcare research. This may explain why it is one of the most commonly used data collection methods. Interviews are used in both qualitative and quantitative research as the primary data collection method or as a supplementary method in mixed methods studies.

Reasons for undertaking interviews

The purpose of undertaking a research interview varies widely. The research aim will dictate the exact nature and form of the interview in terms of structure, direction and depth. Generally the more that is known about a topic beforehand, the more structured and less in-depth the exploration.

A structured interview approximates to a standardised interviewer-administered questionnaire in that the wording and order of questions is the same for all participants. Structured interviews normally generate quantitative data. Some include limited open questions and have some capacity to produce qualitative data. Structured interviews would be used for a survey in order to measure variables in a specific population. They are useful when a certain amount is already known about the subject under examination, and are used to explore differences between people with varying characteristics or experiences (Murphy *et al.* 1998: 112–123). The inclusion of open questions facilitates the collection of data to illuminate survey responses.

The majority of interview-based studies in nursing are qualitative in nature and so adopt a less-structured, more 'in-depth' and flexible approach. Such methods are recommended when the research purpose is to:

- explore a phenomenon about which little is known
- understand context
- generate a hypothesis or theory to explain social processes and relationships
- verify the results from other forms of data collection, for example observation
- illuminate responses from a questionnaire survey
- conduct initial exploration to generate items for questionnaires.

Interviews, therefore, have the capacity to describe, explain and explore issues from the perspective of participants.

Research Examples 28.1, 28.2 and 28.3 illustrate different uses of the research interview. Collins and Reynolds (2008) use semi-structured interviews to

---

RESEARCH EXAMPLE

28.1 Using Interviews as a Single Method of Data Collection in a Qualitative Study

Collins S, Reynolds F (2008) How do adults with cystic fibrosis cope following a diagnosis of diabetes. *Journal of Advanced Nursing* **64**(7): 478–487.

In this study, 22 patients with a diagnosis of cystic fibrosis-related diabetes were interviewed (10 women, 12 men, age range 24–55). Mean time from their diabetes diagnosis was 8 years 4 months (range 1–35 years). The aim was to explore patients' experience of adapting to a diagnosis of diabetes, which, for them, would be a second chronic illness. The semi-structured interviews were conducted and audio-taped. The tapes were transcribed verbatim and analysed using interpretative phenomenological analysis (IPA). Four themes were identified: emotional response to the diagnosis, looking for understanding, learning to live with diabetes and limiting the impact of diabetes. Two challenges emerged for patients adapting to the dual diagnosis. These were managing the conflicting dietary demands of the illnesses and a lack of practical professional advice.

The interviews were able to uncover sensitive and subtle responses to the diagnosis of diabetes. For example, the study revealed more extreme initial feelings of shock and uncertainty at the new diagnosis as well as the way that for some the diagnosis led them to confront and review their feelings about cystic fibrosis. It allowed experiences to be categorised and better understood and indicated how health professionals can better educate patients with cystic fibrosis-related diabetes.

RESEARCH EXAMPLE

28.2 A Study Using Interviews in a Mixed Methods Study

Astin F *et al.* (2008) Primary angioplasty for heart attack: mismatch between expectations and reality. *Journal of Advanced Nursing* **65**(1): 72–83.

This mixed methods study aimed to explore patients' experiences of primary angioplasty and to assess their illness perceptions. A total of 29 patients (16 men and 13 women, age 36–83) were interviewed 3–12 days after hospital discharge. Following the interview participants were asked to complete an Illness Perception Questionnaire (IPQ-R) (Moss-Morris *et al.* 2002). A topic guide was used in the interview, but this contained fairly open questions, for example 'Can you tell me about your recent admission to hospital for your heart problem'. This allowed the patient to lead the focus and content of the interview. The IPQ-R assesses people's perceptions and beliefs about their illness, specifically with regard to illness identity, timeline and consequences. The interview data allowed in-depth exploration of patient experiences from which conclusions were drawn about how patients characterised their illness. The IPQ-R responses were able to support, verify or challenge these findings. For example, the speed with which primary angioplasty occurs can create confusion for people and make it difficult to understand what has happened to them. The IPQ-R was able to affirm that respondents were more likely to see their condition as acute, rather than as an acute episode of a chronic condition. This has implications for their recovery and secondary prevention.

28.3 A Study Using Interviews to Collect Data in a Quantitative Study

Laws R (2004) Current approaches to obesity management in UK primary care: the Counterweight Programme. *Journal of Human Nutrition and Dietetics* **17**: 183–190.

This study aimed to examine obesity management in 40 primary care practices in the UK. A total of 141 general practitioners and 66 practice nurses were interviewed using a structured approach. A researcher-administered questionnaire was used to establish which of five obesity management approaches participants used. The approaches were based on time spent with patients and the nature of advice given. Referral practice and attitudes to obesity management were also recorded. Reported practice in the interviews was compared to recorded practice in the clinical notes.

The approach revealed that obesity was under-reported and under-recognised in primary care. However, it demonstrated the challenge of collecting data from busy clinical staff as one-third of the participants did not complete the questionnaire/interview.

explore the experience of patients with cystic fibrosis in adapting to a diagnosis of diabetes, a second chronic illness (see Research Example 28.1). This study demonstrates how interviews can generate qualitative data to inform care givers of the implications of having this dual diagnosis and their conflict-

ing and complex demands. Astin *et al.* (2008) used interviews in the qualitative component of a mixed methods study to explore UK patients' experience of primary angioplasty (see Research Example 28.2). It demonstrates how interview data can be used alongside a questionnaire to illuminate the patient experience. In this study the questionnaire data were used to verify and inform the qualitative findings. Laws (2004) uses structured interviews to collect quantitative data from doctors and nurses on obesity management (see Research Example 28.3).

The difference between a clinical and research interview

Nurses are trained to use interviews to obtain information from patients in clinical settings. While this clinical experience may be a good preparation, the research context and purpose is different and requires different skills. In research interviews the focus of data collection is broad, as it is necessary to understand meanings about the area of study from the participants' viewpoint.

In the clinical context, data collection is focused on identifying a problem, fitting it into a predetermined category, e.g. diagnosis, and deciding a management or intervention strategy (Britten 1995). This means the clinical situation lends itself to being more controlled by the clinician. In addition, a nurse would freely respond to patients' questions related to the clinical situation. In a research interview, this is not appropriate. To respond to questions may deviate from the interview focus and bias responses by changing the participant's knowledge base. Judgements made by researchers therefore differ from those of the nurse.

TYPES OF INTERVIEW

Structure

Robson (2002) states that the most common distinction made between different types of interview is the degree of structure and standardisation. A continuum exists from completely structured to unstructured interviews (Figure 28.1). In general, the less structured an interview the more in-depth and flexible the questioning. An unstructured interview is likely to be led more by the informant agenda than by the interviewer. It will generate qualitative data.

In structured or standardised interviews the balance of control lies with the interviewer. Such an approach would be adopted for survey purposes or when less in-depth data is required. Structured interviews are also used if it is not possible for the participant to self-administer a questionnaire, for example if the participant does not have the ability or concentration to read or does not have the time to participate. In nursing research, a structured interview may be used to gain some insight where competing work or home demands would make a more in-depth interview impossible. Interviewing nurses on a busy ward might be an example of this.

In many qualitative studies, semi-structured and unstructured interviews are used. Semi-structured interviews will have predetermined topics and open-ended questions laid down in an interview schedule.

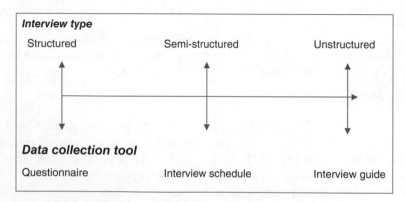

Figure 28.1 The continuum of interview structure and data collection tool required

They retain the flexibility necessary to follow issues raised by participants that had not been anticipated. Control and direction of interviews of this nature still lies with the researcher, but there will be capacity to be responsive to the interviewee's agenda and views. Semi-structured interviews are widely used in qualitative studies adopting a number of methodological approaches in nursing research.

Unstructured interviews are the most in-depth and least directive. The aim here is often to explore in great detail a general area of interest or a phenomenon from the participant's perspective. A few themes may guide the interview, but it will be led by the participant's perspective and viewpoint. Interviews of this nature are very informal and can appear more like a conversation than an interview. The interview guide will comprise a list of topics rather than predefined questions. This approach is more commonly adopted in qualitative research methodologies where little previous knowledge exists regarding the area of study.

The degree of structure employed in an interview will depend on the purpose of the study and the depth of inquiry required. It will also vary according to the resources available. With structured interviews questioning techniques are standardised to ensure the reliability of the data. Unstructured interviews can be labour intensive and expensive. Their informal and unguided structure means they can take a long time to conduct and also to transcribe and analyse. As is always the case with research, it is important to choose the right tool for the job and to make sure the approach adopted is achievable within the time and cost restraints of a study.

Face-to-face versus telephone interviews

The vast majority of individual interviews are conducted face to face. The researcher is able to probe and investigate hidden and suppressed views and experiences. The ability to observe body language and have eye contact helps to interpret what is being said. It also helps to interpret emotion, distress, anxiety and silence, and to respond accordingly. For example, if a respondent displays emotion it may provide an appropriate opportunity to collect data on a sensitive and upsetting experience of great value to the study. On the other hand it may be appropriate to appraise the situation with regard to stopping the interview. Making this judgement is difficult if the interview is not face to face.

Telephone interviews are increasingly being used to conduct structured and semi-structured interviews. In some circumstances it may be a cheaper, more convenient mode of inquiry. Telephone interviews are limited in their ability to detect detailed information, misinformation, and the emotional implications and subtext relating to the interview topic. However, there are situations where telephone interviews have clear advantages, particularly for structured interviews. Midanik and Greenfield (2003) compared the use of telephone and in-person interviews to collect data for a national survey on alcohol use. They found no differences in the number and quality of responses, and so advocate the use of telephone interviews for national surveys. Telephone interviews are cheaper, require less travel and the equipment needed is minimal (a simple connecting cable between the phone and tape recorder).

In a qualitative research project, Garbett and McCormack (2001) were able to capture the views of 26 nurses working in different roles and settings across the UK by using telephone interviews. To undertake face-to-face interviews would have been expensive and involved travelling long distances to. Using the telephone also helped to ensure participants were not under any pressure to participate, as they found it easier to refuse.

Telephone interviews can offer a more sensitive and less-threatening approach when the nature of the research topic may create a risk of participants thinking they will be judged. It also provides a more convenient option if people are busy and have conflicting commitments.

One-off or longitudinal interviews

Numerous studies use interviews as a one-off strategy of data collection where interviews are collected at one point in time. Longitudinal or sequential interviews include the ability to collect data at different time points, for example during the course of a patient's illness. This captures the evolving experience of the participant and tracks changes and gaps, for example in expectations and experiences or in health status.

Sequential interviews can generate richer data. Field and Morse (1985) claim that it is often impossible to collect good-quality data at the first interview. The increased trust that develops over time between researcher and interviewee will also facilitate more in-depth and better-quality data.

UNDERTAKING AN INTERVIEW

On the surface an interview may appear to be a process of asking a few questions. In reality, conducting a sound and rigorous interview can be a testing and complex enterprise (Robson 2002). The researcher has a responsibility to master certain techniques in order to produce results that are meaningful, useful and ensure the interviewee's generous contribution is not in vain.

Developing the data collection tool

It is important to develop the right tools to address the research purpose and answer the research question. Key to this is developing a data collection tool with the right level of structure. Examples are provided in Table 28.1.

A structured interview will require a structured, inflexible schedule akin to a questionnaire. It has to be administered in the same way and the same order, with the same wording for each participant. An unstructured interview will have maximum flexibility and often requires a guide comprising only a few core items. With a semi-structured interview a suitable schedule is essential for achieving the right balance of direction and flexibility. This means the central research question will be addressed, and it will also allow new and interesting responses to be explored further. An unstructured interview has no set of questions and may be more discursive. It may just consist of an opening question or invitation for the participant to share their experience of the issue being explored.

Table 28.1 Examples of interview structure, purpose and questions

Interview structure	Research purpose	Example of a question(s)
Structured or standardised interview	To identify (i) the nature, range and frequency of angina symptoms experienced by the population of a geographical area; and (ii) variation in symptom experience between and within the population according to characteristic, e.g. age, gender, ethnicity	a) Which of the following angina symptoms do you experience? (provide a list of symptoms with boxes to tick) b) How often do you experience them? (provide a scale for participants to indicate frequency of experience)
Semi-structured interview	To explore and identify barriers to angina symptom reporting and diagnosis?	Can you tell me a bit about yourself? How old are you? Are you married? Do you have any children? When did you first notice that there was something wrong with your heart? What symptoms or discomfort did you experience? What did you think was causing these feelings at first?
Unstructured interview	To understand an individual's experience of living with angina and the meaning it has for them in their life	Can you tell me about your experience of living with angina?

A number of factors should be considered when constructing an interview schedule. How important these are may depend on the purpose of the study (i.e. to generate quantitative or qualitative data) and the nature of the questioning (i.e. level of structure and sensitivity of the subject).

First, it is necessary to be clear about the types of questions to be asked. Six main types of questions have been identified (Britten 1995; Patton 1987):

- behaviour or experience
- opinion or belief
- feeling
- knowledge
- sensory experience
- background information such as demographics.

Some are easier to ask about and answer than others. Questions related to behaviour and knowledge may elicit short and specific responses. In comparison, questions about beliefs and feelings are more challenging, complex and potentially sensitive. They may need to be approached gradually and only after non-threatening questions have been asked.

It is common for the sequence of the schedule to be divided into sections, for example introduction, 'warm-up' or opening questions, the main interview questions, 'wind-down' questions and closing the interview (see Table 28.2).

Inappropriate timing of questions can sabotage the interview. If rapport and trust have been established it is possible to ask questions of an extremely sensitive nature. It is necessary continually to judge the appropriateness of an interview question in terms of the timing and how it will be interpreted and received by the interviewee.

Prompts can be built into the interview. These are particularly important in semi-structured interview

Table 28.2 Sequence of questions in an interview

Interview sequence	Type of questions
Introduction	• Introducing the study • Explain the purpose of the interview • Check the participant understands the purpose and nature of the study • Obtain or verify consent • Promote a relaxed atmosphere by making conversation
Warm-up	• Ask neutral, unthreatening questions • Ask for factual background information, e.g. age, children, job • Seek clarification or expansion if necessary
Main interview questions	• Ask questions relating to the main research aim • Ensure sequence follows some logic and sense • Start with broad questions followed by more focused ones • Leave the most sensitive and difficult questions until last • Use prompts and probes to generate deeper and richer data
Wind-down	• Round off with a few simple questions especially if the interview has been tense, emotional or sensitive • Let the interviewee know the interview is winding up, for example say 'to finish with …' • Ask if there is anything else they would like to add
Close of interview	• Check again there is nothing else they want to add • Check people know and remember what will happen to the data • Thank the participant

(Compiled with reference to Robson 2002; Legard et al. 2003)

Box 28.1   Example of questions used in a semi-structured interview

Broad question *(asked at the beginning of the interview to gain an overview of the patient's experience, develop rapport and influence subsequent questioning)*
Can you tell me something about your general health?

Focused question *(asked afterwards to elicit information about diagnosis of angina and any other chronic condition)*
Do you have any long-standing illness or disability?

Structured questionnaire *(administered as a way of verifying the patient has angina)*
Administer the 'Rose Angina Questionnaire' (Rose *et al.* 1977). This is a short questionnaire eliciting information on the patient's chest pain and is an objective measure of angina symptoms.

Prompt *(if not mentioned investigate further whether they have angina)*
Has your doctor told you what is wrong with you, i.e. what causes the chest pain?

(The results of this study are found in Tod *et al.* 2001)

schedules. Prompts have been described as questions that derive from the researcher (Robson 2002). They are intended to test an *a priori* assumption of the researcher or facilitate the interviewee to reflect on or expand on a certain theme issue (Legard *et al.* 2003). They can also be used if participants lose their thread as a way of encouraging them to re-engage with the interview.

Tod *et al.* (2001) used a semi-structured interview schedule to explore patients' experience of angina symptoms in order to identify barriers and facilitators in symptom reporting. Box 28.1 provides examples of broad questions used to start the interview followed by more focused questions with predetermined prompts.

CONDUCTING THE INTERVIEW

Selecting a suitable environment

Maintaining a suitable interview environment will often require a trade-off between accessibility, comfort and level of distraction. If a venue is considered inappropriate or inaccessible, people will be reluctant to take part. Common choices are the interviewee's home or workplace. A more neutral location may be required if people are likely to be distracted by or protective of their personal or professional setting.

The comfort of the environment is essential if interviewees are to feel relaxed, at ease and able to concentrate. On occasions, however, it may be necessary to sacrifice some comfort in order to involve participants from certain groups, for example interviewing patients on bed rest or nurses on or near their ward.

Choosing an environment with minimum risk of disruption is also a concern. There are certain things that a researcher can do to facilitate this, such as turning off telephones and other equipment and putting up a 'do not disturb' sign.

Even the best-laid plans can go astray and sometimes the unpredictable occurs, for example a participant having unexpected childcare commitments resulting in a child being present at the interview. The researcher then needs to make a judgement about whether to proceed with the interview in the knowledge that the quality may be affected, or whether to cancel the interview and risk offending the participant.

Establishing rapport

A successful interview will be reliant on developing a sense of trust and rapport. The attitude and demeanour of the interviewer is key, and it is essential that they appear genuine and interested in the participant's views. Legard *et al.* (2003) suggest that the researcher displaying confidence, tranquillity and credibility facilitates this. Humour and adaptability are also tools. Being organised, efficient and focused, having a well-planned and paced schedule of questions and being responsive to the mood, body language and priorities of the interviewee all help to develop a good interview relationship. The posture and bearing of the researcher should convey attention and interest.

Questioning technique

Techniques used to facilitate questioning need to maintain a balance between direction and flexibility. Where the balance lies will reflect the research aim, method and level of structure. Techniques include active listening, being clear and unambiguous, not leading respondents towards particular views or beliefs and, again, staying interested. The tradition is to advise researchers to say as little as possible because of the risk the interviewer may contaminate, influence or confuse the interviewee. Some researchers argue for more interaction in qualitative interviews on the grounds that it allows the researcher to test out emerging ideas, and discussion helps to explore more complex issues (Melia 2000). One approach to being more interactive is what Melia (2000) refers to as 'verbal memo-ing', where the interviewer investigates initial arguments emerging from analysis. Another option that can be used in both qualitative and quantitative research would be to construct vignettes or scenarios from earlier accounts to draw out opinion in subsequent interviews.

The appropriate use of prompts and probes can help achieve the right balance of breadth and depth in the questioning (Legard *et al.* 2003). In structured interviews they may be used to clarify a question if it is misunderstood. In unstructured and semi-structured interviews some questions lead the respondent to broad statements that may set the stage or reveal a range of issues and dimensions. Probes may then be used to uncover layers of meaning. Probing questions have the capacity to amplify, explore, explain or clarify (Legard *et al.* 2003). The astute use of silence to help participants reflect and respond is a valuable interview technique. An interested look, maintaining eye contact or summarising can all help to prompt a response.

Managing the interview

An interview is a sensitive interaction and needs careful handling. This should start from the outset by considering how the researcher is perceived by the participant. Difference or similarity in age, ethnicity, gender or social status can all make a difference to how people respond. The interviewer's demeanour and appearance may depending on whether they are interviewing a chief executive of a hospital or a teenager. Clarity of introduction both of the researcher and the project itself can also help. This will also minimise any risk of role conflict for a nurse conducting a research interview.

Setting the scene for the respondent is essential. Points to explain include:

- there are no right or wrong answers
- they have the right to withdraw or stop at any time
- they can interrupt or ask for explanations whenever they want
- the interview will be recorded (usually on audio tape) with their permission.

COMMON PITFALLS IN CONDUCTING INTERVIEWS

Field and Morse (1985) include the risk of losing the research role and slipping into that of a teacher, preacher or counsellor. This risk is a particular danger in less-structured interviews where the discussion is more in-depth. On occasions it is difficult to avoid role conflict, especially for nurses and others with a clinical training. The interviewer must avoid putting their own view and perspective forward. This is a particular hazard when the respondent has said something the researcher disagrees with or finds offensive. To explore such views gently will be more productive than challenging them (Legard *et al.* 2003).

Handling a situation that is emotionally charged can be testing if a participant becomes upset, anxious or angry. Sensitive questioning can help, as will communicating empathy and interest with body language and eye contact. However, it is important not to be frightened of such emotional situations. Not only do they often produce the most valuable and insightful data, but the participant may find it a positive experience to discuss the issue in this way.

Selecting the most appropriate way of recording an interview is a key factor in its success. The most common form of recording is audiotape, supplemented by fieldnotes. Other media include video recording, video conferencing or internet chat rooms. In making a decision it is important to consider how intrusive the technology will appear to the participant, ease of use of the technology, reliability, and ethical aspects regarding confidentiality and privacy. It is always important to check that recording equipment is working well before the interview. It may be false economy to skimp on the quality of this technology. Following the interview the recording is normally transcribed verbatim ready for analysis.

Researchers taking fieldnotes need to be aware of how the respondent will interpret this activity. If the researcher appears more absorbed in scribbling notes than in participating in the interview it is easy for the respondent to think that they are not listening or not interested.

Additional challenges in managing an interview can occur if the researcher and participant do not speak the same language and an interpreter is used. Developing rapport and trust can be more difficult if the interview is being conducted through a third person. It is therefore necessary to ensure the interpreter is acceptable to the participant and culturally appropriate, in addition to having good language skills. Maintaining accuracy in collecting data is also difficult. The interpreter should be skilled and practised in research interview work and be able to demonstrate accuracy of translation between interviewee and interviewer.

Managing an interview well is a difficult task and needs practice. Piloting is recommended, especially when the researcher is new to the interview process. Piloting allows questions to be tested and refined, and practice gained in using recording equipment. A novice interviewer is advised to secure good supervision, not just to support the research design and data analysis, but also to aid reflection of the interview experience. Mistakes are inevitable, but it is always worth reflecting on these and discussing ways to avoid the same pitfalls in the future.

ADVANTAGES AND DISADVANTAGES OF INTERVIEWS

Interviewing is a flexible and adaptable method of data collection and can be an efficient way of collecting data on a myriad of subjects, including participants' views, attitudes, behaviours and experiences. The flexibility of the interview format and structure is one of its greatest advantages. The interview is malleable and can be adapted to fit the needs and purpose of different studies from quantitative surveys to detailed phenomenological explorations of individuals' experiences.

Structured interviews have the capacity to generate a large volume of data from a large sample. They are an excellent means of collecting data that is predominantly quantitative but can incorporate qualitative questioning. It is possible to use structured interviews to test the findings of smaller, in depth interview studies with a larger population.

Semi-structured and unstructured interviews have an unrivalled ability to generate data of depth and complexity. The forum of the interview provides the opportunity to explore the intricacy of an issue from the perspective of individual participants.

Interviews may provide the only method of eliciting the views of people who are often 'hard to reach' in terms of research, and who would be reluctant or unable to participate in research using other methods. There is some indication that, while not intentionally having a direct therapeutic effect, people do find the experience of being interviewed a positive one.

Many of the disadvantages are reflected in the challenges referred to earlier, for example the risk of introducing bias by inadequate sampling or questioning. Following the advice and techniques above can avoid this. However, one danger to be considered is that the involvement in the interview itself may change the views or perceptions of the participants. The researcher should be continually vigilant of this risk of a 'Hawthorne effect' throughout data collection and analysis.

Finally, interviewing can be expensive in terms of time and funding. Resources may be required to support the researchers' or participants' involvement, for example travel, care of participants' dependants, reimbursement for loss of earnings, refreshments. The cost of reliable technical recording equipment and transcription are not insignificant and need to be considered when making the decision to use interviews as a data collection method.

VALIDITY AND RELIABILITY

The degree of reliability (the accuracy and consistency of the data collection) required from an interview will vary. In a structured interview, high levels of reliability will be sought. Training and a robust schedule will ensure standardised practice between different researchers. With a more in-depth, semistructured or unstructured interview reliability is less achievable. Such an interview will be flexible and interactive in order to understand the individual's social construction and representation of the research phenomenon. However, a competent researcher with a consistent approach and well-designed schedule will be able to maximise the rigour of the results (Lincoln & Guba 1985).

The validity of a study considers how 'true' the data are. The challenge is to demonstrate that the findings are an accurate account of the participant's representation of the topic, and not due to bias.

Data collection bias may arise in interviews because of the way the sample has been selected, how the interview is conducted or because of the researcher's influence. To protect against these risks it is necessary to monitor and reflect on the following questions.

- Has the sample any inbuilt bias, e.g. are some groups excluded or under-represented?
- Are the questions addressing the participant's concerns, views and experiences?
- Have the interviewees been given the opportunity to adequately present their views?
- Has the researcher led or influenced the participant's responses in any way?

Having clear and well-prepared documentation will help address these questions, for example interview schedules and fieldnotes.

ETHICAL ISSUES WITH INTERVIEWING

Some of the major ethical issues relating to interview based studies are outlined here.

Consent

Chapter 10 gives details of the procedures that need to be followed to obtain informed consent. Potential interviewees should be approached with sufficient time to allow them to reflect on the implications of participation and not feel pressurised into taking part. A signature is required to indicate that informed consent has been given. When this is obtained some time prior to the interview taking place, consent should be verified immediately before the actual interview.

Anonymity and confidentiality

The names and identity of participants should not be revealed as a result of the collection, analysis and reporting of the study, in order to preserve their anonymity and confidentiality. It is important to ensure that first contact with participants about the study is via someone with a legitimate role and right to identify them, for example the consultant or senior nurse involved in a patient's care.

There are circumstances when complete anonymity is not possible to guarantee, for example when reporting the age, gender and medical condition/role would identify a person. In smaller interview-based studies recruiting from a limited sampling frame, this is a real risk. Where this threat occurs it should be pre-empted and included in the informed consent procedure. Sometimes people are prepared to be involved despite the risk of being identified, but they should be given the chance to agree any direct references and quotes from them used in any reports or publications.

To protect anonymity interviewees are sometimes referred to by number or pseudonym. Asking a person to choose their own pseudonym can help them understand the confidentiality implications of participation.

Once an interview tape has been recorded, all identifiable references need to be removed from the tape and transcript. These ought then to be stored in locked, secure storage and in password-protected computers. Tapes are usually destroyed or returned to participants on completion of the study.

Protecting participants' and researchers' rights, and protecting them from harm

Ensuring interviewees' understanding of the study and its requirements is a key concern when protecting them from harm. It is therefore important to make certain people know what subjects will be covered, especially where these are sensitive or distressing in nature. Where necessary, support for the participant may be required and, where available, stated in the information sheet.

When explaining the study, it is important not to raise participants' expectations regarding its impact on their own care, other people's care or the development of services. People often participate in interviews where they share their views and experiences for altruistic reasons. Researchers should endeavour to be realistic in any claims that the study has the capacity to make change.

One major risk in conducting interviews is where a risk to the participant or someone else is revealed. Examples include:

- a patient revealing suicidal thoughts
- a patient or staff member describing an incident of negligence or abuse
- a patient revealing that their medical condition has deteriorated.

These challenging dilemmas should be considered on a case-by-case basis. The risk–benefit balance of reporting what the participant has disclosed or remaining silent may vary tremendously. Where possible, the risk of this should be pre-empted, and a reporting process should be put in place and made clear in the information sheet. For example, the situation might be discussed with a patient's doctor or nurse.

Finally, the researcher has a requirement to protect themselves. If an interview has been particularly emotional, tense or challenging, the availability of experienced, trusted supervision to facilitate reflection is invaluable.

The other main risk for a researcher relates to issues of personal safety. It is standard practice for interviewers to inform an identified person of the time and location of an interview and inform them when it is over and they have left the venue. This is a particular requirement when interviewing in people's own homes or unknown environments. A mobile phone and panic alarms are sometimes carried as additional means of communication if the researcher feels exceptionally threatened.

CONCLUSIONS

Conducting an interview involves sharing an aspect of someone's life. As such, the decision to employ interviews as a data collection method should not be taken lightly. The practical, procedural, ethical and cost implications all have to be considered. However, if these are addressed, and a researcher has the required expertise and support, conducting an interview can be a vehicle to gaining a unique insight into the area of study and a privilege and pleasure to undertake.

References

Astin F, Closs JS, Mclenahchan J, Priestley C (2008) Primary angioplasty for heart attack: mismatch between expectations and reality. *Journal of Advanced Nursing* **65**(1): 72–83.

Britten N (1995) Qualitative research: qualitative interviews in research. *British Medical Journal* **311**: 251–253.

Collins S, Reynolds F (2008) How do adults with cystic fibrosis cope following a diagnosis of diabetes. *Journal of Advanced Nursing* **64**(7): 478–487.

Field PA, Morse JM (1985) *Nursing Research: the application of qualitative approaches*. London, Chapman & Hall.

Garbett R, McCormack B (2001) The experience of practice development: an exploratory telephone interview study. *Journal of Clinical Nursing* **10**: 94–102.

Laws R (2004) Current approaches to obesity management in UK Primary Care. *Journal of Human Nutrition and Dietetics* **17**: 183–190.

Legard R, Keegan J, Ward K (2003) In-depth interviews. In: Ritchie J, Lewis J (eds) *Qualitative Research Practice*. London, Sage, pp 138–169.

Lincoln Y, Guba E (1985) *Naturalistic Inquiry*. London, Sage.

Melia KB (2000) Conducting an interview. *Nurse Researcher* **7**(4): 75–89.

Midanik LT, Greenfield TK (2003) Telephone versus in-person interviews for alcohol use: results of a 2000 National Alcohol Survey. *Drug and Alcohol Dependence* **72**: 209–214.

Moss-Morris R, Weinman J, Petrie KJ, Horne R, Cameron LD, Buick D (2002) The revised illness perception questionnaire (IPQ-R). *Psychology and Health* **17**: 1–16.

Murphy E, Dingwall R, Greatbatch D, Parker S, Watson P (1998) Qualitative research methods in health technology assessments: a review of the literature. *Health Technology Assessment*. Vol 2. No 16.

Patton MQ (1987) *How to Use Qualitative Methods in Evaluation*. London, Sage.

Robson C (2002) *Real World Research*, 2nd edition. Oxford, Blackwell.

Rose GA, McCartney P, Reid DD (1977) Self-administration of a questionnaire on chest pain and intermittent claudication. *British Journal of Preventive and Social Medicine* **31**: 42–48.

Tod AM, Read C, Lacey A, Abbott J (2001) Overcoming barriers to uptake of services for coronary heart disease: a qualitative study. *British Medical Journal* **323**: 214–217.

Website

www.nres.npsa.nhs.uk/rec-community/guidance/ – National Research Ethics Service. For advice on informed consent, participant information sheets and consent forms.

29 Focus Groups

Claire Goodman and Catherine Evans

Key points

- Focus groups are a useful data collection method when the aim is to clarify, explore or confirm ideas with a range of participants on a predefined set of issues.

- Group interactions are an important feature of focus groups and an integral part of the data collection process.

- It requires considerable preparation and skill to run a successful focus group; ideally one person should act as the moderator of the group while a second researcher acts as observer.

- Analysis of focus group data should ask specific questions about the group process and interaction, as well as the content of the discussion.

THE PURPOSE OF FOCUS GROUPS

A focus group is an in-depth, open-ended group discussion that explores a specific set of issues on a predefined topic. Focus groups are used extensively as a research method in nursing research in two ways:

- to obtain the views and experiences of a selected group on an issue (see Research Examples 29.1 and 29.2)
- to use the forum of a group discussion to increase understanding about a given topic (see Research Example 29.3).

Focus groups seldom aim to produce consensus between participants and are unlikely to be the method of choice if this is the study's aim. The key premise of focus groups is that individuals in groups do not respond to questions in the same way that they do in other settings, and it is the group interaction that enables participants to explore and clarify their experience and insights on a specific issue. Participants can share and discuss their knowledge and even revise their original ideas and understanding. This data collection method allows the researcher to expose inconsistency within a group as well as providing examples of conformity and agreement. Focus groups, therefore, have the potential to provide a rich source of data.

Focus groups were first developed for market research at Columbia University in the US and used to gauge audience responses to propaganda and radio broadcasts during the Second World War. Twohig and Putnam (2002), in a review of studies that have used focus groups in healthcare research, did not identify any studies cited by MEDLINE before 1985

29.1 The Use of Focus Groups with Marginalised Groups and to Address Sensitive Topics

Culley L *et al*. (2007) Using focus groups with minority ethnic communities: researching infertility in British South Asian Communities. *Qualitative Health Research* **17**: 102–112.

This study set out to explore community understandings of infertility and involuntary childlessness in British South Asian communities. The study had two phases: the first explored a cross-section of public attributes and perceptions surrounding infertility and provided the context and insight for the second phase, which involved in-depth interviews with individuals who had experienced infertility problems. By not involving people with infertility problems in the focus groups the researchers were able to explore the social context and stigma and ask direct questions about their views of childless couples. Groups were single sex (important for the Muslim groups and older South Asians) and involved people of similar age. There were 14 focus groups that ranged in size from three to ten people, with a mode of six. The involvement of focus group facilitators from the different South Asian ethnic groups to work as translators, group facilitators and advisors on what was said in the discussions was costly. Recruitment to the groups was labour intensive. When leading the group discussions, attempts to 'depersonalise' what was a very sensitive topic by asking about community constructions of infertility were not always successful. Participants often 'repersonalised' the issue and gave examples of personal and family experience. There was concern that this may have led to over-disclosure because there were so few opportunities in these communities to discuss these issues. They also had experience of people attending the groups to seek help for their own fertility problems. This posed ethical dilemmas for the researchers on how they should respond. The researchers concluded that focus groups were a powerful and versatile tool in accessing community attitudes, and allowed them to understand cultural norms and meanings. However, it was time-consuming, costly, and produced complex and messy data that was further complicated because multiple languages were involved.

but noted it has been a widely used method in sociology, education and political science.

Focus groups are not aligned with a particular tradition of qualitative research. It is therefore important that researchers who use this method are sure that it fits with the overall research approach. As the discussion is organised *outside* the everyday experience and there is a pre-set focus to the interaction, there are inevitable tensions in employing focus group methods in studies that have a strong emphasis on naturalistic inquiry and immersion in the participants' lived experience. For example, the researcher would need to justify how the use of focus groups would fit with a study that is based on grounded theory or phenomenology (see Chapters 13 and 15 for more detailed consideration of this issue).

There is considerable variation in how focus groups are reported in nursing research literature and little

agreement about optimum group size and numbers of groups to include within a study. There is also criticism that focus groups encourage a superficial approach to enquiry and therefore have limited value as a stand-alone data collection method.

CONDUCTING A FOCUS GROUP

It is a misconception to regard focus group interviews as a simple way of gathering data from multiple participants. A focus group requires the researcher to give time to preparation and have skills in facilitating group discussion. It is labour intensive and often involves two researchers, one as moderator of the group discussion and the other as observer. Consideration is given here to sampling strategy and

RESEARCH
EXAMPLE

29.2 The Use of Focus Groups to Elaborate Upon Quantitative Research Findings

Kevern J, Webb C (2004) Mature women's experiences of pre-registration nurse education. *Journal of Advanced Nursing* **45**: 297–306.

Government policy in England has targeted the recruitment of mature women into nurse training as a way of addressing the shortage of qualified nurses. This study aimed to follow up a quantitative study of mature female pre-registration diploma students to gain a deeper understanding of their experiences of higher education and to identify appropriate organisational support systems for them. A purposive sample of mature students (n = 40) was invited by letter to participate in the study. Five focus groups were held involving 32 women. The lead researcher moderated the groups; no observer was present. A list of six agenda items formed the broad framework for the focus groups. The group processes were recorded using audiotape and written notes. From the thematic analysis of the transcripts, the experiences of the mature women nursing students formed three major themes.

- 'Didn't know what to expect' described the women's uncertainty about entering nurse training.
- 'Reality shock' encompassed the competing demands of academic study, nursing placements and family commitments.
- 'Learning the game' referred to the strategies the women adopted to remain on the course, for example moderating their academic expectations of themselves.

The authors conclude that ideology and patriarchy restrict women's activities in university. They identified the need to expand the options for women with multiple role demands by providing, for example, more flexible and well-organised student-centred programmes.

group size, developing a topic guide and how to conduct a focus group, including managing the discussion and recording information.

Sampling strategy and group size

Major challenges to using focus groups include identifying, sampling and recruiting participants, group size and composition, and decisions on how many focus groups should be held.

The identification and sampling of members of the target population is guided by the aims or research questions for the study (see Chapter 2). It can be useful to develop a topic-specific sampling strategy to encompass the diversity of people involved in the subject area (Kitzinger & Barbour 1999). For example, to obtain a spread of views of how minority ethnic groups understood infertility and involuntary

childlessness, Culley *et al.* (2007) used a sampling strategy including participants from four main South Asian communities and involved group facilitators fluent in their different languages (Research Example 29.1).

There is an increasing use of focus groups in research with young people and children (Hennessy & Heary 2005). This requires a different approach to sampling and group composition. Gibson (2007) suggests that age should inform how large the group is and recommends only a 1- to 2-year age difference in members of the group, and that limited language ability and skills may mean that a focus group is not a suitable method for children under six years of age.

To gain access to the possible participants from the target population, it is often helpful to approach a stakeholder or group representative. For example, a director of nursing in a health trust is a useful stakeholder to gain access to NHS nurses. Ways of iden-

29.3 The Use of Focus Groups to Increase Understanding of a Given Topic

Burt J *et al.* (2008) Nursing the dying within a generalist caseload: a focus group study of district nurses. *International Journal of Nursing Studies* **45**: 1470–1478.

This study explored how community nurses understood their role in palliative care as one aspect of the care provided to people living at home. The study was informed by previous studies that had considered district nurses' palliative care work but had not considered it within the wider context of care. The aim was to explore with district nurses their perceptions of their palliative care role and their ability to provide end-of-life care as part of a generalist workload. The focus groups were part of a larger study on the needs of patients for palliative care services in primary care settings. The method was chosen as most likely to enable practitioners to share and discuss their experiences and views about their work. To capture different approaches to palliative care provision and recruit district nurses with a range of qualifications and clinical experience, participants were purposively sampled from four primary care organisations in London. There were 51 participants in nine focus groups with four to seven participants in each group. Group discussions lasted for an average of one and half hours and were recorded and later transcribed. Thematic analysis focused on areas of agreement, dissent or expansion of particular themes. The findings confirmed earlier research that showed district nurses valued their palliative care work. It also explained in more depth the difficulties district nurses experienced. Specifically it showed:

- that district nurses felt their contribution was largely overlooked
- the unpredictability of palliative care and how this could unbalance the case load
- the emotional demands of the work and specifically the difficulties of constant role switching between providing palliative care and routine care.

The findings indicated a need for research on different models of working, where generalist nurses can have access to more resources, specialist support and recognition for their contribution.

tifying participants from populations not necessarily associated with an organisation, for example 'healthy' older people, include approaching places they visit, such as a drop-in centre, and advertising the project, and recruiting a pre-existing group.

Non-random sampling techniques such as purposive and convenience sampling (see Chapter 12) are normally used because the intention of the focus group is usually to increase understanding of a phenomenon, not provide evidence directly generalisable to a wider population. Moreover, a randomly selected group may not hold a shared perspective on the research topic, prohibiting meaningful group discussion (Morgan 1997). Purposive sampling is preferable when sampling participants with specific characteristics, experience or knowledge, such as district nurses (see Research Example 29.3). If the target population is small, difficult to identify or difficult to access, convenience sampling can be helpful. When all participants within the target population would be eligible to participate, selection can be based on interest in participating in the study and availability.

Group composition and size are both contentious issues within the focus group literature. Again, decisions are based on the nature of the enquiry, the study design, and the amount of time and funding available. Debates on group composition focus on homogeneity (similar participants) versus heterogeneity (diverse participants) and the use (or not) of pre-existing groups. Homogeneous groups segmented by, for example, a shared experience (see Research Example 29.3), language group or professional position (see Research Examples 29.1 & 29.2) are generally preferable to ensure free discussion and enable cross-group comparisons (Morgan 1997). However, differences between participants in a heterogeneous group are often illuminating and the use of pre-existing groups can enable the context within which ideas are formed and decisions made to be captured (Kitzinger 1994). Using pre-existing groups can also be useful in recruiting people unlikely to come forward to participate in a focus group if they feel marginalised by society or are unwilling to participate with people they do not know. However, in groups where participants are very familiar with each other, existing group norms and hierarchies may inhibit the contributions of members (Kitzinger & Barbour 1999).

The size of a focus group varies typically from between five members to no more than 12. The group must be large enough to ensure diversity of perspectives, and small enough to ensure everybody has a chance to participate. Decisions on group size are informed by:

- the nature of the subject area (the more sensitive the area the smaller the group)
- the level of group structure (the more structure the larger the group)
- the resources available (funding for more than one group, size of room space)
- moderator expertise (the less experienced the moderator the smaller the group).

Generally, it is advisable to invite more than the required number of group members to counter the inevitable problems of no-shows. Telephoning people who have agreed to participate a few days beforehand can reduce this problem. The focus group needs to be conducted at a convenient time in an accessible venue, and there may be value in interviewing people away from the institution they belong to (Kitzinger & Barbour 1999). In practice, it is often the financial resources and time available for the study that influence venue choices.

Focus groups need more preparation and anticipation than individual interviews. On the day of the focus group the moderator should arrive sufficiently early to signpost the location, arrange the room and prepare refreshments for participants. An ideal room is one that is private, large enough to accommodate the group, quiet and comfortable. If working with an observer it is important to talk through the anticipated process and the topic guide, and agree seating arrangements.

Structuring group discussion and developing a topic guide

The level of group structure depends on the intention of the focus group. A structured group using a topic guide is preferable when the research questions are clear, for example using focus groups to inform further research (see Research Example 29.1). A less-structured group framed around one or two topic areas is useful in exploratory research when little is known about the area of study (see Research Example 29.2). Both approaches have advantages and disadvantages. The structured approach ensures consistency across groups, enabling comparisons to be made between groups, but a narrow set of questions may limit the discussion and inhibit contributions on related issues. Less structure often creates a livelier group discussion. A compromise between the two approaches may also be used. Morgan (1997) describes this as a 'funnel-based' approach in which

'each group begins with a less structured approach that emphasizes free discussion and then moves toward a more structured discussion of specific questions' (Morgan 1997: 41)

The research aims and the literature should inform the development of the topic guide (McLafferty 2004). The intention of the guide is to create a natural progression through the topic areas and stimulate group discussion without influencing the responses. A structured guide uses at most five to six questions. A less structured approach is to organise the guide around two or three broad discussion topics, loosely phrased as questions, like, 'We are interested in _____? What can you tell us about this area?' (Morgan 1997). In both instances, the questions are ordered to move from general to specific and non-sensitive to more sensitive, the aim being to enable all group members to participate. The topic area should be familiar to all, not be intimidating or require personal exposure. More sensitive or probing questions come nearer the middle of the interview. This provides participants with time to feel safe to speak within the group. Open-ended questions prefixed by either, how, what, where or why allow participants freedom to respond. Too many 'why' questions can be experienced as confrontational and provoke defensive responses (Nyamathi & Shuler 1990).

Managing the discussion

Sufficient time should be allowed to greet and seat participants. Begin the session by welcoming participants, introducing yourself and the observer, and clarifying the purpose of the session and the anticipated finish time. Ensure participants understand how the discussion will be recorded, who has access to these recordings and how confidentiality will be maintained. Ask if participants have any questions about the interview format and agree ground rules. Ground rules are intended to facilitate group discussion, not confine it. The agreed rules should be concise, few in number and displayed for participants (e.g. on flip chart). They may state:

- issues discussed in the group are confidential to the participants and the researchers
- only one person to speak at a time.

Introductions to the topic should be brief and clear, and instructions kept to a minimum. This helps participants to understand the focus of the session, without directing their thinking, and emphasises that the ownership of the group discussion belongs to both the participants and the moderator. Participant introductions create an opportunity for all to speak and provides identification markers to differentiate participants for the observer and when transcribing the audiotapes. Plan for latecomers and ensure that participants are informed prior to the interview whether or not they will be able to take part if they arrive after the indicated start time.

Moderators should promote debate by asking open questions and probing for more detail on points of interest, reflecting a point made to confirm understanding and summarising points to check that all

areas have been covered, particularly before changing a topic. These techniques reinforce to participants that the points they make are valued and encourage participation in the discussion. The discussion should include all areas in the topic guide, particularly if conducting several focus groups. Incomplete data sets restrict comparative analysis between groups and may compromise the aims of the study.

Moderators need to encourage participation by inviting group members to comment on an individual's views, especially if someone is dominating the discussion. Avoid expressing personal opinions or correcting participants' knowledge to prevent biasing the discussion towards a particular opinion or position (Gibbs 1997). Correcting or supporting participants' knowledge can be addressed at the end of the interview. For example, Roth *et al.* (2003) provided a healthcare worker in HIV at the end of focus group sessions on bilingual health advocacy and antenatal HIV testing to provide further information on HIV.

Group exercises may be used within the session to explore understanding about a particular issue or to indicate preferences. Kitzinger (1994), for example, used cards with statements on them about HIV to explore participants' perceptions of risks. Such exercises encourage participants to focus on each other rather than the moderator. For young people and children, Gibson (2007) suggests that the inclusion of activities and exercises to maintain interest and concentration as well as facilitate a sense of working together can help stimulate discussion and responses to research questions.

Time keeping is essential and shows respect for participants' time. Leave 5–10 minutes to round up the interview. This provides an opportunity for participants to offer further comments and reflect on their experience of participating in the group.

Recording information

Group interactions are the crucial feature of focus groups and mark them as different from individual interviews. Audio tape, video tape and an observer can be used alone or in combination to record the group interaction. Ideally, transcribed audio tape is preferable, with an observer and/or video-taping. Video-tapings can be poor at recording speech and are normally used in combination with an audio tape. An observer is useful for recording, for example, the group's seating arrangement and non-verbal cues of supportive or aggressive behaviour. An observation sheet with headings for particular areas of interest can help to structure the observations.

Audio and video equipment should be reliable and have a high-quality microphone for recording groups rather than individuals. The quality of the tape recording directly influences the precision of the transcribing and the consequent validity of the transcript analysis. Ensure audio tapes are the correct length for the interview and labelled with an identification number, date and time, to prevent recording over data and as a reference point for transcribing (Bramley 2004).

DATA ANALYSIS

The principles and process of analysis for focus group data are very similar to those applied to qualitative data obtained from individual interviews (see Chapters 28 and 34). When undertaking analysis of a focus group discussion it is important, however, to be clear about the purpose of the analysis and whether it is the group discussion as a whole or the range of contributions to that discussion that is of interest. The research question and the rationale for using focus groups guide the analysis, and inform how the data are organised and read.

It is seldom practical to ask focus group participants to check the validity of transcripts or preliminary analysis. It is therefore useful to summarise at the end of the group what the moderator believes to be the main issues to emerge from the discussion for confirmation or clarification by the group. This not only helps understanding, but also represents the first stage in analysis where tentative themes can be identified and subsequently tested within the detailed analysis of the group transcripts. At the end of the focus group it is also good practice for the group's moderator to debrief with the observer to record initial impressions of how the group went and to

identify issues that may directly affect the analysis. Factors such as dominance of the discussion by particular individuals, impressions of how engaged participants were with the issues raised and whether non-participation in the group indicated disagreement or affirmation with what was being said should be noted. These first impressions are useful as memoranda that can subsequently inform analysis.

In contrast to analysis of individual interviews, an important part of the analytic process is identifying areas of agreement and controversy, and how views are modified or reinforced during the group discussion. When coding data it is helpful to think about the data as a group process. It is therefore sensible to organise the data to reflect how the discussion progressed. Most groups will take some time to establish a rapport, and there will be some issues and questions that generate more interest and contributions than others. Coding the data into narrative units can be helpful, as there will be some major issues identified within the group discussion that either generate the most contributions or the strongest responses. This means that individual responses to a particular issue or question, the asides, challenges and elaborations that occur within the group are coded together and in relation to each other. Software that supports qualitative analysis is invaluable as it can track individual contributions as well as interactions and responses and allows interrogation of the data in different ways. Furthermore, by tracing the development and sequence of statements of the discussion on an issue it is possible to judge which of the ideas participants offered as tentative thoughts at the beginning of a focus group became, by the end of the group, established views.

In a review of the use of focus groups as a research method in nursing research, Webb and Kevern (2001) suggest that the approach to analysis of focus group data is often relatively unsophisticated and that the interaction that occurred within groups is rarely reported. They suggest that the analytic procedure should ask specific questions of the group process and interaction to deepen the understanding of the data obtained. In this way the researcher can identify statements that provoked the most emotion, reaction or conflict, how different statements related to each other, and if there were discernable alliances that emerged within the group or particular interests that were emphasised over others.

The use of descriptive statistics to summarise the frequency with which issues were raised and the amount of time spent discussing an issue can be helpful, particularly when comparing responses between different focus groups. When marked differences are identified between groups this should prompt another look at what it was about these groups, their membership or setting, that could explain the variation. However, there should be considerable caution in suggesting that a particular subject or issue was more important or significant because it was raised more frequently than something else. Counting statements made on particular topics will generate a list of what participants said, but attributing meaning to this can be problematic unless the analysis also accounts for how people interacted within the group.

ISSUES OF VALIDITY AND RELIABILITY

Validity is the extent to which a procedure actually measures what it proposes to measure. Typically, focus groups have high face validity as a credible method that can directly capture the views of participants in response to the study focus. Threats to face validity are those that threaten the accuracy of the participants' views on the topic areas of interest. These can include research questions that are unsuitable for a focus group because they are concerned with the narrative on individual experience. Idiosyncratic and opportunistic recruitment from the population of interest can make it difficult to interpret findings. A lack of transparency in how the group discussion was organised, the prompts used, the amount of direction given to the group by the moderator and approaches to analysis can also threaten the confidence with which the results from focus group research can be interpreted.

Reliability concerns the degree of consistency in observing the area of interest over time. For focus groups, reliability is most relevant as it relates to the consistency in the data gathered within each respective group. Threats to consistency across groups include:

- the structure and delivery of the topic guide
- the impact of moderator bias
- differences between the groups' membership, for example regarding gender
- the interview environment
- accuracy in transcribing and analysing audio tapes.

However, in groups where the emphasis is on discovery, the diversity of the participants may enhance the breadth of understanding.

ADVANTAGES OF FOCUS GROUPS

Although focus groups can appear to be a quick and flexible method of data collection, they are not an inexpensive or time-saving method (see Research Example 29.1). Considerable time is required to recruit participants, set up the groups, transcribe and analyse the data generated. There are, however, some clear advantages that focus group methods have over other data collection methods. In the early stages of a study the discussion and data generated by a focus group can identify complex problems and areas that need further exploration and clarification. A group discussion held at the end of the study provides the opportunity for participants to respond to the findings and offer explanations or alternative interpretations. The exploratory and illuminatory function of focus groups can thus extend and challenge how researchers define their research questions and report their findings. Used in conjunction with other methods, such as interviews and observation, focus group data can confirm, extend and enrich understanding and provide alternative narratives of events and beliefs.

Focus groups are frequently used when the opinions of lay people are sought. The method does not require participants to be able to read and write, and people can feel safe within a group. If facilitated well, participants can express their views in relation to the opinions and experiences of others without feeling pressure to respond all the time. It is participant-driven and enables the language, priorities and attitudes of a group to be expressed. It is one of the few data collection methods that allow people to modify their initial thoughts and ideas as part of the data-gathering process. Paradoxically, focus groups can be a good way of researching topics that are taboo or controversial when participants who hold an experience in common can give each other permission to discuss. For example, focus groups may be used to enable people who are HIV-positive to discuss freely their attitudes to sexual health and the issues they encounter as a result of their health status.

The synergy generated from a group discussion often enables participants to consider the topic with more enthusiasm than an individual interview can achieve. However, questions examining feelings or requiring personal reflection may only be suited to a focus group approach when participants have self-selected or they know each other and are comfortable with that level of public self-disclosure such questions require. It is the level of engagement expressed within a group, the range of participation and the ability to develop the discussion around certain issues that are often a good measure of how successful a focus group has been.

LIMITATIONS OF FOCUS GROUPS

Focus groups can have high credibility and face validity, but equally they can be susceptible to researcher manipulation and bias. The limitations of the method are the reliance on the skill of the group moderator, the risk of individual participants dominating discussion and excluding the contributions of others, and the possibility that the structure and format of focus groups excludes certain groups from participation.

Focus group facilitation is difficult. The novice researcher should take the opportunity to observe some focus groups before taking on the moderator role, consider training on group dynamics and talk through with an experienced colleague how they will lead the group. The moderator has to maintain a balance between encouraging discussion and participation, and being careful not to bias responses by giving preference to speakers whose views are perceived as the most 'interesting'. The moderator

also needs the confidence to be able to refocus the group if participants break into two or three separate discussions at the same time, and intervene if the discussion threatens to become destructive or lead to conflict.

Most authors writing on the subject of focus groups raise the spectre of the dominant group member as a major limitation of the method. Participants who are very assertive in their views can discourage participation from those who disagree or who are less certain in their opinions. Where participants have different levels or authority or education this too can affect willingness to participate. Nevertheless, if the focus group is seen as an opportunity to capture how a group of people express their opinions and if certain people can make statements that are unchallenged and allowed to dominate, then the analysis must capture this. Reed and Payton (1997) argue that if one considers focus groups as 'displays of group perspectives' then *how* groups negotiate and develop their views can be as revealing as what is said.

Focus groups can discriminate against an individual's ability to participate. Kitzinger (1994) described including people who had different communication disabilities such as deafness, partial paralysis affecting speech and dementia in a group. They could all converse individually with the researcher, but had difficulty communicating with each other, precluding meaningful interaction in a group setting. Most focus groups also require people to be able to communicate in the language of the researcher, which may exclude some people from minority ethnic groups who do not share a common language. It is possible to involve translators as an earlier example showed (Roth *et al.* 2003), although this can make the discussion more stilted and meanings harder to interpret. Halcomb *et al.* (2007), in a review of studies that had used focus groups with linguistically diverse groups, found that focus groups are particularly useful for studies on service provision and community needs for minority and multicultural groups.

The location of focus groups may also affect the ability to participate and exclude some potential participants. For example, where a focus group is held may favour participation by people who have easy access to transport or live close to the proposed venue.

ETHICAL ISSUES

The particular ethical issues that arise within focus group research are the maintenance of confidentiality, consent, the management of disclosure, and maintaining the respect and feelings of self-worth of each participant. It is important that participants agree that the discussions held within the group are confidential and not shared outside the group. The moderator needs to ensure that each participant agrees to this, especially in situations where the group members know each other.

The discussion format of a focus group can mean that people forget that the reason they are meeting is to participate in a research project. Frequently, discussion will prompt disclosures that may not have been made within the context of an interview. Although this can interrupt the flow of the conversation, it is the moderator's responsibility to remind group members how the discussion will be used and why.

Consent is more problematic; apart from staying silent it is very difficult for an individual within a group to withdraw their consent to participate. The right to withdraw consent should be discussed prior to the focus group, and although silence can be a useful option it may be wrongly interpreted as a form of assent to what others are saying. Researchers should consider offering participants the opportunity to withdraw consent after the group has met if they believe that the discussion did not reflect their views or it was a process they no longer wanted to be associated with. This would mean their contributions could not be reported.

The process of group participation can lead to unanticipated consequences. It can raise consciousness, expose underlying conflicts and falsely create an expectation that something will be done about the issues raised. Owen (2001) has discussed how distinctions between focus groups and therapy groups can become blurred, especially if participants share painful personal experiences. She outlines the challenges of facilitating a group where women shared the experience of having lost a child. Ensuring group members felt 'safe' was as important as obtaining the data; she describes taking the decision to sensitively move the discussion on when participants were becoming distressed.

Although this kind of data is very rich, it is exploitative if people expose their feelings and reveal their needs but there is then no means of offering further support. It is therefore important to have mechanisms in place for individuals to revisit the issues raised and if necessary to discuss them further. As part of this process the moderator also needs to consider their role within the group discussion, ensuring that it is understood by participants, and consider the extent to which they are prepared to disclose their own views.

Finally, the moderator has a responsibility to ensure that participants do not feel devalued by their experience in the group. This can happen when opinions that are expressed are ridiculed or strongly opposed by other group members. In these situations the moderator should reinforce the right of each person to have an opinion and for it to be listened to, even if people are not in agreement. If this is not possible then the moderator should change the focus of the group's discussion or bring it to a close.

CONCLUSIONS

This chapter has provided an overview of the purpose and usefulness of focus groups for nursing research. It has emphasised that this method of data collection requires careful preparation and skill in leading and managing group discussion. The method is particularly useful when researchers wish to understand and clarify thinking on a topic from a group perspective. The need to be transparent about the purpose and process of the focus group, and sensitive to the particular ethical challenges this method poses, has been emphasised throughout. In conclusion, focus groups are a useful and versatile data collection method that can be used within a wide range of study settings and with diverse groups to great effect.

References

Bramley D (2004) Making and managing audio recordings. In: Seale C (ed) *Researching Society and Culture*, 2nd edition. London, Sage, pp 207–223.

Burt J, Shipman C, Addington Hall J, White P (2008) Nursing the dying within a generalist caseload: a focus group study of district nurses. *International Journal of Nursing Studies* **45**: 1470–1478.

Culley L, Hudson N, Rapport F (2007) Using focus groups with minority ethnic communities: researching infertility in British South Asian Communities. *Qualitative Health Research* **17**: 102–112.

Gibbs A (1997) *Focus Groups*. Guilford, University of Surrey Social Research Update.

Gibson F (2007) Conducting focus groups with children and young people: strategies for success. *Journal of Research in Nursing* **12**: 473–483.

Halcomb EJ, Gholizadeh L, DiGiacomo M, Phillips J, Davidson P (2007) Considerations in undertaking focus group research with culturally and linguistically diverse groups. *Journal of Clinical Nursing* **16**: 1000–1011.

Hennessy D, Heary C (2005) Exploring children's views through focus groups In: Greene S, Hogan D (eds) *Researching Children's Experience: approaches and methods*. London, Sage, pp 236–252.

Kevern J, Webb C (2004) Mature women's experiences of pre-registration nurse education. *Journal of Advanced Nursing* **45**: 297–306.

Kitzinger J (1994) The methodology of focus groups: the importance of interaction between research participants. *Sociology of Health and Illness* **16**: 103–121.

Kitzinger J, Barbour RS (1999) Introduction: the challenge and promise of focus groups. In: Barbour RS, J Kitzinger J (eds) *Developing Focus Group Research: politics, theory and practice*. London, Sage, pp 1–20.

McLafferty I (2004) Focus group interviews as a data collecting strategy. *Journal of Advanced Nursing* **48**: 187–194.

Morgan DL (1997) *Focus Groups as Qualitative Research*, 2nd edition. London, Sage.

Nyamathi A, Shuler P (1990) Focus group interview: a research technique for informed nursing practice. *Journal of Advanced Nursing* **15**: 1281–1288.

Owen S (2001) The practical, methodological and ethical dilemmas of conducting focus groups with vulnerable clients. *Journal of Advanced Nursing* **36**: 652–658.

Reed J, Payton V (1997) Focus groups: issues of analysis and interpretation. *Journal of Advanced Nursing* **26**: 765–771.

Roth C, Ahmed S, Feldman R, Sandall J, Sunderland J (2003) *Bilingual advocacy and HIV testing: an evaluation of service in East London*. London, City University.

Twohig PL, Putnam W (2002) Group interviews in primary care research: advancing the state of the art of ritualised research. *Family Practice* **19**: 278–284.

Webb C, Kevern J (2001) Focus groups as a research method: a critique of some aspects of their use in nursing research. *Journal of Advanced Nursing* **33**: 798–805.

Further reading

Barbour R (2008) *Doing Focus Groups* [qualitative research kit], 3rd edition. London, Sage.

Gibbs A (1997) Focus Groups. *Social Research Update*, Issue 19. University of Surrey, Guilford. Available online at http://sru.soc.surrey.ac.uk/SRU19.html

Dawson S, Manderson LA (1993) *A Manual for the Use of Focus Groups: methods for social research in disease*. International Nutrition Foundation for Developing Countries (INFDC), Boston, MA, USA. Complete manual is online at www.unu.edu/unupress/food2/UIN03E/UIN03E00.HTM

30 Questionnaire Design

Martyn Jones and Janice Rattray

Key points

- Questionnaires are a quick, relatively inexpensive method of gathering standardised information that is convenient for both participant and researcher.

- It is important to be aware of the theoretical process in questionnaire design, both for the design of own questionnaires and the appropriate use of existing measures.

- Establishing the reliability and validity of a measure is an important step in using and adapting previously validated questionnaires.

- Developing a new measure is a lengthy process, with key theoretical and psychometric considerations for item generation, scale construction and response format.

- Questionnaire administration is possible via a series of routes. Pilot testing of a new questionnaire is likely to influence the quality of data returned and response rates.

INTRODUCTION

This chapter will provide the reader with an understanding of the key methodological issues involved in the use of questionnaires, particularly regarding the design and administration of this method of quantitative data collection. It will:

- examine the strengths and limitations of the use of questionnaires to gather self-report data
- introduce basic psychometric evaluation methods as a method of evaluating the worth of established questionnaires
- identify an essential set of methods in developing a new questionnaire.

Establishing the worth of a questionnaire and developing new measures of sufficient methodological rigour are of great importance to researchers and practitioners working in healthcare settings. Understanding the process of questionnaire design is critical in allowing the researcher to decide whether results derived from questionnaires are trustworthy, and to evaluate whether a questionnaire is of sufficient quality for use in a study, or not. It is important that nurses understand fully the theoretical issues associated with questionnaire design, so that they can both interpret study findings and generate their own questionnaires.

Questionnaires allow us to collect data in a standardised manner and make inferences to a wider population when that data is obtained from an appropriate sample of the population being studied (see Chapter 12 on sampling). Standardised questionnaires are those that have undergone rigorous psychometric analysis to demonstrate their reliability and validity, and where possible such a standardised measure should be used. However, this is not always possible and the researcher may have to design their own measure.

This method allows for the collection of self-report data that would be difficult to gather in any other manner (Polit & Beck 2004) and has led to an increase in our understanding of health and wellbeing, including patient experiences and outcomes. The use of questionnaires as a method of data collection continues to increase in healthcare research, both nationally and internationally. Many studies that form the basis for good clinical practice make use of this important method of data collection.

THE PURPOSE OF QUESTIONNAIRES

Nurse researchers use questionnaires to measure knowledge (Furze *et al.* 2003), attitudes (McLafferty 2007), emotion (Zigmond & Snaith 1983), cognition (Moss-Morris *et al.* 2002), and intention and behaviour (Conner & Sparks 1995). This approach captures the self-reported observations of the individual and is commonly used to measure patient perceptions of many aspects of healthcare (see Table 30.1 for examples). The main benefits of this method of data collection are that questionnaires are usually relatively quick to complete, are fairly inexpensive to produce and are usually easy to analyse (Bowling 2002). Standardised questionnaires allow data to be gathered

at different levels of specificity. For example, data on quality of life might be gathered using a generic measure such as the Short-Form 36 (Ware & Sherbourne 1992) or a health-specific measure such as the Cardiovascular Limitations and Symptoms Profile (Devlen *et al.* 1989). Questionnaires may also inform a sampling strategy to recruit participants for individual interviews or focus groups (Barbour 2008).

USING AND ADAPTING PREVIOUSLY VALIDATED QUESTIONNAIRES

There are a number of challenges or problems associated with the use of existing questionnaires. It is important to spend time considering and appraising questionnaires to determine their suitability. When choosing a questionnaire, the researcher must consider a number of questions to inform their choice (see Table 30.2).

The process of demonstrating the reliability and validity of a questionnaire is not easily accomplished. It is perhaps not surprising, therefore, that wherever possible, researchers tend to use existing questionnaires with established reliability and validity.

RELIABILITY

Reliability refers to the repeatability of a questionnaire, i.e. that it will measure what it is supposed to measure in a consistent manner. This can be demon-

Table 30.1 Examples of what questionnaires can measure

Area	Questionnaire
Knowledge	The York Angina Beliefs Questionnaire (Furze *et al.* 2003)
Attitude/Beliefs/Intention	Operationalising the theory of planned behaviour (Conner & Sparks 1995)
	Developing a questionnaire to measure nurses' attitudes towards older people (McLafferty 2007)
Cognition	The Revised Illness Perception Questionnaire (Moss-Morris *et al.* 2002)
Emotion/Mood	Hospital Anxiety and Depression Scale (Zigmond & Snaith 1983)
Health status	Short-Form 36 (Ware & Sherbourne 1992)
Quality of life	EQ-5D (EuroQoL Group 1990)
Behaviour	Functional Limitations Profile FLIP (Patrick & Peach 1989)

Table 30.2 Key questions in choosing a questionnaire

Key questions	
Will the questionnaire provide data to answer the research questions?	When evaluating findings from a study that uses a questionnaire or when deciding whether a questionnaire should be used, it is always good practice to keep revisiting the research questions to ensure that this is an appropriate approach
Is there a standardised questionnaire with demonstrated reliability and validity that can be used?	Using an established standardised questionnaire is preferable to having to develop one from first principles. This can allow for findings to be compared with other patient or participant groups and in some instances allow comparisons with population norms, e.g. Short-Form 36 (Ware & Sherbourne 1992)
If so, how was reliability and validity established?	Reliability and validity of the standardised questionnaire should be established by the developers and it is advisable to access original papers to review this. If the questionnaire has been used by other researchers, they too should present such data
How widely used is the questionnaire?	If a questionnaire has been widely used it is likely that it has good psychometric properties. For example the Hospital Anxiety and Depression Scale (Zigmond & Snaith 1983) has been used in many different patient populations throughout the world and continues to be reliable and valid. However, this is not always the case and evidence of good psychometric properties should always be established
Is the questionnaire responsive to change over time and are there ceiling and floor effects?	In a longitudinal study that seeks to identify change over time, responsiveness of a questionnaire is very important. It is important that small changes can be detected. Ceiling effects mean that continued improvement cannot be detected and floor effects that continued deterioration cannot be detected
Is the questionnaire appropriate for the proposed participants?	It may be tempting to use a standardised questionnaire on a different participant group other than the one for which the questionnaire was designed. This may be possible, but further psychometric analysis will be required
If not, can I adapt an existing questionnaire or do I need to develop my own?	This may be the only option in the absence of a suitable standardised measure. Developing a questionnaire is a rigorous process and it is essential that this is planned in a sound, systematic manner

strated statistically in a number of ways: test–retest, inter-rater and internal consistency (Bowling & Ebrahim 2005).

Test–retest reliability refers to consistency over time, i.e. will a questionnaire yield the same results in the same situation when administered twice over a short period of time, such as days or a week (Polgar & Thomas, 2000)? Statistical tests that can demonstrate this include Cohen's kappa co-efficient and Pearson's correlation (Bowling & Ebrahim 2005). A correlation co-efficient exceeding 0.8 indicates good test–retest reliability (Polgar & Thomas 2000). Test–retest reliability is particularly important if the questionnaire is to be used to assess change over time.

Inter-rater reliability is used to establish the degree of agreement between two or more raters or interviewers. The kappa statistic or correlational analysis quantifies this (Bowling & Ebrahim 2005).

Internal consistency reflects how well items are related to each other, i.e. do scale items measure the same concept or construct. Cronbach's alpha (α) statistic calculates average inter-item correlations (Bowling & Ebrahim 2005). A questionnaire is judged to have good internal consistency when α exceeds 0.70 (Mcnee & McCabe 2008). Cronbach's alpha statistic can be reported for the whole questionnaire or separately for each domain or subscale.

As an alternative to Cronbach's alpha statistic, item-total correlations can be used. This provides additional information about how each item is related to the total score from the questionnaire or domain and can be used to identify items that either do not relate to the construct the questionnaire is measuring, or those that are too similar. However, this score can be biased if sample sizes are small. Calculating corrected item-total correlation is recommended where the item score is removed from the total score prior to the correlation. Kline (1993) recommends removing any questionnaire item with a corrected item-total correlation of <0.3. High inter-item correlations (>0.8) suggest that these are repetitions and the removal of the duplicate is indicated (Kline 1993).

VALIDITY

Validity refers to whether the questionnaire measures what it is supposed to measure, and if it measures it correctly and accurately (Mcnee & McCabe 2008). There are different types of validity.

Face validity is a subjective assessment that the items in a scale appear to be relevant, clear and unambiguous.

Content validity is assessed by asking experts to judge whether questionnaire items fully represent the concept or construct to be measured. This relatively weak form of validity is a useful starting point.

Criterion validity establishes the relationship of a questionnaire with an established 'gold standard' measure. Concurrent and predictive validity are two types of criterion validity.

Concurrent validity examines the relationship of a variable that participants are known to differ on, with the questionnaire (Bryman & Cramer 2005). For example, students vary in their levels of course attendance and may be absent for reasons other than illness. Does a measure of course satisfaction relate to such absence, or not? If not, the measure of course satisfaction may be suspect.

Predictive validity examines the utility of a questionnaire in predicting cross-sectional associations, or a criterion variable measured at a point in the future (Bowling 2005).

Construct validity relates to how well the items in the questionnaire represent the underlying conceptual structure. For example, does a measure of disease-specific quality of life capture the domains theorised to exist? Factor analysis is one statistical technique that can be used to determine the constructs or domains within the developing measure. This approach can therefore contribute to establishing construct validity. Related to this, *convergent validity* is demonstrated when the questionnaire correlates with a related measure and does not correlate with dissimilar measure (*discriminant validity*) (Bowling 2005).

The cultural and temporal relevance of the measure must also be considered when deciding whether to use an existing questionnaire. Making use of measures derived in other cultures and developed in the past is not without difficulty. For example, the Hospital Anxiety and Depression Scale (HADS) (Zigmond & Snaith 1983) was developed in the US in the early 1980s for use in non-psychiatric patients. Is this measure appropriate for use in contemporary research settings in the UK? A range of studies has suggested that this is the case. The reliability of the HADS has been established in the UK, and normative data for a community sample is available (Crawford *et al.* 2001). Other studies have established its use in long-term conditions (Wright *et al.* 2003). However, there may be some caveats in its use in particular specialties or patient groups. For example, the HADS contains items that may relate to physical abilities of the person as well as depression, e.g. 'I feel as if I am slowing down' (Martin & Thompson 2000). This makes it important to continue to assess psychometric properties when a questionnaire is used in settings other than those where validity has already been demonstrated. The adaptation of measures for use in other language groups is also likely to require translation and back translation strategies (Lee *et al.* 2002).

A general rule of thumb is that if a questionnaire requires minor amendment to be appropriate for use in a particular sample, this amendment will require the researcher to demonstrate the reliability and validity of the emergent questionnaire as part of their analytic or evaluation plan (Rattray & Jones 2007). Furthermore, it is good practice to present results from any established standardised questionnaire by detailing the reliability, e.g. Cronbach's alpha, or validity of the measure.

DEVELOPING A QUESTIONNAIRE

From deciding to develop a questionnaire to producing the final standardised measure can be a lengthy process. Research Examples 30.1, 30.2 and 30.3 provide three examples of nurse researchers who have undertaken a rigorous process of developing and testing new questionnaires in different fields of inquiry. There are a number of pitfalls to avoid, including how to avoid bias and error. This bias may be non-responder, acquiescence response or measurement error.

Non-responder bias occurs when those who do not consent to take part in the study differ from those who do. For example, the non-responder group might be younger or older than those who consent, or there may be gender differences. This may present difficulties in interpreting and generalising findings. Optimising recruitment is one way to avoid this.

Acquiescent response bias is the tendency for respondents to agree with a statement, or respond in the same way to all items. This may be avoided by including both positively and negatively worded items, although this is not universally accepted.

Measurement error may be reduced by establishing reliability and validity of the measure.

Developing items

When developing a questionnaire, items or questions are generated that require the participant to respond to a series of questions or statements. These responses are generally then converted into numerical form, summed and statistically analysed. This is an important stage, and time must be taken to develop and pilot these items to ensure they reflect the key concepts identified in the research questions. The researcher can use a number of different sources to

---

RESEARCH EXAMPLE

30.1 A Questionnaire Examining Evidence-based Practice in Nurses

Carlson C (2008) Development and testing of four instruments to assess prior conditions that influence nurses' adoption of evidence-based pain management practices. *Journal of Advanced Nursing* **64**(6): 632–643.

This paper reports on the development and psychometric evaluation of four related questionnaires focusing on the setting conditions that influence nurses' decision to adopt evidence-based pain management strategies. The measure was developed in two stages, with the development and testing of content validity preceding an empirical stage that examined the construct validity and reliability of each measure. The item development process included the systematic search of relevant research literature, the use of experts to confirm item relevance and readability. A total of 187 participants (47% response rate) provided data with the four questionnaires comprising the Carlson's Prior Conditions Instruments, each measuring a theoretically derived theme, i.e. (a) previous practice, (b) innovativeness, (c) felt needs/problems and (d) norms of the social system. Frequency of behaviour (a, b) and beliefs (c, d) were measured using differently keyed five-point scales. The psychometric properties of retained items were then tested using item analysis and Cronbach's alpha (0.73–0.83). Exploratory factor analysis established the construct validity of each factor and revealed the uni-dimensional structure of 'felt needs/problems' (six items) and 'norms of the social system' (seven items). 'Previous practice' (11 items) and 'innovativeness' (six items) had three and two factors respectively. The authors clarify the remaining steps needed to the demonstrate stability over time, i.e. test–retest reliability and the predictive validity of the measures in identifying nurses who are the early adopters of evidence-based pain management strategies. This robust, well-developed set of measures has the potential to improve the quality of care provision in this area.

RESEARCH EXAMPLE

30.2 A Questionnaire Examining Children's Views of the Quality of Hospital Care

Pelander T *et al.* (2008) The quality of paediatric nursing care: developing the Child Care Quality of Hospital Instrument for children. *Journal of Advanced Nursing* **65**(2): 443–453.

This paper reports on the three phases of the development of the Child Care Quality at Hospital (CCQH) Instrument for Children. In Phase 1 (content validity), 40 items were generated following a literature review and a series of interviews/drawings by hospitalised children. An expert panel then reviewed the face validity of the measure. Amendments were made following child-provided interviews (n = 7), questionnaires (n = 57) and nurse comments (n = 217) in Phase 2. This pilot testing in a range of settings allowed additional items to be added to the measure and simplified the wording of a single item.

The main empirical evaluation of the measure (Phase 3) involved the completion of the measure by 388 children who had at least one overnight stay in hospital. The resultant 58-item measure consisted of a three-factor structure including 'nurse characteristics', 'nursing activities' (five subcategories, 28 items) and 'nursing environment' (three subcategories, 19 items), plus three open-ended questions and a drawing activity. The CCQH uses a three-point Likert scale (with numbers and smiley faces), with the nursing environment items using an agreement/disagreement format (including teddy bear figures). The reliability of the measure was identified using inter-item correlations and Cronbach's alpha (0.56–0.81). Nurses working in the same settings generated a Content Validity Index for the items in CCQH, suggesting items for inclusion and those for removal. Principal Components Analysis on the 'nursing characteristics' and 'nursing environment' scales revealed a five-factor (52% of variance) and three-factor solution (50% of variance) respectively. The development of the measure highlighted the different ways that nurses and children conceptualise expectations about the quality of care.

develop items and ensure face and content validity. A review of the literature will be helpful, and consulting with experts may generate relevant items (Bowling & Ebrahim 2005). Discussion with proposed respondents will prevent the inclusion of unnecessary items and identify items that may be sensitive or controversial. It is at this stage that the proposed domain or factor structured should be proposed (Ferguson & Cox 1993). It is not common to develop a questionnaire that relies on a response to a single item, and multi-item scales are generally used in preference to avoid bias or misinterpretation and to reduce measurement error (Bowling 1997). For example, the Student Nurse Stress Index (Jones & Johnston 1999) comprises 22 items representing four subscales. However, single items may have some advantage and are used on occasion to assess general perceptions of health status (Bowling 2005). Single items are usually simple to complete and reduce respondent burden.

The developer must also consider relevance and acceptability of the questionnaire to the target group. The items need to be written in language that respondents are either familiar with or find easy to understand. For example, it is important to avoid the use of technical terms when recruiting lay persons, e.g. 'breathing machine' rather than 'ventilatory support'; 'water pill' rather than 'diuretic'. However, care needs to be taken not to oversimplify language, which may offend.

Items or questions should be clearly written to avoid misinterpretation and leading questions should be avoided. Age can be collected as a continuous or categorised variable. If the latter is the case, then the categories must be clearly identified and be mutually exclusive. For example, in question 1a below, a respondent who is 30 years old would identify with the first and second category whereas in question 1b they would identify with only the first category.

30.3 A Questionnaire about Patient Involvement in Myocardial Infarction Care

Arnetz JE *et al.* (2008) Staff views and behaviour regarding patient involvement in myocardial infarction care: development and evaluation of a questionnaire. *European Journal of Cardiovascular Nursing* **7**: 27–35.

This paper reports on the development of a questionnaire to measure views and behaviour of nursing and medical staff on patient involvement in myocardial infarction care. Five phases of the development of this questionnaire are identified: literature review, focus group discussions, development of items, pilot work and main study to establish reliability and validity. Items were developed from the literature review and focus groups. Pilot work of the initial 59 items of this questionnaire confirmed its use (minus two of the original items). This resulted in a 57-item questionnaire, of which seven items were background/demographic data and six 'a priori' proposed factors or domains. A Principal Components Analysis with Varimax rotation was applied to 47 of the questionnaire items collected in a cross-sectional study (n = 488). Five factors emerged from this analysis, and these were renamed according to item content. Items with a factor loading of >0.4 only were included and as a result 17 items were removed. One factor was divided into two to represent two distinct aspects of a specific domain. Cronbach's alpha statistic for each factor was ≥0.69. Further analysis, including second-order factor analysis, identified two dimensions of this questionnaire: staff views, which included two factors; and staff behaviour, which included four factors. Content validity was demonstrated through the literature review and focus group discussions, construct validity by the factor analysis, and discriminative validity by demonstrating differences between professional groups and different departments. This questionnaire should now be further tested to confirm the factor structure and its reliability and validity.

1a What age are   18–30   30–50   50–70   over 70
    you?
1b What age are   18–30   31–50   51–70   71+
    you?

As another example, if a researcher is interested in how social support receipt influences patient adjustment to a long-term condition, the researcher might ask the following questions:

2a Did you receive practical and   Yes/No
    emotional support?
2b Was this support helpful?   Yes/No

On the face of it, the question 2a might be reasonable, but if the patient had received practical rather than emotional support, or vice versa, the item would be ambiguous. A better way would be to ask four questions.

3a Did you receive practical support?   Yes/No
3b If yes, was this practical support   Yes/No
    helpful?
4a Did you receive emotional support?   Yes/No
4b If yes, was this emotional support   Yes/No
    helpful?

Level of data

The type of question, language used, order of items and indeed how the questionnaire is presented may all bias response and influence response rates. Participants need to be clear about the purpose of the questionnaire and understand what they are being asked to do. It is important to engage the participant's interest early on to encourage completion. It is thought best to avoid presenting controversial or emotive items at the beginning of the questionnaire.

To prevent boredom, demographic and/or clinical data may be presented at the end.

Closed questions, where respondents are offered a restricted range of responses, can be viewed as too restrictive by some respondents. There may not be an appropriate response option and therefore consideration should be give to include the option for free text responses or open questions. This is a particularly useful option when developing a questionnaire.

There are a range of scales and response styles that may be chosen which produce different types or levels of data. Probably the lowest level of measurement is *categorical* or *nominal* data, which can be grouped into distinct categories. The most common questionnaire item that provides data at a categorical or nominal level is gender. Participants may be categorised according to clinical condition or demographic data, such as diagnosis or gender.

Ordinal data imply an order to responses, but there is no equal distance between each option. For example, the assumption is often made that the same distances exist between strongly agree and agree as between strongly disagree and disagree. However, this is not the case. A measurable or quantifiable difference between each item on the scale can only exist at the next level of data, which is *interval* or *ratio*. In this instance, the difference in temperature of 37°C and 38°C is the same as between 36°C and 37°C, i.e. 1 degree of temperature. The level of data collected by a questionnaire will influence the nature of subsequent analysis. Therefore when developing a new questionnaire, the developer must be clear which scale and response format should be used. Chapter 35 discusses types of data and their analysis in more detail.

Range of scales

A range of response format scales is available. Most commonly used in research in nursing is the '*Likert-type*' or *frequency* scale. These provide ordinal-level data and Likert-type scales generally measure level of agreement. Respondents may be given a range of five, seven or even nine pre-coded options ranging from strongly agree to strongly disagree. This scale makes the assumption that attitudes can be measured, although there is no assumption that the differences between strongly agree and agree are equivalent to those between strongly disagree and disagree. There is controversy about whether to offer a neutral point, i.e. undecided or no opinion, in such scales of agreement. If the respondent has no opinion about an item, it may cause confusion or irritation not to offer that choice and therefore increase the possibility of non-response bias (Burns & Grove 1997).

Less commonly used in nursing research are Thurstone and Guttman scales. Thurstone scales are constructed following analysis of empirical data, often provided by expert panels, such that attitudes and behaviours measured by the items are equally spaced along a continuum from favourable to unfavourable, and each item is given a weighting. Items included in the final questionnaire usually have a dichotomous response format and are chosen to represent the range of assigned weights. An example of such a scale is the Nottingham Health Profile (Hunt *et al.* 1985). These scales are relatively rare in nursing research. Guttman scaling uses methods that establish a hierarchy of items such that when participants agree with an item, they will also agree with items of a lower ranking, e.g. Katz Index of Activities of Daily Living (Katz *et al.* 1963) and the Rivermead Mobility Index (Collen *et al.* (1991). Further details of the questionnaire development process for Thurstone and Guttman can be seen in Oppenheim (1992).

Response formats

A range of response formats is possible. For example, participants may be asked to indicate an appropriate response from a choice of five boxes. For example:

	All of the time	Most of the time	Some of the time	Rarely	Never
I feel anxious					

Alternatively, a horizontal or vertical, linear scale may be used and the respondent asked to mark where they would position themselves on the line.

I feel anxious

Never   *All of the time*

├─────────────────────────────────┤

What is important is that before deciding on the response format, the researcher must be clear how the data will be analysed.

Certain questions should be avoided, e.g. those that lead or include double negatives or double-barrelled questions (Bowling 2005). A mixture of both positively and negatively worded items may minimise the danger of acquiescent response bias, i.e. the tendency for respondents to agree with a statement or respond in the same way to items.

It may be appropriate to allow respondents to expand on answers and provide more in-depth responses; free text response or open questions may be included. While this approach may be welcomed by respondents and may provide rich data, such material can be difficult to analyse and interpret (Polgar & Thomas 2000). Such problems may be outweighed by the benefits of including this option, particularly in the early development of a questionnaire. Free text comments can inform future questionnaire development by identifying poorly constructed items or new items for future inclusion.

ADMINISTERING QUESTIONNAIRES

Questionnaires can be administered via a variety of routes, i.e. either postal or face to face. In the clinical setting, questionnaires may be self-completed by participants, or be presented by interviewer either face to face or via telephone. Increasingly, questionnaires are being delivered online, i.e. web-based with a request to participate delivered by email.

Presentation and layout of the questionnaire is important and this can affect response rates. Always try to make it easy for the participant to complete. A covering letter and/or a participant information sheet is used to introduce the study to the participant. The purpose of this is to establish the credibility and salience of the study and to convince the participant of the worth of the study (Czaja & Blair 2005). The covering letter must establish what the study is about, why it is important, how findings will be used and how the respondent was selected. It must clarify issues surrounding confidentiality and anonymity and provide a contact number for respondents to contact if they have questions (Czaja & Blair 2005).

Participant information sheets fulfil a similar purpose and are required by ethics committees (Barrett & Coleman 2005).

There are some simple guidelines or principles to follow that will encourage responses and avoid non-completion to reduce the number of missed items.

- Simple instructions before each section of the questionnaire are helpful. This may include a worked example.
- It is always good to thank the respondent for participating in your study.
- The font size should be large enough to be read easily.
- Items or questions should be clearly numbered.
- Avoid the overuse of capital letters, and use lower case wherever possible as it is easier to read.
- If the questionnaire is to be administered by post, it is best to have questions on one side of the paper only.
- Consider the length of your questionnaire and always try to keep it as brief as possible.
- Reminders may be sent to participants. This can increase the response rate, but must be detailed as part of an ethics application and research protocol.

The use of coding systems ensures the confidentiality and anonymity of participants, with the principal investigator maintaining and storing securely a codebook linking the code on a questionnaire to the participant name. This protects the identity of participant, but allows the linking of questionnaire data with other forms of data, which may include data in existing secondary data sets or data held in other health-related records. Questionnaire packs must be adequately prepared and coded and include the covering letter, consent form, return and contact details. If presumed consent was part of the ethical approval, return of the questionnaire may be taken to indicate consent (Czaja & Blair 2005).

Principles of good clinical practice require that the nurse researcher has the requisite experience, supervision and training. Research governance procedures must be adhered to and ethical approval obtained. For less-experienced researchers, support from senior colleagues and the principal investigator on the project must also be available. For example, Polit & Beck (2004) provide an example of a training manual for an interview study. This includes detail of the research study and the research protocol, detailing study procedures and the role of the researcher in either gaining consent and or administering the questionnaire pack by the chosen administration route. Polit & Beck (2004) also detail a data collection protocol, which identifies the conditions necessary for collecting data, the time and setting in which data can be collected and replies to frequently asked questions (revealed during piloting of the questionnaire). Clarity in such matters is particularly important in any study conducted in a clinical situation.

PILOTING

A key stage in the development of the questionnaire is piloting. This allows the pre-testing of the measure ahead of the main study. Piloting allows evaluation of the performance of the measure in meeting the study objectives or research questions. This is an essential stage, particularly if the study is using a newly constructed questionnaire. It allows the researcher to establish whether questions are intelligible and unambiguous. It establishes whether the items are acceptable and inoffensive, and how long the measure takes to complete (Polit & Beck 2004). Such pilots can be relatively informal with small numbers of participants. It is also appropriate at this stage to develop a plan for validation of the measure (Czaja & Blair 2005; Rattray & Jones 2007). The opinion of experts may be sought to establish the face or content validity of the measure.

The measure may be piloted more formally with up to 50 participants to test the acceptability of questionnaire items and should include an initial examination of reliability and validity (Bowling 2002). As part of this evaluation, item analysis provides a strategy to decide on whether all items in the measure should remain. An item-total correlation cut-off of <0.3 can be used to identify items that do not add to the explanatory power of the measure, and that should be discarded (Kline 1993). Questionnaire items that have high endorsement of particular response options

add little to the discriminatory power of the measure and should be deleted (Priest *et al.* 1995). A more detailed discussion of these issues can be found in Rattray and Jones (2007).

RESPONSE RATES

Response rate has been defined as 'the number of eligible sample members to complete, divided by the total number of eligible sample members' (Czaja & Blair 2005: 37). Response rates of 75% and above are considered good (Bowling 2002), although response rates far lower than this are common. Lower response rates are problematic in that those sample members who have not completed may differ from responders. Strategies to establish the nature of any response bias are recommended.

The return route also has an impact on response rates. Response rates for questionnaires presented by interviewer may be increased. This may be because the interviewer can clarify items and motivate the respondent (Polit & Beck 2004).

COMPARISON BETWEEN FACE-TO-FACE STRUCTURED INTERVIEWS AND POSTAL QUESTIONNAIRES

Questionnaires may be self-completed and returned by mail. In a postal survey, the questionnaire may be mailed to participants following receipt of consent forms, for self-completion and return by post. Questionnaires may also be presented on other media, with web-based surveys increasingly seen in the literature. One issue with the internet survey surrounds the process for identifying the sample frame for the study (Czaja & Blair 2005) and establishing the eligibility of participants. Other forms of data collection are possible, including diary data gathered using paper or electronic formats (Johnston *et al.* 2006).

Each method of administration has its own strengths and limitations, and methods of administration may be combined. For example, in a face-to-face study, the researcher may make an initial approach to gain consent, and having given the person time to consider (usually at least 24 hours) may then administer the questionnaire to the participant, either for self-completion and return in the setting, or for the participant to self-complete and return by post. Alternatively, the researcher may administer the questionnaire as a structured interview. Such structured interviews may be delivered face to face or as a telephone survey. Response rates for structured interviews tend to be higher than for postal surveys, fewer missing items are found and the researcher can ensure that the participant filled out the questionnaire in the required sequence (Bowling 2002). Having the interviewer present to clarify any particular questions the participant has may promote a good response. However, one potential disadvantage of interviews is that the interviewer biases or influences the response given by the participant (Polit & Beck 2004). Separation of data collection from intervention delivery and interviewer training may reduce the effects of such bias. The setting in which a participant completes a questionnaire may influence results. Participants providing information in a hospital may be more anxious than those providing information at home (Paul *et al.* 2007).

STRENGTHS AND LIMITATIONS OF QUESTIONNAIRES

The standardised questionnaire has many advantages. It allows the collection of a great deal of data quickly, and relatively cheaply. It is generally convenient, and can be administered in a range of settings. It allows for a count of key issues and occurrences in a systematic and standardised manner, and can be supplemented with routinely gathered information or more objective data from case notes, subject to the requisite governance and ethical consent (Bowling 2002).

Social desirability may also be a limitation of questionnaire data, with participants attempting to influence the impression they provide through their answers (Bowling 2005). Self-completed questionnaires are thought to be less prone to such bias than those administered by researchers/interviewers (Bowling 2002). The researcher may consider the use of a measure of social desirability to evaluate this form of self-presentation bias (Crowne & Marlowe 1960).

Questionnaire data are almost exclusively retrospective based and are gathered by asking a respondent to consider and report on a construct of interest and rate their response considering the recent past. Such accounts are provided retrospectively and rely on autobiographical or semantic memory. Autobiographical memory is affected by the participant's current affective state. Such state-congruent recall effects can systematically bias data, with current depression biasing previous symptom reports (Shiffman & Stone 1998). Such introspection effects create systematic bias, with the attitudes and expectations of the person influencing their retrospective account. Gathering information about thoughts or decisions in a particular situation retrospectively may also be compromised by the person's knowledge of the outcome.

There are additional issues to consider when designing a study with a data collection strategy based on questionnaires. The administration of a questionnaire may by itself change participant behaviour. For example, asking a participant about their alcohol consumption may influence subsequent reports. Repeated use of a measure may also lead to familiarity with the questionnaire, which may make it difficult to discriminate such practice effects from actual change over time. The nurse researcher should be aware of such limitations.

ETHICAL ISSUES ASSOCIATED WITH QUESTIONNAIRES

There is a range of ethical issues relating to the use of questionnaires. Ensuring that informed consent is obtained is vital in any study. Participants must be given sufficient time to consider the research request before being asked to provide information. Questionnaire studies must at least guarantee confidentiality, i.e. that the identity of the respondent will not be revealed in any dissemination of findings and that the respondent's identity will never be linked to the information they provide (Polit & Beck, 2004). Anonymous responses may allow the participant to feel more ready to provide information. However, true anonymity is difficult to achieve, particularly in small surveys, and does not allow linkage of data or sending of reminder letters. In many instances, it is not possible for the participant to remain anonymous. In such situations, all data from survey or face-to-face data gathering must be treated as confidential, and the respondent reassured that only key researchers will be able to access the data (Oppenheim 1992). Some postal survey studies assume implied consent, and that return of the questionnaire has demonstrated informed consent, but this may not be justified in situations involving vulnerable participants (Polit & Beck 2004).

In situations where the subject area might cause distress to the respondent, or where there is an indication of a change or worsening of clinical condition, the researcher must have strategies to deal with this. For example, if a participant's score on a screening measure of depression suggests a potential depressive disorder then it may be appropriate to refer that patient to their general practitioner. Furthermore, questionnaires that include intrusive or offensive items, or that include items that are not needed, or questionnaires that do not have established reliability and validity may all be ethically suspect. Ethics committees will offer guidance in this area.

CONCLUSIONS

This chapter has provided a summary of issues associated with the design and use of questionnaires. The decision process involved in either choosing an established measure or developing a questionnaire has been discussed, and the researcher needs to be assured that using this approach will address the relevant research questions. The use and purpose of questionnaires in quantitative research is increasing and it is essential that practitioners and researchers have a good understanding of design and administration issues if evidence-based care is to be informed by such methods. A logical and systematic approach needs to be adopted when both designing and appraising a questionnaire. This involves consideration of items, developing an 'a priori' factor structure and subsequent analytic confirmation, including demonstration of the reliability, validity and acceptability of a questionnaire appropriate to a particular research setting and participants. Presentation, wording, order and layout are all important factors in influencing validity and response rates. There are a number of strategies to improve this, but good representative responses are important to minimise bias and measurement error. Questionnaires that are administered or designed according to standards required by research governance and ethics lead to high-quality research and ultimately can improve patient care.

References

Arnetz JE, Höglund AT, Arnetz BB, Winblad U (2008) Staff views and behaviour regarding patient involvement in myocardial infarction care: development and evaluation of a questionnaire. *European Journal of Cardiovascular Nursing* **7**: 27–35.

Barbour R (2008) *Introducing Qualitative Research: a student guide to the craft of doing qualitatitve research.* London, Sage.

Barrett G, Coleman M (2005) Ethical and political issues in the conduct of research. In: Bowling A, Ebrahim E (eds) *Handbook of Health Research Methods: investigation, measurement and analysis.* Maidenhead, Open University Press, pp 555–583.

Bowling A (2005) Techniques of questionnaire design. In: Bowling A, Ebrahim S (eds) *Handbook of Health Research Methods: investigation, measurement and analysis.* Maidenhead, Open University Press, pp 394–427.

Bowling A (2002) *Research Methods in Health.* Buckingham, Open University Press.

Bowling A (1997) *Measuring Health: a review of quality of life measurement scales.* Milton Keynes, Open University.

Bowling A, Ebrahim E (eds) (2005) *Handbook of Health Research Methods: investigation, measurement and analysis.* Maidenhead, Open University Press.

Bryman A & Cramer D (2005) *Quantitative Data Analysis with SPSS 12 and 13: a guide for social scientists.* London, Routledge.

Burns N, Grove SK (1997) *The Practice of Nursing Research Conduct, Critique, & Utilization*, 3rd edition. Philadelphia, WB Saunders and Co.

Carlson C (2008) Development and testing of four instruments to assess prior conditions that influence nurses' adoption of evidence-based pain management practices. *Journal of Advanced Nursing* **64**(6): 632–645.

Collen FM, Wade DT, Robb GF, Bradshaw CM (1991) The Rivermead Mobility Index: a further development of the

Rivermead Motor Assessment. *International Disabilities Studies* **13**: 50–54.

Conner M, Sparks P (1995) The theory of planned behaviour and health behaviours. In: Conner M, Norman P (eds) *Predicting Health Behaviour*. Buckingham, Open University Press, pp 121–162.

Crawford JR, Henry J, Crombie C, Taylor E (2001) Normative data for the HADS from a large non-clinical sample. *British Journal of Clinical Psychology* **40**(4): 429–434.

Crowne DP, D Marlowe (1960) A new scale of social desirability independent of psychopathology. *Journal of Consulting Psychology* **24**: 349–354.

Czaja R, Blair J (2005) *Designing Surveys: a guide to decisions and procedures*. Thousand Oaks, Pine Forge Press.

Devlen J, Michaelson S, Maguire P (1989) *Cardiovascular Limitations and Symptoms Profile*. Manchester, Manchester Center for Primary Care Research.

EuroQoL (1990) A new facility for the measurement of health-related quality of life. *Health Policy* **16**: 199–208.

Ferguson E, Cox T (1993) Exploratory factor analysis: a user's guide. *International Journal of Selection and Assessment* **1**(2): 84–94.

Furze G, Bull P, Lewin RJP, Thompson DR (2003) Development of the York Angina Beliefs Questionnaire. *Journal of Health Psychology* **8**(3): 307–315.

Hunt S, McEwen J, McKenna SP (1985) Measuring health status: a new tool for clinicians and epidemiologists. *Journal of the Royal College of General Practitioners* **35**: 185–188.

Johnston D, Beedie A, Jones M (2006) Using computerised ambulatory diaries for the assessment of job characteristics and work-related stress in nurses. *Work and Stress* **20**(2): 163–172.

Jones MC, Johnston DW (1999) The derivation of a brief Student Nurse Stress Index. *Work and Stress* **13**(2): 162–181.

Katz S, Ford A, Moskowitz R (1963) Studies of illness in the aged: the Index of ADL: a standardised measure of biological and psychosocial function. *Journal of American Medical Association* **185**: 914–919.

Kline P (1993) *The Handbook of Psychological Testing*. London, Routledge.

Lee JW, Jones PS, Mineyama Y, Zhang XE (2002) Cultural differences in responses to a Likert scale. *Research in Nursing and Health* **25**: 295–306.

Martin C, Thompson D (2000) A psychometric evaluation of the Hospital Anxiety and Depression Scale in coronary care patients following acute myocardial infarction. *Psychology, Health & Medicine* **5**: 193–201.

McLafferty E (2007) Developing a questionnaire to measure nurses' attitudes towards hospitalized older people. *International Journal of Older People* **2**: 83–92.

Mcnee CL, McCabe S (2008) *Understanding Nursing Research: reading and using research in evidence-based practice*, 2nd edition. Philadelphia, Wolters Kluwer Health/Lippincott Williams & Wilkins.

Moss-Morris R, Weinman J, Petrie K, Horne R, Cameron LD, Buick D (2002) The Revised Illness Perception Questionnaire (IPQ-R). *Psychology and Health* **17**(1): 1–6.

Oppenheim A (1992) *Questionnaire Design, Interviewing and Attitude Measurement*. London, Continuum.

Patrick D, Peach H (eds) (1989) *Disablement in the Community*. Oxford, Oxford University Press.

Paul F, Hendry C, Jones M (2007) The quality of written information for parents regarding the management of febrile convulsion: a randomised controlled trial. *Journal of Clinical Nursing* **6**(12): 2308–2322.

Pelander T, Leino-Kilpi H, Katajisto J (2008) The quality of paediatric nursing care: developing the Child Care Quality of Hospital Instrument for children. *Journal of Advanced Nursing* **65**(2): 443–453.

Polgar S, Thomas S (2000) *Introduction to Research in the Health Sciences*, 4th edition. Edinburgh, Elsevier Churchill Livingstone.

Polit DF, Beck C (2004) *Nursing Research: principles and methods*. Philadelphia, Lippincott, Williams and Wilkins.

Priest J, McColl BA, Thomas L, Bond S (1995) Developing and refining a new measurement tool. *Nurse Researcher* **2**(4): 69–81.

Rattray J, Jones MC (2007) Essential elements in questionnaire design and development. *Journal of Clinical Nursing* **16**: 234–243.

Shiffman S, Stone A (1998) Introduction to the special section: ecological momentary assessment in health psychology. *Health Psychology* **17**(1): 3–5.

Ware J, Sherbourne C (1992) The MOS 36-item short-form health survey (SF-36) I: conceptual framework and item selection. *Medical Care* **30**: 473–483.

Wright C, Barlow J, Turner A, Bancroft G (2003) Self-management training for people with chronic disease: an exploratory study. *British Journal of Health Psychology* **8**(4): 465–476.

Zigmond A, Snaith RP (1983) The Hospital Anxiety and Depression Scale. *Acta Psychiatrica Scandinavica* **67**: 361–370.

31 Observation

Hazel Watson, Jo Booth and Rosemary Whyte

Key points

- The use of observation in research provides a first-hand account of behaviours or events, collected systematically for analysis and theory development.

- Depending on the theoretical approach of the research, observation may range from completely unstructured to highly structured; observer roles may vary from complete observer to full participant.

- Participant observation is more commonly used within the qualitative paradigm and requires immersion of the researcher in the field.

- Structured observation is more common in quantitative research and requires the rigorous use of checklists and categories to record the observed data.

THE PURPOSE OF OBSERVATION

Observation involves using our senses to gather information and develop an understanding of the world around us. It can entail using all of the senses, judging and interpreting what we perceive to enable us to make sense of the information. When providing clinical care for patients, nurses observe patients' physical condition while also observing for signs of pain or emotional and psychological distress.

In nursing research, observation is an active process by which data are collected about people, behaviours, interactions or events. The aim of data collection through observation is to gain detailed information that can contribute to understanding the phenomena being studied. Observational data provide a first-hand account of witnessed behaviours or events, collected systematically to facilitate the development or testing of theories.

Observation can be used as the principal data collection method in both quantitative and qualitative studies. Whyte et al. (2006) used observation in two ways; first by directly observing the ward setting where nurse/patient contact and interaction took place (see Research Example 31.1), and also by verbal exchanges between nurses and patients which were captured through audio-recorded indirect observation. Whyte's study provides an example of how observation can be used with a range of data collection methods in a qualitative study. The studies conducted by Booth et al. (2005) and Ampt et al. (2007) illustrate the use of observation within the context of quantitative research (Research Examples 31.2 and 31.3).

31.1 Using Observation in Qualitative Research

Whyte R *et al.* (2006) Nurses' opportunistic interventions with patients in relation to smoking. *Journal of Advanced Nursing* **55**(5): 568–577.

This study aimed to identify the extent to which nurses recognise and utilise opportunities to provide health education on smoking to patients in hospital. A qualitative case study, using facets of ethnography, evaluated the smoking-related health education role of 12 diplomate nurses. Data were collected through lifestyle questionnaires, tape-recorded nurse–patient interactions and interviews, observation, fieldnotes and examination of patients' nursing documentation. Triangulation of data enabled in-depth exploration of the nurses' health education interactions in acute wards and contributed to rigour in the study.

The findings indicated that smoking was part of nurses' health agenda, as evidenced by their recognition of opportunities to introduce the topic, although the content of their interactions was variable.

31.2 Non-participant Structured Observation in Quantitative Research

Booth J *et al.* (2005) Effects of a stroke rehabilitation education programme for nurses. *Journal of Advanced Nursing* **49**(5): 465–473.

Using non-participant observation of morning care, this study examined the effects of education on nurses' practice in two rehabilitation stroke units. Fifty-one baseline 90-minute observation sessions were recorded. Patient activities, physical interaction styles, contact person and verbal interaction style were coded numerically and recorded every 20 seconds on a standard proforma. Prior testing of the instrument confirmed its reliability and validity. The staff in the intervention unit received 7 hours' education on therapeutic handling in relation to morning care activities. Following this, the same observation method was used to record 49 post-intervention observation sessions. Statistical comparisons were made between units. After the education, staff in the intervention unit showed a change in physical interaction style more in line with therapeutic practice, with the proportion of 'doing for' interventions reducing (44.5% versus 33.2%; $P < 0.05$). The proportion of facilitatory interventions increased (3.9% versus 6.1%); however, this difference was not statistically significant ($P = 0.098$). The change in styles of practice was achieved with no increased demand on nurses' time.

As a preliminary phase in research, observations can be used to identify routines, activities and happenings that occur in settings to provide the basis for more focused observations during the main study. As the exploratory phase of a study of nurse–patient interactions, Whyte *et al.* (2006) conducted non-participant observation to determine the organisation of nursing care in hospital wards and to identify the times of nurse–patient contact (Research Example 31.1). The aim was to collect data about nursing activities in the wards to inform the development of data collection methods for the pilot and main studies.

Observation can be used to confirm or support data that have been collected through other methods, such as questionnaire or interview (see Research Example 31.3). Providing a record of behaviour or events as

31.3   Non-participant Observation in Experimental Design

Ampt A *et al.* (2007) A comparison of self-reported and observational work sampling techniques for measuring time in nursing tasks. *Journal of Health Services Research & Policy* **12**(1): 18–24.

In this study, self-reported and observational work sampling techniques were compared when applied to ward-based nurses. Nine nurses self-reported on their work over an 8-week period, followed by an observational work sampling study over 4 weeks. Fieldnotes were also recorded. A total of 3,910 data points were collected, 667 during the self-report study and 3,243 in the observational study. The two techniques indicated significant differences in registered nurses' work patterns. The observational study showed that, compared with the self-reported study, patient care (40% versus 33%, P < 0.000) and ward-related activities (7% versus 3%; P < 0.001) were recorded significantly more frequently, and documentation less frequently (8% versus 19%; P < 0.000). Both techniques generated similar proportions of time spent in breaks (12%), medication tasks (13%) and clinical discussion (15%). The study concluded that the self-report work sampling technique is not a reliable method for obtaining an accurate reflection of the work tasks of ward-based nurses.

they occur can help to overcome sources of bias, such as the effect of time on memory, or of participants giving socially acceptable answers. Instead, they provide a means of recording what people actually do as opposed to what they say that they do. When used in longitudinal studies, observation methods can uncover processes that evolve over time.

Observer roles

Depending on the theoretical approach of a study, the researcher may be a participant or a non-participant observer. In participant observation, the researcher participates in the activities of those who are being observed, while in non-participant observation the researcher remains detached from those being observed. In a seminal paper, Gold (1969) identified four observational roles that researchers might adopt.

- Complete participant – the researcher participates fully in the activities of those being observed and attempts to act as one of the group. Observation may be conducted overtly or covertly.
- Participant-as-observer – the researcher participates in the activities of those being observed

but the role is made explicit and observation is conducted overtly.

- Observer-as-participant – the researcher participates briefly with those being observed but spends most of the time observing behaviour/events.
- Complete observer – the researcher is chiefly concerned with observing behaviours and has no interaction with those being observed.

This may be seen as a continuum ranging from the researcher's complete participation with the work and activities of those being observed to complete detachment from them (Figure 31.1).

Where the researcher is a participant, irrespective of the extent of the participation, the research approach is generally qualitative, whereas in quantitative research the researcher assumes a non-participant role, i.e. that of complete observer.

The observer role may not be as rigid as Gold's typology would suggest and researchers may find their role changing as a study progresses. For example, during the course of a study the researcher's role of participant-as-observer may change to that of observer-as-participant, depending on the needs of the study (Melnyck & Fineout-Overholt 2005).

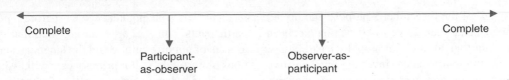

Figure 31.1 Observations roles (from Gold 1969)

There is also the possibility of role confusion, especially when nurse researchers conduct research in their specialist area. Millard *et al.* (2006), in a study on community nursing, adopted the role of observer-as-participant. As a practising community nurse, Millard reported a tendency for nurse participants to involve her in discussions or to seek her advice.

Collecting observational data

Researchers who use observational methods may choose one of two forms of sampling, namely *event sampling* or *time sampling*. Event sampling involves identifying specific events, such as used by Whyte *et al.* (2006). The 'event' in her study was the provision of smoking-related information (Research Example 31.1). In time sampling, the researcher records on an activity sheet behaviours, which have previously been identified within a category system, at regular intervals throughout a specified period of time. Booth *et al.* (2005), for example, observed each participating patient every 20 seconds over a period of 1.5 hours (Research Example 31.2).

Observation data can be collected directly by the researcher 'on the spot' in the research setting, in which case observations are coded using an observation schedule. Alternatively, various forms of equipment may be utilised. The activities to be observed can be video-recorded, with the advantages that the researcher does not need to be present and that a permanent record of the observed phenomena is obtained and can be repeatedly viewed. In this way, multiple layers of analysis can be undertaken, such as an exploration of patients' activities and exploration of nursing activities during the same encounter. Thus a diverse range of activities and interactions can be explored and analysed in great detail from different perspectives (Francis 2004). In addition, both verbal and non-verbal interactions may be captured simultaneously.

Verbal interactions can be audio-recorded, such as verbal exchanges during nurse–patient interactions to identify 'facilitating' and 'blocking' behaviours (Whyte *et al.* 2006). When a range of behaviours is being observed, such as physical activity, non-verbal and verbal interactions, an activity checklist can be used simultaneously with audio-tape recording, allowing the observer to concentrate on a limited range of phenomena at the time.

PARTICIPANT OBSERVATION

This form of observation, associated with the qualitative paradigm, is used to explore, understand and interpret a culture or group from an insider's or *emic* perspective. Participant observation has its origins in social anthropology, where data are collected in the normal surroundings of the people or events being studied. For example, the anthropologists Mead (1935) and Malinowski (1922) studied the lives and traditions of groups of people in their social surroundings by immersing themselves in the cultures of the groups, sometimes for several years (see Chapter 14 for a more detailed account of the use of participant observation in ethnography).

Characteristics and purpose of participant observation

According to Gold's typology (1969) there are three roles the researcher might adopt as a participant observer, namely the complete participant, participant-as-observer and observer-as-participant (see Figure 31.1).

As a complete participant, observation may be conducted covertly to ensure that those being observed are not aware of the researcher's purpose and do not change their behaviour. Covert observation has been used in sociological and anthropological studies, often with the purpose of investigating sensitive topics, thereby promoting an understanding of events and behaviours (Petticrew *et al.* 2007). In a study by Rosenhan (1973), eight participants were admitted to different psychiatric hospitals in America in order to observe the way in which psychiatric wards operated and the behaviour of staff towards psychiatric patients. The participants gained entry to the hospitals by claiming to 'hear voices'. Seven of the participants were diagnosed with schizophrenia and one with manic depressive psychosis. Once admitted, the pseudo-patients stopped pretending to exhibit symptoms and reverted to 'normal' behaviour, although the diagnoses of schizophrenia remained. Through covert participant observation the pseudo-patients recorded their experiences and those of other patients and demonstrated the powerlessness and depersonalisation that was the reality for psychiatric patients at that time. The data collected in the study could not have been obtained had the research been conducted overtly. However, the ethical issues associated with covert observation, such as deception and observing participants without their knowledge and consent, make this a problematic role for nurse researchers.

In participant-as-observer and observer-as-participant the researcher's role is known and consent is obtained from the study participants. The openness of the role allows the researcher to ask group members to explain activities or events that have been observed. The amount of time the researcher spends in participation in each of these roles will depend on the data to be collected, and the researcher may, in fact, switch between roles spending more time on participation or more time on observation as required (Melnyck & Fineout-Overholt 2005).

Negotiating access and building rapport

As discussed in Chapter 10, those who wish to conduct research must obtain permission to access the study site. The process will require approval of the ethics committee, NHS research and development departments and negotiation with local nursing and medical personnel/gatekeepers before potential participants can be approached. Familiarity with aspects of nursing culture and the language and traditions of hospitals and/or primary care will assist nurse researchers when entering a setting for the first time. The researcher may be considered an 'insider', which can facilitate the exploration of practice processes and the understanding of the phenomenon being studied (Carnevale *et al.* 2008). Nonetheless, this is only the first step and the researcher must spend time learning to integrate with people in the setting to gain trust and acceptance.

In an ethnographic study, Simmons (2007) adopted the role of participant-as-observer at a hospital where she was employed as a senior manager. Her managerial role facilitated negotiations with hospital gatekeepers in providing access to the organisation and potential participants. She also found that previously established relationships with many of the potential participants gave her credibility to the extent that they readily consented to participate in her study. Simmons questioned the influence her professional role may have had on potential recruits to the study. She focused on two aspects: participants' trust in her – their belief in the benefits of the study to nursing because of her 'insider' status; her concern that some staff may have found it difficult to decline to participate. However, interviews with participants demonstrated that they felt neither pressured nor coerced to participate in the study.

Negotiating access and building rapport with participants should be considered not as a one-off event, but as a continuing process that requires patience and diplomacy to ensure that essential data are collected (Hammersley & Atkinson 1995; Robson 2002). Without the trust of participants, researchers may find they are not accepted and are unable to access the data they seek.

Working in the field and minimising disruption

Researchers conducting participant observation first enter the setting with a broad idea of what they want to observe. The researcher's intention is to gain a 'feel' for the setting, the participants, how activities are conducted and the context in which they occur. Participation in the work and activities of a group, and a developing rapport with participants enables the researcher to refine the areas of observation, a process that Spradley (1980) referred to as 'forming a funnel'. This allows the observation to become more focused.

Researchers may spend long periods of time working alongside study participants to familiarise themselves with the environment and the culture. This enables them to join in day-to-day activities and to share experiences with participants. Polit and Hungler (2006) call this 'getting backstage' to discover the reality of a group's experiences and behaviour, free from 'protective facades'. How well this is achieved is dependent on the trust and rapport that is developed between researcher and study participants.

Spending time in a site prior to data collection also enables participants to become familiar with the presence of the researcher and any audio- or video-recording equipment that might be used. It is essential that the researchers' presence during data collection causes minimal disruption so that observed behaviours or events accurately reflect normality. While it is not possible to remove the effect of the researcher completely, it is important that researchers try to minimise the extent to which their presence is felt.

Recording observations – fieldnotes

Fieldnotes are a record of the observations the researcher has made and should be recorded as soon as possible after observing an event to ensure accuracy. They may be written in a notebook used specifically for the purpose or may be audio-recorded. Whichever method is used, the security and confidentiality of the material is essential.

As a participant and an observer it may be difficult to record fieldnotes when and where they occur. The researcher may have to move out of an area to do so. It may also be useful to record fieldnotes in a place that is conducive to thinking about and interpreting observed data, away from an area that is busy or noisy.

The way in which fieldnotes are organised may be revised or refocused as observation progresses, or they may reflect themes that have been identified in the course of observation. The material constitutes collected data and, as the researcher attempts to make sense of observations and their contexts, the analytical process begins. An example of recorded fieldnotes is presented in Box 31.1.

Most qualitative researchers keep a diary/journal record of their personal reflections during the periods of participant observation. In it they record their feelings, experiences and thoughts, and acknowledge their position as a research instrument through which data pass.

Researchers as participant observers must recognise their potential effect on the study participants and the setting, and hence the data they collect. This process, called reflexivity, is critical self-reflection on the researcher's experiences, preconceptions, presuppositions and theoretical standpoint (Mantzoukas 2005). Freshwater (2005) describes reflexivity as '… the process of examining and recording the impact of the researcher and intersubjective elements in research' (Freshwater 2005: 311). In qualitative research reflexivity contributes to the trustworthiness of the data.

NON-PARTICIPANT OBSERVATION

In non-participant observation, the researcher assumes the role of complete observer and endeavours to have no influence on the phenomena under observation. In quantitative research, a validated structured schedule is used for data collection, whereas in qualitative research, less structured forms of data collection are used. However, a systematic process to both the collection and analysis of data is equally important for both forms of research.

Recording unstructured observations

As outlined in Research Example 31.1, Whyte *et al.* (2006) assumed a non-participant observer role in a qualitative study of the provision of smoking-related information and used an unstructured approach to observation by audio-recording nurse–patient interactions. The audio-recordings were transcribed verbatim and the data were analysed qualitatively using

Box 31.1   Fieldnotes

Readiness to learn

Assessing readiness to learn is important for any strategy for health education. Fieldnotes made during observation demonstrate a patient's lack of readiness not only to stop smoking but for information about smoking (Whyte, 2004).

Case study 7

11.15am – Nurse B (nurse participant) is working in the ward with a patient who is not in the study. I am in the ward dayroom with Sheila (patient participant).

Sheila is talking with three patients, all of whom are smoking. The talk is about smoking – ways of giving up, feeling like outcasts, problems caused by smoking. Sheila says she has spent a lot of money trying to give up and she wishes she hadn't bothered and just spent it on cigarettes instead. Doctors have been telling her for years that smoking is the cause of her heart trouble but she doesn't believe it as all of her family has had heart trouble and none of them smokes. She thinks it's in her genes and nothing to do with smoking, although she admits that she might be kidding herself. (Observation & fieldnotes)

I don't think Sheila is ready to stop smoking.

2pm – Nurse B and Sheila are sitting talking beside Sheila's bed. They appear quite relaxed.

Nurse B uses the opportunity to introduce the subject of smoking. Sheila's tone of voice becomes defensive when she is asked if she is a heavy smoker and she tries to change the subject. Nurse B talks about the harmful effects of smoking but Sheila eventually stops the conversation by saying: '... nobody nags me to do anything about my smoking because they know what I've been through.' (Observation, fieldnotes and tape-recorded data)

Sheila is not ready to stop smoking – assessment of readiness would have identified that.

---

a framework developed specifically for the study, based on literature on verbal communication and health education.

Observation methods using a structured method of data collection are appropriate for quantitative studies, collecting data about actions and behavioural interactions (see Research Examples 31.2 and 31.3).

Recording structured observations

In studies that use structured observation, the researcher is a non-participant observer who records the phenomena under examination using a framework for data collection. Such a framework is developed prior to commencement of the study. The researcher's aim is to devise a tool that will facilitate the systematic collection of data in a way that will, as far as possible, limit subjectivity and observer bias, thereby enhancing validity and reliability. This involves a process that is similar to that followed when developing a questionnaire or structured interview schedule.

Category system

The first stage is to draw up a category system from which activity checklists and/or rating scales are developed for completion by the observer. A category system comprises a comprehensive list of the behaviours likely to arise within the situation under observation.

In developing the category system, the researcher needs to be clear about the phenomena to be observed.

Expressing these as concise written statements is an important discipline in helping to ensure clarity. This also enables the researcher to identify subcategories for each category.

In observation research the categories often comprise the following:

- location
- time
- activity
- facial expression
- verbal interaction
- personnel.

Each category has within it a range of attributes or subcategories that are amenable to observation (Box 31.2).

In designing observation schedules, it is important that the categories are mutually exclusive so that the observed phenomena can only be coded within one category (e.g. see the example of 'weeping' in Box 31.2).

When the category system has been developed, the next stage is to assess its face and content validity. This can be achieved by seeking the views of a panel of individuals who have expertise in the topic of the investigation. When testing for face validity, the

---

Box 31.2 Category system for structured observation

Location

Bed, bedside, dayroom, treatment room, bathroom

Time

Starting time, finishing time

Activity

Sleeping, eating, walking, reading, watching television

Facial expression

Natural repose, smiling, laughing, grimacing, weeping[*]

Verbal interaction

The nature of the interaction, e.g. question, explanation, reassurance, humorous exchange
The tone of voice, e.g. soft, harsh

Personnel

Patient, nurse, doctor, occupational therapist, family member

[*] Note that the word 'weeping' is used rather than 'crying', which could be interpreted as 'crying out' as, for example in pain or anger. The careful use of descriptive words is crucial in avoiding ambiguity and subsequent errors in coding.

Patient	Sleeping	Eating	Walking	Reading	Watching TV
1		✓			
2	✓				
3	✓				
4			✓		
5					✓

Figure 31.2   A simple activity checklist

Box 31.3   An activity checklist used in structured observation

Walking

1   Unable to walk, even with maximum assistance.
2   Constant assistance of one or two persons is required during ambulation.
3   Assistance is required with reaching aids and/or their manipulation. One person is required to offer assistance/support.
4   The patient is independent in walking up to 50 yards/metres, or may require supervision for confidence or safety.
5   The patient must be able to assume the standing position, sit down and use necessary walking aids correctly. The patient must be able to walk 50 yards/metres without help or supervision.

---

individuals are asked to comment on the appropriateness of the categories and the clarity of the wording. Assessing the content validity involves asking for views of the appropriateness of each item of the category system and whether, in their view, it is sufficiently complete or whether additional behaviours should be recorded.

Activity checklist

Activity checklists are developed from the subcategory systems. These can be simple lists that require

to be coded, as shown in Figure 31.2. Alternatively they can be more complex. Using a numerical coding scheme to rate the activity can provide a more qualitative level of observation, as indicated in Box 31.3, where 'walking' is rated using the criteria given for ambulation in the Modified Barthel Index (Shah *et al.* 1989).

The next stage in the process is to establish the reliability of the schedule. Reliability in observational methods refers to the consistency with which categories of observation are identified and recorded when the same behaviours are observed and recorded, either by different observers or by the same observer on different occasions. There are therefore two aspects of reliability that ought to be tested during the development of the schedule. These are the *inter-observer* reliability, i.e. the level of reliability of the schedule when used by more than one observer, and its *intra-observer* reliability, i.e. the level of reliability of the schedule when used by the same observer on more than one occasion.

If more than one observer is used to collect data on the same phenomena, it is important that they are trained in using the observation schedule and that the *inter-observer* reliability is evaluated. This involves each observer collecting and recording data on the same situation at the same time and using statistical procedures to analyse the results. The Kappa statistic is a measure of agreement based on the proportion of subjects who give the same responses (Armitage & Berry 1994). The value of Kappa can range from zero, which indicates no agreement, to 1.0 for perfect agreement. A value that exceeds 0.75 represents excellent agreement; values less than 0.4 indicate poor agreement. *Intra-observer* reliability can be assessed using the same statistical procedure, but in this case the data are collected and recorded on the same behaviours on two different occasions by the same observers. It may be difficult to ensure that the same behaviours can be observed on separate occasions. This can be overcome by using a video-tape recording of the activity and making recordings during a series of showings.

The observation schedule can be used in conjunction with a diagram of the physical environment and fieldnotes can be made to provide a verbal description to place the quantitative recordings in context.

ADVANTAGES AND DISADVANTAGES OF OBSERVATION

Observational methods have the advantage that they can uncover and describe practice and behaviours as they actually happen, rather than what people think or say they do. Observation also allows researchers to access the context in which study participants are operating, so can help to explain the phenomena that are observed. Unlike studies that rely on self-report data, real-time observational data is not subject to the effects of recall or to misinterpretation by the participant. They are therefore inherently more reliable. Observation can offer verification of self-report data and contribute to the reliability, validity, trustworthiness and rigour of a study.

Using a structured observation schedule helps to minimise observer bias in that the data that are collected are pre-determined, as is the coding scheme (Schnelle *et al.* 2005). An advantage of using a previously validated observation schedule is that it allows researchers to replicate the work of others in different settings or with different populations. Since structured observation offers a means of collecting quantitative data, this method of data collection can be incorporated into descriptive or cross-sectional surveys or experiments (Curtis *et al.* 2003; Booth *et al.* 2005). Designing a schedule provides other researchers with a tool with which to conduct replication studies.

While structured observation schedules undoubtedly have advantages in terms of reliability and validity, highly structured systems for coding and recording behaviour may prevent the capture of complex activities that occur spontaneously. Use of a rating scheme can have the effect of 'pigeon-holing' observed behaviours such that inappropriate judgements are made about events under examination. In addition, any form of interruption during a period of observation is likely to result in incomplete data collection with the consequent need to abandon the unit of observation.

While useful in helping us to understand *what* people do, structured observation offers little insight into *why* they do it. Underlying meanings that are ascribed to behaviours remain inaccessible when structured observation is used as the primary and sole source of data. Participant observation, on the other hand, is intrinsically more flexible.

Participant observation allows the researcher to reflect the reality of events as they occur and can be used to provide in-depth descriptions of behaviours, events and activities (Carnevale *et al.* 2008), thereby contributing to explaining them in their natural contexts (Oeye *et al.* 2007). The opportunity for the researcher to assume a participant role facilitates the development of trust between researcher and those being observed. This may help to break down barriers and lead to enhanced understanding of the subtleties of complex behaviour and dynamic interpersonal interaction. Participant observation offers a means of studying the art of nursing, whereas structured observation can be used to investigate its science. For any form of observation study, however, it has to be remembered that the events observed represent only a 'snapshot' of the overall activity.

Throughout participant observation the researcher has two roles – as both nurse and researcher. This dual role has the potential to be a source of conflict. There is a risk that researchers may become immersed in the culture and fail to maintain sufficient distance between themselves, the culture and the participants, thereby losing their research perspective and threatening the credibility of the data.

One of the strongest criticisms that can be levelled at observation methods is that the presence of the observer, be that a person or a camera, may influence the very behaviours that are the focus of the study. Schnelle *et al.* (2005) have argued that prolonged exposure to observation reduces the likelihood of behaviour resulting from the 'observer effect'. However, this contention is problematic since one cannot know what the behaviour would have been had the subjects not been observed.

Observational methods of data collection are relatively time-consuming, as the researcher needs to be present during the period of direct observation, or when conducting or viewing video tape-recordings, and hence are considered costly to undertake.

VALIDITY AND RELIABILITY

As has been seen, observation can be used in both qualitative and quantitative studies. In qualitative studies, the terms used to encompass the concepts of validity and reliability have been described as 'trustworthiness' or 'rigour' (see Chapter 34).

In structured observation, the terms 'reliability' and 'validity' are pertinent. The use of a carefully designed tool for recording the observations is impor-

tant. Using a structured observation schedule helps to minimise observer bias in that the data that are collected are pre-determined, as is the coding scheme. All personnel who are involved as observers need to undergo training in using the schedule and in coding and recording the data to ensure consistency and inter-observer reliability of the study. Careful piloting can help identify problems such as observer bias so that corrective action can be taken before the main study is conducted.

The trustworthiness or validity of an observation study can be affected if the observer misconstrues certain phenomena, misinterprets their importance or is temporarily distracted or tired. Some behaviours may be outside the range of the observer's field of vision or may not be captured, being outside the observation period. Actions may be misinterpreted because the observer is not sufficiently knowledgeable about the topic of the study, or the observer may be influenced by a preconception of the situation that is observed.

The presence of the observer can also influence the behaviour of those being observed and hence the trustworthiness and validity of the data. The likelihood of this increases when a researcher conducts an observation study within their own workplace (Mulhall 2003).

ETHICAL ISSUES ASSOCIATED WITH OBSERVATION

There are key principles that govern the ethics of nursing research. Adherence to these principles ensures that practitioners involved in undertaking research respect the autonomy and personhood of all participants.

Covert observation

In studies where covert observation is used, researchers should ensure that disclosure is made and debriefing provided for each participant when their participation in the study is completed. However, as a general principle, covert observation is not considered ethical because the autonomy of the individuals who are being observed, their right to information about the study and their right to consent are breached. In cases where covert observation is considered, alternative, more open ways of addressing the problem should be sought.

Overt observation

The researcher should plan the study such that all individuals who may be present during any period of observation are given full information about the study in advance so that they can decide whether or not to take part. However, this may prove difficult if, during the observation, an unanticipated event occurs which necessitates the presence of another individual or group of people. In this instance, the researcher may be required to seek consent retrospectively.

A further dilemma concerns what constitutes 'full information'. It could be argued that failure to provide full information diminishes the autonomy of the individual to make an informed decision regarding consent to participate. On the other hand, by providing full details of the phenomena to be observed, the researcher may risk influencing the participant's behaviour, thereby diminishing the validity of the findings of the study. As it is unethical to undertake research that is rendered less valid by the information that is given, it may be necessary to reach a compromise.

The principle of non-maleficence requires that the research does not cause harm. The researcher may come across an incident where they feel the need to intervene in clinical care, perhaps because of a sense of the need to 'help out' when clinical colleagues are overstretched, or where they observe inappropriate practice. This poses problems on at least two fronts. First, such a distraction will prevent the continuous observation of the focus of the study. And second, it raises ethical issues concerning the professional clinical role of the nurse researcher. The Code of Professional Conduct for Nurses and Midwives (Nursing and Midwifery Council 2008) is clear in stating the necessity for intervention if patient care or safety is compromised. In situations that do not involve patients, researchers may need to discuss what has been observed with members of staff or colleagues. In such cases the researcher's role as a participant observer may be changed to such an extent that the study can no longer continue.

CONCLUSIONS

Recording and analysing observed events and activities as they actually occur in naturalistic settings can enhance a study's scope to provide reliable and valid findings. This method of data collection is appropriate for either qualitative or quantitative studies and, depending on the nature of the study, the researcher's role may involve participation to varying degrees. Importantly, when using observation the researcher must consider the ethical issues associated with this method of data collection.

References

Ampt A, Westbrook J, Creswick N, Mallock N (2007) A comparison of self-reported and observational work sampling techniques for measuring time in nursing tasks. *Journal of Health Services Research & Policy* **12**(1): 18–24.

Armitage P, Berry G (1994) *Statistical Methods in Medical Research*. Oxford, Blackwell Science.

Booth J, Hillier VF, Waters KR, Davidson I (2005) Effects of a stroke rehabilitation education programme for nurses. *Journal of Advanced Nursing* **49**(5): 465–473.

Carnevale FA, Macdonald ME, Bluebond-Langer M, McKeever P (2008) Using participant observation in pediatric health care settings: ethical challenges and solutions. *Journal of Child Health Care* **12**(1): 18–32.

Curtis V, Biran A, Deverell K, Hughes C, Bellamy K, Drasar B (2003) Hygiene in the home: relating bugs and behaviour. *Social Science and Medicine* **57**: 657–672.

Francis D (2004) Learning from participants in field based research. *Journal of Education* **34**: 265–277.

Freshwater D (2005) Writing, rigour and reflexivity in nursing research. *Journal of Research in Nursing* **10**(3): 311–315.

Gold R (1969) Roles in sociological field observation. In: McCall G, Simmons J (eds) *Issues in Participant Observation: a text and reader*. London, Addison Wesley.

Hammersley M, Atkinson P (1995) *Ethnography: principles and practice*, 2nd edition. London, Routledge.

Malinowski B (1922) *Argonauts of the Western Pacific*. London, Routledge & Kegan Paul.

Mantzoukas S (2005) The inclusion of bias in reflective and reflexive research. *Journal of Research in Nursing* **10**(3): 279–295.

Mead M (1935) *Sex and Temperament in Three Primitive Societies*. New York, Morrow.

Melnyck BM, Fineout-Overholt E (2005) *Evidence-Based Practice in Nursing and Healthcare. A Guide to Best Practice*. Philadelphia, Lippincott Williams and Wilkins.

Millard L, Hallet C, Luker K (2006) Nurse–patient interaction and decision-making in care: patient involvement in community nursing. *Journal of Advanced Nursing* **55**(2): 142–150.

Mulhall A (2003) In the field: notes on observation in qualitative research. *Journal of Advanced Nursing* **41**: 306–313.

Nursing and Midwifery Council (2008) *Code of Professional Conduct*. London, NMC.

Oeye C, Bjelland AK, Skorpen A (2007) Doing participant observation in a psychiatric hospital – research ethics resumed. *Social Science and Medicine* **65**: 2296–2306.

Petticrew M, Semple S, Hilton S, Creely KS, Eadie D, Ritchie D *et al.* (2007) Covert observation in practice: lessons from the evaluation of the prohibition of smoking in public places in Scotland. *BMC Public Health* **7**: 204.

Polit D, Hungler B (2006) *Essentials of Nursing Research: methods, appraisal and utilisation*, 6th edition. Philadelphia, Lippincott.

Robson C (2002) *Real World Research*, 2nd edition. Oxford, Blackwell.

Rosenhan D (1973) On being sane in insane places. *Science* **179**: 250–258.

Schnelle JF, Osterweil D, Simmons SF (2005) Improving the quality of nursing home care and medical-record accuracy with direct observational technologies. *The Gerontologist* **45**(5): 576–582.

Shah S, Vanclay F, Cooper B (1989) Improving the sensitivity of the Barthel Index for stroke rehabilitation. *Journal of Clinical Epidemiology* **42**: 703–709.

Simmons M (2007) Insider ethnography: tinker, tailor, researcher or spy? *Nurse Researcher* **14**(4): 7–17.

Spradley JP (1980) *Participant Observation*. New York, Holt, Rinehart & Winston.

Whyte RE (2004) The provision of health education on smoking to patients in hospital: a critical evaluation of the role of diplomate nurses. Unpublished PhD thesis, Glasgow Caledonian University.

Whyte R, Watson HR, McIntosh J (2006) Nurses' opportunistic interventions with patients in relation to smoking. *Journal of Advanced Nursing* **55**(5): 568–577.

32 Think Aloud Technique

Tracey Bucknall and Leanne M Aitken

Key points

- Think aloud is a technique that allows for the examination of an individual's thinking processes and decisions that are being considered at that point in time. Participants are asked to think aloud while carrying out specific tasks such as problem solving, diagnosis or patient management.

- Think aloud can be used in both simulated and natural settings, as well as conducted concurrently during the task and/or retrospectively during follow-up interviews.

- When planning to conduct a study using think aloud it is necessary to consider the study setting, recruitment plans, data collection, and data analysis processes and strategies to optimise validity and reliability of the data.

- Think aloud technique can be used as a single method or in a combination of methods.

INTRODUCTION

The process of comparing and evaluating information to form an opinion or decision about future actions is fundamental to human behaviour. Not surprisingly, making sound clinical decisions is a key attribute required of clinicians. Clinical decisions are usually made in a climate of uncertainty and with incomplete information. They frequently consist of a combination of factual information and value judgements, and as a result practices may vary among clinicians even when similar information is available to them. The variation in clinical practice has been the subject of much debate, particularly with the growing interest in evidence-based practice. Patient, clinician and organisational characteristics have been shown to

alter the context of a situation, thus changing the availability of information and subsequent patient outcomes (Bucknall *et al.* 2008). Yet in spite of a growing knowledge on the influence of context on clinical decision making, there remains limited understanding of the decision-making processes underlying clinical practice decisions. The think aloud technique, also referred to as verbal protocols, has been widely used in research to elicit information underlying thinking processes and actions.

WHAT IS THINKING ALOUD?

Thinking aloud is a technique that allows for the examination of an individual's thinking processes and decisions that are being considered at that point in time. Subjects are asked to think aloud while carrying out specific tasks such as problem solving, diagnosis or patient management. Participants may be unaware of the topic of interest and are required to report only the information being considered and their intentions as they actually occur (Payne 1994).

Think aloud reports provide a sequential record of the subject's thinking and behaviour while completing the specific task. They supply the cues, context, processes, goals and strategies that comprise the affective and behavioural responses mediated by thinking (Schragen *et al.* 2000). In particular, it measures alternative information choices accessed and their sequence of selection, identifying the decision rules that guide an individual's search patterns (Johnson 1993).

BACKGROUND TO THINKING ALOUD

As early as 1890, William James noted the importance of introspection as a method of scientific inquiry (James 1890). Verbal protocols were collected by behavioural psychologists to gather detailed descriptions of subjects' thinking. However, the validity of this approach was highly criticised as the subjects required prior training in introspective techniques in order to specify and interpret their own thinking as they proceeded. Then about 40 years ago, Newell and Simon (1972) used the think aloud part of introspection to pioneer verbal protocol analysis. Think aloud research has since been guided by the highly regarded work of Ericsson and Simon (1984, 1993), who assumed that verbal reports could be analysed like other behaviours.

Based on the principles of information theory, think aloud was used to report concurrently on subjects' thinking during problem-solving tasks (Newell & Simon 1972). Describing an interaction between the problem solver and the specified task, information processing assumes that decisions are based on information that has been processed and transformed by the human brain. This information may be stored in short- or long-term memory. Although short-term memory is readily accessible, it holds limited information for a short duration. In contrast, long-term memory is less accessible but has an unlimited capacity for storing information and is a combination of factual information and personal experiences. Using a complex system of integrated nodes, information is retrieved from long-term memory and transferred to short-term memory for quick response. A clinician's performance is then dependent on the acquisition, storage and retrieval of basic and updated knowledge, and the integration of experience into long-term memory (Schmidt *et al.* 1990).

In clinical practice, health professionals are constantly confronted with large volumes of information that can only be partially processed at any one time. Clinical research based on information-processing theory has attempted to describe the process clinicians use to adapt to differing task complexities. Many believe clinicians adapt to task complexity and storage limitations by reducing information into workable chunks in order to quickly process information and focus on priorities (Baumann & Deber 1987; Newell & Simon 1972).

APPLYING THINK ALOUD IN NURSING RESEARCH

Close analysis of verbal protocols obtained from problem solvers as they worked out diagnostic or treatment decisions has provided valuable evidence of information use in clinical settings. In nursing, much of the research originally focused on the approaches that nurses used to decide on a diagnosis, with little emphasis on the management of patient problems. More recently researchers have applied think aloud to study nurses' decision making during patient assessment and patient care as a means of improving patient outcomes (Aitken & Mardegan 2000). Think aloud research helps us to understand how nurses use information on which to base their practice decisions. As well as understanding the cognitive processes and inferences being drawn at the time, it can also be used to identify faulty reasoning (Offredy & Meerabeau 2006). Payne (1994) also suggests that think aloud may be useful:

■ in providing early insight into behaviours
■ for pre-testing questionnaires to improve clarity

- to compare it with data collected by other methods
- to test hypothesis about behaviour
- to build and test models of behaviour, such as expert systems.

Think aloud can be used in both simulated and natural settings, as well as conducted concurrently during the task and/or retrospectively during interviews following observation.

Think aloud has also been used in combination with other methods to offer greater insight into a phenomenon than a single method alone. Given that all research methods have strengths and weaknesses, think aloud may be used to reinforce or offer alternative viewpoints from the findings of other approaches. For example, a recent study by Bucknall and colleagues used participant think aloud following observation of clinical nurse handover, observations from a non-participant observer, and a ward environment assessment that included staffing resources and patient profiles (Forbes *et al.* 2009). From this data we could analyse the type of information given in handover, the type of data sought following handover, the influencing contextual characteristics and the use of the information in planning nursing care.

Research Example 32.1 provides an overview of six studies that illustrate the different uses of the think aloud methodology in gaining an understanding of the decision-making processes and products of nursing across different clinical settings.

HOW TO USE THINK ALOUD

When planning to conduct a study using think aloud it is necessary to consider a variety of questions about the aims of the study, which will influence the specific method that is used. These questions concern the study setting, recruitment plans, data collection and analysis processes, and strategies to optimise validity and reliability of the data.

Possibly the most fundamental question regarding method is whether the work can be conducted in the natural setting or whether a simulated setting provides an environment that will adequately answer the questions being considered. Natural settings enable you to study your research question in the usual practice environment, thereby enhancing the external validity of your findings. However, it is limited by needing to conform to the limitations of usual practice and does not allow you to control the research setting (Aitken & Mardegan 2000).

In contrast, simulated settings allow easy control and reproducibility of the decision scenario, and the ability to preselect the task that you wish to study in order to optimise the relevance to the research question and to compress the elements of the decision task, thereby reducing the time and resources required (Aitken & Mardegan 2000; Fonteyn *et al.* 1993). However, depending on the research question being investigated and the level of complexity of the simulated environment, it may not truly replicate the characteristics that influence practice or allow for interaction between the participant and either patients or colleagues, thereby limiting the external validity of findings (Lutfey *et al.* 2008). Where simulations are used, it is essential that they are developed through thorough review of real practice, with extensive review by experts in the field to ensure content validity (Fonteyn *et al.* 1993; Goransson *et al.* 2007).

RECRUITMENT

Elements to determine when developing a plan for recruitment of participants into a study using think aloud include the number of participants, any particular levels or types of experience or expertise of the participants and the process to be used to recruit participants.

Participant numbers in think aloud studies are generally relatively low due to the depth and richness of data that is usually gained from each participant, with some reports suggesting that as few as five or six participants produce reasonably stable results (Van Den Haak *et al.* 2003). As participant numbers increase, there is the ability to synthesise findings from individual participants and make some comparisons across the participants, as well as to draw some inferences about the overall reasoning process (Fonteyn *et al.* 1993). Large participant numbers are more likely to be found in short decision

32.1   Different Approaches to Using Think Aloud

Study 1: Using think aloud in simulations

Tanner CA, Padrick KP, Weastfall UE, Putzier DJ (1987) Diagnostic reasoning strategies of nurses and nursing students. *Nursing Research* **36**(6): 358.

In a study of nurses and nursing students, Tanner *et al.* (1987) examined their diagnostic reasoning strategies using the verbal protocol method. Subjects (n = 43) were asked to think aloud as they progressed through their problem solving following three simulated patient situations. These situations included: (a) a verbal change of shift report; (b) a video with a patient showing signs and symptoms suggesting one or more problems; and (c) additional data containing past history and current health data. It was concluded that the diagnostic reasoning processes of nurses are similar to those of physicians. Subjects generated early hypotheses and directed subsequent data collection to confirm or eliminate hypotheses. The findings also suggested that the more experienced and knowledgeable nurses were more specific in data collection and diagnostic accuracy.

Study 2: Using think aloud in natural settings

Han K-J, Kim HS, Kim M-J, Hong K-J, Park S, Yun S-N *et al.* (2007) Thinking in clinical nursing practice: a study of critical care nurses thinking applying the think-aloud, protocol analysis method. *Asian Nursing Research* **1**(1): 68–82.

Five critical care nurses consented to think aloud while they were carrying out patient care in a Korean hospital that contained five different types of critical care unit. Han and colleagues (2007) aimed to discover the type of information, the sequence and use of data collection, and the processes involved in the nurses' thinking. Following a practice routine in non-clinical situations, the participants were told to verbalise all their thoughts as they cared for the patients for a 40–50 minute duration. All thinking aloud was audio-recorded at the beginning of a shift following handover. A researcher followed each participant to prompt them when they failed to speak after several seconds. All care was conducted under normal circumstances except that the nurse was speaking into a lapel microphone. Data analysis used three phases: recording and transcribing verbalisations; encoding; and analysis of sequential patterns. The findings from this study highlighted the sequences and patterns of thinking, types of problems encountered and the breadth of thinking.

Study 3: Using think aloud concurrently and retrospectively in natural settings

Aitken LM (2003) Critical care nurses' use of decision making strategies. *Journal of Clinical Nursing* **12**(4): 476–483.

The purpose of this study was to investigate the decision making of eight Australian critical care nurses who had critical care qualifications and at least five years' experience. Using the think aloud approach Aitken (2003) studied the nurses while they cared for critically ill patients, with pulmonary artery pressure monitoring over a 2-hour period. All patients had had recent cardiac surgery and were in a similar stage of recovery. Nurses were asked to describe the data they were collecting and their responses to that data. They were advised not to try and explain their thinking as that information would be followed up during the interviews. Data analysis used the transcripts from both concurrent and retrospective think aloud sessions. This paper highlights the occurrence and frequency of hypothesis generation, and the stage of deactivation when the hypotheses are redundant to the clinical situation. Nurses used the hypotheses to link information and concepts, continually updating hypotheses to guide future data collection and revision.

Study 4: Using think aloud to compare nurses' decision-making accuracy

Goransson KE, Ehnfors M, Fonteyn ME, Ehrenberg A (2008) Thinking strategies used by Registered Nurses during emergency department triage. *Journal of Advanced Nursing* **61**(2): 163–172.

This study of 16 Registered Nurses was set in an emergency department triage area in Sweden. The aim of this study was to describe and compare nurses' thinking processes, strategies and triage accuracy. Nurses were preselected from the results of a previous study examining triage accuracy. Five scenarios based on real patient situations were developed. Participants read the scenario aloud and verbalised their thinking as if they were actually reviewing a triage patient. Content analysis was used to analyse verbatim transcripts. The research demonstrated a wide variety of thinking strategies being used by nurses, with surprisingly little difference between nurses based on the previous study of accuracy.

Study 5: Using think aloud to compare nurse practitioners and general practitioners

Offredy M, Meerabeau E (2006) The use of 'think aloud' technique, information processing theory and schema theory to explain decision-making processes of general practitioners and nurse practitioners using patient scenarios. *Primary Health Care Research and Development* **6**(1): 46–59.

Using six patient scenarios, 11 nurse practitioners and 11 general practitioners in England explored the cognitive overlap between participants. Information processing and schema theories frame the exploration of decision-making processes in the two groups. The study used schema theory to explain correct and incorrect responses to the scenarios, as well as areas of concurrence. Of interest is the ability of thinking aloud and information processing theory to identify errors in decision making. In a time of increased emphasis on patient safety, this approach will facilitate clinician education in decision making.

Study 6: Using think aloud to validate patient management tools

Hagen N, Stiles C, Nekolaichuk C, Biondo P, Carlson L, Fisher K, Fainsinger R (2008) The Alberta breakthrough pain assessment tool for cancer patients: a validation study using a Delphi process and patient think-aloud interviews. *Journal of Pain and Symptom Management* **35**(2): 136–152.

Breakthrough pain in cancer patients is difficult for clinicians to manage. To measure the effectiveness of interventions requires a standardised validated tool that can be appropriately used by patients. This study used think aloud by patients as an additional measure of validating a questionnaire on pain assessment. Nine patients completed the survey. They were told to talk about what they were thinking as much as possible while completing the form. The information provided specific feedback on areas of improvement with revisions being made when multiple patients reported similar difficulty. The think aloud method was reported to be useful in providing both clarity and feasibility of tool completion.

scenarios studied in the simulated setting (Lutfey *et al.* 2008).

Consideration of whether participants' prior experience or expertise might influence the study question is essential. A number of studies using think aloud have limited investigation to participants with specific expertise, for example novices or experts, or specific experience, for example extensive triage experience. Alternatively, groups of participants at opposing ends of the spectrum have been included to allow comparison of findings to determine common and unique cognitive processes.

DATA COLLECTION

The process used for data collection in think aloud studies will vary depending on the research question being answered, the setting for the study and the time frame needed to collect sufficient data to answer the question. Despite these differences the common principles of audio recording, training of participants, provision of instructions and interaction with the participant will need to be considered for all think aloud studies.

Data collected from the participant will be recorded on an audio recorder (in some instances video recording will also be used). It is essential that the audio recorder is an appropriate size and placed to avoid interruption to the participant's usual processes. A small lapel-mounted microphone attached to a pocket-size recorder is often ideal. Pilot work using the study equipment within the study environment is essential to determine the quality of the audio recording and the amount of background noise, so as to ensure the think aloud can be heard adequately for transcription purposes.

Training participants in the technique of think aloud is an important component of data collection and provides an opportunity for the researcher to explain to participants that they should only be attempting to verbalise, not rationalise, their thought processes. Training also allows participants to practise the process and ask any questions they might have, particularly those regarding what elements of information should be verbalised (Li 2004). One of the most common exercises given to participants to train them in the method of think aloud is to ask them to 'count the number of windows in their home', as it requires sequential progression through various rooms in their home while being a simple exercise that most participants are able to complete rapidly, thereby giving confidence in the technique. Other exercises include counting the number of dots on a page or performing an arithmetic exercise. Some investigators consider that it is important to select practice tasks where the researcher can verify the accuracy of the verbalisations (Nicholls & Polman 2008).

Other advice given to participants prior to beginning data collection includes the need to keep talking as long as the participant is thinking, as well as the lack of need to provide an explanation or rationale for thoughts or actions, or to make thoughts rational (Aitken & Mardegan 2000; Nicholls & Polman 2008). If a follow-up interview is being conducted it is useful to emphasise that this interview can be used for clarification of decision processes. The clarity and simplicity of instructions to participants are particularly important in limiting the bias to participants' cognitive processing. Wherever possible, participants should not be told the explicit hypotheses being investigated in the study, but instead be given general information. For example, in a series of studies investigating critical care nursing practice, participants have been given general information about the focus of the study (how the participants cared for critically ill patients) rather than advice on the specific focus of haemodynamic monitoring (Aitken 2000) or sedation assessment and management (Aitken *et al.* 2009). Such strategies help to reduce the likelihood that participants will be tempted to concentrate on a specific area of practice in a way that does not reflect usual processes.

Interaction with the participant should be minimal during data collection, preferably limited to prompts to 'keep talking' or 'keep thinking aloud' when the participant stops verbalising (Ericsson & Simon 1993; Van Den Haak *et al.* 2003). This guidance is intended to reduce any influence or change to the usual cognitive processes. Throughout the data collection session it is helpful if the researcher takes notes on the activities that are being undertaken.

These notes will help to inform a follow-up interview if one is being used, and also to provide clarity and context during data analysis.

DATA ANALYSIS

Analysis of think aloud data generally consists of three steps – transcribing, segmenting and coding.

Transcribing

The first stage of data analysis requires converting the verbal data from an audio recording to a verbatim transcription. Depending on whether the think aloud process was conducted within the natural or simulated setting, this transcription may be time-consuming and problematic if there is significant background noise, poor-quality recording or lack of clarity of the participant's speech. Transcription may be more accurate if it is carried out by someone who is familiar with the content area (Fonteyn *et al.* 1993); however, care must be taken that they transcribe only the words that were actually verbalised rather than what the transcriber might be expecting.

Segmenting

This phase of data analysis involves dividing the transcription into meaningful components so that each segment deals with a single, but complete, decision process (Yang 2003). At this point most investigators remove data that are not relevant to the decision task, for example social interaction with colleagues.

Coding

Coding involves assigning categories or concepts to each of the identified segments. These codes may consist of a single level or alternatively incorporate multiple levels of categories and subcategories. Within the coding component of analysis there is a requirement to develop the coding schemes and protocols – this may be undertaken prior to data collection with categories determined *a priori* based on current literature or practice (Ericsson & Simon 1993) or may be developed inductively throughout data analysis, with the data informing development of categories (Fonteyn *et al.* 1993; Yang 2003; Bloem *et al.* 2008; Nicholls & Polman 2008).

There are two perspectives regarding how to approach coding, with Ericsson and Simon (1993) recommending that segments are coded in random order, thereby reducing the possibility of introducing bias as a result of the contextual information provided prior to and following the segment. Using this process is believed to increase the likelihood that the analysis is an accurate reflection of what was actually said, rather that what the analyst believed the participant was thinking or how the analyst would have thought in a similar situation.

The alternative, and most common, perspective is to code the data in sequential order, thereby allowing the contextual information to inform the interpretation of the data. Throughout this process the analyst builds up an overall understanding of the data, including different patterns between individual participants. To reduce the chance of bias, strategies such as dual coding by two analysts and limited knowledge of the study hypotheses and participants' background should be used (strategies discussed under 'Issues of validity and reliability').

Detailed steps within the coding phase have been described, with one of the most clear processes put forward by Fonteyn and colleagues (1993). These authors propose a three-step coding process involving:

- referring phrase analysis – identification of all nouns and noun phrases to allow identification of the concepts used by the participant
- assertional analysis – identification of the assertions made by participants to determine the relationships between concepts
- script analysis – identification of the operators used by participants and how they structured the problems, made choices and progressed through the decision process.

Box 32.1 demonstrates an example of think aloud analysis.

401

Box 32.1   An example of think aloud analysis

Think aloud transcript

She has a fair bit of pain because she has had a cut in her neck from the operation last night and that hurts … she can open her eyes and all of that stuff … But she is a lot more awake than yesterday and that is because we have taken one of the sedation drugs away … her BP is a bit high, she seems to be a bit rigid, [to patient] Natalie – do you have pain? [patient responds with nod], [to patient] Is that pain in your neck? [patient responds with nod] … I am just going to give 2 ml of fentanyl for pain relief. She has a bit of bruising around her neck.

Phrase	Category	Cues used
She has a fair bit of pain because she has had a cut in her neck from the operation last night and that hurts	Evaluation	Pain, wounds
she can open her eyes and all of that stuff	Assessment	Eye opening
But she is a lot more awake than yesterday	Evaluation	Wakefulness
that is because we have taken one of the sedation drugs away	Evaluation	Sedative administration
her blood pressure is a bit high	Assessment	BP
she seems to be a bit rigid	Assessment	Rigidity
[to patient] do you have pain? [patient responds with nod]	Assessment	Patient's experience of pain
[to patient] Is that pain in your neck? [patient responds with nod]	Assessment	Patient's experience of pain
I am just going to give 2 ml of fentanyl for pain relief	Management	Fentanyl
She has a bit of bruising around her neck	Assessment	Wound, bruising

VALIDITY AND RELIABILITY

There has been limited investigation of the reliability and validity of think aloud as a data collection technique within various settings, including healthcare. Considerations to optimise validity and reliability include specifying what level of verbalisation is being sought from participants, the timing of data collection and processes to optimise each phase of data analysis.

Ericsson and Simon (1993) describe three levels of verbalisation.

1 Vocalisation of covert articulation that requires no intermediate processes and the subject is not required to expend special effort to achieve this.

2 Description and explication of the thought content that does not require bringing new information, but simply explicating or labelling information that is held in a compressed internal format.

3 Explanation and discussion of thought processes, which involves linking information from both short- and long-term memory.

Ericsson and Simon (1993) argue that levels 1 and 2 verbalisation do not change the sequence of information; however, level 3 verbalisation requires an additional process of information retrieval that changes the sequence of heeded information and therefore no longer reliably reflects the usual cognitive processes. This view is supported by a number of other researchers in the field (Yang 2003; Nicholls & Polman 2008), but argued against by others (Davison *et al.* 1995; Nielsen & Yssing 2004; Guan *et al.* 2006). The opposing view, although in the minority in the literature, does suggest that practitioners think faster than they speak, have difficulty verbalising the complexity of their thought processes and consider that think aloud interferes with their usual problem-solving process (Nielsen & Yssing 2004).

The reliability of data collection through think aloud may be affected by the timing of the data collection. Concurrent think aloud is often considered to accurately and completely reflect the usual cognitive processes used in performing the task (Fonteyn *et al.* 1993), while retrospective think aloud is more likely to be open to error through either inaccurate memory of the decision task or the requirement to explain a procedure and therefore access long-term memory (Yang 2003). Despite this, a benefit of retrospective think aloud is that it does not require the participant to verbalise until after the task is complete, therefore reducing the interference with usual task processes (Guan *et al.* 2006). A combination of concurrent and retrospective think aloud is considered as a potential strategy to provide the most accurate and full description of the reasoning used during a particular problem-solving task (Fonteyn *et al.* 1993) and has been used in a number of studies into nursing practice (Aitken 2000; Goransson *et al.* 2008; Aitken *et al.* 2009) as well as other fields (Bloem *et al.* 2008).

Each phase of the data analysis should be checked by a second person to ensure inter-coder reliability. In the transcribing phase this is relatively easy and involves someone other than the transcriber listening to the audio-tapes as they check the content against the transcription, and should be carried out on all the data from each participant. Within the segmenting phase reliability testing can be achieved by having a second coder segment a component of the transcriptions, with segments compared between the coders (Ericsson & Simon 1993). If significant differences are present between the two versions of analysis, further discussion and clarification of the rules guiding this phase of the analysis are required before repeating the process. Reliability testing of the coding phase of data analysis should also be undertaken, using a similar process to that outlined for the segmenting phase. Assessment of inter-coder reliability for the segmenting and encoding phases is usually carried out on 10–20% of the study data (Goransson *et al.* 2008).

Bias in data analysis may also occur, generally as a result of the data coders having prior knowledge of the research question or hypotheses under investigation and therefore subconsciously wanting to support or disprove the hypotheses. Alternatively, data coders may expect participants to think in the same way that they do, and therefore add meaning to the analysis that is not explicit in the data. As far the first source of bias is concerned, data coders should, if possible, be limited in their knowledge of the explicit hypotheses under investigation and group membership, for example if there are both novice and expert participants in the study (Goransson *et al.* 2008). The second source of bias can be limited by coders randomly coding segments of information rather than coding them in sequential order, by having coders without domain specific knowledge (Li 2004) or alternatively by computerising as much of the analysis as possible (Li 2004; Goransson *et al.* 2007).

One technique that has been suggested to improve the trustworthiness of think aloud data is to return the analysis to each participant to verify whether the protocols compiled for them truly reflect their cognitive processes (Li 2004; Nicholls & Polman 2008). The value of this process may be limited as it is unlikely that participants will be able to accurately recall their cognitive processes (Fonteyn *et al.* 1993), or participants may actually proceed through a decision scenario in a different manner to how they believe, although it is reasonable to expect they may be able to confirm broad concepts.

ETHICAL ISSUES

Earlier studies by nursing researchers were mostly conducted in simulated settings due to ethical concerns about disruption to the subject's thinking, which may potentially lead to patient care errors in real clinical settings. However, there is evidence to suggest that the talking that occurs is similar to discussions that routinely take place between students and educators or doctors and nurses, and therefore should not compromise patient care (Fonteyn *et al.* 1993; Greenwood & King 1995; Aitken 2000; Aitken & Mardegan 2000).

Two processes can be followed to reduce the risk of harm to patients. First, an explanation of the process to the patients and families prior to commencing data collection. In this situation, they are usually given an explanation about the process and a reassurance that the data collection will be stopped if they find it upsetting. Second, the subjects are encouraged not to verbalise any information that they believe would be upsetting for the patient to hear. Information can be discussed either away from the bedside or later, during the interview process (Greenwood & King 1995; Aitken & Mardegan 2000).

Other ethical considerations regarding privacy and anonymity of patient information can be addressed by deleting from the written transcripts any identifying information that is audio-recorded inadvertently. Given that the focus of the study is on the individual nurse's thinking and the low level of risk for patients, then patient consent may not always be required.

Other ethical issues concerning recruitment and data collection are not unique to think aloud. Similar concerns were documented in an observational study by Bucknall (2000; 2003) where audio recordings of an observer following a nurse were collected. However, in think aloud it is particularly important that participation is voluntary in order to minimise the chance that participants strive to provide data that they believe is being sought and to be truthful in their responses (Li 2004). Ensuring that the conduct, particularly the recruitment and data analysis, is not undertaken by anyone in a management role within the study setting will also help to increase the truthfulness of the data provided.

STRENGTHS AND LIMITATIONS

Think aloud provides a unique opportunity to study decision making in the natural clinical setting in that it offers a greater understanding of observed behaviour compared with the same subject working under silent conditions (Ericsson & Simon 1993). In particular, it makes available detailed information concurrently being processed by the decision maker. Although it is relatively inexpensive to collect the information, data analysis is detailed and very time-consuming.

Importantly, participants do not need to be trained in the process of introspection to carry out the task, as interpretation is not required. Subjects need to be instructed only to verbalise their thoughts as they arise, not to try and explain them (Ericsson & Simon 1993). Retrospective recall during interviews and field observations can later be used for this purpose. However, retrospective reports are subject to recall bias, where reconstruction of the decision process may occur, rather than the actual processing, and as a result are less valued than concurrent reports. Nevertheless, Ericsson and Simon (1998) have recognised that when subjects are asked to retrospectively explain their thinking, their performance is changed and indeed, mostly improved. Such cases offer an educational opportunity to improve student reasoning and have been likened to researchers expressing their analysis in writing.

However, three main concerns have been raised about think aloud reports. These are: the validity of reports equating to thinking; the reactivity of subjects when reporting their thinking; and the objectivity of the reports compared with other behavioural research (Crutcher 1994).

Critics of think aloud argue that verbalisations may reflect the norms for behaviour rather than verification of the underlying processes because people are unable to report on higher-order mental processes. It is also recognised that heavy cognitive loads may limit verbalisations, although their completeness may depend on conscious processing of information (Ericsson & Simon 1993).

In addition, think aloud has been criticised for increasing reaction times for task performance and changing the outcomes of decisions. In using cognitive resources to verbalise thinking, think aloud may alter the process or at the very least focus the person on information that is more readily available to report. However, Barber and Roehling (1993) found that think aloud reports using two different mediums (written or verbal reports) did not affect task performance of information requested or decision outcomes. They also investigated the effect of prompts on task performance and found no discernable differences between the control and experimental groups. Similarly, Williamson and colleagues (2000) argued that prompts do not lead to reactivity but rather encourage the subject to articulate their thoughts in more detail. Sudden insight from the subject may, in fact, be the retrieval of prior knowledge from long-term memory, reorganised into new schemata (Smagorinsky 1998).

Similar to all research, the quality and objectivity of the research is dependent on the process. Apart from deciding if think aloud is the most appropriate method for studying the decision task, the objectivity of reports depends on the preparation of the subject in the think aloud process and the quality of the data collection process. Evidence to support the validity of think aloud was demonstrated in a study by Biggs *et al.* (1993) comparing data from concurrent verbal protocols with a computer search. Although think aloud increased the time to process, it did not affect the type of information, the amount selected or the accuracy of the decision.

More generally, a criticism of the approach is one levelled at most qualitative research methods, i.e. that a consequence of using small numbers means the results are not generalisable outside the study population. Although think aloud generally uses small numbers, the analysis of many decision-making instances are similar to repeating an experiment multiple times over, this is also known as replication logic. This process does allow for theoretical generalisation to existing theory rather than generalisation to other populations.

CONCLUSIONS

The think aloud approach provides a unique way of eliciting information about the cues, context, proc- esses, goals and strategies that comprise an individual nurse's response to information in clinical or simu- lated settings. Identifying alternatives and their sequence of selection offers researchers an opportu- nity to view and understand the decision rules that guide clinicians during patient care. Think aloud can be used concurrently or retrospectively, as a single method or in a combination of methods. Data analysis can comprise both qualitative and quantitative tech- niques depending on the focus of the study. Notably the think aloud technique is a low-risk, economical way of increasing our understanding of clinical deci- sion making and offers greater insight into problem solving than methods where behaviour is viewed in silence.

References

Aitken LM (2003) Critical care nurses' use of decision making strategies. *Journal of Clinical Nursing* **12**(4): 476–483.

Aitken LM (2000) Expert critical care nurses' use of pul- monary artery pressure monitoring. *Intensive and Critical Care Nursing* **16**(4): 209–220.

Aitken LM, Mardegan KJ (2000). 'Thinking aloud': data collection in the natural setting. *Western Journal of Nursing Research* **22**(7): 841–853.

Aitken LM, Marshall A, Elliott R, McKinley S (2009) Critical care nurses' decision making: sedation assess- ment and management in intensive care. *Journal of Clinical Nursing* **18**(1): 36–45.

Barber AE, Roehling MV (1993) Job postings and the deci- sion to interview: a verbal protocol analysis. *Journal of Applied Psychology* **78**(5): 845–856.

Baumann A, Deber R (1987) Decision making in critical care: implications for future development. In: Hannah KJ, Reimer M, Mills W, Letourneau S (eds) *Clinical Judgement and Decision Making: the future with nursing diagnosis: proceedings of the International Nursing Conference*. New York, John Wiley and Sons.

Biggs SF, Rosman AJ, Sergenian GK (1993) Methodological issues in judgment and decision-making research: con- current verbal protocol validity and simultaneous traces of process. *Journal of Behavioral Decision Making* **6**(3): 187-206.

Bloem EF, van Zuuren FJ, Koeneman MA, Rapkin BD, Visser MR, Koning CC, Sprangers MA (2008) Clarifying quality of life assessment: do theoretical models capture the underlying cognitive processes? *Quality of Life Research* **17**(8): 1093–1102.

Bucknall TK (2003) The clinical landscape of critical care: nurses' decision-making. *Journal of Advanced Nursing* **43**(3): 310–319.

Bucknall TK (2000) Critical care nurses' decision-making activities in the natural clinical setting. *Journal of Clinical Nursing* **9**(1): 25–36.

Bucknall TK, Kent B, Manley K (2008) Evidence use and evidence generation in practice development. In: Manley K, McCormack B, Wilson V (eds) *International Practice Development in Nursing and Healthcare* Oxford, Wiley-Blackwell, pp 84–104.

Crutcher R (1994) Telling what we know: the use of verbal report methodologies in psychological research. *Psychological Science* **5**(5): 241–243.

Davison GC, Navarre SG, Vogel RS (1995) The articulated thoughts in simulated situations paradigm: a think-aloud approach to cognitive assessment. *Current Directions in Psychological Science* **4**(1): 29–33.

Ericsson KA, Simon HA (1998) How to study thinking in everyday life: contrasting think-aloud protocols with descriptions and explanations of thinking. *Mind, Culture, and Activity* **5**(3): 178–186.

Ericsson KA, Simon HA (1993) *Protocol Analysis: verbal reports as data*, 2nd edition. Cambridge, MA, MIT Press.

Ericsson KA, Simon HA (1984) *Protocol Analysis: verbal reports as data*, 1st edition. Cambridge, MA, MIT Press.

Fonteyn ME, Kuipers B, Grobe SJ (1993) A description of think aloud method and protocol analysis. *Qualitative Health Research* **3**(4): 430–441.

Forbes H, Bucknall T, Smenda H, Legg S (2009) Using thing aloud to study nurses' decision making after clinical handover. *Conference Proceedings Nursing a Sound Investment for Healthy Returns*. Royal College of Nursing Australia, p 66.

Goransson KE, Ehnfors M, Fonteyn ME, Ehrenberg A (2008) Thinking strategies used by Registered Nurses during emergency department triage. *Journal of Advanced Nursing* **61**(2): 163–172.

Goransson KE, Ehrenberg A, Ehnfors M, Fonteyn M (2007) An effort to use qualitative data analysis software for analysing think aloud data. *International Journal of Medical Informatics* **76**(Suppl 2): S270–273.

Greenwood J, King M (1995) Some surprising similarities in the clinical reasoning of 'expert' and 'novice' orthopaedic nurses: report of a study using verbal protocols and protocol analyses. *Journal of Advanced Nursing* **22**(5): 907–913.

Guan Z, Lee S, Cuddihy E, Ramey J (2006) The validity of the stimulated retrospective think-aloud method as measured by eye tracking. Paper presented at the Proceedings of ACM CHI 2006 Conference on Human Factors in Computing Systems, Montreal, Canada.

Hagen N, Stiles C, Nekolaichuk C, Biondo P, Carlson L, Fisher K, Fainsinger R (2008) The Alberta breakthrough pain assessment tool for cancer patients: a validation study using a Delphi process and patient think-aloud interviews. *Journal of Pain and Symptom Management* **35**(2): 136–152.

Han K-J, Kim HS, Kim M-J, Hong K-J, Park S, Yun S-N *et al.* (2007) Thinking in clinical nursing practice: a study of critical care nurses thinking applying the think-aloud, protocol analysis method. *Asian Nursing Research* **1**(1): 68–82.

James W (1890) *The Principles of Psychology*. New York, Holt.

Johnson M (1993) Thinking about strategies during, before, and after making a decision. *Psychology and Aging* **8**(2): 231–241.

Li D (2004) Trustworthiness of think-aloud protocols in the study of translation processes. *International Journal of Applied Linguistics* **14**(3): 301–313.

Lutfey KE, Campbell SM, Renfrew MR, Marceau LD, Roland M, McKinlay JB (2008) How are patient characteristics relevant for physicians' clinical decision making in diabetes? An analysis of qualitative results from a cross-national factorial experiment. *Social Science & Medicine* **67**(9): 1391–1399.

Newell A, Simon HA (1972) *Human Problem Solving*. Englewood Cliffs, NJ, Prentice-Hall.

Nicholls AR, Polman RC (2008) Think aloud: acute stress and coping strategies during golf performances. *Anxiety Stress Coping* **21**(3): 283–294.

Nielsen J, Yssing C (2004) *Working Paper: the disruptive effect of think aloud*. Copenhagen, Department of Informatics, Copenhagen Business School.

Offredy M, Meerabeau E (2006) The use of 'think aloud' technique, information processing theory and schema theory to explain decision-making processes of general practitioners and nurse practitioners using patient scenarios. *Primary Health Care Research and Development* **6**(1): 46–59.

Payne JW (1994) Thinking aloud: insights into information processing. *Psychological Science* **5**(5): 241–248.

Schmidt HG, Norman GR, Boshuizen HP (1990) A cognitive perspective on medical expertise: theory and implications. *Academic Medicine* **65**(10): 611–621.

Schragen J, Chipman S, Shalin V (eds) (2000) *Cognitive Task Analysis*. Mahwah, NJ, Lawrence Erlbaum Associates.

Smagorinsky P (1998) Thinking and speech and protocol analysis. *Mind, Culture, and Activity* **5**(3): 157–177.

Tanner CA, Padrick KP, Weastfall UE, Putzier DJ (1987) Diagnostic reasoning strategies of nurses and nursing students. *Nursing Research* **36**(6): 358.

Van Den Haak MJ, De Jong M, Schellens PJ (2003) Retrospective vs concurrent think-aloud protocols: testing the usuability of an online library catalogue. *Behaviour and Information Technology* **22**(5): 339–351.

Williamson J, Ranyard R, Cuthbert L (2000) A conversation-based process tracing method for use with naturalistic decisions: an evaluation study. *British Journal of Psychology* **9**(2): 203–221.

Yang SC (2003) Reconceptualizing think-aloud methodology: refining the encoding and categorizing techniques via contextualized perspectives *Computers in Human Behavior* **19**(1): 95–115.

33 Outcome Measures

Peter Griffiths and Anne Marie Rafferty

Key points

- Selecting outcome measures is a vital part of designing a study.

- Researchers need to be clear about the intended outcomes of care before identifying outcomes.

- Having identified the intended outcomes appropriate measures with evidence of reliability and validity must be selected or developed.

- Researchers need to consider the sensitivity of the outcome to change and the timing of outcome measurement.

- Researchers need to carefully assess the properties of research instruments and not simply accept the claims of others that a measure is valid.

INTRODUCTION

Nursing care is complex and has many facets. However, at its core is the attempt to make a difference in some way to the lives of the people who receive care. Consequently, research exploring the 'outcomes' of care has a central role in the history of the discipline. Florence Nightingale is often credited with developing the modern profession of nursing. What is less often recognised is her contribution to research through her use of outcome data to demonstrate variations in the quality of care in field hospitals in the Crimea and, on her return, hospitals in England. Working with a statistician, John Farr, Nightingale identified the extremely high mortality rates that existed in hospitals and demonstrated the impact of reforms to the system of care, including

basic hygiene measures and provision of space, which dramatically improved the situation.

In a Crimean field hospital the division of labour between surgeons and the nurses could be crudely describe in the following terms. The surgeon's intervention would generally be immediate and often crude (not extending far beyond setting bones, ligation and amputation). Because of the risk of infection, even relatively minor wounds could be life threatening. There the surgeon's job ended. Subsequent recovery was more a matter of accident than design, with little done to prevent secondary complication and actively promote recovery. So poor was the basic standard of care that death was a very frequent outcome. Nightingale's work showed that the relatively simple nursing interventions that she implemented could do much to improve the situation and this was demonstrated by improving mortality. Where the benefits of change are so dramatic and the outcome as clear-cut as death, there is little more required than to measure the outcome of interest over a period of time and watch it change. Because the main change was in the organisation of nursing it was easy to attribute this outcome to nursing.

Fortunately, in modern healthcare systems, while death rates may still be a key measure of success, we can turn our attention to other aspects of care and aim to promote health and better or faster recovery, alleviate suffering and generate positive experiences for patients. But modern healthcare is far more complex than it was in Nightingale's day. In an equivalent modern situation there is no easy division of labour and death rates are unlikely to vary greatly. The initial surgical procedure is likely to be far more sophisticated, giving the patient an improved chance of recovery and shifting the focus to the speed and extent of return of function. Variation in mortality will have far more to do with the underlying prognosis of the patient than anything else, with only a few being at significant risk of death. Most people will recover, but variations in recovery after surgery will be affected by many factors, including nutrition, speed of remobilisation, infection prevention measures, early identification and correct treatment of complications, and a patient's sense of wellbeing. These factors are in themselves important, since infections, for example, are costly to treat and distressing to patients in their own right, irrespective of their overall contribution to the speed of recovery.

Nurses might play a significant part in all these areas, but they will not do so alone. Furthermore, these outcomes are less clear-cut and present more challenges than the observation and recording of death. Issues include how we might measure the speed and extent of recovery and at what point it would be best to do so? How can experiences such as 'distress' and 'wellbeing' be measured? How can we be sure if relatively small differences in a patient's condition are due to nursing when so many other professions contribute and the underlying condition of patients matters so much?

We have somewhat simplified our description of the situation in the Crimea (and no doubt taken some historical liberties) in order to make a single point: in most situations it is not so easy to identify the outcomes of care. In this chapter we aim to examine the key principles in identifying, selecting and using outcome measures to research the impact of nursing care. We emphasise that these are principles only since the potential 'outcomes' of nursing care are too vast to be enumerated.

NURSE-SENSITIVE OUTCOMES

The introduction has already identified that it is unlikely that any change in a patient's condition will be the sole result of the intervention of nurses. Many factors contribute to the outcome of care for a particular patient, including care given by other professionals, organisational, environmental and demographic variables. To this we must add changes in patient wellbeing (positive or negative) that may occur irrespective of external intervention. For a researcher then, the challenge is to identify outcomes that are sensitive to the inputs of nursing. This can be defined as:

'... a variable patient or family caregiver state, behaviour, or perception responsive to nursing intervention' (Maas *et al.* 1996: 296).

There are two key aspects to identifying a nurse-sensitive outcome for a particular study. First, if a researcher intends to examine the impact of a specific nursing intervention they need to be clear about what the intended consequence of that intervention is. While this might sound self-evident it is not always a straightforward endeavour. Sometimes there can be a lack of clarity about what the intended outcome is. In these cases the remedy is clear. The researcher needs to examine critically what might be realistically achieved by a given intervention. Such theory must be strong and not general, in the sense that there should be a clear and plausible hypothesis about the mechanism that links an intervention to a particular outcome. It is not sufficient to simply suppose that doing 'X' will 'make someone better'. For example, a programme of meditation and relaxation during the postoperative recovery period might be introduced mainly because it is thought that it might reduce pain and hence reduce the use of analgesics and promote earlier mobilisation. The link between these outcomes and the intervention is clear. If we added 'quality of life' to the list of possible outcomes the link becomes general and somewhat tenuous and speculative. Equally if the only outcome measured were 'relaxation', then the purpose of implementing such an intervention would be missed.

However, in many cases the relevant outcomes are quite general. For example, there is a growing literature that links aspects of good-quality nursing organisation and leadership to quality of care as measured by mortality (Kazanjian *et al.* 2005). However, mortality is not the only outcome that could be measured, and as we shall see later, may not be the best measure to use for a variety of reasons, not least that it might not be as sensitive to nursing as other outcomes. In these cases researchers wishing to study the results of variation and change need to consider a wide range of outcomes that might result.

There are many possible outcomes and not all will apply in all circumstances. A recent review of possible outcome measures for nursing quality (Griffiths *et al.* 2008) revealed the huge diversity of phenomena that have been considered as nurse sensitive. Table 33.1 shows those most frequently identified, but many other phenomena have been considered and supported as nurse sensitive. This list is by no means exhaustive but it does give an indication of the diverse and diffuse impacts of nursing.

Degrees of sensitivity

A researcher will need to consider just how sensitive to nursing a particular outcome is. This will vary across different settings and according to the precise focus of a study. A study examining the effectiveness of a programme of pressure ulcer prevention would clearly be designed in the expectation that this outcome is sensitive to it. A well-designed controlled trial would ensure that the nursing intervention was the only *difference* in professional input that patients received. However, other factors would still be important in determining whether or not a patient actually acquired a pressure ulcer. An examination of previous literature and local data is necessary to give some indication of baseline rates of the problem.

Table 33.1 Frequently identified nurse sensitive outcomes (based on Griffiths *et al.* 2008)

Indicator	Type
Cardiac arrest/shock	Safety
Communication and successful giving of information	Effectiveness/experience
Complaints	Patient experience
Confidence and trust	Patient experience
Continence	Effectiveness
Failure to rescue	Safety
Falls	Safety
Infection	Safety
Instrumental activities of daily living and self-care	Effectiveness
Knowledge of condition and treatment	Effectiveness/experience
Length of stay	Effectiveness/safety
Medication administration errors	Safety
Mortality	Safety/effectiveness
Nutrition	Effectiveness/safety
Pain	Effectiveness
Pulmonary embolus/Deep vein thrombosis	Safety
Pressure ulcer	Safety
Respiratory failure	Safety
Satisfaction with care	Patient experience
Symptom control	Effectiveness

Problems that are more frequent or severe have more potential for improvement and are thus potentially more sensitive. Existing literature may also give an indication of how much change might be expected. For example, if other programmes of pressure ulcer prevention have shown only small benefits, a researcher might be alerted to the likelihood that changes will be relatively small.

This issue is even more significant where a study is focused on something that is intended to alter quality of care more generally. Clearly a study of pressure ulcer prevention *must* consider pressure ulcers. But what if the study is exploring something more general, such as the impact of levels of nurse staffing on patient outcomes? A recent systematic review of the association between nurse staffing and patient outcomes in acute hospitals illustrates this (Kane *et al.* 2007). A number of outcomes were identified as consistently associated with staffing levels, but the degree of sensitivity to nursing varied considerably across outcomes and care settings (see Table 33.2).

Table 33.2 Percentage reduction in the odds of adverse outcomes associated with an increase of one Registered Nurse per patient day (based on Kane *et al.* 2007)

All patients	
Cardiopulmonary resuscitation	28%
Hospital-acquired pneumonia	9%
Mortality	4%
Pulmonary failure	6%
Intensive care patients	
Cardiopulmonary resuscitation	28%
Hospital-acquired pneumonia	30%
Mortality	9%
Pulmonary failure	60%
Relative change in length of stay	24%
Unplanned extubation	51%
Surgical patients	
Cardiopulmonary resuscitation	28%
Failure to rescue	16%
Hospital-acquired bloodstream infection	36%
Mortality, surgical patients	16%
Relative change in length of stay	31%
Surgical wound infection	85%

OUTCOMES VERSUS PROCESS

A focus on outcomes appears to be an obvious one. To put it bluntly, if nursing is intended to deliver benefit to patients then the best way of studying interventions and care delivery is to demonstrate improvement in those patient outcomes that are influenced by nursing. However, there are many circumstances where this is not possible or is not the highest priority. Outcomes of care can be distinguished from the processes of care: the acts undertaken to deliver care and treatments (Donabedian 1978). The aim of many interventions is to change the *process* of care on the assumption that the process will lead to better outcomes. Clearly such research has a purpose and is of considerable importance. If an intervention is designed to improve care processes it is important to examine if the changes did in fact occur.

However, it should not be assumed that changes in process lead to improvements in outcomes. Because of the complexity of nursing it is often unclear which (if any) particular aspects of care processes are important in delivering outcomes. For example despite their widespread use, there is no clear evidence that using pressure ulcer risk assessment tools has an impact on ulcer incidence (Pancorbo-Hidalgo *et al.* 2006). Researchers designing studies need to assure themselves of the relative importance and priority of assessing outcomes and should certainly not assume that many cherished nursing processes are validated by a link with outcomes. Assessment of process alone is only sufficient when the evidence base for the link to outcomes is clear.

CHARACTERISTICS OF MEASURES

So far we have talked about outcomes in a quite general way. We have offered some examples and illustrated their diversity. Outcomes can be broadly classified as relating to effectiveness (positive impacts), safety (prevention of harm) and patients' experience of care (Griffiths *et al.* 2009). Table 33.1 gives examples of these types of outcome. In this section we will explore characteristics of measures in more depth.

Measuring subjective states

Subjective measures are generally areas where there is self-report of individual interpretations and assessments. Many such outcomes are of great importance and the role of subjective measurement extends to areas beyond what is typically considered 'experience' into evaluations of the effectiveness of care. For example, pain is a subjective state that must largely rely on patient report. To examine changes and to research interventions researchers must often attempt to turn such subjective assessments into measures so that comparison can be made.

There is a variety of approaches to measuring such subjective states. A single concept (for example pain, happiness, satisfaction) can be assessed using a single item with various approaches taken to quantifying it. One frequently used approach, particularly in pain assessment, is the use of a visual analogue scale. Typically, a visual analogue scale is a line 100 mm long, with anchors at either end describing extremes of the state. The patient is asked to mark a position on the line to indicate their current state. The researcher can then measure the line to get a numerical estimate (see Figure 33.1). Some versions will have additional descriptors at intermediate points. Such approaches generally work well for pain assessment and have been widely used in nursing research, but they may not be suited to everyone or in all circumstances. For example, visual analogue scales cannot be used over the telephone and there is some question over their use with children and those with cognitive impairment. A frequently used alternative is the numerical rating scale where patients are asked to give a number (generally from 0 to 10) with similar anchors given. Alternatively, descriptions of pain intensity can be used to form a verbal rating scale

(e.g. no pain, mild pain, moderate pain, severe pain, excruciating pain) or a series of faces indicating increasing distress can be used.

A commonly used alternative to this approach is the Likert scale. With a Likert scale respondents are asked to rate the extent to which they agree or disagree with a statement (e.g. 'my pain is well controlled'). Typically, there are five response categories offered ranging from 'strongly agree' to 'agree' through to 'disagree' and 'strongly disagree'. There is some controversy about the most appropriate middle response category but 'undecided' or 'neither agree nor disagree' are typical. The most positive response is conventionally assigned a score of 5, running down to 1 for the most negative response.

Measurement scales and batteries

For other outcomes there may not be a simple, single item that can be measured directly, even where there might be directly observable elements. Outcomes such as independence (or dependence) in activities of daily living or stress are complex. For example, while stress could be measured by a single question (are you feeling stressed?), the subjective response to this question would not properly capture the more complex theoretical underpinning of what psychologists understand and define as stress. In these cases a series of items are needed to assess the underlying concept. These items form a scale that aims to give an overall measure. To do this there needs to be a clear conceptual basis for the underlying (or latent) variable and a clear basis on which the items on a scale can be summed to give an overall score. See Table 33.3 for examples of measurement scales commonly used in nursing and healthcare research or practice.

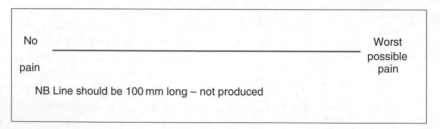

Figure 33.1 Visual analogue pain scale

Table 33.3 Examples of measurement scales

Outcome	Scale	Source
Anxiety	State-Trait Anxiety Inventory (STAI)	(Spielberger *et al.* 1970)
Anxiety and depression	HADS (Hospital Anxiety and Depression Scale)	(Zigmond & Snaith 1983)
Functional dependence	Barthel Index	(Mahoney & Barthel 1965)
Functional independence	Functional Independence Measure (FIM)	(Linacre *et al.* 1994)
Health status	Short Form Medical Outcomes Survey 36 (SF36)	(Ware & Sherbourne 1992)
Pressure sore risk	The Braden Scale	(Bergstrom *et al.* 1987)
Quality of life	EuroQual	(EuroQol Group 1990)
Self-esteem	Rosenberg Self-esteem Scale	(Rosenberg 1979)
Stress	The Perceived Stress Scale	(Cohen *et al.* 1983)

Inclusion on this list is not intended to imply that the scale is conceptually clear, reliable or valid.

Developing scales requires rigorous testing to ensure that the items selected genuinely reflect and relate to the underlying construct. Procedures used include assessing the extent to which each item correlates with the overall score, and the statistical procedure of factor analysis to determine whether meaningful groupings of items emerge that are clearly related to the construct.

It is important that researchers distinguish such scales, where individual items have little significance on their own, from batteries where a series of questions each represent an outcome or item of interest. Since there are likely to be numerous 'outcomes' of nursing care it is important to be clear if a series of questions (for example, 'Was your pain well controlled?, Were you given explanations about your medications you could understand?') are seen as part of a scale or not. If these items are seen as a scale measuring a single outcome, then it is the summary score from the group of questions that is of interest. If each is a question in its own right then issues of the relationship of one question to a 'score' is not relevant. Each item must be considered in its own right.

Objective measurement

Measures of a person's own psychological state and perceptions are of necessity subjective, and this in itself is not a problem for researchers. However, in other cases subjective judgement may be incorporated into an attempt to rate what might be regarded as an objective characteristic. An objective characteristic or measure is one that can be directly measured or assessed. While absolute 'objectivity' is never attainable, there is considerable difference between assessing (say) whether or not someone has been discharged from hospital compared to grading a pressure sore.

In the former case any judgements made can be clearly verified and there is little room for inconsistency. In the latter case there are fine judgements to be made. There must be precise and clear definitions of the parameters to be assessed and the characteristics that define whether a pressure sore is to be graded at one given level or another. These need to be specified in such a way as to ensure that the definitions are interpreted in the same way by different observers (see Research Example 33.1). Other examples may be where patients or clinicians report on a patient's performance in activities of daily living. Interpretations of whether or not a task can be performed can be confused with how difficult it is. Furthermore, if rating is not based on direct observation there is also a problem caused by inexact recall or other sources of error.

While more objective measures of theoretically objective outcomes such as pressure sores might be desirable, this is not always the case. Some subjective states such as pain or stress may have objective correlates, such as physiological measurements that are associated with these states. For example, both pain and stress are associated with elevated serum cortisol and elevated blood pressure. Pain is associated with

33.1 Comparison of Pressure Sore Grading Systems

Pedley GE (2004) Comparison of pressure ulcer grading scales: a study of clinical utility and inter-rater reliability. *International Journal of Nursing Studies* **41**(2): 129–140.

This study measured inter-observer agreement of three different grading systems for pressure sores. All three classified pressure sores into four stages and were apparently very similar. Thirty-five observations were made by two Registered Nurses on 35 recorded ulcers on 30 adult inpatients using all three systems. The two nurses agreed on presence of an ulcer in 29/35 cases. One or other nurse identified a pressure ulcer in 34 cases and both agreed that there was no ulcer in one case. However, when it came to grading the ulcer they agreed in only 54% of cases for the best system and 49% for the worst. Qualitative data identified problems with scale construction relating to visualisation of the base of the wound, discolouration of the skin, abrasions and shallow ulcers. The authors concluded that while refinements in scale construction may improve agreement between raters, there is a need to develop objective measures of pressure induced tissue damage.

a raised pulse. Although it might seem appealing to avoid 'subjective' measures and use these measures instead, such physiological measures are not themselves measures of the subjective state and should not be given precedence because of their seeming objectivity. Such objective measures are of most significance when they are of interest in their own right (e.g. blood pressure).

VALIDITY AND RELIABILITY

No measurement of outcomes can ever be perfect. In many cases measurement is direct and fairly precise, but even then there can be a small margin of error. For example, length of hospital stay, while reasonably clear-cut, is based on an assessment of when a stay begins (arrival in A&E?, admission to the ward?) and is recorded with a degree of precision (hours or minutes) that is never absolutely precise. In general the level of precision in these measurements is sufficient for the likely purposes of research, although the potential of different definitions means that care needs to be taken when looking across studies to ensure that like is being compared with like. Similarly, if studies are conducted across different sites it is important that definitions and approaches to assess-

ment are standardised. However, in many cases outcome assessment is considerably more problematic.

In selecting outcomes it is important to determine both the reliability and validity of the assessment. For clinical outcomes there are a number of issues to be considered. We will consider validity first. In essence, validity refers to the extent to which we are measuring what we desire to measure.

Often consideration of validity focuses on the extensive procedures for validating scales where a subjective state (latent construct) is assessed by a series of items. Some similar issues apply to single item ratings scales, for example a global rating of satisfaction. There needs to be a careful assessment that the answer (or score) 'means' exactly what we think it means. The process of validation begins with an assessment of face and content validity. Face validity is a subjective assessment that items are relevant and clear. Content validity is a more formal judgement that the content of an instrument logically and comprehensively covers the domain of interest. Factor analysis is often used to select an initial set of items from a wider pool and to assess the extent to which a final set of items reflects theoretically meaningful underlying variables. However, of far more significance is evidence of 'criterion validity', which demonstrates that theoretically expected relationships do in fact exist. This can take the form of showing a strong correlation with another, similar outcome or scale (concurrent validity) or that the scale predicts future events in the way that would be expected (predictive validity). For example, a functional status measure examining people's abilities in activities of daily living would be expected to predict ability to live independently at home.

Ideally, to validate a measure there should be an objective 'gold standard' for the outcome, and while this is not always available the issue needs to be considered. Where an outcome measure is the presence or absence of disease or disorder it is often necessary to use a less-than-perfect measure in research because a full diagnostic procedure is complex or unfeasible for another reason. This is often the case with psychological states or condition. For example, the Edinburgh Postnatal Depression Scale (EPDS) is often used to assess the outcomes of supportive and preventative interventions by midwives and health visitors in the antenatal and postnatal period. Validating such a scale is problematic and often researchers simply compare the results of the EPDS to another, similar scale. However, the criterion used to validate the outcome measure should be the 'gold standard' approach to making the diagnosis or assessment. This will of course vary, but in the case of postnatal depression it is a full, standardised psychiatric assessment.

Where the criterion is a category, generally presence or absence of disease or a problem as opposed to some measure of 'amount' of a problem, the researcher needs to seek evidence of *sensitivity* and *specificity*. These relate to the extent to which the instrument misclassifies people using the gold standard as a reference. Sensitivity is the percentage of people who have the diagnosis (according to the gold standard) who are correctly identified by the instrument. Specificity is the percentage of people who do not have the diagnosis (according to the gold standard) who are correctly classified. For research purposes researchers must seek evidence that these figures are sufficiently high in a population similar to that currently being investigated. To do this, researchers must look at the description of the population in previously published research and consider in particular if the frequency and severity of the disorder is likely to be similar in the population at hand.

Reliability refers to the extent to which the same measure of the same outcome can vary irrespective of changes in the underlying outcome. Any measure is subject to some degree of imprecision and many human characteristics vary naturally over time without any underlying changes. Variation can occur because of imprecision in the measure, either because of the measurement equipment or procedure itself (for example a device to measure blood pressure), or because of variation in the way the measure is applied (for example variation in the way the operator of the device uses it). Often in research studies different people conduct measurements and they too may vary in their approach. In such cases the same measurement applied at the same time would give different results. The outcome itself may also vary somewhat over time, irrespective of change in a person's underlying state. For example, blood pressure varies from moment to moment but these changes do not necessarily reflect alterations in an underlying condition leading to hypertension.

Typically two forms of evidence are sought for reliability. One is inter-rater reliability – where a measure is taken at approximately the same time by two different people. The assumption is made that the underlying characteristic (say blood pressure) has not changed during any brief interval between assessments. Over a series of ratings (covering the full range of possible values) the extent to which the two ratings agree is assessed. The other approach is test–retest reliability. This is when the measurement is repeated over time. Again the assumption is made that the underlying 'outcome' has not varied during the interval between measures. This approach to reliability assessment is primarily designed to assess unreliability due to 'natural' variation, although it would also be influenced by unreliability in the measurement procedure itself.

The approach taken to assessing reliability will depend on the outcome to be measured. Test–retest reliability is unlikely to be particularly relevant if measuring a fixed or slow-changing characteristic such as height, but inter-rater reliability is important in that there is scope for variation in the measurement procedure. In other cases both assessments are important. There is natural variation in blood pressure over the course of the day. If the outcome 'hypertension' is to be assessed by a single measure, it is important to explore how reliable this single measure is by assessing agreement between measures over a period of weeks, when the underlying condition will not change but blood pressure will. The individual measurement is also subject to unreliability due to the measurement procedure itself and so in this case both forms need to be assessed. For most patient-completed scales (for example psychological measurement based on questionnaires) test–retest reliability is the key, because asking the same person to complete the same questionnaire twice at the same time is logically impossible, but it is important to establish that the measure is constant over periods when it is thought that the outcome is also constant.

BIAS IN MEASUREMENT

In addition to error, which is random, there is also the potential for *systematic* differences in measurement, also referred to as bias (although this is not intended to reflect deliberate or motivated misreporting). For example, where two observers are making measurements (or where two devices are used to assess the same measurement) there is potential for *systematic* differences arising from different approaches and interpretations. One observer might consistently (perhaps subconsciously) round a pulse measurement up to the nearest 5. There is certainly ample evidence that some 'terminal digits' are preferred to others, with numbers ending in 5 or 0 being recorded far more frequently than others (Wen *et al.* 1993). Such an observer would give a rating that was consistently higher than one who rounded down. Assessment of agreement between raters on interval measures needs to consider more than just correlation. It needs to explore the extent to which the assessment of two raters or repeated measures using the same instrument might differ consistently. Correlation coefficients do not give any indication of such systematic difference (Brennan & Silman 1992).

Because of the linked issues of error and bias, the oft-quoted solution of using a single observer to undertake outcome assessment creates a false sense of security. It is indeed likely that a single observer will be less prone to random 'error' because they are likely to be consistent with themselves. However, they are still subject to observer drift, where criteria or procedures are applied differently over time as fatigue or carelessness sets in, leading to systematic differences in recordings at the beginning compared to the end of observation periods. More significantly, having a single observer does nothing to protect against systematic 'bias', where that one rater uses the measures in a way that consistently over- or under-represents the true value. The key solution is to pick instruments with known reliability, train observers properly and consistently, and check their levels of agreement. If there is considerable disagreement further training and standardisation of administration must be sought.

SELECTING OUTCOME MEASURES

In selecting outcomes and measures to assess them, researchers should never simply rely on the previous use of a measure as evidence of validity or reliability. Furthermore, they should be wary of taking other researchers' claims of validity at face value. Selecting an outcome measure requires a full assessment of the current evidence of validity. The complexity of validation and reliability testing means that the process is a significant undertaking in itself – the development of a new instrument should not be undertaken lightly, without considerable resource. However imperfect, researchers with limited resources are generally advised to use an existing instrument. There are a number of key questions to consider in assessing the suitability of existing instruments.

- Is the outcome of interest clearly linked to the goal of the study (e.g. intervention)?
- Is the conceptual basis of any instrument clear?
- Does it match the outcome of interest?
- Does the measure have face validity (as assessed by the local research team, not the originators)?

- What evidence of criterion and predictive validity is there?
- Are the criteria used to assess the instrument meaningful and valid?
- Is there evidence that the measure is reliable?

Formal claims about content validity have little meaning in the absence of evidence of criterion or predictive validity. However, they may be of relevance in selecting items for a battery of questions (see above) or a battery of outcome measures. We identified above that in some cases the outcomes to be assessed follow directly and logically from the goal of the intervention. In many cases this may not be clear-cut. Few interventions have a single object. Even the treatment of life threatening disease aims to do more than simply save life, and the 'outcome' or effectiveness of treatment has many dimensions and can be defined differently from different perspectives.

In many research studies a 'battery' of measures and outcomes are used and researchers must often select a range of outcomes to measure. Certainly theory should inform the selection of measures. Increasingly, service users, those who have experienced care themselves, are involved in identifying appropriate domains of outcome measurement. However, simply measuring all possible outcomes is not an acceptable approach because there are problems associated with using multiple measures. The burden of measurement (on research participants and researchers) is a vital consideration. Furthermore, taking multiple measures risks the possibility of making type 1 errors where it is concluded that a result is 'statistically significant' even when it is the product of chance alone. Such chance relationships occur due to random variation in the measurements or because of chance variation between groups. Such errors occur with a known frequency when one outcome is measured – the frequency is 5 times in 100, when statistical significance is set at 0.05 (see Chapter 36). However, if a study includes tests of several outcomes that are independent of each other the probability of making a type I error increases dramatically because each relationship tested carries an additional chance of error and so the overall chance of making at least one such error is increased.

OTHER CONSIDERATIONS IN IDENTIFYING OUTCOMES

We have already identified many issues to be considered when selecting outcome measures to use in a study. We identified that it is likely that a given study will have several outcomes. In such cases it is important to clearly identify a *primary* outcome – that is the single most important outcome. Earlier we described a hypothetical relaxation intervention for reducing postoperative pain. If pain relief were the main goal this would be the most appropriate primary outcome, with outcomes such as relaxation and recovery time identified as secondary outcomes. The primary outcome should be identified before the study commences and certainly before data are analysed.

Defining a single primary outcome has a number of purposes. It identifies for future readers what the researcher saw as the most important *question* before data began to provide answers, which is important in maintaining objectivity. Procedures to assess the required sample size should be based on the primary outcome. Emphasis on the results from the primary outcome in framing conclusions helps to avoid making type 1 errors because conclusions based on secondary outcomes alone should be more tentative, as the risk of these errors is higher.

There is little point in identifying a primary outcome that is not sufficiently sensitive to change to show a difference in a study. For example, many studies show a relationship between levels of nurse staffing and mortality, but it is unlikely that introducing a new nurse on one ward would show a measurable difference in death rates. A study on a single ward would thus be destined to fail unless a meaningful primary outcome could be identified (perhaps impact on staff sense of wellbeing and effectiveness).

Another key issue to consider is the timing of outcome assessment. Often the same outcome will be assessed after several different periods of time. It is often easy to demonstrate an immediate effect of an intervention, but such immediate effects are often of less interest than longer-term ones. Researchers need to decide how long benefit must be sustained in order to be truly important. For example, studies of relaxation therapy may show a reduction in anxiety and blood pressure. However, unless this reduction is sustained in some way beyond the immediate period of relaxation the outcome may be relatively trivial if the concern is (say) hypertension, although such short-term benefits may be sufficient if the therapy is designed to help people cope with a transient stress, such as undergoing a painful or uncomfortable procedure. In deciding the primary outcome the appropriate follow-up period must also be defined.

USING CLINICAL DATA AND OTHER ROUTINELY COLLECTED DATA IN RESEARCH

Clinical records and many administrative systems contain rich data that can be used in research. In England, the Hospital Episode Statistics (HES) contain details of all admissions to NHS hospitals in England based on an abstract from the medical record. Each HES record contains a wide range of information about an individual patient admitted to an NHS hospital. For example:

- clinical information about diagnoses and operations
- information about the patient (such as age, gender and ethnic category)
- administrative information, such as time waited and date of admission
- geographical information on where the patient was treated and the area in which they lived.

Some of this information is readily available in aggregated forms and under some circumstances detailed information is available to researchers. The NHS Information Centre also provides detailed information on NHS staffing, which can be accessed and used for research. Local administrative systems and audits can often give even richer data from the medical and nursing records. Some important nursing research has been undertaken using this sort of data, including a series of highly influential studies linking nurse staffing to patient outcomes (see Research Example 33.2).

RESEARCH EXAMPLE

33.2 Using Routinely Collected Data in Research

Rafferty AM, Clarke SP, Coles J, Ball J, James P, McKee M, Aiken LH (2007) Outcomes of variation in hospital nurse staffing in English hospitals: cross-sectional analysis of survey data and discharge records. *International Journal of Nursing Studies* **44**(2): 175–182.

There is an increasing body of research in nursing that has used routinely collected patient and/or workforce data to assess the impact of variation in nurse staffing on patient outcomes. Rafferty *et al.* (2007) explored whether English hospitals in which nurses care for fewer patients have better outcomes, building on growing evidence from the United States. They used hospital administrative data to look at patient mortality and failure to rescue (mortality risk for patients with complicated stays). They also conducted a survey to explore nurse job dissatisfaction, burnout and nurse-rated quality of care. The use of existing data meant that 118,752 patients in 30 English acute trusts could contribute. They found that patients and nurses in the quartile of hospitals with the most favourable staffing levels (the lowest patient-to-nurse ratios) had consistently better outcomes than those in hospitals with less favourable staffing. Patients in the hospitals with the highest patient-to-nurse ratios had 26% higher mortality (95% CI: 12–49%); and the nurses in those hospitals were approximately twice as likely to be dissatisfied with their jobs, to show high burnout levels, and to report low or deteriorating quality of care on their wards and hospitals.

However, use of these data is not without problems. Although researchers can often access data on a scale that they would not otherwise be able to do, it is important to consider that these data were not gathered for research purposes. Before embarking on such a study researchers need to consider the quality of the data. While some objective outcomes, such as mortality or place of discharge, are likely to be accurately recorded, others are not. For example, a study of pressure ulcer incidence using nursing records would be dependent on accurate and timely identification of the ulcer, and accurate, timely and correct recording and classification of ulcer severity using one of several systems. Researchers would not have the opportunity to train observers and so issues of unreliability and bias in observations could be severe. Errors and inconsistencies in recording would also add further to both error and bias.

CONCLUSIONS

There are many issues to be considered when selecting outcome measures for a study. Careful thought and selection of measures prior to commencing a study can do much to enhance the usefulness of study's findings by reducing error and ensuring a valid measure of outcome is offered. Researchers should be wary of accepting the previous use of a measure as evidence of its reliability, validity or utility for a particular study. Nursing care has the potential to make significant changes in people's lives and it is a key task for research to measure and demonstrate those changes properly.

References

Bergstrom N, Demuth PJ, Braden BJ (1987) A clinical trial of the Braden Scale for predicting pressure sore risk. *Nursing Clinics of North America* **22**(2): 417–428.

Brennan P, Silman A (1992) Statistical methods for assessing observer variability in clinical measures. *British Medical Journal* **304**: 1491–1494.

Cohen S, Kamarck T, Mermelstein R (1983) A global measure of perceived stress. *Journal of Health and Social Behavior* **24**(4): 385–396.

Donabedian A (1978) The quality of medical care. *Science* **200**: 856–864.

EuroQol Group (1990) EuroQol-a new facility for the measurement of health-related quality of life. *Health Policy* **16**: 199–208.

Griffiths P, Jones S, Maben J, Murrells T (2008) *State of the Art Metrics for Nursing: a rapid appraisal.* London, King's College London.

Kane R, Shamliyan T, Mueller C, Duval S, Wilt T (2007) The Association of Registered Nurse staffing levels and patient outcomes: systematic review and meta-analysis. *Medical Care* **45**(12): 1195–1204.

Kazanjian A, Green C, Wong J, Reid R (2005) Effect of the hospital nursing environment on patient mortality: a systematic review. *Journal of Health Services Research and Policy* **10**: 111–117A.

Linacre J, Heinemann A, Wright B, Granger C, Hamilton B (1994) The structure and stability of the Functional Independence Measure. *Archives of Physical Medicine and Rehabilitation* **75**(2): 127–132.

Maas ML, Johnson M, Moorhead S (1996) Classifying nursing-sensitive patient outcomes. *Journal of Nursing Scholarship* **28**(4): 295–302.

Mahoney FI, Barthel DW (1965) Functional evaluation: the Barthel Index. *Maryland State Medical Journal* **14**: 61–65.

Pancorbo-Hidalgo PL, Garcia-Fernandez FP, Lopez-Medina IM, Alvarez-Nieto C (2006) Risk assessment scales for pressure ulcer prevention: a systematic review. *Journal of Advanced Nursing* **54**(1): 94–110.

Pedley GE (2004) Comparison of pressure ulcer grading scales: a study of clinical utility and inter-rater reliability. *International Journal of Nursing Studies* **41**(2): 129–140.

Rafferty AM, Clarke SP, Coles J, Ball J, James P, McKee M, Aiken LH (2007) Outcomes of variation in hospital nurse staffing in English hospitals: cross-sectional analysis of survey data and discharge records. *International Journal of Nursing Studies* **44**(2): 175–182.

Rosenberg M (1979) *Conceiving the Self.* New York, Basic Books.

Spielberger CD, Gorsuch RL, Lushene R (1970) *STAI Manual.* Palo Alto, CA Consulting Psychologists Press.

Ware JE, Sherbourne CD (1992) The MOS 36-item short-form health survey (SF-36). *Medical Care* **30**(6): 473–483.

Wen S, Kramer M, Hoey J, Hanley J, Usher R (1993) Terminal digit preference, random error, and bias in routine clinical measurement of blood pressure. *Journal of Clinical Epidemiology* **46**(10): 1187.

Zigmond AS, Snaith RP (1983) The Hospital Anxiety and Depression Scale. *Acta Psychiatrica Scandinavica* **67**(6): 361–370.

Further reading

Doran D (2003) *Nursing-sensitive Outcomes: state of the science*. Sudbury, MA, Jones and Bartlett.

McDowell I (2006) *Measuring Health: a guide to rating scales and questionnaires*, 3rd edition. New York, Oxford University Press.

Waltz C, Strickland O, Lenz E (2005) *Measurement in Nursing and Health Research*. New York, Springer Publishing Company.

Making Sense of the Data

Section 5 is short, but the processes it describes are of critical importance in any research study. Without analysis of data it would be impossible to convey with any clarity or precision what exactly the research has discovered. It is also the stage in the research process that is often the most taxing and confusing, as the researcher wades through a mass of statistical or narrative data and wonders how to bring order out of the seeming chaos.

Chapter 34 tackles qualitative data analysis. Many of the chapters dealing with qualitative methods have already given some guidelines for analysis, but here a clear overview of the broad principles of qualitative analysis is presented, with the aim of getting the novice researcher started. A choice can then be made between major methods such as narrative analysis, framework analysis and grounded theory. The chapter builds on the earlier chapters in Section 3 (Chapters 13–16), and the reader is encouraged to use the five chapters in parallel, and to pursue the suggestions for further reading in particular areas as necessary.

Chapters 35 and 36 are designed to be read together, as they are written by the same authors and use a consistent worked example (updated for this edition) throughout. Chapter 35, however, may be sufficient for some readers who need only to be able to present and describe quantitative data in a basic way. For those wishing to test hypotheses or analyse relationships in data, Chapter 36 takes the reader further into statistical analysis and provides some basic methods of making inferences from data. Recommendations for further reading are given for the student who wishes to pursue statistical analysis in more depth.

34 Qualitative Analysis

Judith Lathlean

Key points

- There are a number of different approaches to qualitative analysis depending on the research design and nature of the data.

- Qualitative data analysis is usually ongoing and iterative throughout the research process; as such it can inform the research design as well as provide an interpretation of the findings.

- The validity of the analysis, triangulation and reflexivity are all important concepts when undertaking qualitative analysis.

- Different frameworks and software packages exist to assist in the practical process of qualitative data analysis.

INTRODUCTION

For the qualitative researcher in nursing, the process of analysing data is not linear or even predictable. Qualitative research studies do not follow the traditional route of hypothesising or identifying a research problem, doing a literature review to clarify what is already known about the proposition or problem, collecting some data and only then analysing these data. Indeed, the actual analytical process can start at the very beginning and inform all the aspects and stages of the research. Furthermore, there is no one 'right' way of doing the analysis and no standard recipe for success. It depends as much on what one wants to achieve as the view of what would lead to the production of a rich account and a deep understanding about the phenomena being studied.

Despite the relative lack of prescription, much has been written about qualitative data analysis and there is general agreement that there are some helpful principles to consider as well as some tried-and-tested schematic approaches and practical aids. This chapter explores these principles and discusses several more popular methods of analysis in some detail. It also looks at the practicalities of qualitative data handling and analysis, including the growing use of software packages.

PRINCIPLES OF QUALITATIVE ANALYSIS

Objectivity or subjectivity?

In thinking about the nature of qualitative research, the discussions have frequently been presented as dichotomous choices. Are objective or subjective data being generated and are the analysis processes lending themselves to objective or subjective descriptions? Is the aim for replication (that is, if a finding holds true in one setting, does it also in another comparable setting) or for authenticity (is this an authentic and credible portrait of what is being examined)? Is the aim to study representative samples or is there more interest in purposely selected samples? Is the ability to generalise conclusively being sought or is it accepted that all situations are unique, and therefore only tentative theoretical generalisations are possible? In reality these distinctions are not clear-cut, although the qualitative analyst will tend to lean more towards the right-hand position in these dichotomies.

Building theory

Qualitative researchers almost invariably agree that theory (or theorisation) should be the primary goal of research. Nevertheless, they frequently reject the formulation of theories in advance of their fieldwork, considering this to be unduly constraining. The process of developing and testing theory is often said to proceed in tandem with data collection, and the main methods of analysis, such as analytic induction and grounded theory, offer fruitful strategies for theory building. So, for example, in analytic induction the analyst tries to formulate generalisations that hold true across all of their data, and when adopting a grounded theory approach, the theory is inductively derived from the study of the phenomenon it represents.

Eisenhardt (1989) provided a useful description of how to build theories from case study research. In doing so she drew on grounded theory building and the analytical methods described by Miles and Huberman (1994). Her logical, step-by-step approach to developing theory includes tips on entering the field, analysing within-case data, searching for cross-case patterns, shaping hypotheses, comparing emergent concepts and theory with the existing literature, and reaching closure (the point when the analyst ceases to add cases and stops going back and forth between theory and data).

Concurrent data collection and analysis

It is common in qualitative research for data that are analysed early on in research to inform the rest of the data collection, the research design and sometimes even the actual research questions. This is illustrated by a study I undertook of the implementation and development of lecturer practitioner roles in nursing (Lathlean 1997). At the outset, I had anticipated using an action research approach where I tried to find out 'how' these new roles should be developed and what processes were necessary to enhance their effectiveness. Following initial data collection and analysis, it quickly became obvious that the prime question was not to do with 'how' but rather 'what', i.e. 'what is the nature and reality of the job of lecturer practitioner?' So I chose an ethnographic research design with a number of different stages, each being thoroughly analysed before proceeding to the next one.

Another reason for analysing data as a study progresses is to identify when the data have reached 'theoretical' saturation (see Chapter 13).

Validation by respondents or researchers

In qualitative research the distinction is sometimes made between internal validity (the extent to which research findings represent reality) and external validity (the extent to which abstractions and concepts are applicable across groups). The qualitative analyst has strategies that can be used to ensure or at least facilitate both. These include giving the original data (e.g. an interview transcript) to the interviewee and asking them to clarify the meaning of their responses. Participant observation (which is common in ethnographic studies) allows data to be collected over a prolonged period and this is accompanied by continual data analysis. In this way, constructs can be refined and checked out with participants. A crucial test of qualitative research accounts is whether those people whose beliefs and behaviour are supposedly presented in the accounts actually recognise the validity of the accounts. However, it is necessary to be cautious about the process of respondent validation, since it cannot be assumed that any actor is a privileged commentator on their actions, in the sense that the intentions, motives and beliefs involved are accompanied by a *guarantee* of truth.

Triangulation

Data-source triangulation (Denzin 1970) involves the comparison of data relating to a phenomenon that have been derived from, for example, separate phases of the fieldwork or the accounts of various participants including the researcher. The claim is that if different kinds of data lead to the same conclusion, this increases confidence in the conclusions. This approach should not be confused with '*methodological* triangulation' when methods either from within the same paradigm or across paradigms are used to study the same phenomena. This type of triangulation has relevance to mixed methods research (see Chapter 27) where, for example, the results of interviews are compared with the researcher's observations or with data from very structured questionnaires relating to the same phenomenon. This can be problematic, however, since it assumes that there is a single 'reality' that is waiting to be discovered, a suggestion that is anathema to most qualitative researchers.

In my research on lecturer practitioners, the presentation of my accounts of their lives to the participants was a way of 'validating' those accounts and a form of triangulation (Lathlean 1997). The accounts generated at the three different stages over three years were compared and contrasted for each participant, as well as being examined for consistency across cases. However, I needed to be careful to distinguish between differences that occurred as a result of the way the data had been collected (for example, the interviews may have thrown up different points about the experiences of the lecturer practitioners than I gleaned in my role as observer) and differences that were the result of real disparities in their lives at separate points in time.

Following the ethnographic study, I surveyed the perspectives of all lecturer practitioners who were in post in one health authority at that time, using a structured questionnaire. Conducting this separate study could have been construed as a form of triangulation as the intention was to achieve a fuller and more penetrating understanding of the lecturer practitioners. But I had to be cautious about interpreting the results. A match or mismatch between the perceptions of the participants in the survey and the 'reality' of the lecturer practitioners as observed in the ethnographic study did not necessarily confirm or put into question the validity of either study. Rather it could simply mean that there were differences between the lives of lecturer practitioners and other people's understandings of those lives.

Reflexivity

Qualitative research stresses the importance of reflexivity, whereby the researcher recognises that they have a social identity and background that has an impact on the research process. Reflexivity is especially relevant in nursing research because often the researcher is also a nurse. In such circumstances the researcher needs to think carefully – to reflect – on the impact that being a member of the same professional group as study participants may have on all aspects of the research process, especially interpretation of research findings. So, for example, in a qualitative study that was undertaken of community mental health nurses' experience of taking part in a clinical trial of treatment for patients with common mental health problems (see Simons *et al.* 2008), the researcher – a nurse herself – had to make a conscious effort to expose and make clear what biases she brought to the research so that the analyses could be viewed in that light. Simons' use of narrative analysis in her study, with its emphasis on the nurses' talk and the *way* they told their stories, was also helpful in this respect.

EXAMPLES OF METHODS OF ANALYSIS

Two particular general strategies for analysis are frequently cited: analytic induction and grounded theory. In addition there are other approaches that are especially suited to more open-ended forms of textual data, such as discourse, conversation and narrative analysis. Finally, since policy and applied research is increasingly important in nursing, analytical methods such as the 'Framework' approach have been developed.

Analytic induction

Analytic induction is a process of analysing data where the researcher tries to find explanations by carrying on with the data collection until no cases (referred to as deviant or negative cases) are found that are inconsistent with a hypothetical explanation of a phenomenon. The process of analytic induction is illustrated in Box 34.1.

From this brief description it can be seen that the analytic induction method shares attributes of 'positivism' or a 'realist' stance in research, for example the setting up of a 'hypothesis' and the confirmation or refutation of that hypothesis. However, it is based on a case study research design, whereby cases are not selected to be representative and therefore theoretical rather than statistical generalisation occurs. Furthermore, the final explanations that result from analytic induction may specify the conditions that are *sufficient* for a phenomenon to occur, but rarely those that are *necessary*. So, for example, studies have shown that certain people in particular circumstances become drug or alcohol dependent, but analytic induction will not shed light on why other people with the same characteristics in similar circumstances do *not* become addicted. Also, in analytic induction, there are no hard-and-fast rules as to how many cases need to be investigated before the absence of negative cases and the validity of the hypothesis can be confirmed.

Grounded theory

For a detailed discussion of grounded theory, see Chapter 13. However, it is referred to briefly here since it is one of the most widely cited approaches to the analysis of qualitative data. While there is some disagreement about the precise nature of the grounded theory approach, most consider that there are usually four aspects in the analytical process: theoretical sampling, coding, theoretical saturation and constant comparison (see Box 34.2).

Some studies claim to be using a grounded theory methodology, when what they really mean is that they are employing some of the stages or principles of analysis, such as theoretical saturation or constant comparison. This is not necessarily a problem but, in these instances, it needs to be recognised that only parts of the approach are being adopted.

Analysing narrative

The most common approaches to analysing narrative are conversation analysis, discourse analysis and narrative analysis. Conversation analysis is based on an attempt to describe people's methods for producing orderly social interaction and has a relatively long history. It is concerned with the sequential organisation of talk – how talk overlaps and the lengths of pauses in a conversation are key attributes. Silverman (1998) says that it is important in conversation analysis to try to identify sequences of related talk, to examine how speakers take on certain roles or identities through their talk, such as 'client-professional',

---

Box 34.1   Steps in analytic induction

1   Set up a definition of a problem
2   Provide a hypothetical explanation of the problem
3   Investigate a number of cases
  a   Find that these cases are in line with the hypothesis – hypothesis is confirmed
  b   Find cases that deviate from hypothesis
    i   reformulate hypothesis and go back to step 3 or
4   Redefine hypothetical explanation to exclude deviant cases and end data collection

Box 34.2   Key aspects in a grounded theory approach to analysis

Theoretical sampling – this is 'the process of data collection for generating theory whereby the analyst jointly collects, codes and analyses his (sic) data and decides what data to collect next and where to find them, in order to develop his theory as it emerges' (Glaser & Strauss 1967).

Coding – this is where data are broken down into component parts and names are given to the parts.

Theoretical saturation – this refers to the point when no further coding is necessary because no new instances are required to confirm a category, and/or when no new data collection is required as there is sufficient confidence about the nature of the emerging concepts.

Constant comparison – this is the process whereby the data and the subsequent conceptualisations from it are compared to ensure that there is a good fit. This happens throughout data analysis.

and to look for particular outcomes in talk, such as laughter, and then work back from there to see how it was produced. For an introduction to conversation analysis, see Heritage (2004).

Discourse analysis is very similar to conversation analysis in that it seeks to analyse the activities present in talk. However, unlike conversation analysis, discourse analysis possesses the following three features:

- it is concerned with a far broader range of activities, such as gender relations or social control
- it does not always use analysis of ordinary conversation as a baseline for understanding talk in organisational settings
- it works with far less precise transcripts than conversation analysis.

A good example of the use of discourse analysis is to be found in the study of violent behaviour in an acute mental health setting by Benson *et al.* (2003) (see Research Example 34.1). In this study, discourse analysis was found to be illuminative because of

'its capacity to reveal constructions of the self, the other and the world, and the ways in which actors understand social actions and interactions' (Benson *et al.* 2003: 918)

In this respect, the authors are referring to the work of Potter and Wetherell (1995), which is a good reference source for discourse analysis, as is Potter (2004).

There are numerous definitions and conceptualisations of narrative research and narrative analysis, which leads to differing views and methods of analysis. Lieblich *et al.* (1998) suggested the dimensions of holism and category as important differentiations, wherein the first approach analyses a narrative in its entirety and the latter supports the extraction of text for thematic classification. Reisman (2008), in a good source book, offers four approaches – thematic, structural, visual and performative analysis. Smith and Sparkes (2008) present a helpful typology of narrative analysis predicated by the use of systematic and rigorous strategies and techniques designed to identify, explain and think about the features of the story. They divide story analysis between investigating the 'whats' and 'hows'. This involves questions being asked of the stories such as why was the narrative told in that way and in that order? How is the narrator located in relation to other characters and to the audience? What are the identity claims and how are these performed?

Bingley *et al.* (2008) claim that qualitative analysis methods applied to narratives and narrative analysis

34.1   A Study Using Discourse Analysis

Benson A, Secker J, Balfe E, Lipsedge M, Robinson S, Walker J (2003) Discourses of blame: accounting for aggression and violence on an acute mental health inpatient unit. *Social Science and Medicine* **57**: 917–926.

This study was based on 16 semi-structured interviews in one mental health unit and aimed to address the paucity of research on how all involved in such a setting understand the attributed meaning to violent or aggressive situations and how these attributions justified individual perceptions, reactions and actions. Although the analysis was based on only two incidents involving one client (the other clients being unwilling or unable to give retrospective accounts), it clearly demonstrates how discourse analytic techniques can be used to examine client accounts and those of staff members engaged in the incidents. The findings reveal that participants discussed key themes in terms of dilemmas, e.g. whether the violent or aggressive behaviour was 'mad' or bad'; predictable or unpredictable; and had resulted from a personality disorder or mental illness. It also indicated that discourses of staff and clients were remarkably similar and had at their core the attribution of blame.

34.2   A Narrative Study

Brown J, Addington-Hall J (2008) How people with motor neurone disease talk about living with their illness: a narrative study. *Journal of Advanced Nursing* **62**(2): 200–208.

This study was based on longitudinal narrative interviews conducted at three-monthly intervals over 18 months with 13 people suffering from motor neurone disease. Narrative case studies were used, with the unit of analysis being the person (patient) in their own home or a care home. The interviews were analysed by focusing on the form and content of the narrative. Four types of narrative or storyline were found: sustaining (relating to living life and keeping active); enduring (where a person feels disempowered and unable to fight); preserving (where the essence is survival); and fracturing (with its concern with loss and fear of what is to come). The paper concluded that 'storylines' help make sense of complex narratives by encouraging listening – on the part of the 'interviewer' – as well as being organising threads to assist professionals and families to better understand what it is like for someone to live with motor neurone disease. The paper also includes a useful diagram of the iterative process for analysis of narratives, including the stages of immersion, analysis of narratives, trial framework, framework mapping, and narrative types and storylines.

are distinct approaches. In the former, general methods of qualitative analysis such as thematic, discourse and conversation analysis may be applied to the interpretation of narratives as well as other sources of data. In the latter, specific analytic techniques have been developed which are devoted to narratives. Bingley *et al.*'s paper offers a summary table of different narrative analysis approaches when the emphasis is on content, structure and/or form.

A commonality across narrative analysis methods is that the focus of inquiry lies on the narrative, regardless of whether the emphasis is on content, structure and/or form. A good example of the use of form in narrative is found in the study investigating how patients talk about living with motor neurone disease (Brown & Addington-Hall 2008) (see Research Example 34.2).

Framework analysis

Ritchie and Spencer (1994) developed 'framework' as a method of data analysis particularly suited to policy and applied research. It involves a number of distinct, though interconnected, stages (see Box 34.3). An example of a project in healthcare where framework analysis was used is a study by Elkington *et al.* (2004) (see Research Example 34.3). A worked example of how codes are attached and how a coding

---

Box 34.3 Five key stages of data analysis in the 'framework' approach

Familiarisation – immersion in the data (e.g. listening to tapes, reading transcripts, studying notes, etc.) to get an initial feel for the key ideas and recurrent themes.

Identifying a thematic framework – the process of identifying key issues, concepts and themes, and the setting up of an index or framework. This can be used for sifting and sorting data including *a priori* issues (used to inform the focus of the research and the data collection guides), emergent themes raised by respondents and analytical themes that are evident through recurring patterns in the data.

Indexing – the process of systematically applying the index or framework to the text form of the data, by annotating the text with codes in the margin.

Charting – data are 'lifted' from their original context and rearranged according to themes in chart form. There may be separate charts for each major subject or theme and they will contain data from several different respondents. This process involves considerable synthesis and abstraction.

Mapping and interpretation – the charts are used to define concepts, map the range and nature of phenomena, create typologies and find associations between themes in order to provide explanations for the findings. This process is guided by the original research questions as well as themes and relationships emerging from the data.

RESEARCH EXAMPLE

34.3 A Study Using the Framework Approach to Analysis

Elkington H, White P, Addington-Hall J, Higgs R, Pettinari C (2004) The last years of life of COPD: a qualitative study of symptoms and services. *Respiratory Medicine* **98**: 439–445.

This study set out to assess the symptoms experienced and their impact on patients' lives in the last year of chronic obstructive pulmonary disease (COPD), and to assess patients' access to and contact with health services. The framework approach was used for the qualitative analysis of in-depth interviews with 25 carers of COPD patients who had died in the preceding 3–10 months. Five phases of the approach are described: familiarisation, identification of a thematic framework, indexing, charting and mapping, and interpretation. The paper presents two key areas to emerge from this process – the first relating to the symptoms experienced and their impact on patients' lives and the second relating to patients' contact with health services in the community.

framework is developed when adopting this strategy is given in Research Example 34.4.

PRACTICALITIES

Recording and transcribing data

To be able to analyse data from interviews, a verbatim record of the interview should be gained. By far the best approach is to tape- or video-record the interaction and then transcribe the tape. Some researchers use a transcription service, but wherever possible it is better for the interviewer to do this themselves, since it is a good opportunity to start the process of 'immersion' in the data. The extent to which every single word is extracted, and every pause and emphasis noted, will depend on the particular approach to analysis. So, for example, if thematic analysis is chosen, then pauses are not essential to record, whereas with discourse and narrative analyses, there are conventions that must be followed in preparing the transcript. Transcription is a very lengthy process, with a 60-minute interview needing several hours for transcription.

Fieldnotes in observation can follow a structure, according to the purpose of the observation, or they can be more free-flowing. If a structure is used, this can form the basis for the analysis. On the other hand, a pre-determined structure may be unduly constraining. Sometimes it is a good idea to take a few notes during an interview as well, even when it is being tape-recorded. This can be helpful both as a prompt for further questioning in a relatively unstructured or semi-structured interview and as a back-up, should the tape recorder fail or the tape run out.

RESEARCH EXAMPLE

34.4   Analysis Using the Framework Approach

As part of a study of out-of-hours health services (Lattimer *et al.* 2005) a postal survey of patient satisfaction with the services was undertaken, resulting in both quantitative and qualitative data. The qualitative data were in the form of open-ended comments which were analysed using the framework approach. First, extracts from three comments related to the telephone contact are presented with codes attached. Second, an excerpt is given from the coding frame, and third, the chart shows how these can be compared across different sites.

Comment A: 'I was quite happy with phone service;   *generally satisfied (2.1)*

I'd seen notices about it in the doctor's surgery and I read   *well advertised (2.1.1)*
about it in the local paper;

but there was one small aspect that I found irritating and it   *repeated questioning (2.2.1)*
could be improved – different people asking the same
questions *(balanced – 1.1)*

Comment B: Can't fault [the phone service]; got to speak to   *put straight through to nurse/*
nurse immediately which was good *(all positive – 1.3)*   *doctor (2.1.7)*

Comment C: Didn't realise that I'd have to phone GP and   *ringing doctor and then NHSD*
NHS Direct as well; so I was not pleased and then the   *(2.1.10) person spoke too fast*
operator spoke so fast I couldn't take it in *(all negative
– 1.2)*

Extract from coding framework (with examples of codes)

Balance of comments overall:	1
Balanced comments	1.1
All negative comments	1.2
All positive comments	1.3

Theme: Ease of access over the phone:	2
Positive	2.1

General
Well advertised	2.1.1
Good recommendation of other services	2.1.2
Continuity of information between services	2.1.3, etc.

Waiting time
Put straight through to nurse/doctor	2.1.7, etc.
Negative	2.2

Questioning
Repetitive questioning	2.2.1
Repetitive questioning causing delay	2.2.2
Perceived irrelevant questioning	2.2.3, etc

Clarity of process
Ringing doctor and then NHSD	2.2.10
Emergency doctors with no access to information	2.2.11, etc.

Communication problems
Person spoke too fast	2.2.19
Difficulty communicating with call handler	2.2.20, etc.

Extract from chart comparing responses across sites

	Code	Site 1		Site 2		Site 3	
		n	%	n	%	n	%
Balance of comments	1						
Mixed comments	1.1	47	29.4	31	26.1	30	29.1
All negative comments	1.2	47	29.4	35	29.4	27	26.2
All positive comments	1.3	66	41.3	53	44.5	46	44.7
All comments coded		160		119		103	
Returned questionnaires		332		274		249	
Theme: Ease of access over the phone	2						
Positive	2.1	23	35.9	9	25.0	7	35.0
Negative	2.2	41	64.1	27	75.0	13	65.0
Total		64	40.0	36	30.3	20	19.4

Doing qualitative analysis

The most usual way of condensing or grouping data is to attach codes to it. These codes may have been decided on in an *a priori* way or they may emerge as the fieldwork unfolds. Different approaches to analysis use the word 'code' to mean slightly different things, so the best plan when following one particular type of analysis is to be clear about what constitutes a 'code' in that approach. All the forms of analysis refer to the development of themes and categories, but the way in which they are derived or they emerge is again related to the analytical method.

A thematic analysis process is illustrated by a study of prisoners' views of a telepsychiatry service, conducted by Sarah Leonard (Leonard 2004). She undertook 20 tape-recorded, semi-structured interviews with prisoners after they had participated in an experimental telepsychiatry initiative. The questioning focused on the experience of the prisoners being assessed in terms of their mental health by a video-recorded link with a remote psychiatrist in a setting far from the prison. While their feelings about the experience of assessment using this process were central to the interview, the prisoners also talked graphically about their lives in prison.

These interviews were analysed using the stages outlined by Creswell (2007). First, each interview was transcribed by the researcher and the transcription was then shared with the interviewee. This was to check with them her understanding of the language they used – which tended to rely quite heavily on prison 'jargon' – rather than to 'validate' the transcripts. She then imported the text of the transcripts into a software package (see below). The second stage involved familiarisation with the range, depth and diversity of the data by listening to the tapes, reading the transcripts several times and reflecting on each interview. During this 'immersion' in the data, 'memos' – consisting of initial impressions, key ideas and recurring themes – were written in the margins of the transcript. The next stage entailed description, the identification of codes and the clustering of similar ones under theme headings. Examples relating to the prisoners' life in prison included: 'lack of structure and meaningful activity', 'routines and lack of change' and 'rigid system', and 'predictability'.

Finally, the data clustered under these themes were again scrutinised and presented within a framework of main headings. Thus the aforementioned became subthemes under the main heading of 'factors that help or hinder adaptation' to prison life. Verbatim comments were used to provide evidence of the participants' experience.

EXAMPLES OF ANALYSES

As referred to previously, different types of analytical approach require the transcribed data to be presented in particular ways. Two contrasting examples are given to illustrate this – a narrative analysis (see Research Example 34.5) and a piece of analysis using the 'framework' approach (see Research Example 34.4). It should be noted that while these are quite different strategies, for example the narrative analysis requires the data to be presented with every single utterance, repetition and pause and with lines identified, whereas the framework analysis works on chunks of verbatim quotes with undue repetition left out, there are still similarities. Thus the analyst in both works from the transcripts, identifying key concepts and producing an analytical framework, which can then be used to compare across other cases.

Analysing qualitative data is never easy, despite the impression given by many published studies that the results flow effortlessly from an obvious process, and it is often not possible to stick slavishly to one particular approach. A helpful sourcebook of methods, which is as much for the novice as for the more experienced researcher, is that of Miles and Huberman (1994). They define analysis as 'consisting of three concurrent flows of activity: data reduction, data display, and conclusion drawing/verification' (Miles & Huberman 1994: 10). Data reduction refers to the process of selecting, focusing, simplifying, abstracting and transforming the data found in fieldnotes and transcriptions, and it occurs throughout the project – not just at the end of a data collection period. The second type of activity is data display, which can mean the presentation of an extended quantity of text – or at the very least copious snippets of verbatim quotes. Miles and Huberman provide examples of different types of display, such as charts, graphs,

34.5   Narrative Analysis

This example is from Lucy Simons' qualitative study of community mental health nurses' experiences of treating patients with common mental health problems within a randomised trial (Simons *et al.* 2008). It is in three parts: first a story described by Len about his experience, presented using the conventions of narrative analysis (see Reisman 2002); second, the detailed analysis of this story; and third, the template that this story is placed in so that it can be compared and contrasted with the other narratives in the study.

	Line No.
The story: 'Len, the most rewarding of all'	
Er:::m (1) but I think actually one of the most rewarding ones was	*105*
the e:r (,) um was a relatively young guy (.) who worked in a local Bank	*106*
who um (1) lived I think with his sister so a single guy um (.) and um	*107*
who actually not only told me that his problems were resolved by the end	*108*
but actually said you know how how he now understood about tackling his	*109*
future problems you know in view of you know (.) that he not only not	*110*
only resolved his current problems but had learnt had learnt a way of	*111*
tackling (.) um how he perceives things in the future you know um which I	*112*
I find that (.) actually the most rewarding of all um (.) erm: you know	*113*
because hopefully you know not only has has it resolved during the time	*114*
that I saw him but he will be able to do it himself next time which is	*115*
what of course was said on the on the course itself but um (.) he	*116*
actually he actually came out with that himself and when he when he did	*117*
it um you know that was quite encouraging.	*118*

‑ ‑ ‑ ‑ ‑ ‑ ‑ ‑ ‑ ‑ ‑ ‑ ‑

I think like	508
I said it was great when that guy said to me you know that he got	509
something he got something (.) for himself for the future he could use	510
you know and how to perceive things differently if you know I think that	511
was ur extremely good.	512

The detailed analysis of the story

Narrative characters and how Len wants them to be known

Len provided an introduction to the patient at the start of this narrative. He is constructed as a single young man who held a respectable job and lived with his sister (lines 106–107). Within this narrative Len hardly features and little is learnt about his character. This narrative featured some time into the interview and Len had already made identity claims earlier on.

Social positioning

The patient has the most dominant social position in this narrative in that all the actions that take place are attributed to him. The patient's actions are related to what he tells Len about the outcome of the encounter – that his problems were resolved (line 108) and that he had learnt to manage better in the future (lines 109–110). These ideas were then repeated twice (lines 110–112, 114–5). The patient had also offered this information to Len without prompting (line 117). When Len returned to the narrative much later in the interview the actions taken

Continued

were still the patients' actions of telling Len that he had learnt for the future (lines 509–510).

In contrast Len did not attribute any actions to himself during the narrative. He described how he felt about the encounter: it was 'rewarding' (line 105), which he found 'quite encouraging' (line 118) and 'extremely good' (line 512), but it was not clear what actions Len had actually taken to help bring about the problem resolution and the skills that the patient told him he had acquired. Len was the passive recipient in this narrative, as the patient told him what the outcome of the encounter was and even where Len refers to the problem-solving training course he frames this as what was said to him rather than what he learnt (line 116).

Although the patient was the most active and agentic character in the narrative, the activity attributed to him is about telling Len the result of the treatment encounter. The problems were described as being 'resolved' (lines 108, 111, 114) by the end of the encounter without any clear idea who or what was responsible for this outcome.

Other narrative/discursive devices

Repetition

Len repeated the main idea of the narrative on three occasions throughout the whole narrative but rather than build on or add detail to the idea, at each repetition he simply restated what happened.

Analytical framework

Who are the characters in the story?	Patient (dominant): young, single guy
Are they dominant or subordinate?	Len (subordinate): on receiving end of action
Type of story?	Change achieved and possibly successful PST*
What action takes place?	*Patient*:
	108: told Len problems were resolved
	109: told Len understood how to tackle problems
	111: had resolved current problems
	117: identified learning from the encounter
	509: told Len what he had got from the encounter
	Len: none
Does the patient achieve change?	Yes, problems resolved
Social positioning of characters:	*Patient*:
	108: problems resolved (no action taken)
	110–112: resolved problems (taken action) and learnt how to in future
	114: resolved during the time (no action)
	115: future action indicated
	Len:
	108, 117, 509: informed by patient
	118, 512; encouraged by events of this encounter
Other narrative devices used:	Repetition
	Main idea returned to much later in interview
Blame (if no change achieved)	N/A

(*Problem-solving technique used to treat patients randomised to this intervention) matrices and networks, which can work well to begin to show relationships and connections. The third 'stream' of activity is that of conclusion drawing and verification. This process does in fact start in the data collection stage when the researcher begins to note possible patterns, explanations and propositions. However, 'final' conclusions may not be apparent until the data collection is completed. Then the conclusions need to be 'tested' and 'verified' lest the analyst is left with an interesting story of what happened but one of unknown truth and utility.

USING COMPUTER SOFTWARE FOR QUALITATIVE DATA ANALYSIS

The use of dedicated software packages for analysing qualitative data has become increasingly popular. The early software of the late 1980s was designed mainly for the analysis of text. However, more recently software to handle a variety of data, including visual and multi-media non-numerical material, has been developed. They software now also has many more functions than initially, such as both coding and retrieval, and theory building categories. Computer Assisted Qualitative Data Analysis (or CAQDAS) provides tools to identify and code themes, concepts, processes and contexts to build theories or enlarge upon existing theories. Two of the most popular packages currently are: ATLAS.ti6 (www.atlasti.com/index.html) and QSR NVivo8 (www.qsrinternational.com). The reader is directed to Lewins and Silver (2007), which provides a very helpful step-by-step guide to using these two packages and five others. Up-to-date information can also be gained from the company websites and those detailed below.

Above all, software packages can help with the process of analysing data, but they are not shortcuts to rigorous analysis and they still require the researcher to make decisions about categorisation. As such they are tools to facilitate the analytical process, but many would say that they are no substitute for immersing oneself in the data, and really getting a feel for the nature of the data and the inter-relationships between different aspects. In essence,

they are geared more to medium-sized to larger projects where there are reasonable amounts of data, Conversely, where the beginning researcher has perhaps a few short interviews, they can provide learning opportunities for use in future projects.

CONCLUSIONS

In conclusion, qualitative data analysis in nursing research is a complex, creative process that is ongoing, interactive, inductive and reflexive. It occurs throughout the study from the initial conception of the idea to the production of the final report or account. While it can be quite different from the processes used to analyse quantitative data, nevertheless it still needs to be rigorous, systematic and transparent.

References

Benson A, Secker J, Balfe E, Lipsedge M, Robinson S, Walker J (2003) Discourses of blame: accounting for aggression and violence on an acute mental health inpatient unit. *Social Science and Medicine* **57**: 917–926.

Bingley AB, Thomas C, Brown JB, Reeves J, Payne S (2008) Developing narrative research in supportive and palliative care: the focus on illness narratives. *Palliative Medicine* **22**(5): 653–658.

Brown JB, Addington-Hall J (2008) How people with motor neurone disease talk about living with their illness: a narrative study. *Journal of Advanced Nursing* **62**(2): 200–208.

Creswell JW (2007) *Qualitative Inquiry and Research Design: choosing among five epproaches*, 2nd edition. Thousand Oaks, Sage.

Denzin NK (1970) *The Research Act in Sociology: a theoretical introduction to sociological methods*. London, Butterworth.

Eisenhardt K (1989) Building theories from case study research. Academy of Management Review **14**(4): 532–550. Reprinted in Huberman AM, Miles MB (eds) (2002) *The Qualitative Researcher's Companion*. Thousand Oaks, Sage, pp 5–35.

Elkington H, White P, Addington-Hall J, Higgs R, Pettinari C (2004) The last years of life of COPD: a qualitative study of symptoms and services. *Respiratory Medicine* **98**: 439–445.

Glaser B, Strauss A (1967) *The Discovery of Grounded Theory*. Chicago, Aldine.

Heritage J (2004) Conversation analysis and institutional talk: analysing data. In: Silverman D (ed) *Qualitative Research: theory, method and practice*. London, Sage, pp 161–182.

Lathlean J (1997) *Lecturer Practitioners in Action*. Oxford, Butterworth-Heinemann.

Lattimer V, Turnbull J, Burgess A, Surridge H, Gerard K, Lathlean J *et al.* (2005) Effect of introduction of integrated out-of-hours care in England: observational study. *British Medical Journal* **331**: 81–84.

Leonard S (2004) The successes and challenges of developing a prison telepsychiatry service. *Journal of Telemedicine and Telecare* **10**: 69–71.

Lewins A, Silver C (2007) *Using Software in Qualitative Research: a step-by-step guide*. London, Sage.

Lieblich A, Tuval-Mashiach R, Zilber T (1998) *Narrative Research: reading, analysis and interpretation*. Thousand Oaks, Sage.

Miles MB, Huberman AM (1994) *Qualitative Data Analysis: an expanded sourcebook*, 2nd edition. Thousand Oaks, Sage.

Potter J (2004) Discourse analysis as a way of analysing naturally occurring talk. In: Silverman D (ed) *Qualitative Research: theory, method and practice*, 2nd edition. London, Sage, pp 144–160.

Potter J, Wetherell M (1995) Discourse analysis. In: Smith JA, Harre R, Van Langenhove L (eds) *Rethinking Methods in Psychology*. London, Sage, pp 80–92.

Reissman CK (2008) *Narrative Methods for the Human Sciences*. Thousand Oaks, Sage.

Reissman C K (2002) Narrative analysis. In: Huberman AM, Miles MB (eds) *The Qualitative Researcher's Companion*. Thousand Oaks, Sage, pp 217–270.

Ritchie J, Spencer L (1994) Qualitative data analysis for applied policy research. In: Bryman A, Burgess R (eds) *Analysing Qualitative Data*. Routledge, London. Reprinted in Huberman AM, Miles M B (eds) (2002) *The Qualitative Researcher's Companion*. Thousand Oaks, Sage, pp 305–331.

Silverman D (1998) *Harvey Sacks and Conversation Analysis* (Polity Key Contemporary Thinkers Series). Cambridge, Polity Press.

Simons L, Lathlean J, Squire C (2008) Shifting the focus: sequential methods of analysis with qualitative data. *Qualitative Health Research* **18**(1): 120–132.

Smith B, Sparkes AC (2008) Narrative and its potential contribution to disability studies. *Disability & Society* **23**(1): 17–28.

Further reading

Bryman A (2008) *Social Research Methods*, 3rd edition. Oxford, Oxford University Press (especially chapters on Qualitative Data Analysis and Computer-Assisted Data Analysis).

Miles MB, Huberman AM (1994) *Qualitative Data Analysis: an expanded sourcebook*, 2nd edition. Thousand Oaks, Sage.

Pope C, Ziebland S, Mays N (2006) Analysing qualitative data. In: Pope C, Mays N (eds) *Qualitative Research in Health Care*. Oxford, Blackwell, pp 63–81.

Silverman D (2006) *Interpreting Qualitative Data: methods for analyzing talk, text and interaction*, 3rd edition. Thousand Oaks, Sage.

Websites

http://caqdas.soc.surrey.ac.uk – CAQDAS Networking Project. University of Surrey, ESRC Researcher Development Initiative Project including Qualitative Innovations in CAQDAS (QUIC) programme. It provides:

- training and support in use of a range of CAQDAS packages
- comprehensive bibliography relating to use of CAQDAS packages
- links to online journals and articles
- links to software development and distributor sites, including free and low-cost packages
- reports on funded research.

http://onlineqda.hud.ac.uk – Online CAQDAS and Qualitative Date Analysis. University of Huddersfield and University of Surrey, ESRC Research Methods Project.

www.cardiff.ac.uk/socsi/qualiti – QUALITI: Qualitative Research Methods in the Social Sciences: Innovation, Integration and Impact. School of Social Sciences, Cardiff University, ESRC National Centre for Research Methods Project.

35 Descriptive Analysis of Quantitative Data

Stephen Walters and Jenny Freeman

Key points

- Different types of quantitative data need to be handled, presented and described in appropriate ways.

- Data checking and cleaning are essential first steps in recording and entering data for analysis.

- Tables and graphs are commonly used to display data, but attention needs to be paid to presentation.

- Summary statistics such as means, medians and standard deviation are used to describe quantitative data.

INTRODUCTION

The prospect of collecting and analysing quantitative data can be daunting, especially the first time. However, it need not be, and the purpose of this and the next chapter is to demystify the process and introduce some basic statistical ideas in preparation for conducting a study. This chapter describes the basic data types encountered in quantitative analysis and some simple ways of describing and displaying them. The following chapter introduces the concept of hypothesis testing and describes some basic methods for testing hypotheses. To provide continuity, data from the same study will be used throughout the two chapters to illustrate key concepts. This study is described in Research Example 35.1, but briefly, it is a randomised controlled trial (see Chapter 17) of community versus hospital rehabilitation followed by telephone or conventional follow-up in 161 patients with the lung condition chronic obstructive pulmonary disease (COPD). Patients were assessed at entry to the study, eight weeks after randomisation and then at six-monthly intervals until the final follow-up at 18 months. Outcome measures included exercise capacity, health-related quality of life and use of healthcare resources.

DATA TYPES

To collect and analyse data as part of the research process it is necessary to understand what the different types of data are. Figure 35.1 shows a basic hierarchy of data types. Data are either *quantitative* or *categorical*. Quantitative variables can be either *count* or *continuous*. Count data are also known as

35.1 Case Study of a Randomised Controlled Trial

JC Waterhouse, SJ Walters, Y Oluboyede, RA Lawson (2010) The CoHoRT study: a randomised 2 x 2 trial of community versus hospital rehabilitation followed by telephone or conventional follow up; impact on quality of life, exercise capacity and use of health care resources. *Health Technology Assessment* 2010: 14.

This study comprised a randomised controlled trial to test whether pulmonary rehabilitation undertaken in a community setting was more effective than that undertaken in a hospital setting (standard care), as assessed by exercise capacity and health-related quality of life. In addition, it looked at whether a further telephone follow-up produced a greater persistence of effect of pulmonary rehabilitation compared to standard care.

Two hundred and forty patients with chronic obstructive pulmonary disease (COPD) were randomised to receive pulmonary rehabilitation in either a community (n = 111) or hospital setting (n = 129). Following standardised pulmonary rehabilitation for six weeks patients were followed up over 18 months (with assessments post-rehabilitation approximately eight weeks post-randomisation, and 6, 12 and 18 months after rehabilitation). Analysable data were obtained for exercise capacity post-rehabilitation for 161 patients, 85/129 (66%) in the hospital group and 76/111 (68%) in the community group. Patients were further randomised to telephone or standard follow-up, with analysable data for n = 40, 34, 25 and 36 respectively in hospital rehabilitation/telephone follow-up, hospital rehabilitation/standard follow-up, community rehabilitation/telephone follow-up and community rehabilitation/standard follow-up groups. The primary outcome was distance walked post-rehabilitation on the endurance shuttle walk test.

The mean baseline endurance shuttle test walking distance was 280.5 m and 278.9 m for the community and hospital groups respectively. Post-rehabilitation the mean distance walked was 496.6 m and 557.7 m for the community and hospital groups respectively. The baseline-adjusted mean difference in walking distance immediately post-rehabilitation was not significantly different at 67.8 m in favour of the hospital group (95% CI, −41.8 to 176.6, p = 0.22). Over the long-term 18 months post-rehabilitation follow-up, the mean difference in endurance shuttle walking test distance between the hospital and community groups, after adjustment for baseline distance walked, time and factorial design, was not significantly different at 52.3 m (95% CI −31.7 to 136.3, p = 0.22). Furthermore, there was no significant difference in endurance shuttle walking distance in telephone versus standard follow-up groups, with a mean difference, after adjustment for baseline distance walked, time and factorial design, in post-rehabilitation walking distance of 65.1 m (95% CI −19.4 to 149.6, p = 0.131).

discrete data and occur when the data can only take whole numbers, such as the number of children in a family or the number of visits to a GP in a year. Continuous data are data that can be measured, and they can take any value on the scale on which they are measured. They are limited only by the scale of measurement, and examples include height, weight, blood pressure and distance walked.

Data are described as categorical when they can be categorised into distinct groups, such as ethnic group or disease severity. Although categorical data may be coded numerically, for example gender may be coded 1 for male and 2 for female, these codes have no intrinsic numerical value; it would be nonsense to calculate an average gender. Categorical data can be divided into either *nominal* or *ordinal*. Nominal data have no natural ordering, and examples include eye colour, marital status and area of residence. *Binary* data is a special subcategory of nominal data, where there are only two possible values, for example (male/female, yes/no, treated/not treated). Ordinal data occur when there can be said to be a natural ordering

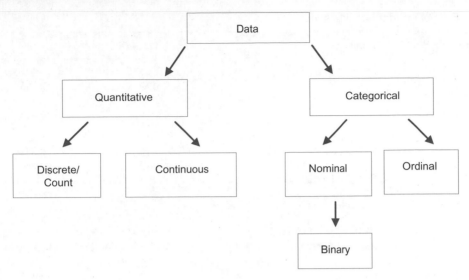

Figure 35.1 Types of data

of the data values, such as better/same/worse grades of breast cancer or social class.

RECORDING DATA

Data may be collected using either *forms* or *questionnaires*. Forms are used to record factual information, such as a subject's age, ethnic group or blood pressure. They are often completed by the study investigator(s) and thus need to be clearly laid out and familiar to all investigators. Although questionnaires may ask about basic demographic information, they are generally used to measure more personal, subjective attributes such as attitudes and opinions, or levels of pain. When designing the layout of questionnaires it is usual for the data to be recorded in a series of boxes, as this aids data entry.

In addition to using forms and questionnaires, a *data coding sheet* may also be useful. This document is a link between the data collected on paper and the data stored on a computer as it contains information about how the individual variables are to be named, labelled and coded in the chosen computer package or spreadsheet. It should also have details of any special codes that are to be used for data that are missing or not applicable. It is a common convention when coding data to reserve 9, 99, 999, etc. as codes for missing data. Table 35.1 is an example of a data coding sheet.

Use of spreadsheets and statistical packages

Once the data have been collected and the questionnaires and forms completed, the information recorded can be input directly to the computer ready for analysis. Two of the most commonly used packages for data storage and basic statistical analysis are Excel and SPSS® (Statistical Package for the Social Sciences). Both are Windows packages with easy-to-follow pull-down menus. Excel is a spreadsheet with some statistical functions. It also has good facilities for producing graphs. However, if more than the most basic statistical analyses are planned, it is better to use SPSS as this has more comprehensive and flexible statistical analysis and data management facilities. Data can be entered into either package and, most usefully, it is possible to transport files and data between the two, should this be necessary. SPSS will read Excel files, while it is possible to save SPSS files as Excel files. As stated previously, all data should be coded numerically when being entered into the computer, unless it is free text. Free text is data that

Table 35.1 Example of data coding sheet

Variable	Label	Values	
ID	Patient ID number		
Age	Age (years)	999	Missing
Sex	Sex	0	Male
		1	Female
		9	Missing
Height	Height (metres)	999	Missing
Weight	Weight (kg)	999	Missing
BMI	Body mass index	999	Missing
Group	Rehabilitation group	0	Community
		1	Hospital
Withdrawn	Withdrawn from study	0	No
		1	Yes
Reason2	Reason for withdrawal	string	
Reason2	Recoded reason for withdrawal	1	Completer
		2	Deceased
		3	Lost to follow-up
		4	Now unsuitable
		5	Protocol violator
		6	Withdrawn

is entered as a string of words. For example, in the rehabilitation trial, for those patients who withdrew, data were recorded on their reason for withdrawal. These would have been entered into a single variable as a string of words, which could then be recoded into numeric categories. In SPSS it is possible to label both variables and the individual values of a categorical variable to ensure that all output is appropriately labelled and readily understandable.

Data entry and data storage

When entering data into the computer, either into a spreadsheet or a statistical package, it is conventional for each column to represent a different variable and each row to represent the data for an individual subject. For categorical variables the different categories should be input as distinct numerical values. This is because the standard statistical packages can have problems handling non-numerical data. They are not able to test for a difference between the two groups 'male' and 'female'; they would, however, be able to test for a difference between groups 1 and 2. Figure 35.2 shows the data view window of SPSS for

the rehabilitation trial data (see Research Example 35.1). Each row contains the data for a particular patient, identified by their (unique) patient id number (STUDYNUMBER) and each column contains the data for a particular variable. For example, the first column contains patient id number (STUDYNUMBER), the second column contains information on the group the patient was randomised to (GROUP01) and so on. Although the latest version of SPSS will allow variable names longer than eight characters, in general, statistical packages including older versions of SPSS restrict the length of variable names to eight characters. Thus the data coding form can be useful in linking the variable names on the computer to a longer more informative label.

Data checking

Errors in recorded data are common. Errors can be made when measurements are taken (data collection), when the data are originally recorded, when they are transcribed from the original source (such as from hospital notes) or when being typed into a computer (data transfer). It is not always possible to know what

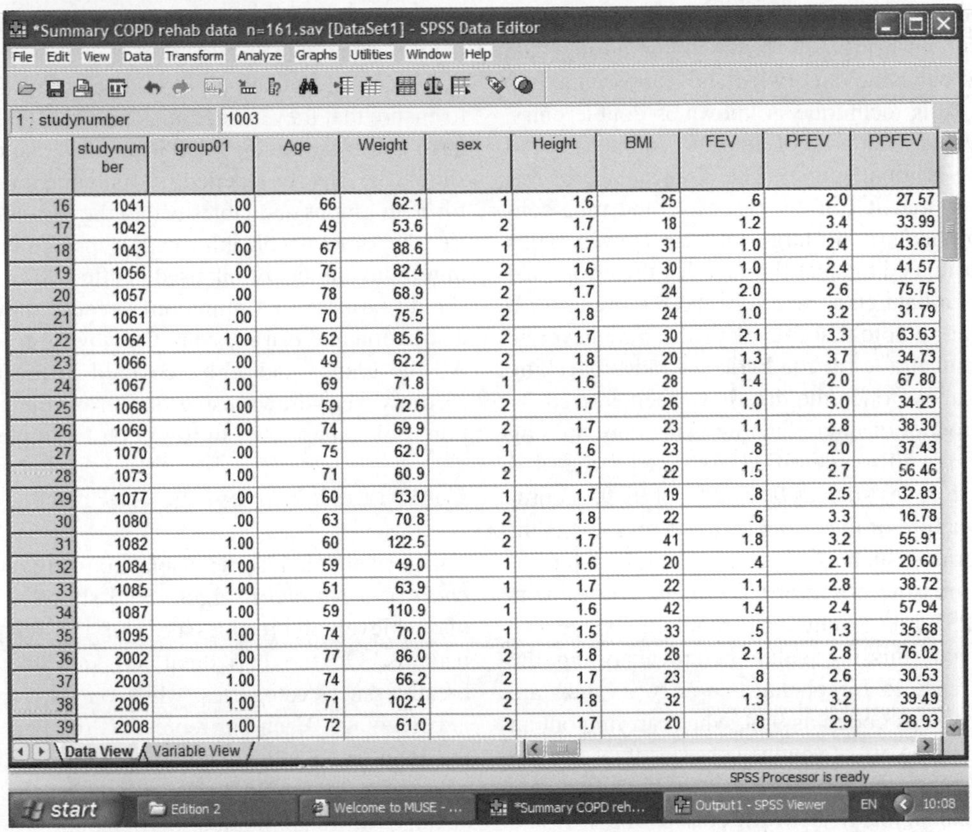

	studynumber	group01	Age	Weight	sex	Height	BMI	FEV	PFEV	PPFEV
16	1041	.00	66	62.1	1	1.6	25	.6	2.0	27.57
17	1042	.00	49	53.6	2	1.7	18	1.2	3.4	33.99
18	1043	.00	67	88.6	1	1.7	31	1.0	2.4	43.61
19	1056	.00	75	82.4	2	1.6	30	1.0	2.4	41.57
20	1057	.00	78	68.9	2	1.7	24	2.0	2.6	75.75
21	1061	.00	70	75.5	2	1.8	24	1.0	3.2	31.79
22	1064	1.00	52	85.6	2	1.7	30	2.1	3.3	63.63
23	1066	.00	49	62.2	2	1.8	20	1.3	3.7	34.73
24	1067	1.00	69	71.8	1	1.6	28	1.4	2.0	67.80
25	1068	1.00	59	72.6	2	1.7	26	1.0	3.0	34.23
26	1069	1.00	74	69.9	2	1.7	23	1.1	2.8	38.30
27	1070	.00	75	62.0	1	1.6	23	.8	2.0	37.43
28	1073	1.00	71	60.9	2	1.7	22	1.5	2.7	56.46
29	1077	.00	60	53.0	1	1.7	19	.8	2.5	32.83
30	1080	.00	63	70.8	2	1.8	22	.6	3.3	16.78
31	1082	1.00	60	122.5	2	1.7	41	1.8	3.2	55.91
32	1084	1.00	59	49.0	1	1.6	20	.4	2.1	20.60
33	1085	1.00	51	63.9	1	1.7	22	1.1	2.8	38.72
34	1087	1.00	59	110.9	1	1.6	42	1.4	2.4	57.94
35	1095	1.00	74	70.0	1	1.5	33	.5	1.3	35.68
36	2002	.00	77	86.0	2	1.8	28	2.1	2.8	76.02
37	2003	1.00	74	66.2	2	1.7	23	.8	2.6	30.53
38	2006	1.00	71	102.4	2	1.8	32	1.3	3.2	39.49
39	2008	1.00	72	61.0	2	1.7	20	.8	2.9	28.93

Figure 35.2 Example of the data view window in SPSS

is correct and so attention must be restricted to making sure that the recorded values are plausible. The data should be scrutinised for potential errors and omissions, and if possible these should be corrected, either by checking the original questionnaire or remeasuring the variable. This process is known as *data checking* (or *data cleaning*). Since the data will be analysed on a computer, this checking should take place after the data have been entered into the computer.

Initial checks should be made that the values are logical and that there are no missing or clearly implausible values. For categorical variables this can be as basic as tabulating the values (i.e. calculating the frequency for each value and putting these into a table) and checking that they are all possible. If, for example, sex can only take the numerical values 1 (male), 2 (female) and 9 (missing), then any values outside these three are clearly wrong.

For continuous measurements, it should be possible to specify lower and upper limits on what is reasonable for the variable concerned. For example, for age, limits of 0 and 100 may be used. Age values above 100 should be checked, because although these are possible they are unlikely. Equally, if adults are being studied, values below 18 should be checked. Values that lie away from the main body of the data are known as *outliers*. They may be genuine observations from individuals with extreme values of the measurement, or they may be erroneous. As with all error checking, once outliers have been checked they should only be changed if they are known to be wrong, and values remaining outside a pre-specified range must be left as they are, or recorded as 'missing'. Values should never be removed from the data set simply because they are higher or lower than would be expected, although the presence of these outlying values may influence the choice of statistical technique used (as outlined in the following chapter). One method for ensuring few errors occur during data entry is to enter the data twice and compare the two data sets. This technique is known as double entry, and any values that are not the same can be checked against the original source. The disadvantage of this approach is that it can be expensive and time-consuming, particularly for large data sets. However, this must be balanced against the fact that the errors that can occur in data entry will have been minimised. It is important to note that this method should never be used as a substitute for the logic and range checking described above once the data have been entered.

A by-product of data cleaning is that any missing observations will be identified. As stated earlier it is usual to use codes such as 9, 99, 999 or 99.9, according to the nature of the variable, although some computer programs, such as SPSS, allow a full stop (.) to indicate a missing observation. If a numeric value is used in SPSS it is essential to identify the value as a 'user-defined' missing value before analysing the data. It is easy to forget that one or two values are missing, perhaps coded as 999, when carrying out an analysis, and the effects on the subsequent results can be severe.

As a final point, it is worth considering why the data are missing. In particular, is there a reason related to the nature of the study? If this is the case it can have serious implications for the generalisability of the study results. Frequently, however, values are missing essentially at random for reasons not related to the study. As with impossible values, it may be possible to check with the original source of the information that missing observations are really missing.

PRESENTING DATA IN GRAPHS

As a first step to any analysis it is useful to plot the data and examine them visually. This will show any extreme observations (outliers) together with any interesting patterns. In addition to being a useful preliminary step to analysis, information can also be displayed pictorially when summarising the data and reporting results. Graphs are useful as they can be read quickly and are of particular help when presenting information to an audience. However, when using graphs for presentation purposes care must be taken to ensure that they are not misleading. A graph should have a title explaining what is displayed and the axes should be clearly labelled. A fundamental principle for both graphs and tables is that they should maximise the amount of information presented for the minimum amount of ink used (Tufte 1983). Gridlines should be kept to a minimum because they act as a distraction and can interrupt the flow of information. All the graphs and tables covered in the following sections were drawn using data from the rehabilitation trial as described in Research Example 35.1.

Basic graphs for categorical data

Categorical data may be displayed using either a *bar chart* or a *pie chart*. Figure 35.3 shows a bar chart of the level of breathlessness of the rehabilitation patients. On the horizontal axis are the different breathlessness categories, while on the vertical axis is percentage. Each bar represents the percentage of the total population in that category. For example, examining Figure 35.3, it can be seen that the percentage of rehabilitation participants who walked slower than their contemporaries on level ground due to breathlessness was about 30%.

Figure 35.4 shows the same data displayed as a pie chart. Generally pie charts are to be avoided as they can be difficult to interpret, particularly when the number of categories is greater than five. In addition, unless the percentages in the individual categories are displayed (as here) it can be much more difficult to estimate them from a pie chart than from a bar chart. For both chart types it is important to include the number of observations on which it is based, particularly when comparing more than one chart. And finally, neither of these charts should be displayed in three dimensions as this makes them especially difficult to read and interpret (Huff 1991; Freeman *et al.* 2008).

Basic graphs for quantitative data

There are several graphs that can be used for quantitative data. *Dot plots* are one of the simplest ways of

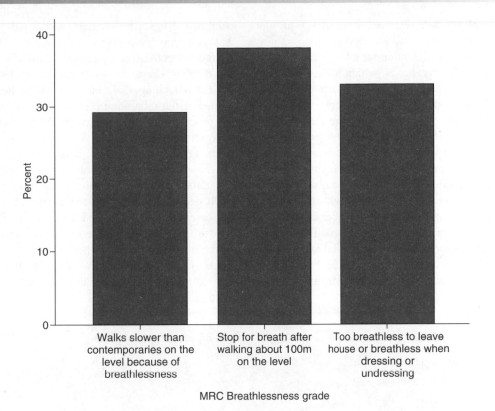

Figure 35.3 Bar chart of breathlessness status for the rehabilitation patients (n = 161)

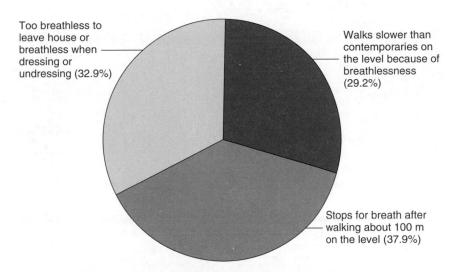

Figure 35.4 Pie chart of breathlessness status for the rehabilitation patients (n = 161)

displaying all the data. Figure 35.5 shows a dot plot of the heights for the rehabilitation patients, by sex. Each dot represents the value for an individual and is plotted along a vertical axis, which in this case represents height in metres. Data for several groups can be plotted alongside each other for comparison; for example, data for men and women are plotted separately in Figure 35.5 and the differences in height between men and women can clearly be seen.

The most common method for displaying continuous data is a *histogram*. To construct a histogram the data range is divided into several non-overlapping equally sized categories and the number of observations falling into each category counted. The categories are then displayed on the horizontal axis and the frequencies are displayed on the vertical axis, as in Figure 35.6. The way that data are distributed can be examined using a histogram. Occasionally the percentages in each category are displayed on the vertical axis rather than the frequencies, and it is important that if this is done, the total number of observations that the percentages are based on is included in the chart. For the rehabilitation data there are a total of 161 observations (73 females and 88 males) and it is convention to write this as 'n = 161'.

The choice of number of categories is important: too few categories and much important information is lost, too many and any patterns are obscured by too much detail. Usually between 5 and 15 categories will be enough to gain an idea of the distribution of the data. One useful feature of a histogram is that it makes it possible to see whether the distribution of the data is approximately *Normal*. The histogram of Normally distributed data will have a classic 'bell'

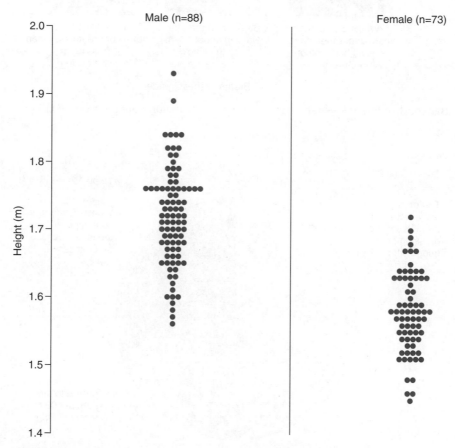

Figure 35.5 Dot plot of height by sex for (n = 161) rehabilitation patients

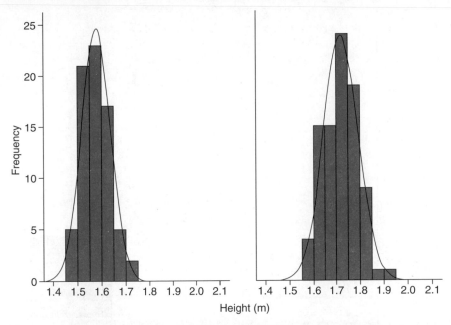

Figure 35.6   Histograms of height for male and female rehabilitation patients

shape, with a peak in the middle and symmetrical tails, such as those in Figure 35.6 for the height of men and women, displayed here with a theoretical Normal distribution curve. The *Normal distribution* (sometimes known as the Gaussian distribution) is one of the fundamental distributions of statistics, and its properties underpin many of the methods explored in the following chapter.

Another extremely useful method of plotting continuous data is a *box-and-whisker* or *box plot*. Box plots can be particularly useful for comparing the distribution of the data across several groups. The box contains the middle 50% of the data, with the lowest 25% of the data lying below it and the highest 25% of the data lying above it. In fact, the upper and lower edges represent a particular quantity called the interquartile range (described later, see Box 35.2). The median is shown by the horizontal line across the box (described later, see Box 35.1, but briefly it is the value such that half of the observations lie below this value and half lie above it). The whiskers extend to the largest and smallest values, excluding the outlying values. The outlying values are those values more than 1.5 box lengths from the upper or lower edges, and are represented as the dots outside the whiskers.

Figure 35.7 shows box plots of the heights of the men and women in the rehabilitation trial. The gender differences in height are immediately obvious from this plot and this illustrates the main advantage of the box plot over histograms when looking at multiple groups. Differences in the distributions of data between groups are much easier to spot with box plots than with histograms.

The association between two continuous variables can be examined visually by constructing a *scatter plot*. The values of one variable are plotted on the horizontal axis (sometimes known as the x-axis) and the values of another are plotted on the vertical axis (y-axis). If it is known (or suspected) that the value of one variable (independent) influences the value of the other variable (dependent), it is usual to plot the independent variable on the horizontal axis and the dependent variable on the vertical axis (the reason for this will be explained in the following chapter). Figure 35.8 shows the scatter plot of forced expiratory vital capacity (in litres) against height (in metres), and each dot represents the height and forced expiratory vital capacity values for an individual. As height determines forced expiratory vital capacity to an extent, and not the other way round, it is plotted on

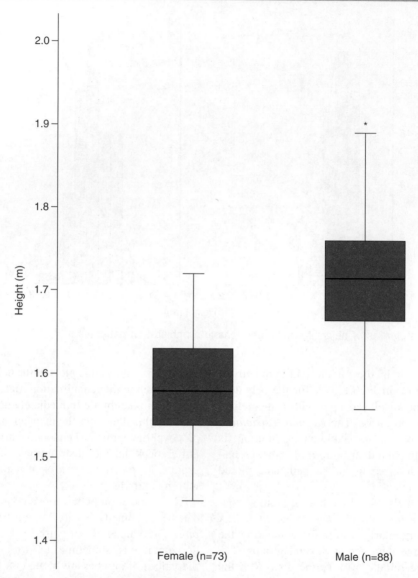

Figure 35.7   Box plot of height for men and women

the horizontal axis, although the variables could legitimately be plotted the other way round.

DESCRIBING DATA

Describing categorical data

A first step in analysing categorical data is to count the number of observations in each category and express them as percentages of the total sample size. For example, as part of the rehabilitation trial the participants were asked about their level of breathlessness. There were three categories, as displayed in Table 35.2. The first column shows category names, while the second shows the number of individuals in each category and the third shows its percentage contribution to the total. In addition to tabulating each variable separately, it might be of interest to compare two categorical variables at the same time, and in this case the

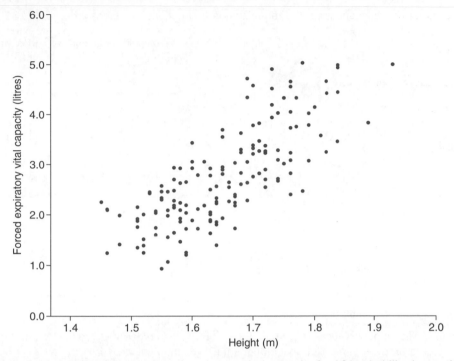

Figure 35.8   Scatter plot of height and forced expiratory vital capacity for 161 rehabilitation patients

Table 35.2   Level of breathlessness for the rehabilitation trial patients (n = 161)

MRC Breathlessness grade	n	%
Walks slower than contemporaries on the level because of breathlessness	47	(29.2)
Stops for breath after walking about 100 m on the level	61	(37.9)
Too breathless to leave house or breathless when dressing or undressing	53	(32.9)

data can be *cross-tabulated*. Table 35.3 shows the distribution of level of breathlessness by study group; in this case it can be said that breathlessness status has been cross-tabulated with study group. Table 35.3 is an example of a contingency table with three rows (representing level of breathlessness) and two columns (representing treatment group). This table suggests that the distribution of breathlessness status is broadly similar between the two study groups and in the following chapter this will be formally tested.

Describing quantitative data

As it can be difficult to make sense of a large set of numbers, an initial approach would be to calculate summary measures, to describe the *location* (a measure of the 'middle value') and the *spread* (a measure of the dispersion of the values) of each variable. These are of great interest, particularly if a comparison between groups is to be made or the results of the study are to be generalised to a larger group, and so it is necessary to find reliable ways of determining their values.

Measures of location

There are several commonly used measures of location, as summarised in Box 35.1. The simplest is the *mode*. This is simply the most common observation and is the highest bar of the histogram. Looking at the histograms (Figure 35.6) for height, 1.70 to 1.75 m

447

Table 35.3 Level of breathlessness for the rehabilitation trial patients, by study group (n = 161)

	Community group n (%)	Hospital group n (%)
MRC Breathlessness grade:		
Walks slower than contemporaries on the level because of breathlessness	20 (26.3)	27 (31.8)
Stops for breath after walking about 100 m on the level	29 (38.2)	32 (37.6)
Too breathless to leave house or breathless when dressing or undressing	27 (35.5)	26 (30.6)
Total	76 (100)	85 (100)

Box 35.1   Measures of location

Mode   Most common observation

Median   Middle observation, when the data are arranged in order of increasing value. If there is an even number of observations the median is calculated as the average of the middle two observations.

Mean $\dfrac{\text{Sum of all observations}}{\text{Number of observations}}$

For example, consider the ages (in years) of five patients recruited to the rehabilitation trial: 81, 58, 72, 85 and 72.

The most common observation is: 72, which occurs twice, thus the **mode** is 72. However, it is sometimes the case that no single number occurs more frequently then other numbers and then there is no unique mode. If there are several numbers that occur with equally high frequency, the data are said to be multi-modal.

The five ages in ascending order are: 58, 72, 72, 81 and 85. The **median** is the middle or third value of the ranked or ordered ages, i.e. 72 years.

The **mean** is: 58 + 72 + 72 + 81 + 85 = 368 divided by the number of observations, 5, i.e. 73.6 years.

---

is the modal height category for men, as this is the height category with the highest bar on the histogram, and 1.55 to 1.60 m is the modal category for women. However, the mode is rarely used because its value depends on the accuracy of the measurement. If, for example, the height intervals were 10 cm wide rather than 5 cm, the mode would change to 1.6 to 1.70 m. In addition, it can be difficult to determine if there is

more than one distinct peak, such as that for the height of all patients (Figure 35.9). In this case the presence of two peaks is a reflection of the differing distribution of height between men and women.

Two other more useful and commonly calculated measures are the *median* and the *mean*. The median is the middle observation, when the data are arranged in order of increasing value. It is the value that divides

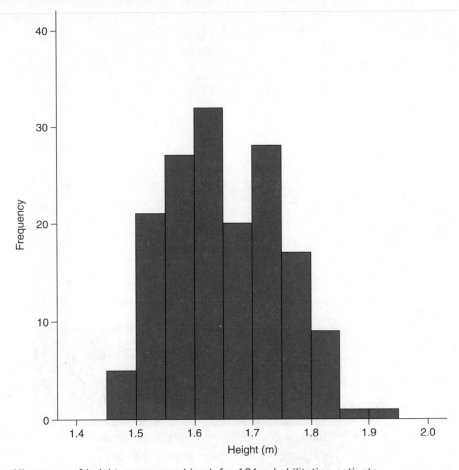

Figure 35.9 Histogram of height, sexes combined, for 161 rehabilitation patients

the data into two equal halves. If there is an even number of observations then the median is calculated as the average of the two middle observations. For example, if there are 11 observations the median is simply the sixth observation, but if there are 10 observations the median is the (5th + 6th observation)/2. The median is not sensitive to the behaviour of outlying data, thus if the smallest value was even smaller, or the largest value even bigger it would have no impact on the value of the median.

Generally the most useful measure of the central value of a set of data is the *mean*. It is calculated as the sum of all observations divided by the total number of observations. Each observation makes a contribution to the mean value and thus it is sensitive to the behaviour of outlying data; as the largest value

increases this causes the mean value to increase and conversely, as the value of the smallest observation becomes smaller the value of the mean decreases.

Both the mean and median can be useful, but they can give very different impressions when the distribution of the data is *skewed*, because of the relative contributions (or lack of, in the case of the median) of the extreme values. Skewed data are data that are not symmetrical. This is best illustrated by examining the shape of the histogram for the percentage of rehabilitation sessions attended (Figure 35.10). There are few observations at lower end of the scale, while the majority of observations are clustered at the top end of the scale, showing clearly that the majority of participants attended most of their rehabilitation sessions. This is described as being negatively skewed,

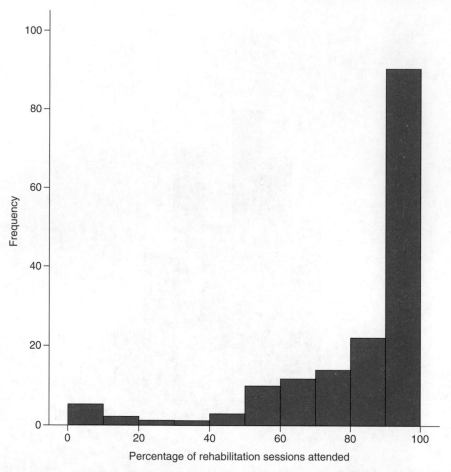

Figure 35.10 Histogram of the percentage of rehabilitation sessions attended showing negative skew of the percentage for this sample (long tail of lower percentages and clustering of values at the higher percentages) for 161 rehabilitation patients

as there is a long left-hand tail at lower values. Data that have a long right-hand tail of higher values, but where the majority of observations are clustered at lower values, are called positively skewed. The forced expiratory volume data in Figure 35.11 are an example of positively skewed data. There are no firm rules about which to use, but when the distribution is not skew it is usual to use the mean. However, if data are skew then it is better to use the median, as this is not influenced by the extreme values and may not be as misleading as the mean.

Measures of spread

In addition to finding measures to describe the location of a data set, it is also necessary to be able to describe

its spread. Just as with the measures of location, there are both simple and more complex possibilities (as summarised in Box 35.2). The simplest is the *range* of the data, from the smallest to the largest observation. The range of age for the rehabilitation patients is 49 to 86 years (or 36 years as a single number). The advantage of the range is that it is easily calculated, but its drawback is that it is vulnerable to *outliers*, extremely large and extremely small observations. A more useful measure is to take the median value as discussed above and further divide the two data halves into halves again. These values are called the quartiles and the difference between the bottom (or 25% percentile) and top quartile (or 75th percentile) is the interquartile range (IQR). This is the observation

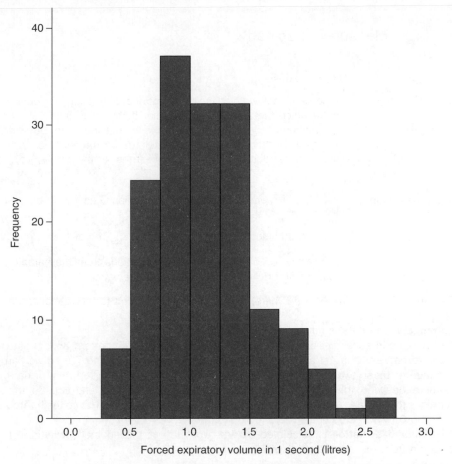

Figure 35.11 Histogram of forced expiratory volume in one second in litres for 160 rehabilitation patients showing positive skew

below which the bottom 25% of the data lie and the observation above which the top 25% lie. The middle 50% of the data lie between these limits. Unlike the range it is not as sensitive to the extreme values. The IQR for the age of the 161 patients involved in the rehabilitation trial is 63 to 75 years or 12 years. Strictly speaking the range and IQR are single numbers, but frequently the two values, minimum and maximum, or the 25% and 75% percentiles respectively, are reported as this can be more informative.

However, the most common measure of the spread of the data is the standard deviation (see Box 35.2). It provides a summary of the differences of each observation from the mean value. The standard deviation has units on the same scale as the original measurement (e.g. metres if height is being measured).

As with the measures of location, when deciding which measure of spread to present, it is necessary to know whether the data are skewed or not. This will also have a bearing on how the data will be analysed subsequently, as will be seen in the following chapter. When the distribution is not skew it is usual to use the standard deviation. However, if data are skew then it is better to use the range or interquartile range.

PRESENTING DATA AND RESULTS IN TABLES

Some basic graphs for displaying data have been described earlier in this chapter. As stated, plotting

Box 35.2 Measures of spread

Range Minimum observation to the maximum observation.

Interquartile range Observation below which the bottom 25% of data lie and the observation above which the top 25% of data lie. If the value falls between two observations, e.g. if 25th centile falls between the 5th and 6th observations then the value is calculated as the average of the two observations (this is the same principle as for the median).

Standard deviation $\sqrt{\dfrac{\sum\limits_{i=1}^{n}(x_i - \bar{x})^2}{n-1}}$ where $\bar{x}$ is the sample mean, x_i is the ith observation,

n is the sample size and the notation $\sum\limits_{i=1}^{n}$ represents the addition

or summing up of all the squared deviations from the sample mean from the first ($i = 1$) to the last (n^{th}) observation.

For example, consider the ages (in years) of five patients recruited to the rehabilitation trial: 85, 72, 81, 72 and 58.

The **range** of the data is from 58 to 85 years or 27 years.

The five ages in ascending order are: 58, 72, 72, 81 and 85. The bottom 25% of data, falls somewhere between the 1st and 2nd ordered observations, i.e. 58 and 72, so we can take the average of these two observations 58 + 72 = 130/2 = 65.0. The top 25% of data, falls somewhere between the 4th and 5th ordered observations, i.e. 81 and 85. So the 75th percentile is the average of the two observations 81 + 85 = 166/2 = 83. Hence the **interquartile range** is 65.0 to 83 years or 18 years.

The **standard deviation** is calculated by first working out the squared deviation of each observation from the sample mean of 75.6 years, i.e.

$(85 - 73.6)^2 + (72 - 73.6)^2 + (81 - 73.6)^2 + (72 - 73.6)^2 + (58 - 73.6)^2 = 433.2$ years^2.

This result is divided by the number in the sample minus one (i.e. 5 − 1 = 4), i.e. 433.2/4 = 108.30 years^2. Finally, we take the square root of this number to give us a standard deviation of 10.41 years.

data can be a useful first stage to any analysis as it will show extreme observations together with any interesting patterns. Graphs are useful as they can be read quickly, and are particularly helpful when presenting information to an audience, such as in a seminar or conference presentation. Although there are no hard and fast rules about when to use a graph and when to use a table, when presenting the results in a report or a paper it is often best to use tables so that the reader can scrutinise the numbers directly. Tables can be useful for displaying information about many variables at once, while graphs can be useful for showing multiple observations on groups or individuals (such as a dot plot or a histogram). As with graphs, there are a few basic rules of good presentation.

■ Numerical precision should be consistent throughout and summary statistics such as means and standard deviations should not have more than one extra decimal place compared to the raw data. (Spurious precision should be avoided, although when certain measures are to be used for further calculations or when presenting the results of analyses greater precision may be necessary.)

■ Gridlines can be used to separate labels and summary measures from the main body of the data in a table. However, their use should be kept to a minimum, particularly vertical gridlines, as they can interrupt eye movements and thus the flow of information. Elsewhere, white space can be used to separate data, for example different variables from each other.

■ The information in tables is easier to comprehend if the columns (rather than the rows) contain like information, such as means and standard deviations, as it is easier to scan down a column than across a row.

■ Tables should be clearly labelled and a brief summary of the contents of a table should always be given in words, either as part of the title or in the main body of the text.

When summarising categorical data, both frequencies and percentages can be used, but if percentages are reported it is important that the denominator (i.e. total number of observations) is given.

For summarising numerical data, the mean and standard deviation may be used, or if the data have a skewed distribution, the median and range. As with categorical data, the number of observations should be stated.

CONCLUSIONS

This chapter has looked at the different types of data encountered in quantitative analysis, and ways of displaying these different data types. Basic summary measures of both location and spread have been discussed and advice given on the best way of presenting these statistics. In the next chapter some basic

approaches to the analysis of these types of data will be examined.

References

Freeman JV, Walters SJ, Campbell MJ (2008) *How to Display Data*. Oxford, BMJ Books, Blackwell.

Huff D (1991) *How to Lie with Statistics*. London, Penguin Books.

Tufte ER (1983) *The Visual Display of Quantitative Information*. Connecticut, Graphics Press.

Waterhouse JC, Walters SJ, Oluboyede Y, Lawson RA (2010) A randomised 2×2 trial of community versus hospital rehabilitation followed by telephone or conventional follow up; impact on quality of life, exercise capacity and use of health care resources. *Health Technology Assessment* **14** (00).

Further reading

Altman DG (1991) *Practical Statistics for Medical Research*. London, Chapman & Hall.

Altman DG, Machin D, Bryant TN, Gardner MJ (2000) *Statistics with Confidence. Confidence intervals and statistical guidelines*, 2nd edition. London, BMJ Books.

Bland M (2000) *An Introduction to Medical Statistics*. Oxford, Oxford Medical Publications.

Campbell MJ, Machin D, Walters SJ (2007) *Medical Statistics: a text book for the health sciences*, 4th edition. Chichester, Wiley.

Field A (2000) *Discovering Statistics using SPSS for Windows*. London, Sage.

Hart A (2001) *Making Sense of Statistics in Healthcare*. Oxford, Radcliffe Medical Press.

Kinnear PR, Gray CD (2004) *SPSS for Windows Made Simple*. Release 12, Hove, Psychology Press.

Petrie A, Sabin C (2000) *Medical Statistics at a Glance*. Oxford, Blackwell Science.

Swinscow TDV, Campbell MJ (2002) *Statistics at Square One*, 10th edition. London, BMJ Books.

Websites

http://peltiertech.com/Excel/Charts/statscharts. html#BoxWhisker Excel charts (biostatistics, charting and graphing data, charting data, Excel charting tutorials, charts for statistics, box and whiskers plots. Statistics tutorial DISCUSS (Discovering Important Statistical Concepts Using Spread Sheets).

www.bettycjung.net/ – Betty C Jung – quality information on the web for public health and healthcare researchers.

www.coventry.ac.uk/discuss/ – provides web-based interactive spreadsheets, designed for teaching elementary statistics.

www.statsoftinc.com/textbook/stathome.html – StatSoft electronic textbook. An electronic statistics textbook offering training in the understanding and application of statistics.

www-users.york.ac.uk/%7Emb55/pubs/pbstnote.htm – statistics notes in the *British Medical Journal*.

36 Examining Relationships in Quantitative Data

Jenny Freeman and Stephen Walters

Key points

- There are two basic approaches to statistical analysis: hypothesis testing using P-values and estimation using confidence intervals.

- Appropriate statistical methods for analysing relationships in quantitative data include tests for differences between groups and tests for relationships between variables.

- When choosing the correct statistical test for the purpose of the study, the nature of the research question and the type of data collected are crucially important.

INTRODUCTION

The previous chapter looked at the different types of data encountered in quantitative analysis and ways of displaying them. Basic summary measures of both location and spread were discussed and advice given on the best ways of presenting these statistics. This chapter will examine the two basic approaches to statistical analysis, *hypothesis testing* (using P-values) and *estimation* (using confidence intervals), and consider some elementary approaches to analysing the types of data outlined in the previous chapter, including the use of statistical techniques for investigating differences between groups. Example outputs from SPSS will be shown, but formulae and mathematical detail will be kept to a minimum, and the interested reader is referred to the more advanced texts listed at the end of Chapter 35 and this chapter. All the example analyses will be based on data from the

COPD rehabilitation trial outlined in Box 35.1 of Chapter 35.

STATISTICAL ANALYSIS

It is rarely possible to obtain information on an entire population and usually data are collected on a sample of individuals from the population of interest. The main aim of statistical analysis is to use the information from the sample to draw conclusions (*make inferences*) about the population of interest. For example, the COPD rehabilitation trial (see Box 35.1) was conducted because it was not possible to study the rehabilitation of all individuals with COPD and so instead a sample of affected individuals was studied to estimate the effect of community compared to hospital rehabilitation for patients with COPD. The two main approaches to statistical analysis, hypothesis testing and estimation, are outlined in the following section.

Hypothesis testing (using P-values)

Before examining the different techniques available for analysing data it is essential to understand the process of hypothesis testing and its key principles, such as what a P-value is and what is meant by the phrase 'statistical significance'. Figure 36.1 describes the steps in the process of hypothesis testing. At the outset it is important to have a clear research question and know what the outcome variable to be compared is. Once the research question has been stated, the null and alternative hypotheses can be formulated. The null hypothesis (H_0) assumes that there is no difference in the outcome of interest between the study groups. The study or alternative hypothesis (H_1) states that there is a difference between the study groups. In general, the direction of the difference (for

example that treatment A is better than treatment B) is not specified. For the rehabilitation trial, the research question of interest is:

> For patients with COPD does rehabilitation in a community setting rather than rehabilitation in hospital affect exercise capacity (distance walked on an endurance shuttle test)?

The null hypothesis, H_0, is:

> There is no difference in exercise capacity (distance walked on an endurance shuttle test) between the hospital and community rehabilitation groups.

And the alternative hypothesis, H_1, is:

> There is a difference in exercise capacity (distance walked on an endurance shuttle test) between the hospital and community rehabilitation groups.

Having set the null and alternative hypotheses the next stage is to carry out a significance test. This is done by first calculating a *test statistic* using the study data. This test statistic is then used to obtain a *P-value*. For the comparison above, patients in the hospital group could, on average, walk 65.7 m more post-rehabilitation than the community group, and the P-value associated with this difference was 0.292. The final and most crucial stage of hypothesis testing is to make a decision, based on the P-value. To do this it is necessary to understand what a P-value is and what it is not, and then to understand how to use it to make a decision about whether or not to reject the null hypothesis.

So what does a P-value mean? *A P-value is the probability of obtaining the study results (or results more extreme) if the null hypothesis is true.* Common misinterpretations of the P-value are that it is either the probability of the data having arisen by chance or the probability that the observed effect is not a real one. The distinction between these incorrect definitions and the true definition is the absence of the phrase 'when the null hypothesis is true'. The omission of 'when the null hypothesis is true' leads to the incorrect belief that it is possible to evaluate the probability of the observed effect being a real one. The observed effect in the sample is genuine, but what is true in the population is not known. All that can be known with a P-value is, if the null hypothesis is true,

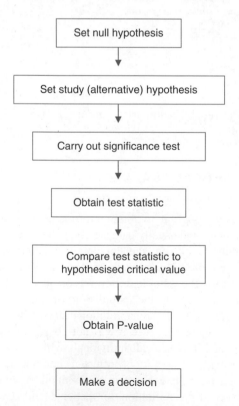

Figure 36.1 Hypothesis testing: the main steps

how likely is the result obtained (from the study data). For the current example the null hypothesis is that there is no difference in the distance walked, thus the P-value tells us how likely it is that we would have found a difference at least as large as the one that we have got if there truly was no difference in distance walked between the two rehabilitation groups.

It is important to remember that a P-value is a probability and its value can vary between 0 and 1. A 'small' P-value, say close to zero, indicates that the results obtained are unlikely when the null hypothesis is true and the null hypothesis is rejected. Alternatively, if the P-value is 'large', then the results obtained are likely when the null hypothesis is true and the null hypothesis is not rejected. *But how small is small?* Conventionally, the cut-off value or *significance level* for declaring that a particular result is *statistically significant* is set at 0.05 (or 5%). Thus if the P-value is less than this value the null hypothesis (of no difference) is rejected and the result is said to be statistically significant at the 5% or 0.05 level (Box 36.1). For the example above, the P-value for the difference in the distance walked is 0.292. As this is more than the cut-off value of 0.05 the difference in exercise capacity is said to be non-significant between the two groups at the 5% level.

If we were to ignore the effect of the type of rehabilitation (hospital/community) and instead ask the question 'does rehabilitation affect the exercise capacity of an individual with COPD?', we have the following null and alternative hypotheses.

Null hypothesis: *Rehabilitation makes no difference to the exercise capacity of patients with COPD.*

Alternative hypothesis: *Rehabilitation makes a difference to the exercise capacity of patients with COPD.*

When we compare the results in exercise capacity, as measured by distance walked, from before rehabilitation to after, there is a mean difference of 251 m. Before rehabilitation, on average patients could only walk 280 m, whereas after rehabilitation the distance walked had increased to 531 m and the P value associated with this change was less than 0.001. As this is less than 0.05, we can conclude that there is a statistically significant change in the distance walked following rehabilitation at the 5% level.

Though the decision to reject or not reject the null hypothesis may seem clear-cut, it is possible that a mistake may be made, as can be seen from the shaded cells of Table 36.1. Whatever is decided, this decision may correctly reflect what is true in the population: the null hypothesis is rejected when it is in fact false; or the null hypothesis is not rejected when in fact it is true. Alternatively, it may not reflect what is true in the population: the null hypothesis is rejected when it is in fact true (*false positive* or *Type I error*, α); or

---

Box 36.1   Statistical significance

We say that our results are statistically significant if the P-value is less than the significance level (α) set at 5% or 0.05.

	P ≤ 0.05	**P > 0.05**
Result is	Statistically significant	Not statistically significant
Decide	That there is sufficient evidence to reject the null hypothesis and accept the alternative hypothesis	That there is insufficient evidence to reject the null hypothesis

We cannot say that the null hypothesis is true, only that there is not enough evidence to reject it

Table 36.1 Making a decision

		The null hypothesis is actually:	
		False	**True**
Decide to:	Reject the null hypothesis	Correct	Type 1 error (α) (False positive error)
	Not reject the null hypothesis	Type 2 error (β) (False negative error)	Correct

the null hypothesis is not rejected when in fact it is false (*false negative, Type II error*, β).

The probability that a study will be able to detect a difference of a given size, if one truly exists, is called the *power* of the study and is the probability of rejecting the null hypothesis when it is actually false. It is usually expressed in percentages, so for a study that has 80% power, there is a likelihood of 80% of being able to detect a difference, of a given size, if there genuinely is a difference in the population.

Estimation (using confidence intervals)

Statistical significance does not necessarily mean the result obtained is clinically significant or of any practical importance. A P-value will only indicate how likely the results obtained are when the null hypothesis is true. It can only be used to decide whether the results are statistically significant or not, it does not give any information about the likely effect size. Much more information, such as whether the result is likely to be of clinical importance, can be gained by calculating a *confidence interval*. A confidence interval may be calculated for any estimated quantity (from the sample data), such as the mean, median, proportion or even a difference, for example the mean difference in distance walked between the two rehabilitation groups. It is a measure of the precision (accuracy) with which the quantity of interest is estimated (in this case the mean difference between the community and hospital groups in exercise capacity – the distance walked post-rehabilitation).

Technically, the 95% confidence interval is the range of values within which the true population

quantity would fall 95% of the time if the study were to be repeated many times. Crudely speaking, the confidence interval gives a range of plausible values for the quantity estimated; although not strictly correct, it is usually interpreted as the range of values within which there is 95% certainty that the true value in the population lies. For the rehabilitation trial above, the quantity estimated was the mean difference in the distance walked between the hospital and community groups following rehabilitation, 65.7 m (see Figure 36.3, explained fully below). The 95% confidence interval for this difference was −56.9 m to 188.2 m. Thus, while the best available estimate of the mean difference was 65.7 m, it could be as low as −56.9 m or as high as 188.2 m, with 95% certainty. This range clearly does include the value for no difference (in this case 0). So the confidence interval is consistent with there being no difference in distance walked post-rehabilitation between the groups. The P-value associated with this difference was 0.292 and in the previous section it was concluded that this difference was not statistically significant at the 5% level. While the P-value will give an indication of whether the result obtained is statistically significant or not, it gives no other information. The confidence interval is more informative as it gives a range of plausible values for the estimated quantity. Provided this range *does not* include the value for no difference (in this case 0) it can be concluded that there is a difference between the groups being compared.

Statistical versus clinical significance

So far we have considered the processes of hypothesis testing and estimation. However, in addition to statistical significance it is useful to consider the concept of clinical significance. While a result may be statistically significant it may not be clinically significant (relevant/important), and conversely, an estimated difference that is clinically important may not be statistically significant. For the example above, while there is no statistically significant difference between the two rehabilitation groups in terms of the distance walked, the confidence interval for the difference is rather large, it ranges from −56.9 m to 188.2 m. Thus it is possible that the difference could be as great as 188 m, a difference that could be (clinically) important to some individuals with COPD. To conclude that there truly was no difference between the two groups we would want a confidence interval that not only included 0, but was also narrow enough to exclude any difference of importance. For example, if we were to decide that a difference of more than 30 m was clinically important, then in order to state that there was no clinically important difference between the groups we would want to see that not only did the confidence interval include 0, but that it lay between the limits −0.30 and 30 m.

This is not just a trivial point. Often in presentations or papers, P-values alone are quoted and inferences are made based on this one statistic. It may be possible to have a P-value greater than the magic 5% but for there to be a genuine difference between groups. Conversely, statistically significant P-values may be masking the fact that differences have little clinical importance: absence of evidence is not evidence of absence.

CHOOSING THE STATISTICAL METHOD

What type of statistical analysis is carried out depends on the answers to five key questions (Box 36.2). Once these questions have been answered, an appropriate approach to the statistical analysis of the data collected can be decided on. The type of statistical analysis depends fundamentally on what the main purpose of the study is. In particular, what is the main question to be answered? The data type for the outcome variable will also govern how it is to be analysed, as an analysis appropriate to continuous data would be completely inappropriate for binary data. The distri-

> **Box 36.2 Five key questions to ask**
>
> 1 What are the aims and objectives?
> 2 What is the hypothesis to be tested?
> 3 What type of data are the outcome data?
> 4 How are the outcome data distributed?
> 5 What is the summary measure for the outcome data?

> **Box 36.3 Three most common problems in statistical inference**
>
> 1 Comparison of independent groups, e.g. groups of patients given different treatments.
> 2 Comparison of the response for paired observations, e.g. in a cross-over trial or for matched pairs of subjects.
> 3 Investigation of the relationship between two variables measured on the same sample of subjects.

bution of the data is also important, as is the summary measure to be used. Highly skewed data require a different analysis compared to data that are *Normally* distributed.

The choice of method of analysis for a problem depends on the comparison to be made and the data to be used. This chapter outlines the methods appropriate for the three most common problems in statistical inference as outlined in Box 36.3. Before beginning any analysis it is important to examine the data, using the techniques described in Chapter 35; adequate description of the data should precede and complement the formal statistical analysis. For most studies and for randomised controlled trials in particular, it is good practice to produce a table or tables that describe the initial or baseline characteristics of the sample.

Comparison of two independent groups

Before comparing two independent groups it is important to decide what type of data the outcome is and how it is distributed, as this will determine the most appropriate analysis. This section describes, for different types of data, the statistical methods available for comparing two independent groups, as outlined in Figure 36.2.

Independent samples *t*-test for continuous outcome data

The independent samples *t*-test is used to test for a difference in the mean value of a continuous variable between two groups. For example, one of the main questions of interest in the rehabilitation trial was whether there was a difference in distance walked post-rehabilitation between the hospital and the community groups. As the distance walked is continuous data and there are two independent groups, assuming the data are Normally distributed in each of the two groups, then the most appropriate summary measure for the data is the sample mean, and the best comparative summary measure is the difference in the mean distance walked post-rehabilitation between the two groups.

When conducting any statistical analysis it is important to check that the assumptions that underpin the chosen method are valid. The assumptions underlying the two-sample *t*-test are outlined in Box 36.4. The assumption of Normality can be checked by plotting two histograms, one for each sample; these do not need to be perfect, just roughly symmetrical. The two standard deviations should also be calculated, and as a rule of thumb, one should be no more than twice the other.

Figure 36.3 shows the SPSS output for comparing distance walked post-rehabilitation (endurance shuttle walk test) between the two groups using the two independent samples *t*-test. It can be seen that there is no significant difference between the groups: *the 95% confidence interval for the difference* suggests that, on average, patients in the hospital group might be able to

> ### Box 36.4 The assumptions underlying the use of the independent samples *t*-test
>
> 1. The groups are independent.
> 2. The variables of interest are continuous.
> 3. The data in both groups have similar standard deviations.
> 4. The data is normally distributed in both groups.

walk up to 188.2 m further than patients in the community group; equally patients in the community group might, on average, be able to walk up to 56.9 m further than patients in the hospital group (with 95% certainty) and the best estimate is a mean difference of 65.7 m. Clearly the confidence interval includes a zero difference and the result is equivocal.

Mann-Whitney *U* test

There are several possible approaches when at least one of the requirements for the *t*-test is not met. The data may be transformed (e.g. the logarithm transformation can be useful particularly when the variances are not equal) or a *non-parametric method* can be used. Non-parametric or distribution-free methods do not involve distributional assumptions, i.e. making assumptions about the manner in which the data are distributed (for example that the data are Normally distributed). An important point to note is that it is the test that is parametric or non-parametric, not the data.

When the assumptions underlying the *t*-test are not met, then the non-parametric equivalent, the Mann-Whitney *U* test, may be used. While the independent samples *t*-test is specifically a test of the null hypothesis that the groups have the same mean value, the Mann-Whitney *U* test is a more general test of the null hypothesis that the distribution of the outcome variable in the two groups is the same. It is possible for the outcome data in the two groups to have similar

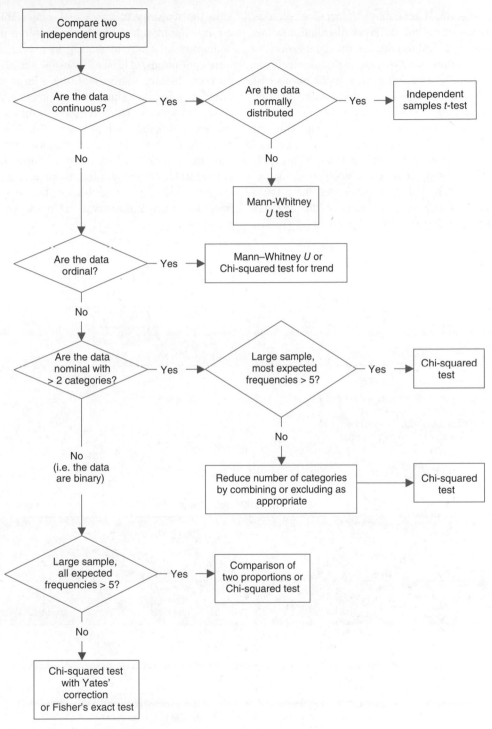

Figure 36.2 Statistical methods for comparing two independent groups or samples

measures of central tendency or location, such as mean and medians, but different distributions. The Mann-Whitney U test requires all the observations to be ranked as if they were from a single sample. From this the statistic U is calculated; it is the number of all possible pairs of observations comprising one from each sample for which the value in the first group precedes a value in the second group. This test statistic is then used to obtain a P-value.

Examining the output from the Mann-Whitney U test in SPSS (Figure 36.4) there is insufficient evidence to *reject the null hypothesis* that there is no difference in distribution of data for the distance walked between the hospital and community groups.

In the majority of cases it is reasonable to treat *discrete data*, such as number of children in a family or number of visits to the GP in a year, as if they were continuous, at least as far as the statistical analysis goes. Ideally, there should be a large number of different possible values, but in practice this is not always necessary. However, where ordered categories are numbered, such as stage of disease or social class, the temptation to treat these numbers as statistically meaningful must be resisted. For example, it is not sensible to calculate the average social class or stage of cancer, and in such cases the data should be treated in statistical analyses as if they are ordered categories.

Group Statistics

	Rehabilitation Group	N	Mean	SD	SE
Endurance Distance Walked (m) - post rehabilitation	Hospital	85	562.2	411.7	44.7
	Community	76	496.6	371.1	42.6

As the standard deviations for the two groups are similar, results from the 'Equal variance assumed' row in the table below can be used.

Independent Samples Test

		Levene's Test for Equality of Variances		t-test for Equality of Means						
							Mean Difference	SE Difference	95% Confidence Interval of the Difference	
		F	Sig.	t	df	Sig. (2-tailed)			Lower	Upper
Endurance Distance Walked (m) - post rehabilitation	Equal variances assumed	1.643	.202	1.058	159	.292	65.7	62.1	-56.9	188.2
	Equal variances not assumed			1.064	158.987	.289	65.7	61.7	-56.2	187.5

The P-value is 0.292. Thus the results are likely when the null hypothesis (that there is no difference between the groups) is true. The result is said to be *not statistically significant* because the P-value is greater than the significance level (α) set at 5% or 0.05 and there is insufficient evidence to reject the null hypothesis and accept the alternative hypothesis that there is a difference in mean distance walked between the hospital and community rehabilitation groups.

Figure 36.3   SPSS output from the independent samples *t*-test

Non-parametric tests

Mann-Whitney test

Ranks

	Rehabilitation Group	N	Mean Rank	Sum of Ranks
Endurance Distance Walked (m) - post rehabilitation	Community	76	77.76	5910.00
	Hospital	85	83.89	7131.00
	Total	161		

Test Statistics[a]

	Endurance Distance Walked (m) - post rehabilitation
Mann-Whitney U	2984.000
Wilcoxon W	5910.000
Z	-.833
Asymp. Sig. (2-tailed)	.405

P-value: probability of observing the test statistic under the null hypothesis. As the value of 0.405 is greater than the significance level (α) set at 0.05 or 5% this means that the result obtained is likely when the null hypothesis is true and it is said to be not statistically significant. Thus there is insufficient evidence to reject the null hypothesis and accept the alternative hypothesis that there is a difference in the distribution of endurance distance walked after rehabilitation between the hospital and community and groups.

a. Grouping Variable: Rehabilitation group

Figure 36.4   SPSS output from the Mann-Whitney *U* test

Comparing more than two groups

The methods outlined above can be extended to more than two groups. For the independent samples *t*-test, the analogous method for more than two groups is called the *Analysis of Variance (ANOVA)* and the assumptions underlying it are similar. The non-parametric equivalent for the method of ANOVA when there are more than two groups is called the *Kruskall-Wallis test*. A fuller explanation of these methods is beyond the scope of this chapter and the interested reader is referred to the more advanced statistical textbooks listed at the end of this chapter and Chapter 35.

Chi-squared test for categorical outcome data

When comparing two independent groups, sometimes the outcome variable is categorical rather than continuous. For example, in the rehabilitation trial it was of interest to know whether patients increased their exercise capacity after rehabilitation or if it remained the same or deteriorated, and if there was a difference between the groups with respect to the

proportions with increased exercise capacity post-rehabilitation. With two independent groups (hospital and community) and a binary (exercise capacity increased versus no change/decreased) rather than a continuous outcome, the data can be cross-tabulated as in Table 36.2. This is an example of a 2 × 2 contingency table with two rows (for treatment) and two columns (for outcome), i.e. four cells in total. The most appropriate summary measure is simply the proportion in the sample whose exercise capacity increased and the best comparative summary measure is the difference in proportions with increased exercise capacity between the two groups. The most appropriate hypothesis test, assuming a large sample and all expected frequencies >5, is the *chi-squared test*.

The null hypothesis is that the two classifications (e.g. group and increased exercise capacity) are unrelated in the relevant population (patients with COPD). More generally, the null hypothesis, H_0, for a contingency table is that there is no association between the row and column variables in the table, i.e. they are independent. The general alternative hypothesis, H_1, is that there is an association between the row and column variables in the contingency table, i.e. they are not independent or unrelated. For the chi-squared

Table 36.2 Cross-tabulation of treatment group versus post-treatment increase in exercise capacity

	Treatment group		
	Hospital rehabilitation	Community rehabilitation	Total
Increase in exercise capacity:			
No change or deteriorated	22 (28.9%)	17 (20.0%)	39 (24.2%)
Improved	53 (71.1%)	68 (80.0%)	122 (75.8%)
Total	76	85	161

Box 36.5 Guidelines for the Chi-squared test to be valid

1 At least 80% of cell should have an expected frequencies greater than 5.
2 All cells should have expected frequencies greater than 1.

test to be valid, two key assumptions need to be met, as outlined in Box 36.5. If these are not met, Fisher's exact test can be used for 2×2 tables.

Figure 36.5 shows the results of analysing Table 36.2 in SPSS. The P-value of 0.255 indicates that there is little evidence of a difference in the proportion of patients with increased exercise capacity post-rehabilitation between the community and hospital groups.

Two groups of paired observations

When there is more than one group of observations it is vital to distinguish the case where the data are paired from that where the groups are independent. Paired data may arise when the same individuals are studied more than once, usually in different circumstances, or when individuals are paired, as in a case-control study. For example, as part of the rehabilitation trial, data were collected on exercise capacity (distance walked on the endurance shuttle test) at base-

line and post-rehabilitation (approximately eight weeks post-baseline). We have already demonstrated that there is no statistically significant difference in distance walked between the hospital and community groups. However, Figure 36.5 shows that 75.8% (122/161) of the combined sample increased their exercise capacity. Suppose we want to test whether the change in distance walked pre- to post-rehabilitation is different from zero, i.e. that rehabilitation makes a difference to exercise capacity, irrespective of where it is delivered. Methods of analysis for paired samples are summarised in Figure 36.6.

Paired t-test

Distances walked at baseline and post-rehabilitation are both continuous variables and the data are paired, as measurements are made on the same individuals at baseline and post-rehabilitation (approximately eight weeks). Therefore, interest is in the mean of the differences, not the difference between the two means. If we assume that the paired differences are Normally distributed, then the most appropriate comparative summary measure is the mean of the paired difference in distance walked between baseline and post-rehabilitation. Given the null hypothesis (H_0) that there is no difference (or change) in mean distance walked at baseline and post-rehabilitation follow-up, the most appropriate test is the paired t-test.

There were 161 patients with both pre- and post-rehabilitation distance walked data. Examining the SPSS output for the comparison of distance walked for these 161 patients pre- and post-rehabilitation shows that the result is statistically significant (Figure 36.7). *The 95% confidence interval of the difference*

Crosstabs

Increase in exercise capacity post-rehabilitation * Rehabilitation group Crosstabulation

			Rehabilitation group Hospital (n=85)	Rehabilitation group Community (n=76)	Total
Inrease in exercise capacity post-rehabilitation	No change or deteriorated	Count	17	22	39
		% within Rehabilitation group	20.0%	28.9%	24.2%
	Yes	Count	68	54	122
		% within Rehabilitation group	80.0%	71.1%	75.8%
Total		Count	85	76	161
		% within Rehabilitation group	100.0%	100.0%	100.0%

To improve the approximation for a 2 x 2 table, Yates' correction for continuity is sometimes applied. Altman (1990) recommends the use of Yates' correction for all chi-squared tests on 2 x 2 tables. In a 2 x 2 table when expected cell counts are less than 5, or any are less than 1, even Yates' correction does not work and thus Fisher's exact test is used. When comparing frequencies amongst groups that have an ordering (e.g. group by pain score), any difference among the groups would be expected to be related to the ordering and the Mantel-Haenszel test for linear association or trend can be carried out. Although the Mantel-Haenszel statistic is displayed, it should not be used for purely nominal data, like we have here.

Chi-Square Tests

	Value	df	Asymp. Sig. (2-sided)	Exact Sig. (2-sided)	Exact Sig. (1-sided)
Pearson Chi-Square	1.750[b]	1	.186		
Continuity Correction[a]	1.296	1	.255		
Likelihood Ratio	1.750	1	.186		
Fisher's Exact Test				.202	.127
Linear-by-Linear Association	1.739	1	.187		
N of Valid Cases	161				

a. Computed only for a 2x2 table

b. 0 cells (.0%) have expected count less than 5. The minimum expected count is 18. 41.

This suggests that the Chi-squared test is valid as all the expected counts are greater than 5.

The P-value of 0.255 indicates that the results obtained are likely if the null hypothesis (of no association between the rows and columns of the contingency table above) is true. Thus there is insufficient evidence to reject the null hypothesis and the results are said to be not statistically significant.

Figure 36.5 SPSS output for Crosstabs procedure and Chi-squared test

suggests that we are 95% confident that distance walked has changed or increased by between 196.9 m and 306.2 m between baseline and post-rehabilitation, and the best estimate is a mean change of 251.6 m.

The assumptions underlying the use of the paired *t*-test are outlined in Box 36.6. If these are not met a non-parametric alternative, the *Wilcoxon signed rank sum test*, can be used.

THE RELATIONSHIP BETWEEN TWO CONTINUOUS VARIABLES

Many statistical analyses are undertaken to examine the relationship between two continuous variables within a group of subjects (Table 36.3). Two of the main purposes of such analyses are:

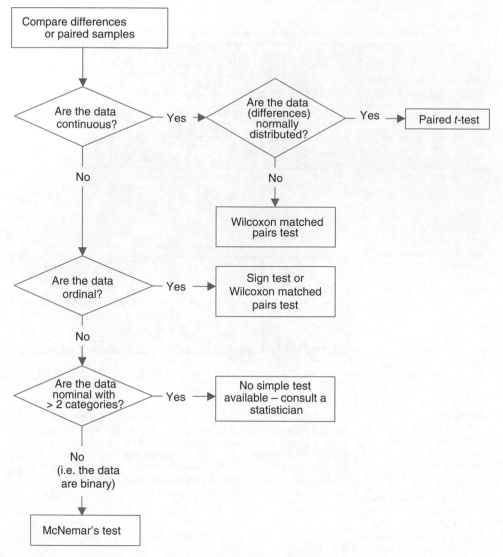

Figure 36.6 Statistical methods for differences or paired samples

Box 36.6 The assumptions underlying the use of the paired *t*-test

1 The paired differences are plausibly normally distributed (it is not essential for the original observations to be normally distributed).
2 The paired differences are independent of each other.

T-test

Paired Samples Statistics

		Mean	N	SD	SE Mean
Pair 1	Endurance Distance Walked (m): baseline	279.7	161	138.3	10.9
	Endurance Distance Walked (m) - post rehabilitation	531.2	161	393.2	31.0

Paired Samples Test

		Paired Differences					t	df	Sig. (2-tailed)
					95% Confidence Interval of the Difference				
		Mean	SD	SE Mean	Lower	Upper			
Pair 1	Endurance Distance Walked (m): baseline - Endurance Distance Walked (m) - post rehabilitation	251.6	351.1	27.7	196.9	306.2	-9.091	160	.000

In SPSS if the P-value is less than 0.001, it is written as 0.000, thus here the P-value is < 0.001 (not 0.000 as could be misinterpreted from this table), indicating that the results obtained are unlikely when the null hypothesis is true. The result is statistically significant because the P-value is less than the significance level (α) set at 0.05 or 5% and there is sufficient evidence to reject the null hypothesis. The alternative hypothesis, that there is a difference in distance walked before and after rehabilitation is accepted.

Figure 36.7 SPSS output for paired *t*-test

Table 36.3 Statistical methods for relationships between two variables measured on the same sample of subjects

	Continuous, normal	Continuous, non-normal	Ordinal	Nominal	Binary
Continuous	Regression Correlation: (Pearson's r)	Regression Rank correlation: (Spearman's r_s)	Rank correlation: (Spearman's r_s)	One-way Analysis of Variance	Independent samples *t*-test
Continuous, non-normal		Regression Rank correlation: (Spearman's r_s)	Rank correlation: (Spearman's r_s)	Kruskall-Wallis test	Mann-Whitney U test
Ordinal			Rank correlation (Spearman's r_s)	Kruskall-Wallis test	Mann-Whitney U test Chi-squared test for trend
Nominal				Chi-squared test	Chi-squared test
Binary					Chi-squared test Fisher's exact test

- to assess whether the two variables are associated. There is no distinction between the two variables and no causation is implied, simply *association*
- to enable the value of one variable to be predicted from any known value of the other variable. One variable is regarded as a *response* to the other *predictor (explanatory)* variable and the value of the predictor variable is used to *predict* what the response would be.

For the first of these, the statistical method for assessing the association between two *continuous* variables is known as *correlation*, while the technique for the second, prediction of one continuous variable from another, is known as *regression*. Correlation and regression are often presented together and it is easy to get the impression that they are inseparable. In fact, they have distinct purposes and it is relatively rare that one is genuinely interested in performing both analyses on the same set of data. However, when preparing to analyse data using either technique it is always important to construct a scatter plot of the values of the two variables against each other. By drawing a scatter plot it is possible to see whether or not there is any visual evidence of a straight line or linear association between the two variables.

Correlation

As stated previously, as part of the rehabilitation trial, distance walked on the endurance shuttle test was measured at baseline (pre-rehabilitation) and follow-up (post-rehabilitation). Plotting the distance walked at baseline and follow-up indicates that there is a positive linear relationship between baseline and follow-up distance walked (Figure 36.8). Unsurprisingly, distance walked post-rehabilitation is generally related to distance walked pre-rehabilitation, i.e. short distances walked at baseline generally correspond with shorter distances walked after rehabilitation, and longer distanced walked at baseline seem to correspond with greater distances at follow-up. To examine whether there is an association between the two variables, the *correlation coefficient* can be calculated. At this point, no assumptions are made about whether the relationship is causal, i.e. whether one variable is influencing the value of the other variable. The standard method (often ascribed to Pearson) leads to a statistic called r. In essence r is a measure of the scatter of the points around an underlying *linear trend*: the closer the spread of points to a straight line the higher the value of the correlation coefficient; the greater the spread of points the lower the correlation. Pearson's correlation coefficient r must be between -1 and $+1$, with -1 representing a perfect negative correlation, $+1$ representing perfect positive correlation and 0 representing no linear trend.

The assumptions underlying the validity of the hypothesis test associated with the correlation coefficient are outlined in Box 36.7. The easiest way to check the validity of the hypothesis test is by examining a scatter plot of the data. This plot should be produced as a matter of routine when correlation coefficients are calculated, as it will give a good indication of whether the relationship between the two variables is roughly linear and thus whether it is appropriate to calculate a correlation coefficient. If the data do not have a Normal distribution, a non-parametric correlation coefficient, Spearman's rho (r_s), can be calculated.

Box 36.7 The assumptions underlying the validity of the hypothesis test associated with the correlation coefficient

1 The two variables are observed on a random sample of individuals.
2 The data for at least one of the variables should have a normal distribution in the population.
3 For the calculation of a valid confidence interval for the correlation coefficient both variables should have a normal distribution.

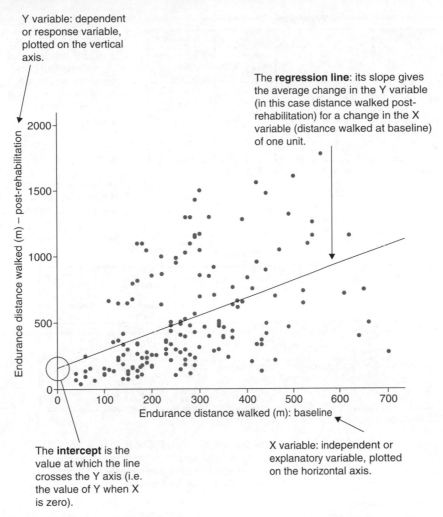

Figure 36.8 Scatter plot of pre- (baseline) and post-rehabilitation distance walked on endurance shuttle test for 161 patients with COPD

From Figure 36.9 it can be seen that the Pearson correlation coefficient between pre- and post-rehabilitation distance walked on the endurance shuttle test is 0.464 and this is statistically significant.

Regression (including multiple regression)

Often it is of interest to quantify the relationship between two continuous variables, and given the value of one variable for an individual, to predict the value of the other variable. This is not possible from the correlation coefficient as it simply indicates the strength of the association as a single number; to describe the relationship between the values of the two variables, a technique called *regression* is used. Thus, using regression, the value of baseline distance walked could be used to predict the post-rehabilitation distance walked. Baseline pre-rehabilitation distance walked is regarded as the X variable; it is also called the independent, predictor or explanatory variable and it should be plotted on the horizontal axis of the scatter plot. Post-rehabilitation distance walked is regarded as the Y variable; it is also known as the dependent or response variable and is plotted on the vertical axis of the scatter plot (Figure 36.8). Three

Correlations

		Endurance Distance Walked (m): baseline	Endurance Distance Walked (m) - post rehabilitation
Endurance Distance Walked (m): baseline	Pearson Correlation	1	.464**
	Sig. (2-tailed)		.000
	N	161	161
Endurance Distance Walked (m) - post rehabilitation	Pearson Correlation	.464**	1
	Sig. (2-tailed)	.000	
	N	161	161

**. Correlation is significant at the 0.01 level (2-tailed).

The Pearson correlation coefficient between distance walked at baseline and distance walked post-rehabilitation is 0.464. Its associated P-value is given underneath it; in this case its value is 0.000 indicating that the result is statistically significant and there is sufficient evidence to reject the null hypothesis of no linear relationship between distance walked at baseline and post-rehabilitation. It can be concluded that the two are correlated.

Correlations

			Endurance Distance Walked (m): baseline	Endurance Distance Walked (m) - post rehabilitation
Spearman's rho	Endurance Distance Walked (m): baseline	Correlation Coefficient	1.000	.558**
		Sig. (2-tailed)	.	.000
		N	161	161
	Endurance Distance Walked (m) - post rehabilitation	Correlation Coefficient	.558**	1.000
		Sig. (2-tailed)	.000	.
		N	161	161

**. Correlation is significant at the 0.01 level (2-tailed).

The Spearman correlation coefficient is 0.558 (P-value = 0.000). This is very similar to the results for the Pearson correlation coefficient, though this will not always be the case.

Figure 36.9 Output of correlation analysis in SPSS

Box 36.8 Assumptions underlying regression analysis

1 The values of the response variable Y should have a normal distribution for each value of the explanatory variable X.
2 The variance (or standard deviation) of Y should be the same at each value of X, i.e. there should be no evidence that as the value of Y changes, the spread of the X values changes.
3 The relationship between the two variables should be linear.

---

important assumptions underlie regression analysis as outlined in Box 36.8.

Regression slopes can be used to predict the response of a new patient with a particular value of the predictor/explanatory/independent variable. However, it is important that the regression model is not used to predict outside of the range of observations. In addition, it should not be assumed that just

Variables Entered/Removed[b]

Model	Variables Entered	Variables Removed	Method
1	Endurance Distance Walked (m): baseline [a]	.	Enter

a. All requested variables entered.

b. Dependent Variable: Endurance Distance Walked (m) - post rehabilitation

Model Summary

Model	R	R Square	Adjusted R Square	Std. Error of the Estimate
1	.464[a]	.215	.210	349.4431

a. Predictors: (Constant), Endurance Distance Walked (m): baseline

R^2 is a number which gives the percentage of variability explained by the predictor variable, X, and gives an indication of how well the model explains the data.

ANOVA[b]

Model		Sum of Squares	df	Mean Square	F	Sig.
1	Regression	5321185	1	5321184.728	43.577	.000[a]
	Residual	2E+007	159	122110.483		
	Total	2E+007	160			

a. Predictors: (Constant), Endurance Distance Walked (m): baseline

b. Dependent Variable: Endurance Distance Walked (m) post rehabilitation

Coefficients[a]

Model		Unstandardized Coefficients		Standardized Coefficients			95% Confidence Interval for B	
		B	Std. Error	Beta	t	Sig.	Lower Bound	Upper Bound
1	(Constant)	162.465	62.284		2.608	.010	39.455	285.476
	Endurance Distance Walked (m): baseline	1.319	.200	.464	6.601	.000	.924	1.713

a. Dependent Variable: Endurance Distance Walked (m) - post rehabilitation

Regression coefficient for the value of the intercept. The value of 162.465 indicates that when distance walked at baseline is zero, distance walked post rehabilitation is 162.465 m.

Regression coefficient for the slope of distance walked at baseline. The value of 1.319 indicates for every increase of a metre in distance walked at baseline, there is an increase in distance walked post rehabilitation of 1.319 m.

The P value for the intercept is 0.010, which indicates that the value of the intercept (162.465) is unlikely when the null hypothesis (that the true value is zero) is true. Thus the result is said to be statistically significant. This is also the case for the regression coefficient for the slope: distance walked at baseline.

Figure 36.10 SPSS output from regression analysis

because an equation has been produced it means that X causes Y. The results of regressing post-rehabilitation distance walked on baseline distance walked are displayed in Figure 36.10. Looking at the table for the coefficients at the bottom of the figure it can be seen that the slope coefficient for baseline distance walked is 1.32 (P-value = 0.000), indicating that baseline distance walked has a significant effect on post-rehabilitation distance walked. The value of r^2 is often quoted in published articles and indicates the proportion (sometimes expressed as a percentage) of the total variability of the outcome variable that is

471

Model Summary

Model	R	R Square	Adjusted R Square	Std. Error of the Estimate
1	.474[a]	.225	.210	349.5416

a. Predictors: (Constant), Gender, Age (years), Endurance Distance Walked (m): baseline

Coefficients[a]

Model		Unstandardized Coefficients		Standardized Coefficients	t	Sig.	95% Confidence Interval for B	
		B	Std. Error	Beta			Lower Bound	Upper Bound
1	(Constant)	320.995	280.860		1.143	.255	-233.756	875.746
	Endurance Distance Walked (m): baseline	1.211	.215	.426	5.646	.000	.787	1.635
	Age (years)	-3.305	3.697	-.065	-.894	.373	-10.608	3.998
	Gender	63.635	57.511	.081	1.106	.270	-49.960	177.231

a. Dependent Variable: Endurance Distance Walked (m) - post rehabilitation

Figure 36.11 SPSS output from multiple regression analysis

explained by the regression model fitted. In this case, 21.5% of the total variability in post-rehabilitation distance walked is explained by pre-rehabilitation distance walked.

Regression, as described above, involves the investigation of the effect of a single explanatory variable on the outcome of interest. However, there is usually more than one possible explanatory variable influencing the values of the outcome variable, and the method of regression can be extended to investigate the influence of more than one variable. In this case it is referred to as *multiple regression*, and the influence of several explanatory variables on the outcome of interest are investigated simultaneously. For example, in the rehabilitation trial, apart from baseline distance walked, age and gender may have a role to play in post-rehabilitation distance walked and these may be fitted into the model to examine what their influence on distance walked is, over and above that exerted by baseline distance walked. Figure 36.11 shows the results of this multiple regression analysis. Age and gender are not significantly associated with post-rehabilitation distance walked, so the simpler model of Figure 36.10, with baseline distance walked as the only predictor variable is to be preferred.

Regression or correlation?

Regression is more informative than correlation. Correlation simply quantifies the degree of linear association (or not) between two variables. However, it is often more useful to *describe* the relationship between the two variables, or even *predict* a value of one variable for a given value of the other, and this is done using regression. If it is sensible to assume that one variable may be causing a response in the other, then regression analysis should be used.

CONCLUSIONS

In summary, this chapter has outlined the process of testing hypotheses and emphasised the usefulness of confidence intervals when drawing conclusions from the results of studies. In addition, it has covered some of the basic statistical tests for the types of data outlined in the previous chapter. Armed with this information, for a given set of such data it should be possible to decide on the most appropriate analysis, carry out the chosen method and draw conclusions from the results.

Reference

Altman DG (1990) *Practical Statistics for Medical Research*. London, Chapman & Hall.

Further reading

Huff D (1991) *How to Lie with Statistics*. London, Penguin Books.
Kinnear R, Gray CD (2004) *SPSS for Windows Made Simple: Release 12*. Hove, Psychology Press.
See Chapter 35 for further references.

Putting Research into Practice

The final section of this book moves on from the practical process of doing research to consider how research can make a difference to nursing and healthcare practice.

Chapter 37 deals with the very important stage of moving a research study on from an investigation into a piece of new knowledge, accessible to other members of the profession and the wider public. It is a practical guide to writing research reports, journal articles, presenting at conferences and other means of dissemination.

Chapters 38 and 39 take the next logical step of considering how healthcare practice integrates (or does not) the new knowledge generated by research. These two chapters, now both written by the same author, are designed to be read together, but each also stands complete in itself. Chapter 38 looks at the theory underpinning evidence-based practice and assesses different models of research utilisation relevant to nursing. Chapter 39 builds on this foundation to discuss knowledge translation and the different ways in which research products can be used in practice. The difficult process of implementing change is fundamental to this process and is given some consideration in the last section of the chapter.

The book ends with a chapter that continues the discussion begun in Chapter 1 about the policy context of building research capacity in nursing in the four countries that make up the UK. Five imperatives are identified and appraised, each of which is essential if nursing is to move forward in its quest to increase its research base, to establish nursing research as a viable career option and to increase the impact of nursing knowledge on healthcare policy. Ultimately, the success or otherwise of this quest will impact, for better or worse, on patient outcomes, and it is this which really underlines the value of nursing research.

37 Disseminating Research Findings

Kate Gerrish and Anne Lacey

Key points

- Research findings need to be disseminated in various ways for different audiences.
- Journal articles and research reports are the main written forms of dissemination and each needs to be written in an appropriate style.
- Presentations at conferences, verbally or in poster format, are effective ways of disseminating results and networking with other researchers.
- Websites, workshops and clinical guidelines can be used by researchers to tell others about their work.

INTRODUCTION

Although research may be an interesting and intellectually satisfying activity in its own right, there is little point in carrying out research unless it is disseminated to those who can make use of the new knowledge generated. Public funding of research by bodies such as the Department of Health and Research Councils is done on the understanding that results will be made known to the public and, where appropriate, used to improve healthcare. Having said this, it is still true that many research reports never get far beyond the desks of those carrying out the study and those funding it. Even publication in a journal does not guarantee that the appropriate community, professional or public will hear about the research. So how do we ensure optimum communication from the research community to the professionals involved in healthcare, the users of healthcare and the wider public?

COMMUNICATING WITH DIFFERENT AUDIENCES

The same piece of research may be disseminated in different ways. First, a report is likely to be written as a permanent record of the research and to satisfy the needs of those commissioning, funding and supporting the study. If the research was undertaken as part of an education programme, the report will take the form of a dissertation or thesis.

The research may also be reported as an article in a high-status academic journal such as the *Journal of Advanced Nursing* or the *British Medical Journal*, where it is likely to be read by nurses and other health professionals in academic roles and by some students and advanced practitioners. Such journals have strict guidelines for the reporting of research (see for example www.journalofadvancednursing.com, www.bmj.com) that need to be followed. The research findings may be picked up from high-profile journals and reported in the media, if they are of public interest or controversial.

Research findings may also be written up, perhaps in a different form, in a popular professional journal such as *Nursing Standard*. Here, they will be read by a wider range of practising nurses who are not necessarily engaged in academic study. Furthermore, there is an increasing expectation that research findings should be disseminated to those who participated in the study. A succinct summary written in a suitable language may need to be prepared for patients and the wider public.

Increasingly, research is disseminated via dedicated websites, which may have links to other websites of a similar nature. Websites allow more visual and interactive communication, and so provide opportunities for creative presentation.

Finally, the research may be communicated verbally or as a poster at international, national and local conferences, workshops and seminars, at journal clubs and research interest groups in the workplace.

Each of these ways of disseminating research findings requires a different style and different resources, and serves a different audience. We will address each of these means of dissemination in turn.

THE RESEARCH REPORT

A research study is not complete until a report has been written and submitted to interested parties. The report serves as a complete record of what was done, how it was undertaken, details of results and conclusions. Implications for practice may also be included, where relevant. The report will provide an account of the research to those who commissioned and funded it, but can also become a means of dissemination to those who can make use of the findings. The length and style of the research report is highly variable. Where research is conducted for an education degree, the report is the dissertation or thesis, written in academic language and, in the case of a doctoral thesis, running to 100,000 words or more. In contrast, a small project carried out in clinical practice may be reported in 20 pages or less. Whatever the length and style, however, the content is likely to be similar in format. It should be noted that universities produce guidelines on the presentation and content of a thesis and these should be adhered to.

The writing of a research report follows conventions that closely mirror the research process itself. These are outlined in Box 37.1. Sections of the report will vary according to the intended audience.

WRITING AN ARTICLE FOR PUBLICATION

Publishing research in an academic or professional journal provides a means of disseminating the

---

Box 37.1 Sections of a research report

Abstract or executive summary

This should orientate the reader to the whole study. It is best written at the end after the detailed report is complete.

Introduction

This section describes the background to the study and the context in which it was undertaken.

Aims of the research

The aims, research questions and any hypotheses to be tested should be stated clearly.

Literature review

A comprehensive literature review will set out the available knowledge before the research commenced. The length and depth of this review will depend on the audience of the report. An academic dissertation requires a substantial section critically appraising the available evidence, whereas policy makers are likely to require a more concise summary.

Research design

A clear description of the conceptual framework used, the methodology adopted and data collection methods selected is required to give the reader an understanding of the research design.

Access and ethical approval

All research conducted in a healthcare context should have obtained ethical and research governance approval, and a statement to this effect should be included. Other access negotiations and procedures for recruiting and gaining consent from research participants will be given. Copies of consent forms and information sheets may be included in an appendix.

Sampling

This section will provide details of how sampling was done, sample size calculations, and the composition and characteristics of the sample obtained.

Data collection

A full account of how data were collected, data collection tools and outcome measures used will be given here.

Data analysis

A description of how the data were analysed is necessary, as well as a full presentation of the results. For quantitative research, this will be in the form of tables and figures, with a narrative commentary. For qualitative research, the results will be presented in words, with verbatim quotations from interviews, fieldnotes, etc., as supporting evidence. Qualitative research reports often include discussion within the presentation of the results, rather than keeping the two sections separate as suggested below.

Discussion and conclusion

This section gives the researcher the opportunity to reflect on the findings in the light of previous literature, and to draw conclusions. Implications for practice, suggested further research and any limitations of the study are commonly included.

findings to a wide, possibly international, audience. Authors also gain considerable personal satisfaction from seeing their work in print.

A published article on a research study will generally follow the same structure as a research report referred to in the previous section, albeit in a more condensed format. However, the content of the paper and writing style will vary according to the target audience for the journal. An academic journal normally requires a detailed account of the research in which the author demonstrates rigour in carrying out the study as well as showing how the research contributes to advancing knowledge in the field. The style of writing tends to be formal. By contrast, the account of the research methodology in a professional journal is normally concise, with more emphasis placed on the findings and implications for policy and practice. A journalistic approach that seeks to engage the reader's attention may be used.

Preparing an article for submission

Selecting an appropriate journal for publication requires careful groundwork. The first step is to become familiar with the journal by reading some back issues. This will provide insight into the types of article the editor seeks to publish, the intended audience and the writing style. Most journals provide detailed guidance for contributors, and this may be published in the journal or available on the publisher's website. This guidance frequently provides information on the aims and scope of the journal to help authors decide whether their work is appropriate for a particular journal. A useful website run by the Medical College of Ohio (http://mulford.meduohio.edu/instr/) provides an index of all instructions for authors for healthcare journals.

Once familiar with the types of article published in different journals, a decision can be made about which one to pursue. This decision should be informed by an objective appraisal of the match between the type of article published in the journal and the nature of the research to be reported. If in doubt, advice should be sought from someone who is experienced at writing for publication, or from the journal editors themselves.

The guidelines for authors normally provide details of the expected content and format of the article, and should be followed closely. Increasingly, journals are moving towards electronic submission via a manuscript tracking system that enables the publication process to be managed electronically and gives authors the opportunity to check on the progress of their paper.

Having decided on the journal and studied the guidance for authors, writing can begin. A novice will find it beneficial to co-author with someone with a track record of publication. Once a draft version of the paper has been written it is advisable to seek feedback from colleagues who can provide constructive advice on how it might be improved. A paper is likely to require several revisions before it reaches the stage where it is ready for submission. Before submitting the paper it is important to undertake a final proofread, check all references are correctly cited in the text and the reference list, and ensure that it is presented in the required format.

The review process

All papers submitted to editors undergo some form of assessment to ascertain whether they are suitable for publication in a particular journal. Academic journals and an increasing number of professional journals seek an independent review (peer review) of the paper by one or more people who are judged to be experts in the field. Before a decision is made to send a paper for review, the editor usually undertakes an initial assessment and it may be that the paper is considered unsuitable and rejected at this stage.

Usually a paper is reviewed 'blind', in other words the reviewer does not know the identity of the author and the feedback from the reviewer to the author is anonymised. However, there are increasing calls for a more open review process and some editors are now considering making authors and reviewers aware of each other's identity (Smith 1997).

Many journals provide guidance to reviewers on the areas they should consider when assessing a paper. Whereas journals differ in terms of their aims and readership, the criteria used to assess a paper are often similar. An example of general criteria used by reviewers is given in Box 37.2.

Box 37.2 General criteria used to review an article

- Relevance of topic to journal aims
- Potential interest to readership
- Originality and contribution to knowledge and/or practice
- Scientific rigour
- Clarity and coherence of the article
- Style of writing, angle, level of presentation

It will normally take several weeks for an author to receive feedback from the editor. The reviewers' comments are usually sent to authors together with an editorial decision. In exceptional circumstances the paper may be accepted as submitted. However, it is more common for authors to be asked to revise their paper on the basis of the feedback from reviewers. Where a paper is rejected outright the reviewers' feedback should provide an indication as to why it was considered unsuitable. Suggestions may also be made on how to develop the paper for publication elsewhere.

When revising a paper the author should give serious consideration to the reviewers' recommendations. Where an author disagrees with a reviewer, the editor needs to be informed of the reasons why the author has not taken the recommendations on board. Indeed, many journals ask authors to submit a separate report providing details of how they have responded to the reviewers' comments. A revised paper may need to be sent out for further review, so authors should anticipate a time delay.

The publication process

Once a paper has been accepted for publication the editor will notify the author and often provides an indication of the anticipated publication date. Some journals now publish articles 'online' a couple of months before they appear in the paper version of the journal. Before the paper is published authors will be asked to sign a copyright declaration form that assigns the copyright of the article to the publisher. Whereas assigning copyright imposes certain restrictions on the author's future use of the material, it is designed to protect the interests of the author, for example should others plagiarise their work.

A few weeks before publication the author is sent the page proofs to check. These are presented in the format in which the article will appear in the journal and provide a clear indication of what it will look like in print. It is important that authors check the page proofs carefully for accuracy. However, only essential changes can be made at this stage as more extensive editing is costly and will delay publication. Authors need to be aware that minor changes may have been made to their original manuscript. Usually this is to correct minor errors, but some editors of professional journals may make more significant changes. If an author is unhappy with any changes that have been made to the article it is essential that the editor is informed. After all, it is the author's work and they have the right to decide the ultimate content of the article.

Many journals are now published in electronic, as well as paper, format and some are only produced electronically. These 'e-journals' appear on the internet and articles can be downloaded, but they never appear in print form. This form of publication reduces the time taken for an article to be disseminated. Many e-journals have a stringent system of ensuring quality, just as print journals do. Such journals commonly have no subscription system; however, authors may be asked to pay for publication of their article. The *International Electronic Journal of Health Education* is an early example of such a journal, running since 1998 (www.aahperd.org/iejhe/).

Political issues in the publication process

It may be necessary to seek permission to publish from the funding body that has commissioned the research. This requirement is usually written into the research contract. The research funder may wish to see the paper before it is sent for publication and may require a disclaimer to be included, which states that the views expressed in the paper are those of the authors and not the research funding body.

It is also good practice to acknowledge those who have contributed to the research but are not co-authors of the paper. This may include the funding body, individuals who have granted special permissions, for example agreeing to a questionnaire they have developed being used in the study, or who have provided particular support, such as a supervisor or Project Advisory Group members.

Where a team has undertaken a study it is generally appropriate for all members to be co-authors of the article. This should be agreed in advance, as there can be difficulties if a member of the research team feels they were not given an opportunity to contribute to a paper. Disagreements about whose name will appear first are likely if this is not made clear from the outset. Supervisors often co-author papers with their students, and normally the student's name appears as first author. Anyone who co-authors a paper should have made a significant contribution to the research study and/or to writing the paper. Increasingly, editors require each author to sign a declaration confirming their contribution.

Researchers who are based in academic institutions in the UK may be required to submit their publications as part of the Research Assessment Exercise (RAE). This is a periodic assessment by national and international experts of the quality of research in a particular discipline, for example, nursing. The quality of published research is the main criterion used to judge the overall quality of research within a university. Numerical ratings of research quality ranging from 1* (national significance) to 5* (world-leading) are linked to funding allocations and therefore universities take the RAE most seriously. High-status academic journals are regarded by many disciplines as the most appropriate avenue for research outputs to be included in the RAE. Whereas the RAE Nursing Panel has tended to be more eclectic, valuing a range of possible outputs, new researchers in university settings would do well to seek advice from more experienced colleagues on the most suitable journals in which to publish. Following the 2008 RAE, the process was replaced by the Research Excellence Framework (REF). At the time of going

to press the criteria for judging the quality of nursing research in this new framework have yet to be clarified.

PREPARING A REPORT FOR THE PUBLIC

Increasingly, researchers are expected to feed back their findings to those who have participated in the study and to make their findings more widely accessible to the general public. The researchers will still need to present an account of what they set out to achieve, how they went about undertaking the study, what they found and what conclusions they were able to draw, but the traditional headings of 'aims', 'methodology', 'results' and 'conclusions' may not be easily understandable to the general public, who have little knowledge of the research process. Instead, researchers should write a summary, in plain English, which gives a clear overview of the study. It should be written in a style that engages the reader. Technical terms should be avoided, or where these are necessary, an explanation should be given. It may be helpful to ask lay members of a Project Advisory Group, or even family and friends to comment on drafts to ensure that they are readily understandable to the general public. Details of the full project report or links to a website for further information may also be included for people who are interested in finding out more.

PRESENTING RESEARCH AT A CONFERENCE

Presenting research at a conference helps to disseminate the findings more quickly than is possible by publication. Research findings can be presented in the form of an oral presentation or a poster at national or international conferences. Increasingly, health authorities and NHS trusts host conferences that provide the opportunity to disseminate research across the local health community and facilitate networking with colleagues who share similar interests. Such conferences provide an ideal opportunity for the novice presenter to hone their skills. Many national and international conferences focus on a particular area of nursing, for example clinical practice, management or education, and presentations need to address the conference theme. However, some conferences, such as the Royal College of Nursing Annual International Research Conference, focus specifically on research and invite presentations on a broad range of topics.

Conference organisers may invite lead researchers to present their work, but most researchers are required to submit an abstract for an oral or poster presentation for consideration by a selection panel. When deciding where to submit an abstract it is worth considering the material to be presented and the intended audience. For example, a study examining a new form of treatment for the management of leg ulcers by community nurses might form the basis of an abstract for a conference on community nursing, wound management or a research conference. If the intention is to disseminate the findings to a large number of clinical nurses then a conference related to a particular area of nursing may be most suitable. Research conferences, by contrast, provide the opportunity to discuss aspects of the research process as well as the findings with an audience who have a particular interest in research.

Writing a conference abstract

A major factor in having an abstract accepted for presentation is whether the author has followed the guidelines provided in the published 'call for abstracts'. This normally specifies:

- the conference themes
- the deadline date for submission
- the format and content of the abstract, including the maximum word length
- whether there is an option to present the work either as an oral presentation or a poster
- the criteria by which the abstract will be judged.

The abstract provides the only information the selection panel has to make its decision about whether a proposed presentation is relevant and of suitable quality. It is essential to present information in a concise and informative way that grabs the interest of the reviewer, and ultimately the conference delegate. Box 37.3 gives an example of the criteria by which an abstract may be judged.

Abstracts that exceed the word length or which do not use the specified headings may be automatically rejected. Despite these constraints it is possible to

---

Box 37.3 Abstract submission checklist

**ROYAL COLLEGE OF NURSING OF THE UNITED KINGDOM
ANNUAL INTERNATIONAL NURSING RESEARCH CONFERENCE**

Abstract submission checklist (for concurrent session and poster presentation)

Abstracts submitted to the RCN's annual international nursing research conference are peer reviewed by an international panel. The criteria against which reviewers make their recommendations are detailed in the online abstract submission form. These criteria are listed here in the form of a checklist for you to use prior to submitting your abstract. You may also like to invite a 'critical friend' to review your abstract against these criteria before you submit it. If you have any ticks in the 'no' column you can then amend your abstract before you submit it and hence increase the potential for your abstract to be accepted and included in the conference programme.

Continued

		yes	no	n/a
1	The abstract is about a research project or a research-related issue (for example policy or a methodological issue)			
2	Material presented in abstracts must be concise and coherent, with the focus of the abstract stated clearly			
3	The authors must make explicit what they intend to present			
4	The abstract title should be short and clearly declare the content of the abstract			
5	Abstracts of empirical studies must outline the research process and the focus of the analysis, they must indicate when the data was collected and provide an indication of the results (NB an abstract will not be accepted if data has not already been collected)			
6	Abstracts reporting on the results of research studies should be structured: background, aims, methods, results, discussion and conclusions			
7	Statistics including sample size and sampling method used must be supplied where appropriate			
8	Relevant contextual information must be given			
9	Authors must specify how the paper will contribute to the development of knowledge and policy and practice within health and healthcare			
10	The word limit must be adhered to and authors are required to declare that their abstract is within the limit (a) For **concurrent** and **poster** submissions the word limit is 300 (excluding references) (b) For **symposium** submissions the word limit is 300 for each of the individual papers to be included in the symposium (excluding references, authors details and principal authors' CV) (c) For **workshop** submissions 1000 words (excluding references, authors details and principal authors' CV)			
11	Abstracts for poster and concurrent presentations must not contain information which could identify the author/s, as these are reviewed blind			
12	For poster and concurrent presentations, up to three references may be cited and these must be provided using the Harvard referencing system			
13	Symposium and workshop abstracts must be accompanied by a CV demonstrating the principal author's competence to deliver			
14	All abstracts must be written in English			

The RCN Research Society has published guidance on research ethics and is committed to promoting ethical research and ethical research practice. It is assumed that those submitting an abstract have ensured that all relevant ethical standards have been met. In addition it is assumed that the owner(s) of the intellectual property of any research submitted for presentation have granted their express permission for the research to be submitted for presentation.

Misrepresentation of the same material as original in more than one publication will be discouraged and the World Association of Medical Editors guidance will be applied.

Reproduced with permission from the RCN Research Society and R&D Co-ordinating Centre

37.1 A Conference Abstract

Participatory community research: reflections on a study of the socio-cultural factors influencing an understanding of TB within the Somali community

Participatory community research provides a framework whereby researchers work in partnership with members of the community in which they are undertaking research. The principal features of this approach include collaboration, mutual education and acting on results developed from research questions that are relevant to the community. The knowledge, expertise and resources of the community are key to the success of the research (Macaulay *et al.* 1999). This presentation will provide a reflexive account of the learning that occurred from undertaking a participatory ethnographic study of the socio-cultural factors influencing an understanding of TB within the Somali community. Partnerships were established between academic researchers, healthcare professionals and the Somali community. Data were collected through fieldwork, in-depth interviews and focus groups with Somali TB patients, members of the wider Somali community and healthcare professionals.

Consideration will be given to the nature of the community involvement in the research process. This ranged from collaboration in developing the research proposal, through gaining access to the field, undertaking data collection and analysis, interpreting the findings and disseminating the results using culturally appropriate methods. Key issues that will be discussed include:

- the role of opinion leaders as advocates for the Somali community, custodians of community knowledge, gatekeepers in facilitating access to participants and champions for promoting the study.
- the complementary roles of members of the research team, which included Somali community researchers and a TB specialist nurse in addition to an academic researcher
- the practicalities of involving Somali community researchers
- recognising and responding to cultural and ethnic diversity in the research team
- the place of reciprocity in the research partnership
- the challenge of managing the different expectations of the various collaborators.

The paper will conclude with recommendations for further developing participatory community research approaches.

Macaulay A *et al.* (1999) Participatory research maximises community and lay involvement. *British Medical Journal* **319**: 774–778.

(Oral presentation at the RCN International Research Conference 2009 by K Gerrish, M Ismail, A Naisby)

convey a considerable amount of information in relatively few words. For example:

'A survey by self-completed questionnaire was undertaken with a random sample of ward-based nurses working in a large teaching hospital in England. Content validity and reliability of the questionnaire were established. Of a random sample of 700 nurses, 563 responded.'

This covers the design, method, sample and setting in just 40 words. An example of an abstract is given in Research Example 37.1.

Deciding whether to present an oral paper or a poster is to some extent a matter of personal choice. Whereas novice presenters may feel more comfortable with a poster presentation, they should not underestimate the considerable effort and resources required to produce a high-quality poster and the time required during the conference to be available to discuss the poster. Although the idea of an oral presentation may appear daunting, with careful planning and the opportunity to practise by presenting the paper to colleagues beforehand, the novice researcher can get an enormous amount of personal satisfaction from delivering an oral presentation.

Oral presentations

The letter confirming acceptance of an oral presentation will normally include information about the time allocated for the paper, where it appears on the conference programme and what audiovisual facilities will be available. However, presenters may not be notified in advance of the size and layout of the room in which they will present. There may be no indication of the likely size of the audience, so they will need to plan for different eventualities.

Some presenters may feel that they need to read verbatim from a paper. Whereas this provides the opportunity to produce a coherent, well-constructed presentation, it can be difficult for the audience to concentrate on someone reading for any length of time. A presenter who uses notes or written prompt cards for guidance and who maintains eye contact with the audience is more likely to keep their attention.

The key to presenting a successful paper is to be realistic on how much information can be included within the time available. If planning to read a paper verbatim, a reasonable conversion rate is to consider 500 words as equivalent to five minutes' speaking time. If using PowerPoint slides, it is reasonable to prepare about one slide per two minutes of presentation. This means that only limited information on some aspects of a research study can be included.

Deciding what to include is probably the most difficult task. Delegates at a conference that attracts clinical nurses are likely to be interested in research findings and their implications for practice, whereas those attending a research conference are likely to be interested in the methodology used. Many conferences request that presenters allow time at the end of their paper for the audience to ask questions. Ensure that this is planned into the allotted time.

Including audiovisual aids enhances the presentation and helps maintain the audiences' attention. It is essential to check in advance what facilities are available. Overhead projectors and slide projectors have largely been replaced by computer projection using PowerPoint. When planning to use PowerPoint presentations it is essential to check which version of the software is available. Animation features that have been developed in the most recent version may not work with older versions. Advice should be sought from the conference organisers about how the computer file should be prepared, for example on CD or flash drive. Assistance with preparing audiovisual aids may be available locally in NHS trusts or universities, and can also be found on the internet.

Once the content has been decided upon and audiovisual aids prepared, it is essential to rehearse, preferably in front of friendly colleagues. Keeping to time should be the most important priority. Conference programmes often run to a tight schedule and it can be frustrating for delegates when a paper is cut short because the presenter has run out of time. It is also essential to practise using the audiovisual equipment to ensure a smooth transition in the presentation.

Once at the conference, check out the venue and the audiovisual facilities as far in advance of the presentation as possible, seeking help from a technician if required. In terms of the actual delivery it is important to consider:

- posture, movement and hand actions – face the audience, stand rather than sit, avoid excessive movements and fiddling with paper clips, etc.
- eye contact and facial expression – look at the audience, adopt a relaxed facial expression and try to smile!
- voice – aim to achieve clarity and variety, speak clearly and slowly, and use appropriate intonation by raising, lowering and altering the tone of voice.

Poster presentations

Preparing a poster requires considerable time, so it is essential to think about the presentation well in advance of the conference. Many NHS trusts and universities have departments that can help with both design and production. The cost of producing a poster ranges from a few pounds to several hundred. Although a professionally presented poster produced with the assistance of a graphic designer is impressive, there is no reason why someone with a more modest budget cannot produce a very effective poster. Advice on designing posters is readily available via the internet. Computer software (such as MS Word, PowerPoint and Desktop publishing) is increasingly available in the workplace and can be used to produce posters.

Details of the amount of space available will be provided with the letter confirming acceptance of the abstract. It is essential that the poster fits the parameters given. A poster should not be overcrowded with information as this will detract from its impact and delegates will quickly tire. The noise and bustle of a poster viewing hall is rarely conducive to a serious read. Text should be sufficiently large to be read easily from a distance of at least one metre, although the title should be larger to attract interest from a distance. There should be a balance between text and other visual stimuli such as graphs, figures or photographs. Material should be sequenced in a logical manner with the reader clearly guided through the content. Numbered headings or arrows can help here.

There is a tendency when planning the content of a poster to be over-ambitious in terms of content. The key is to present information succinctly – short phrases rather than full sentences will often suffice. The title needs to be short and snappy to attract attention. The name and contact details of members of the research team should be included. It is usual to provide a brief introduction to the topic or project. Other areas to include depend on the poster topic. If the poster is about a research study, it needs to include information on the aims, sample, methods, findings and conclusions. Supporting materials that delegates can take away can also be produced. For example, a scaled-down version of the poster can be printed on A4 paper, or alternatively a more detailed written account of the research project prepared as a handout.

When designing a poster on a tight budget there may be a tendency to take the easy option of printing out a series of A4 PowerPoint slides and mounting these on the poster board. Although this kind of display can convey the essential information, its visual impact is not as great as a large poster. Many computer software packages allow for a larger format than A4 to be designed. Once the poster has been designed on the computer, it may be possible to have it printed within a local NHS trust or university. Alternatively, a number of high street print companies will produce the poster from disc on to suitably sized paper and laminate it for a reasonable price. However, before the material is taken for printing it is essential to proofread carefully as errors cannot be rectified.

Consideration should be given to transporting the poster to the conference. It is recommended that it is taken as hand luggage in a waterproof container. Although conference organisers may provide materials to mount the poster on the presentation board it is advisable to take an 'emergency kit', including, for example, Velcro, double-sided tape, drawing pins and scissors.

Finally, it is important to remember that presenters are normally required to spend time beside the poster discussing it with interested parties. This is often during meal breaks and presenters need to think about how to manage their time. When it is necessary to leave a poster unattended during a specified conference viewing time it is helpful to leave a note beside the poster indicating when the presenter will be available to answer questions, together with a phone number or email address.

NETWORKING OPPORTUNITIES, RESEARCH PARTNERSHIPS AND COLLABORATIONS

In addition to the more traditional means of dissemination through publications and conference presentations there are several other ways of disseminating research.

Websites

Large-scale, funded research projects often have a dedicated website that will include regular updates with progress of the study and may post interim findings before they are more widely available. University department or professional web pages in a NHS trust may provide the opportunity for a synopsis of ongoing or recently completed research to be posted.

Workshops and seminars

Both NHS trusts and universities may have research interest groups that meet regularly to provide a forum for local researchers to present their work. A seminar, in which the audience is encouraged to discuss a paper in some detail, calls for a more participatory form of presentation than a traditional conference paper. Workshops enable participants to engage more actively in discussion and contribute their own ideas, often through working on specific tasks in small groups. This can be particularly useful for researchers who wish to work with potential 'users' of their research, such as patient groups, healthcare providers, educators and policy makers, in order to consider the implementation of their findings.

Practice guidelines

Chapter 39 considers how research findings can be used to develop clinical guidelines and care pathways. Such guidance is normally based on a systematic review of several studies on a particular topic. However, the findings from an individual study may have important implications for practice. One way of making this information accessible to practitioners is to produce practice guidelines. These are normally concise documents that identify how the research findings can be applied locally. For example, a study examining nurses' attitudes towards the use of IT in a large hospital may identify particular education needs that can be incorporated into in-service training initiatives or used to inform curriculum development of nursing courses in a local university.

CONCLUSIONS

Dissemination of research, while it is being undertaken and after its completion, is essential if the knowledge generated is going to be used by the nursing profession. Dissemination also gives an opportunity for researchers to learn from one another's experience and to engage in networks with others working in a similar field. There are many forms of communication available to researchers, ranging from academic journal articles to informal local discussion groups. The mode of presentation needs to take account of these differing audiences.

References

Macaulay A *et al.* (1999) Participatory research maximises community and lay involvement. *British Medical Journal* **319**: 774–778.

Smith R (1997) Peer review: reform or revolution? Time to open up the black box of peer review. Editorial. *British Medical Journal* **315**: 759–760.

Further reading

Canter D, Fairbairn G (2006) *Becoming an Author: advice for academics and other professionals*. Buckingham, Open University Press.

Gerrish K (2005) Getting published: practicalities, pitfalls and plagiarism. *Journal of Community Nursing* **19**(8): 13–15.

Hardicre J, Devitt P, Cod J (2007) Ten steps to successful poster presentation. *British Journal of Nursing* **16**(7): 398–400.

Jackson K, Sheldon L (2000) Demystifying the academic aura: preparing a poster. *Nurse Researcher* **7**(3): 70–73.

Johnstone M (2004) *Effective Writing for Health Professionals: a practice guide to getting published*. Oxford, Routledge.

Murray R (2008) *Writing Up Your University Assignments and Research Projects*. Buckingham, Open University Press.

Murray R (2006) *How to Write a Thesis*. Buckingham, Open University Press.

Murray R (2004) *Writing for Academic Journals*. Buckingham, Open University Press.

Websites

http://mulford.meduohio.edu/instr/ – the Medical College of Ohio website that lists all instructions for authors for journals in the health and medical sciences.

www.rcn.org.uk/development/researchanddevelopment/ dissemination – the RCN Research and Development Coordinating Centre contains tips and advice on getting published and information on different nursing and health journals with links to their websites.

www.vitae.ac.uk/1298/Publishing-your-research.html – the researchers' portal of the 'vitae realising the potential of researchers' website provides practical advice on presenting research for different audiences and on publishing research findings.

38 Evidence-based Practice

Kate Gerrish

Key points

- Evidence-based practice involves integrating the best available research evidence with professional expertise while also taking account of patient preferences.

- Evidence-based practice is a complex undertaking that involves identifying and appraising different sources of evidence, translating evidence into clear guidance for practice, implementing and finally evaluating the impact of change.

- Research findings may be applied directly to practice in the form of clinical protocols or practice guidelines, used indirectly to inform nurses' understanding of practice or used persuasively to present a case for changes in policy or practice.

- Barriers to achieving evidence-based practice relate to the nature of the evidence, the way in which the evidence is communicated, the knowledge and skills of the individual nurse and the organisational context.

INTRODUCTION

Evidence-based practice has, over the past two decades, become a major concern of healthcare policy makers, care providers and professional groups. Nurses, alongside other healthcare practitioners, recognise that high quality care is dependent on being able to use robust evidence to underpin clinical interventions. Yet achieving evidence-based care is a complex undertaking. It requires considerable skill in identifying and appraising evidence in order to decide whether it is appropriate to use. The evidence then needs to be translated into guidance that can be understood and used by practitioners before being introduced into everyday practice. However,

introducing change is far from straightforward. Commitment is needed from individual nurses, together with support from colleagues within the multidisciplinary team and from managers. Finally, the impact of the change in practice needs to be evaluated. This activity needs to be supported by appropriate resources and take place in an environment where practitioners are comfortable with questioning practice and willing to embrace change.

This chapter examines the concept of evidence-based practice. The debates about what constitutes 'good' evidence are explored and consideration is given to different models of research utilisation and factors influencing evidence-based practice. This sets the scene for the following chapter, which examines the implementation of evidence-based practice.

THE NATURE OF 'EVIDENCE' IN EVIDENCE-BASED PRACTICE

There is considerable debate within the nursing literature about whether the 'evidence' in evidence-based practice should relate solely to research evidence or if a broader definition is more appropriate, bearing in mind that there may be insufficient research evidence to support some nursing interventions. The potential contribution of different forms of evidence is identified in one of the most frequently used definitions of evidence-based practice (Sackett *et al.* 1996). They define the concept of evidence-based medicine as follows.

> The conscientious, explicit and judicious use of current best evidence in making decisions about the care of individual patients. The practice of evidence-based medicine means integrating individual clinical expertise with the best available external evidence from systematic research.

While this definition focuses on the care required by individual patients, the concept of evidence-based practice can be extended to groups of patients, health-care services and policy initiatives (Muir Gray 2004).

It is worth examining the above definition in more detail. The emphasis on *current best evidence* draws attention to the changing nature of evidence. As more research is undertaken on a particular topic, a body of knowledge is built up; however, this knowledge base is constantly evolving. Nurses need to keep up to date with research findings in order to provide the best possible care. The reference to *external evidence from systematic research* implies that research evidence should be in the public domain and accessible. Furthermore, the process whereby the evidence was generated should be clearly stated and open to scrutiny. Sackett *et al.*'s definition also emphasises the part that *clinical expertise* should play in making decisions about the most appropriate care. This is particularly important in situations where research evidence is lacking or the findings are inconclusive or contradictory. Clinical expertise is the proficiency that practitioners gain through experience, and is reflected in effective assessment and thoughtful and compassionate use of individual patient's preferences in making decisions about their care (Sackett *et al.*

1996). Thus evidence-based practice should take account of the preferences of patients and their carers, who will have their own views about the care they should receive.

Let us now consider the different components of evidence-based practice.

Research findings as evidence

As the previous chapters of this book have demonstrated, the systematic nature of research means that it should be possible to use research findings with a reasonable degree of confidence. However, all research has limitations. It is essential, therefore, that research reports are subject to critical scrutiny in order to decide whether or not the quality of the research is sufficient to support the conclusions drawn. Chapter 7 provides guidance on how to undertake a critical appraisal of published research. However, the skills of critical appraisal cannot be viewed in isolation from knowledge of the research process. To undertake a rigorous review of a research report it is essential to have a good understanding of different research designs, and methods of data collection and analysis, and also to be aware of ethical considerations.

Evidence provided from a single research study is generally considered insufficient grounds to justify changing practice. Rather, a body of research evidence on a particular topic needs to be established. Ideally, a systematic review of relevant research (as outlined in Chapter 24) should be undertaken in order to draw an overall conclusion about the cumulative evidence. This activity is time-consuming and requires a sound understanding of research methodologies. It is therefore beyond the scope of many practising nurses unless undertaken as part of an education course. However, there are several organisations that publish systematic reviews of clinical interventions that can be accessed by nurses or which translate the information provided from systematic reviews into evidence-based guidelines (see Box 38.1).

Even when a systematic review has been published it may still not provide conclusive evidence to guide practice. Gerrish *et al.* (1999) describe how their

Box 38.1 Organisations publishing information to support evidence-based practice

Systematic reviews

Bandolier – www.medicine.ox.ac.uk/bandolier/
NIHR Centre for reviews and dissemination – www.york.ac.uk/inst/crd
The Cochrane collaboration – www.cochrane.org/index.htm
The Joanna Briggs Institute – www.joannabriggs.edu.au/about/home.php

Evidence-based guidelines

National Institute for Health and Clinical Excellence (NICE) – www.nice.org.uk
NHS Evidence Health Information Resources – www.library.nhs.uk
Royal College of Nursing – www.rcn.org.uk/development/practice/clinicalguidelines

plans to work with managers and practitioners to implement long-awaited guidance on the prevention and treatment of pressure sores (Effective Health Care 1995) were thwarted when the systematic review concluded that there was insufficient evidence to guide practice, and what evidence there was proved contradictory. They then had to draw on professional expertise to identify best practice to supplement tentative research findings. More recently, NICE guidance on nutrition support of adults based many of the recommendations on best practice as there was a lack of robust research evidence (NICE 2006). Thus in concluding this section it needs to be acknowledged that although the evidence base for some interventions may be extremely well-founded, such as a meta-analysis across a number of clinical trials that finds a consistent effect, other interventions are not underpinned by this level of robust research evidence (Dopson 2007). Moreover, as Bucknall (2007) points out, scientific facts derived from research only become evidence when the practitioner decides that the information is relevant to a particular situation.

Professional expertise as evidence

There is debate within the nursing literature as to whether professional expertise should be considered

'evidence'. Closs (2003), for example, argues that although clinical expertise is essential to the delivery of high-quality care, it does not constitute evidence *per se*. From her perspective, evidence is derived from research findings that have been validated through the process of peer review and resulted in publication. She also cautions against assuming that experience will lead to excellence in practice. Although experienced nurses may be able to predict problems and needs that other nurses may not, they may hold personal opinions that have no factual basis and which do not form reliable evidence.

Other commentators take a much broader view of evidence derived from professional experience. Eraut (1994) describes this form of evidence as 'practical knowledge' and differentiates it from the 'technical' or 'propositional knowledge' derived from research. It is the knowledge that is embedded in practice and which is often tacit or intuitive. It is acquired by nurses working alongside role models or others considered to be experts. Recent research has highlighted the extent to which nurses draw on the knowledge gained experientially in the workplace, for example from specialist nurses, members of the multidisciplinary team and professional networks (Thompson *et al.* 2001; Milner *et al.* 2005). Indeed, nurses draw on these sources of knowledge more frequently than formal sources of knowledge such as published research reports (Gerrish *et al.* 2008).

Liaschenko and Fisher (1999) provide a useful way of conceptualising the knowledge that nurses use within the context of evidence-based practice. They identify three different forms of knowledge.

- *Scientific knowledge* is largely biomedical knowledge derived from research and includes, for example, nurses' knowledge of disease processes and treatment regimes.
- *Patient knowledge* includes knowledge about how an individual becomes identified as a patient, how the person responds to treatment, how to get things done for the patient and who else may be involved in providing services for the patient. Nurses use this practical 'know-how' knowledge gained through experience alongside research-based knowledge to guide their practice.
- *Person knowledge* is gained through viewing a patient as an individual with a personal biography and who occupies a particular social space. Knowing a person means understanding something of what living with the disease or disability is like for the individual and seeing that individual as more than a patient in a healthcare system.

Liaschenko and Fisher indicate that experienced nurses draw on these different forms of knowledge, especially when there may be conflict between an individual patient's preferences and the opinions of healthcare professionals or among the professionals themselves. For example, they use it to justify an alternative approach to disease management and to defend their actions to support an individual patient's choice, even when this may conflict with established biomedical or institutional practices.

The experiential forms of knowledge (patient and person) identified above can have a reciprocal, reinforcing relationship with scientific evidence. Ferlie *et al.* (1999) have shown that research evidence is more influential when it tallies with clinical experience; conversely, when research evidence and clinical experience do not match, its use in practice can be variable. They describe how the use of a drug was influenced by the beliefs of a group of orthopaedic surgeons that were based on their experience. There

was a disparity between the research evidence and clinical expertise and as a result the uptake of the new drug was 'patchy'.

Patient experience as evidence

The third source of evidence that contributes to clinical practice is that derived from the patient experience. Farrell and Gilbert (1996) draw a distinction between *individual* and *collective* involvement of patients and carers in healthcare that provides a useful means of viewing patient experience as a form of evidence. *Individual* involvement concerns individual patients and their contact with particular practitioners during episodes of care, whereas *collective* involvement entails the participation of groups or communities in healthcare planning or service delivery.

To involve *individual* patients and their carers effectively in decisions about their care, it is important that their views and preferences are taken into account. Patients and carers will tend to draw on their knowledge of their physical and psychological 'self', their social lives and their previous experiences of care. Integrating the experiential knowledge of patients with scientific knowledge requires considerable skill. Closs (2003) proposes that nurses should share their knowledge of research findings underpinning clinical interventions with patients, so that patients understand the appropriateness of the intervention and can exercise an informed choice when there are alternative courses of action available. Patients are also becoming more informed about healthcare. Access by the general public to health information has increased significantly in recent years, supported by a number of government initiatives and consumer organisations that provide information via the internet. Some of these initiatives, for example health talk online (http://healthtalkonline.org/), link patients' experiences with research information. However, nurses may encounter a mismatch between the best research evidence and patient preferences. Rycroft-Malone *et al.* (2004) provide an example whereby robust research evidence that recommends the use of compression bandaging to treat venous leg ulcers may not tally with a patient's experience of discomfort caused by the bandaging. The individual practitioner's skills in identifying these issues and negotiating the most appropriate course of action would be essential to improving patient outcomes.

There are various means whereby a *collective* view of patient and carer perspectives can inform evidence-based practice initiatives. For example, at a national level, NICE ensures patient and carer representation on its committees and involvement in the development of national guidelines. The annual national survey of NHS patients undertaken by the Care Quality Commission gathers feedback from patients on different aspects of their experience of care across a variety of services/settings. At a more local level, clinical audit and patient satisfaction surveys undertaken by NHS organisations provide a means whereby a collective view of patient perspectives can be gleaned through patient feedback.

In summary, evidence-based practice requires a blending of the research-based and experiential knowledge of professionals with the individualised personal knowledge of patients and their carers. Indeed, a consensus statement on evidence-based practice produced by an international group of experts in the field placed the patient at the centre of the process, claiming that evidence-based practice decisions should be made by those receiving care, informed by the best available, current, valid and relevant evidence, together with the tacit and explicit knowledge of those providing care (Dawes *et al.* 2005). Such a stance recognises that no single person is the expert as of right, but that everyone has expertise of a differing kind. Figure 38.1 illustrates how these three elements of evidence-based practice are

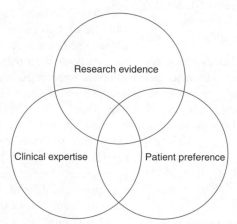

Research evidence
Compression bandaging has improved healing rates compared to treatments using no compression
Compression therapy is more cost-effective because the faster healing rates saved nurses time
High compression achieves better healing rates than low compression
Multi-layer compression systems are more effective than single-layer systems

Research evidence

Clinical expertise   Patient preference

Clinical expertise
Practitioner is:
• informed of benefits of compression bandaging
• trained in applying compression bandaging
• skilled in patient education to promote patient understanding of leg ulcer management and concordance with treatment regime

Patient preference
Willingness to try techniques offered
Readiness to comply with treatment regime
Experience of other treatment programmes

Research evidence drawn from:
Effective Health Care Bulletin (1997) *Compression Therapy for Venous Leg Ulcers*. Centre for Reviews and Dissemination, University of York.
Royal College of Nursing (2006) *The Nursing Management of Patients with Venous Leg Ulcers* . London, RCN.

Figure 38.1 An example of the inter-relationship between three elements of evidence-based practice

inter-related in regard to the use of compression bandages to treat venous leg ulcers. Where there is a lack of congruence, for example between the research evidence, the practitioner's skills to apply the bandages correctly, or in the patient's willingness to try a new treatment, the outcomes for the individual patient are likely to be affected.

HIERARCHIES OF EVIDENCE

If it is accepted that evidence-based practice involves drawing on the different types of evidence outlined above, how then are decisions made about what constitutes the 'best' evidence? Muir Gray (1997) provides a classification that groups different sources of research evidence into five categories and ranks them in order of the strength of the evidence (see Box 38.2).

This form of classification, commonly known as a 'hierarchy of evidence', ranks different research designs in terms of the extent to which they prevent bias from influencing the findings of the research. The randomised controlled trial (RCT) in which the researcher seeks to minimise the effects of bias is judged to be the most robust form of evidence, whereas expert opinion and descriptive studies are considered to be the weakest.

Hierarchies of evidence have played an important role in guiding the systematic reviews undertaken by the Cochrane Collaboration and the National Institute of Heath Research (NIHR) Centre for Research and Dissemination, and in informing the guidance pro-

---

Box 38.2 Hierarchies of evidence

I Systematic review of multiple randomised controlled trials
II Randomised controlled trial
III Non-randomised trials
IV Non-experimental studies
V Descriptive studies, expert committees

(Muir Gray 1997)

---

duced by NICE. However, this approach has been criticised for devaluing the contribution of qualitative and participatory forms of research. Although some of this criticism may be justified, it is important to recognise that the hierarchy of evidence was developed to assist in judging the robustness of evidence examining the *outcomes* of different clinical interventions and treatments, and in this respect it can be a useful tool for deciding which sources of evidence are best able to link cause and effect. If a district nurse wants to know which type of dressing is most effective in healing venous leg ulcers, then an RCT that compares different types of dressing while at the same time seeking to reduce the effect of other factors that might influence wound healing will clearly provide more robust evidence than the professional opinion of nurses who have experience of using different dressings.

However, where evidence is sought to provide guidance for practice on an aspect of care that is not focused on measurable outcomes, the hierarchy of evidence is inappropriate. For example, if a nurse wants to understand what the transition from independence to dependence is like for an older person in order to provide sensitive and appropriate care, then high quality qualitative research is likely to provide appropriate evidence to inform practice. As the contribution of qualitative research becomes more valued, guidance is being developed on how to judge the robustness of evidence derived from this approach and use it to inform the development of clinical guidelines (see Chapters 7 and 24).

What needs to be emphasised is the value of different research methodologies in providing guidance for practice and the need to acknowledge the contribution of different sources of knowledge where research evidence is lacking. In this regard, Smith and Pell (2003) provide an amusing illustration of the inappropriateness of placing too much emphasis on evidence derived from RCTs (see Research Example 38.1).

RESEARCH UTILISATION

The different forms of evidence identified in the hierarchy of evidence lend themselves to different models

RESEARCH
EXAMPLE

38.1   A Cautionary Note on RCTs

Smith G, Pell J (2003) Parachute use to prevent death and major trauma related to gravitational challenge: systematic review of randomised controlled trials. *British Medical Journal* **327**: 1459–1461.

Abstract

Objectives To determine whether parachutes are effective in preventing major trauma related to gravitational challenge.

Design Systematic review of randomised controlled trials.

Data sources Medline, Web of Science, Embase and The Cochrane Library databases; appropriate internet sites and citation lists.

Study selection Studies showing the effects of using a parachute during free fall.

Main outcome measure Death or major trauma, defined as an injury severity score >15.

Results We were unable to identify any randomised controlled trials of parachute intervention.

Conclusions As with many interventions intended to prevent ill health, the effectiveness of parachutes has not been subjected to rigorous evaluation by using randomised controlled trials. Advocates of evidence-based medicine have criticised the adoption of interventions evaluated by using only observational data. We think that everyone might benefit if the most radical protagonists of evidence-based medicine organised and participated in a double blind, randomised, placebo controlled, crossover trial of the parachute.

of research utilisation. Much of the literature on evidence-based practice focuses on the direct application of research findings to practice, often in the form of clinical protocols, practice guidelines or care pathways. Estabrooks (1998) refers to this as *instrumental* research utilisation. Quantitative research, and in particular the RCT, is most suited to such direct application. The hierarchy of evidence referred to earlier is generally used to determine the robustness of evidence used in this model of research utilisation.

The difficulties of implementing research findings in practice have also been demonstrated most clearly through this approach. Hunt's (1987) influential action research study that sought to introduce research guidance on pre-operative fasting was unsuccessful, not because nurses and anaesthetists were not persuaded of the need to reduce the time that patients fasted pre-operatively on physiological grounds, but because the complex healthcare organisation in which they worked was not able to accommodate an individualised approach to patient fasting. The context in which the research findings were being implemented was the influencing factor, not the research findings themselves or the attitudes of the practitioners concerned. Interestingly, some 30 years later implementing evidence in relation to pre-operative fasting remains a challenge (Lorch 2007).

In recognising the importance of context, an alternative model of research utilisation is proposed by Weiss and Bucuvalas (1980). They suggest that research findings may be utilised, but not necessarily always in a direct way that the instrumental model implies. Research findings may exert an influence through a process of subliminal diffusion that informs a person's understanding. In this model of *indirect* research use, practitioners become aware of research findings, internalise them and use them to inform their practice in ways that are often not explicit (Estabrooks 1998). Qualitative research findings tend to be used more indirectly.

Research findings may also be used persuasively to argue for a change in policy or practice. Florence Nightingale's collation of epidemiological data during the Crimean War, which she then used to persuade government officials of the need for radical reform in the British military, is an example of the persuasive use of research at a macro level. However, nurses use research as a means of persuasion in much more modest ways. For example, Gerrish *et al.* (1999) describe how a team of nurses in the operating theatres department in the hospital in which they worked used research examining the risk assessment of pressure damage to change surgeons' perceptions and gain support for the introduction of new theatre mattresses to minimise such risk.

The three models of research utilisation referred to above are helpful in thinking about different approaches to evidence-based practice. The instrumental model of research utilisation is reflected in the standard linear process of evidence-based practice outlined in Box 38.3, whereas the other two models identify how evidence can be used in more subtle ways to inform practice.

Box 38.3 The stages of evidence-based practice

- Identify a problem or issue from practice
- Formulate an answerable question
- Identify the available evidence
- Appraise the evidence
- Develop guidance for practice
- Plan strategy for introducing change
- Implement change
- Evaluate the impact of change

THE PROCESS OF EVIDENCE-BASED PRACTICE

As Box 38.3 shows, there are a number of stages involved in evidence-based practice. Guidance on how to achieve the first four stages can be found in earlier chapters of this book (Chapter 6, 7 and 24), while Chapter 39 deals with the implementation of evidence-based practice in more detail.

Although individuals or small groups of nurses may choose to take forward evidence-based initiatives, the implementation of evidence-based practice often forms part of a broader agenda in healthcare organisations to promote clinical effectiveness. The Department of Health has defined clinical effectiveness as follows.

> The extent to which specific clinical interventions when deployed in the field for a particular patient or population do what they are intended to do, i.e. maintain and improve health and secure the greatest possible health gain from the available resources (NHSE 1996)

Clinical effectiveness involves using sound evidence to improve care. However, this is a complex undertaking. Appleby *et al.* (1996) identify four steps involved.

- The generation of evidence by undertaking rigorous, large-scale clinical and economic evaluations of healthcare interventions.
- Evidence from multiple studies is systematically reviewed and brought together in a way that allows recommendations to be made for practice.
- The findings from systematic reviews are disseminated to those involved in the area in a format they can use.
- The evidence is used to change behaviour and influence decision making by practitioners, managers and policy makers.

This approach to evidence-based practice is concerned primarily with process, that is ensuring that practitioners utilise the best available evidence to inform their practice, rather than with the outcome of that evidence for the patient. However, to use evidence to underpin practice and not to evaluate its effect on patients is short sighted. Clinically effective practice can only occur when practitioners use the best available evidence to maximise patient outcomes. Evaluation is essential to monitoring outcomes of care (Department of Health 2007).

BARRIERS TO ACHIEVING EVIDENCE-BASED PRACTICE

Translating the aspirations of evidence-based practice into reality is far from straightforward and nurses need to be aware of what is entailed. There are barriers to achieving evidence-based practice that need to be overcome and certain conditions are necessary for the implementation of evidence-based practice. These will be considered in turn.

A number of research studies have sought to identify barriers to evidence-based practice by using an anglicised version of the Barriers to Research Utilisation scale developed by Funk *et al.* (1991) in the US (Nolan *et al.* 1998; Parahoo 2000; Bryar *et al.* 2003; Hutchinson & Johnson 2004; Boström *et al.* 2008). Other studies have developed specific instruments to examine different barriers to evidence-based practice (for example McKenna *et al.* 2004; Upton & Upton 2006; Gerrish *et al.* 2007). The collective findings from these studies have identified barriers that can be grouped into four categories.

Barriers to do with the nature of the evidence

Although there has been a considerable increase over the past decade in the amount of research conducted by nurses and/or examining nursing practice, the lack of appropriate clinically relevant research to underpin some nursing interventions is still an issue. Researchers have been accused of not asking questions that are relevant to clinical practice and there is a plethora of small-scale studies that focus on local need as opposed to large-scale definitive studies. The findings from such research may not be generalisable. Nursing research also varies considerably in terms of its quality and not all published research may have been carried out sufficiently rigorously.

Barriers to do with the way the evidence is communicated

Research is often published in academic journals rather than the more popular professional journals that clinical nurses are more likely to read. Evidence suggests that nurses tend not to read research journals (McCaughan *et al.* 2002; Gerrish *et al.* 2008), preferring instead to access research information via a third party, such as specialist nurses and medical staff, or through attending in-service training events and conferences (Gerrish *et al.* 2008). However, opportunities for practising nurses to attend conferences where up-to-date research is presented are limited. It can also be intimidating for practitioners who lack confidence in research to question researchers in a public forum.

The language of research can also act as a barrier. Research papers often use complex terminology and are written in a style that is not particularly accessible. Researchers may also fail to draw out the implications of their research for practice, leaving it to the reader to do the hard work. Nurses may also encounter problems with interpreting and working with research products that are seen to be too complex. They perceive that research reports lack clinical credibility and fail to provide sufficient clinical direction (McCaughan *et al.* 2002; Thompson *et al.* 2005).

Barriers to do with knowledge and skills of the individual nurse

Although nurses may be willing to use research they may lack the skills to do so. Studies examining barriers to research utilisation have consistently identified that nurses do not know how to access and appraise research information. In the past, the main concern has been whether nurses knew how to use library resources effectively. The increasing availability of evidence-based information on the internet means that nurses now need to be competent in using IT in the workplace. Yet, research has shown that nurses appear to lag behind other professional groups in their use of IT (Estabrooks *et al.* 2003; Gerrish *et al.* 2006; Bertulis 2008). One of the challenges of using the internet is coping with information overload. A seemingly straightforward search may result in a baffling array of research and other sources of evidence, some of which may be contradictory. Making sense of all this information is a daunting task even for the most determined practitioner.

Nurses have also been shown to lack skills in evaluating different sources of evidence and in drawing out the implications of research findings for practice. As Chapter 7 shows, critical appraisal of research findings demands considerable knowledge about the research process and is very time consuming. Whereas these skills now form part of both pre- and post-registration nurse education, many nurses still do not consider themselves to be competent in this area (Pravikoff *et al.* 2005; Gerrish *et al.* 2008).

Barriers to do with the organisation

Major obstacles that nurses encounter in implementing evidence-based practice relate to insufficient time to access and review research reports together with lack of authority and support to implement findings. Organisational factors have been identified as a major impediment to achieving evidence-based practice. In particular, lack of support from managers and doctors, problems with dissemination of information within the organisation, difficulties in the management of innovations including the time necessary to implement change and resource constraints are all seen to hinder the successful implementation of evidence-based practice (Closs & Cheater 1994; Newman *et al.* 1998). Additionally, practitioners may experience restricted local access to information, for example library resources or the internet. Encouragingly, recent research (Gerrish *et al.* 2008) has suggested that progress is being made in overcoming some of these organisational barriers, although there remains much to be achieved.

IMPLEMENTING EVIDENCE-BASED PRACTICE

Whereas there is general consensus about what the barriers to evidence-based practice are, there is less agreement about how they might be overcome.

Evidence-based practice requires complex actions on the part of organisations to facilitate its implementation, including high-level management commitment, and putting in place systems for managing information and innovation and for individual skills development (Newman *et al.* 1998; Estabrooks *et al.* 2008). Kitson *et al.* (1998) propose that the implementation of evidence-based practice depends on three factors. First, the nature of the evidence is important, and this has been discussed earlier in this chapter. Second, structures and mechanisms are required to facilitate change. External and internal change agents can support the process of change, although consideration should be given to the personal characteristics of the facilitator, the style of facilitation and the role of the facilitator in terms of authority. Finally, consideration of the context draws attention to the importance of the ward/team culture in terms of patient centeredness; valuing team members and promoting a learning environment; the leadership styles of senior clinical nurses; and the audit and review procedures in place. Successful implementation of evidence-based practice is also dependent on the resources available. These are many and varied and include the availability and access to library and IT resources, finances to support new treatments, an adequate number of nurses with appropriate skills, sufficient time for gathering and appraising research evidence and implementation activities, and finally co-operation from peers, managers and other professionals.

CONCLUSIONS

It is crucial that nurses and other healthcare practitioners use the best available evidence to inform their practice in order to provide high-quality patient care. Evidence derived from rigorous research is fundamental to the process of evidence-based practice but is not sufficient in its own right. Research evidence may be lacking or the findings may be inconclusive or contradictory. In recognising that knowledge derived from research is never absolute, nurses need to draw on their own expertise and that of more experienced nurses to inform decisions about the most appropriate care for a particular patient. Clinical expertise should not be seen as a substitute for research evidence but rather as contributing to the decision-making process. It should be remembered that evidence-based practice is about providing care to patients, and both patients and their carers will have their own views about the care they wish to receive. Nurses, therefore, have a responsibility to share their knowledge of the best available evidence with patients to help them to make informed choices.

Achieving evidence-based practice is a complex undertaking that involves identifying and appraising different sources of evidence, translating evidence into clear guidance for practice, implementing change and finally evaluating the impact of change. Earlier chapters of this book have examined the knowledge and skills nurses need to be able to critically appraise research findings in order to identify the best available evidence. The following chapter considers how the best available evidence can be implemented in practice.

References

Appleby J, Walshe K, Ham C (1996) *Acting on the Evidence*. Birmingham, The NHS Confederation.

Bertulis R (2008) Barriers to accessing evidence-based information. *Nursing Standard* 22(36): 35–39.

Boström AM, Kajermo K, Nordström G, Wallin L (2008) Barriers to research utilization and research use among registered nurses working in the care of older people: does the BARRIERS Scale discriminate between research users and non-research users on perceptions of barriers? *Implementation Science* 3: 24 (www.implementationscience.com/content/3/1/24).

Bucknall T (2007) A gaze through the lens of decision theory toward knowledge translation science. *Nursing Research* 56: S60–S66.

Bryar R, Closs SJ, Baum G, Cooke J, Griffiths J, Hostick T *et al.* (2003) The Yorkshire BARRIERS project: diagnostic analysis of barriers to research utilisation. *International Journal of Nursing Studies* 40: 73–85.

Closs SJ (2003) Evidence and community-based nursing practice. In: Bryer R, Griffiths J (eds) *Practice Development in Community Nursing*. London, Arnold, pp 33–56.

Closs SJ, Cheater F (1994) Utilisation of nursing research: culture, interest and support. *Journal of Advanced Nursing* 19: 762–773.

Dawes M, Summerskill W, Glasziou P, Cartabellatta A, Martin J, Hopayian K *et al.* (2005) Sicily statement on evidence-based practice. *BMC Medical Education* 5: 1.

Department of Health (2007) *Report of the High Level Group (HLG) on Clinical Effectiveness* (Chair Professor Sire John Tooke). London, Department of Health.

Dopson S (2007) A view from organisational studies. *Nursing Research* 56: S72–S77.

Effective Health Care (1995) The prevention and treatment of pressure sores. *Effective Health Care* 2: 1.

Effective Health Care Bulletin (1997) *Compression Therapy for Venous Leg Ulcers*. Centre for Reviews and Dissemination, University of York.

Eraut M (1994) *Developing Professional Knowledge and Competence*. London, Falmer Press.

Estabrooks C (1998) Will evidence-based nursing practice make practice perfect? *Canadian Journal of Nursing Research* 30: 15–36.

Estabrooks C, O'Leary K, Ricker K, Humphrey C (2003) The Internet and access to evidence: how are nurses positioned? *Journal of Advanced Nursing* 42: 73–81.

Estabrooks C, Scott, S, Squires J, Stevens B, O'Brien-Pallas L, Watt-Watson J *et al.* (2008) Patterns of research utilisation on patient care units. *Implementation Science* 3: 31 (www.implementationscience.com/content/pdf/1748-5908-3-31.pdf).

Farrell C, Gilbert H (1996) *Health Care Partnerships*. London, Kings Fund.

Ferlie E, Wood M, Fitzgerald L (1999) Clinical effectiveness and evidence-based medicine: some implementation issues. In: *Clinical Governance: making it happen*. London, The Royal Society of Medicine Press, pp 49–60.

Funk S, Champagne M, Weise R, Tornquist E (1991) BARRIERS: The Barriers to Research Utilisation Scale. *Applied Nursing Research* 4: 39–45.

Gerrish K, Ashworth P, Lacey A, Bailey J (2008) Developing evidence-based practice: experiences of senior and junior clinical nurses. *Journal of Advanced Nursing* 62: 62–73.

Gerrish K, Ashworth P, Lacey A, Bailey J, Cooke J, Kendall S, McNeilly E (2007) Factors influencing the development of evidence-based practice: a research tool. *Journal of Advanced Nursing* 57(3): 328–338.

Gerrish K, Clayton J, Nolan M, Parker K, Morgan L (1999) Promoting evidence-based practice: managing change in the assessment of pressure damage risk. *Journal of Nursing Management* 7: 355–362.

Gerrish K, Morgan L, Mabbott I, Debbage S, Entwistle B, Ireland M *et al.* (2006) Factors influencing use of information technology by nurses and midwives. *Practice Development in Health Care* **5**: 92–101.

Hutchinson A, Johnson L (2004) Bridging the divide: a survey of nurses' opinions regarding barriers to, and facilitators of, research utilisation in the practice setting. *Journal of Clinical Nursing* **13**: 304–315.

Hunt M (1987) The process of translating research findings into nursing practice. *Journal of Advanced Nursing* **12**: 101–110.

Kitson A, Harvey G, McCormack B (1998) Enabling the implementation of evidence-based practice: a conceptual framework. *Quality in Health Care* **7**: 149–158.

Liaschenko J, Fisher A (1999) Theorising the knowledge that nurses use in the conduct of their work. *Scholarly Inquiry for Nursing Practice: An International Journal* **13**: 29–40.

Lorch A (2007) Implementation of fasting guidelines through nursing leadership. *Nursing Times* **103**(18): 30–31.

McCaughan D, Thompson, C, Cullum, N, Sheldon T, Thompson D (2002) Acute care nurses' perceptions of barriers to using research information in clinical decision making. *Journal of Advanced Nursing* **39**: 46–60.

McKenna H, Ashton S, Keeney S (2004) Barriers to evidence-based practice in primary care. *Journal of Advanced Nursing* **45**: 178–189.

Milner M, Estabrooks C, Humphrey C (2005) Clinical nurse educators as agents for change: increasing research utilisation. *International Journal of Nursing Studies* **42**: 899–914.

Muir Gray JA (2004) Evidence-based policy making. Editorial. *British Medical Journal* **329**: 988–989.

Muir Gray JA (1997) *Evidence-based Health Care.* Edinburgh, Churchill Livingstone.

National Health Service Executive (1996) *Promoting Clinical Effectiveness: a framework for action in and through the NHS.* London, NHS Executive.

Newman M, Papadopoulos I, Sigsworth J (1998) Barriers to evidence-based practice. *Clinical Effectiveness* **2**: 11–20.

NICE (2006) *Nutrition Support in Adults: oral nutrition support, enteral tube feeding and parental nutrition.* Clinical Guideline 32. London, NICE.

Nolan M, Morgan L, Curran M, Clayton J, Gerrish K, Parker C (1998) Evidence-based care: can we overcome the barriers? *British Journal of Nursing* **7**: 1273–1278.

Parahoo K (2000) Barriers to, and facilitators of, research utilisation among nurses in Northern Ireland. *Journal of Advanced Nursing* **31**: 89–98.

Pravikoff D, Tanner A, Pierce S (2005) Readiness of US nurses to evidence-based practice: many don't under stand or value research and have had little or no training to help them find evidence on which to base their practice. *American Journal of Nursing* **105**(9): 40–51.

Royal College of Nursing (2006) *The Nursing Management of Patients with Venous Leg Ulcers.* London, RCN.

Rycroft-Malone J, Seers K, Titchen A, Harvey G, Kitson A, McCormack B (2004) What counts as evidence in evidence-based practice? *Journal of Advanced Nursing* **47**(1): 81–90.

Sackett DL, Rosenburg WM, Muir Gray JA, Haynes RB, Richardson WS (1996) Evidence-based medicine: what it is and what it isn't. *British Medical Journal* **312**: 71–72.

Smith G, Pell J (2003) Parachute use to prevent death and major trauma related to gravitational challenge: systematic review of randomised controlled trials. *British Medical Journal* **327**: 1459–1461.

Thompson C, McCaughan D, Cullum N, Sheldon T, Mullhall A, Thompson D (2001) The accessibility of research-based knowledge for nurses in United Kingdom acute care settings. *Journal of Advanced Nursing* **36**: 11–22.

Thompson C, McCaughan D, Cullum N, Sheldon T, Raynor P (2005) Barriers to evidence-based practice in primary care nursing: why viewing decision-making as context is helpful. *Journal of Advanced Nursing* **52**: 432–444.

Upton D, Upton, P (2006) Development of an evidence-based practice questionnaire for nurses. *Journal of Advanced Nursing* **53**: 454–458.

Weiss C, Bucuvalas M (1980) *Social Science Research and Decision Making.* New York, Columbia University Press.

Further reading

Cullum N, Ciliska D, Hayes B, Marks S (2008) *Evidence-based Nursing: an introduction.* Oxford, Blackwell.

Journals

Evidence-based Nursing, BMJ Publishing.
World Views on Evidence-Based Nursing, Blackwell Publishing.

Websites

www.cochrane.org/index.htm – The Cochrane Collaboration is an international not-for-profit and independent organisation, dedicated to making up-to-date, accurate information about the effects of healthcare readily available worldwide. It produces and disseminates systematic reviews of healthcare interventions and promotes the search for evidence in the form of clinical trials and other studies of interventions.

www.library.nhs.uk – NHS Evidence Health Information Resources (formerly National Library for Health) is an online resource accessible to healthcare professionals and patients. The resource provides up-to-date evidence on a broad range of clinical topics. It comprises NHS-funded services across the country and a digital hub, plus commissioned information services and products.

www.shef.ac.uk/scharr/ir/netting/ – Netting the Evidence is designed to facilitate evidence-based practice by providing access to organisations and learning resources, such as an evidence-based virtual library, software and journals.

39 Translating Research Findings into Practice

Kate Gerrish

Key points

- Knowledge translation is the complex process of taking what is learned through research and applying such knowledge in different practice settings and circumstances.

- Clinical guidelines are recommendations on the most appropriate care of people with specific conditions, based on the best available evidence; they provide a means of translating research findings into practice.

- Where possible, existing published guidelines should be adapted for local use. Published guidelines should be appraised so that an assessment can be made of their quality and appropriateness for the local context.

- Strategies for translating research findings into practice should be carefully planned and executed. There are a number of frameworks and tools that can assist at different stages of the process to enhance the likelihood of success.

INTRODUCTION

As discussed in the previous chapter, evidence-based practice involves practitioners in making decisions about the care they provide based on the integration of research evidence with clinical expertise and the patients' preferences and circumstances. It is a complex undertaking that involves identifying and appraising different sources of evidence, translating the evidence into clear guidance for practice, implementing change and finally evaluating the impact of change. Despite a strong commitment to evidence-based practice in nursing and other areas of healthcare, the uptake of research findings in practice continues to be lacking (Gerrish & Clayton 2004). This problem has led to increased recognition that the

process of translating research findings into practice is complex. Attempts have been made to understand how it might be achieved and strategies developed to increase its success.

The term 'knowledge translation' is used increasingly to describe the complex process of taking what is learned through undertaking research and applying such knowledge in a variety of practice settings and circumstances (Sudsawad 2007). Whereas evidence-based practice is concerned with using the best available evidence to inform what practitioners actually do, knowledge translation is a much broader concept and encompasses the whole of the research process. The Canadian Institutes of Health Research (CIHR) is attributed with first using the term knowledge translation and define it as:

'The exchange, synthesis and ethically sound application of knowledge within a complex system of interactions among researchers and users ... to accelerate the capture of the benefits of research for Canadians through improved health, more effective services and products and strengthened health care systems' (CIHR 2005, para 2)

There is often a tendency to assume that knowledge translation occurs at the end of a project, once the findings are known. However, the CIHR (2007) propose that researchers should consider a more integrated approach to knowledge translation, with interactions between researchers and users of research spanning the whole of the research process. As Box 39.1 shows, there are five opportunities within the research cycle during which interactions between researchers and users can facilitate the transfer of knowledge into practice. These range from defining research questions, selecting appropriate research methods, conducting the research itself, disseminating the findings, contextualising research findings and applying the research to resolve practical problems (CIHR 2007). Earlier chapters (in particular Chapters 4, 23 and 37) have outlined strategies that can be used to engage the users of research more actively in the research process (stages 1, 2, 3 and 4 in Box 39.1). The focus in this chapter will be on how research findings can be applied in practice (step 5 in Box 39.1).

Knowledge generated by a particular research study contributes to the overall knowledge base about a specific topic or issue. However, before the findings can be applied in practice they need to be considered within the context of what is already known about the topic (step 3). For example, do the findings support or refute current knowledge or do they provide new insights into practice that indicate the need for change? Systematic reviews provide a mechanism for integrating knowledge from several studies on a particular topic and this is an important step in contextualising knowledge. However, before the findings of a systematic review can be applied there is a need to take account of the context in which the findings will be implemented. This involves consideration of individual and organisational socio-cultural norms, which may influence how the findings might be used. Research findings that reflect closely current practice are more readily accepted and incorporated into everyday practice than findings that challenge existing practice and indicate the need for significant change. Once research findings have been contextualised there is a need to think about how they can most readily be applied in practice (step 4). Relying solely on practitioners to apply research findings to practice is unrealistic. Practitioners may interpret the implications for practice arising from research study differently and this will lead to variability in the standard of care. To avoid such inconsistencies, research findings need to be translated into research tools and products that can be applied in practice.

TRANSLATING RESEARCH FINDINGS INTO RESEARCH PRODUCTS

In most instances it is inappropriate to change practice based on the findings from a single study. Rather,

---

Box 39.1 Opportunities for knowledge translation within the research process

1 Defining research questions and methodologies
2 Conducting research (as in the case of participatory research)
3 Placing research findings into the context of other knowledge and socio-cultural norms
4 Publishing research findings in plain language and accessible formats
5 Making decisions and taking action on research findings

(CIHR 2007)

the findings from several studies on the same topic need to be evaluated and brought together in the form of a systematic review (see Chapter 24). Where there is a range of sources of evidence (not just research), then a realist synthesis (Chapter 25) may be undertaken. Whichever approach is used the intention is to provide a comprehensive account of the knowledge on a particular topic, which will include a statement of the strength of the evidence as a quality indicator. The next step is to translate the evidence synthesis into a 'product' that practitioners can use to inform their practice. Clinical guidelines are the most common research product used by nurses and other healthcare professionals.

CLINICAL GUIDELINES

Clinical guidelines are:

'systematically developed statements to assist practitioner and patient decisions about appropriate health care for specific clinical circumstances' (Lohr & Field 1992)

Guidelines are based on the best available evidence and make explicit recommendations with the intention of influencing what practitioners do (Hayward *et al*. 1995). However, they do not replace a practitioner's knowledge and skills (Pearson *et al*. 2007). Developing robust clinical guidelines requires considerable expertise and resources, so where possible existing guidelines should be adapted for local use.

Several government agencies and professional organisations in the UK and internationally develop clinical guidelines through a structured process of reviewing and synthesising international research literature, drawing on renowned experts in the field and conducting a meta analysis to generate guidelines based on the best available evidence. In the UK, the National Institute for Health and Clinical Excellence (NICE) and the Scottish Intercollegiate Guidelines Network (SIGN) produce guidelines on a range of clinical topics, and professional bodies such as the Royal College of Nursing and some of the medical Royal Colleges also develop guidelines. There are equivalent organisations in many other countries, some of which focus on nursing topics, such as The Joanna Briggs Institute in Australia.

There may be several guidelines on the same topic produced by different organisations and it is worthwhile undertaking a thorough search to identify key ones. Guideline developers may make their guidelines available via the World Wide Web as this reduces dissemination costs and also enables rapid updating as new evidence becomes available (Graham *et al*. 2003). Therefore guidelines may not easily be identified through bibliographic databases such as CINAHL and MEDLINE. Clearly, the websites of organisations such as NICE, SIGN, the Royal College of Nursing and some medical Royal Colleges are a useful starting point for locating existing guidelines. It is also advisable to search the web for guidelines using search engines such as Google. However, there is no guarantee that guidelines published on the web will have been developed through the same rigorous approach adopted by NICE or SIGN. Moreover, even where national guidelines have been produced by one of the organisations identified above, it cannot be assumed that they can be applied directly to the local context. It is important that guidelines are evaluated so that an assessment can be made of their quality and appropriateness for use locally.

There are a number of guideline appraisal tools that can help in the process, with the Appraisal of Guidelines Research and Evaluation (AGREE) instrument (AGREE Collaboration 2001) generally accepted as the gold standard for guideline appraisal (Graham & Harrison 2008). It was developed by an international group of researchers to assess the quality of clinical guidelines by considering the process of guideline development and the extent to which the process has been reported. Although the instrument provides an assessment of the likelihood that the guideline will achieve its intended outcome, it does not assess the impact of the guideline on patient outcomes. It can be used to assess guidelines developed by local, national or international groups and applied to new guidelines or when updating existing guidelines. Ideally, at least two reviewers should independently appraise the guideline.

The AGREE instrument comprises 23 items grouped into six domains, with each domain addressing a separate dimension of guideline quality. Each

Box 39.2 The Appraisal of Guidelines Research and Evaluation (AGREE) Instrument quality criteria

Scope and purpose

1 The overall objectives(s) of the guidelines is (are) specifically described
2 The clinical question(s) covered by the guideline is (are) specifically described
3 The patients to whom the guideline is meant to apply are specifically described

Stakeholder involvement

4 The guideline development group includes individuals from all the relevant professional groups
5 The patients' views and preferences have been sought
6 The target users of the guideline are clearly identified
7 The guideline has been piloted among target users

Rigour of development

8 Systematic methods were used to search for evidence
9 The criteria for selecting the evidence are clearly described
10 The methods used for formulating the recommendations are clearly described
11 The health benefits, side effects and risks have been considered in formulating the recommendations
12 There is an explicit link between the recommendations and the supporting evidence
13 The guideline has been extensively reviewed by an expert panel prior to publication
14 A procedure for updating the guideline is provided

Clarity and presentation

15 The recommendations are specific and unambiguous
16 The different options for management of the condition are clearly presented
17 Key recommendations are easily identifiable
18 The guideline is supported with tools for application

Applicability

19 The potential organisational barriers in applying the guideline have been discussed
20 The potential cost implications of applying the recommendations have been considered
21 The guideline presents key review criteria for monitoring and/or audit purposes

Editorial independence

22 The guideline is editorially independent of the funding body
23 Conflicts of interest of guideline development members have been recorded

(AGREE Collaboration 2001)

item is rated on a four-point Likert scale ranging from 'strongly agree' to 'strongly disagree', which measures the extent to which the item has been addressed. The reviewer is also required to provide an overall assessment of the quality of the guideline, taking each of the appraisal criteria into account, and decide whether the guideline should be 'strongly recommended', 'recommended with provisos' or 'not recommended'. The AGREE quality criteria are shown in Box 39.2.

Once a guideline has been appraised and recommended for use, it may be appropriate to adopt it as it stands, or it may require some adaptation for the local context. For example, some recommendations may not apply to the types of patient seen in the practice setting; alternatively, contextual factors or resource considerations may make it impractical to implement some of the recommendations (Graham & Harrison 2008).

Guideline adaptation involves taking the most appropriate recommendations and repackaging them to form a new local guideline. Modifications to evidence-based recommendations should not be made unless the supporting evidence has changed since the guideline was first developed. Where modifications are made, the rationale for such changes needs to be made explicit (Graham & Harrison 2008).

Following adaptation, the guideline should be reviewed by local practitioners and other stakeholders, such as managers and patients, to test its relevance to the local context in which it will be implemented. The people who will ultimately use the guideline will be able to comment on how relevant the content is to the local setting and identify factors that may influence its uptake. Final adjustments can then be made to the guideline and decisions made as to when and how it will be reviewed and updated before it is officially endorsed by the organisation. Many healthcare organisations have mechanisms set up to approve guidelines prior to implementation and to oversee the review process.

In situations where there are no national guidelines that can be adapted it may be necessary to develop a local guideline. The work involved in developing a guideline cannot be underestimated and it is important that as rigorous a method as possible is used (Campbell *et al.* 2006). A guideline development group should be formed to take collective ownership for the development and subsequent implementation of the guideline. The composition of the group will vary depending on the clinical topic, but as a general principle it is beneficial to involve members of the multidisciplinary team. For example, if developing a nursing care guideline to provide oral nutrition support for patients at risk of malnutrition, it would be prudent to involve nurses who will be involved in using the guideline, a dietitian, a medical consultant with expertise in nutrition, and a speech and language therapist with expertise in dysphagia. Consideration should also be given as to how the patient perspective can be incorporated. This might be through involving a representative in the guideline development group, or through consulting with relevant patient groups at key points in the development process.

Developing local guidelines has been made easier by the availability of high-quality published systematic reviews. However, there are a limited number of systematic reviews on specific nursing topics – in part because robust research evidence to inform many nursing interventions is still lacking. Where there is insufficient research evidence it will be necessary to rely more heavily on expert professional opinion, for example from members of the multidisciplinary team with specialist expertise in the clinical area. In such situations, it is important to acknowledge limitations that may arise from the nature of the evidence on which the guideline is based and the process whereby the guideline was developed (Fedder *et al.* 1999).

As the preceding discussion has shown, there are several steps involved in developing or adapting clinical guidelines. The Practice Guidelines Evaluation and Adaptation Cycle developed by Graham and colleagues (2003) captures each of these steps and provides a useful framework to guide clinical guideline development (Figure 39.1). An example of how the cycle can be applied to the adaptation of national and international clinical guidelines on leg ulcer management for local use is given in Research Example 39.1.

Once a guideline has been formally approved by the organisation, consideration should to be given to how it will be implemented. This is likely to be far from straightforward. As discussed in Chapter 38, there are many barriers to implementing research

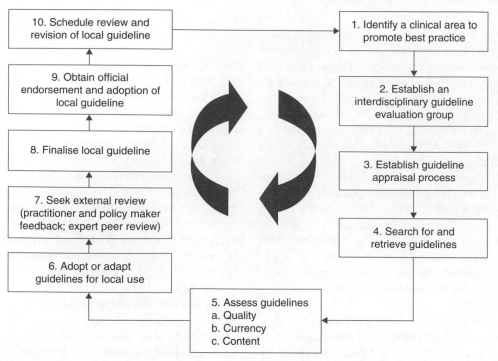

Figure 39.1 Practice guidelines evaluation and adaptation cycle
This figure was published in Graham I, MB Harrison, Brouwers M (2003) Evaluating and adapting practice guidelines for local use: a conceptual framework. In: Pickering S, Thompson J (eds) *Clinical Governance and Best Value*, p 215. Copyright Churchill Livingstone. Reproduced with permission from Churchill Livingstone–Elsevier.

findings in practice. There are several factors that influence the adoption of clinical guidelines, including the characteristics of the guideline, the attributes of the intended users and aspects of the practice setting or organisational context in which the guideline is to be implemented (Grol 2001). Bearing in mind the complexity of behaviour change, there is growing recognition that implementation activities should be guided by a conceptual framework (Graham *et al*. 2008).

KNOWLEDGE TRANSLATION FRAMEWORKS

There are several frameworks that can help guide the translation of research findings into practice. Four of the most common ones are outlined in Box 39.3. The diffusion of innovations theory (Rogers 2003), the

Promoting Action on Research Implementation in Health Services (PARIHS) (Kitson *et al*. 1998, Rycroft-Malone 2004) and the Diffusion of Innovations in Service Organisation (Greenhalgh *et al*. 2004) vary in their level of complexity and focus. However, they all share a common purpose in clarifying the many and varied factors to be considered when seeking to implement research findings in practice. A limitation of these frameworks is that although they describe comprehensively the factors that may influence the uptake of research evidence, they do not in themselves provide guidance on how change might best be achieved. By contrast, the Knowledge to Action framework (Graham *et al*. 2006) provides a series of inter-related stages to progress through in seeking to implement research findings in practice. This framework also considers the creation of knowledge as well as the application of knowledge to practice. It is for these reasons that the Knowledge to Action framework is discussed in more detail.

RESEARCH EXAMPLE

39.1 Adapting National and International Guidelines for Local Use

Buchannan *et al.* (2005) Adapting national and international leg ulcer practice guidelines for local use: the Ontario leg ulcer community care protocol. *Advances in Skin and Wound Care* **18**(6): 307–318.

The increasing need to devote resources to individuals requiring community care for leg ulcers led to the development of a dedicated community-based leg ulcer service in Ontario, Canada. In order to provide up-to-date evidence-based care, existing leg ulcer clinical practice guidelines were identified and appraised for quality and suitability for the new service. The Practice Guideline Evaluation and Adaptation Cycle was used to guide the development of a local protocol for leg ulcer care. This involved:

(i)   systematically searching for practice guidelines
(ii) appraising the quality of identified guidelines using a validated guideline appraisal instrument
(iii) conducting a content analysis of guideline recommendations
(iv) selecting recommendations to include in the local protocol
(v)   obtaining practitioner and external expert feedback on the proposed protocol.

Only guidelines that were treatment focused, written in English and developed after 1998 were included. Of the 19 guidelines developed only five met the inclusion criteria. Of these, three were fairly well developed and made similar recommendations. The level of evidence supporting specific recommendations ranged from randomised clinical trials to expert opinion. The guidelines were assessed for quality and content and a consensus reached regarding recommendations appropriate for local application.

THE KNOWLEDGE TO ACTION FRAMEWORK

The Knowledge to Action framework (Graham *et al.* 2006) was developed following a detailed review of 31 published frameworks for promoting research use and provides a comprehensive account of the stages involved in translating knowledge derived from research through to sustainable changes in practice. It has two components: knowledge creation and an action cycle, and each component has several phases (see Figure 39.2).

Knowledge creation – within the framework, 'knowledge' includes not just knowledge derived from research, but also the tacit knowledge held by patients as well as procedural knowledge derived from clinical expertise. The process of moving from research findings to research products and tools suitable for application is depicted as an inverted funnel, where multiple sources of knowledge are reduced in number through knowledge synthesis and then developed into an even a smaller number of tools or products to facilitate implementation in practice.

The *action cycle* depicts the activities needed for the successful application of knowledge. It starts with a problem or issue being identified by an individual or group who then seek out knowledge relevant to solving the problem and appraise it in terms of its validity and usefulness. Alternatively, an individual or group may start by identifying the new knowledge (e.g. a clinical guideline) and then decide whether there is a knowledge–practice gap that needs bridging. 'Generic' knowledge (such as that derived from a systematic review) is seldom taken directly off the shelf and applied without some sort of tailoring to the local context. The knowledge is therefore assessed in terms of its usefulness in the particular setting and circumstances, and then adapted to fit the local context. The next step is to assess potential barriers that may impede or limit uptake of the knowledge so that these barriers

507

Box 39.3 Common frameworks for knowledge translation

Diffusion of innovations (Rogers 2003)

First developed in the 1950s, Rogers draws on the broader principles of communication theory to propose four main elements that influence the spread of ideas. These are:

1 the characteristics of the innovation itself
2 the channels of communication
3 the time it takes individuals to accept new ideas
4 the characteristics of the social system itself, including the role of opinion leaders and change agents and whether the decisions around the innovation are voluntary or imposed.

Promoting action on research implementation in health services framework (PARIHS) (Kitson et al. 1998; Rycroft-Malone et al. 2004)

According to the PARIHS framework successful implementation of research findings into practice is a function of the interplay of three core elements:

1 the level and nature of the evidence used
2 the context or environment in which the research is to be placed
3 the method by which the research implementation process is facilitated.

Evidence is defined as a combination of research, clinical experience, patient experience and local information. Context refers to the setting in which the proposed change is to be implemented. The framework specifies three themes under context: (i) culture, (ii) leadership and (iii) evaluation. Facilitation has a key role in helping individuals and teams understand what and how they need to change to apply evidence to practice. According to the framework there are three aspects of facilitation: (i) purpose, (ii) roles and (iii) skills and attributes.

Knowledge to action process (Graham et al. 2006)

The Knowledge to Action framework has two components. Knowledge creation involves knowledge inquiry, knowledge synthesis and the production of knowledge tools or products. The action cycle involves a set of eight logically interrelated steps:

1 identifying the problem that needs addressing
2 identifying, reviewing and selecting knowledge relevant to the problem
3 adapting the knowledge to the local context
4 assessing barriers to using the knowledge
5 designing transfer strategies to promote the use of knowledge
6 monitoring how the knowledge diffuses throughout the user group
7 evaluating the impact of the users' application of the knowledge
8 sustaining the ongoing use of knowledge by users.

Determinants of diffusion, dissemination and implementation of innovations in health service delivery and organisations (Greenhalgh et al. 2004)

Greenhalgh and colleagues undertook a systematic review examining the spread and sustainability of innovations in health service organisation and delivery. The complex model identifies eight determinants affecting the diffusion, dissemination and implementation of innovations. These include:

1 the characteristics of the innovation
2 the process of adoption by individuals
3 assimilation of the innovation into the healthcare system
4 the process of diffusion and dissemination
5 the characteristics of the organisation (both structural and cultural)
6 the readiness of the system for innovation
7 the external context in terms of external networks and collaborations
8 implementation and rountinisation.

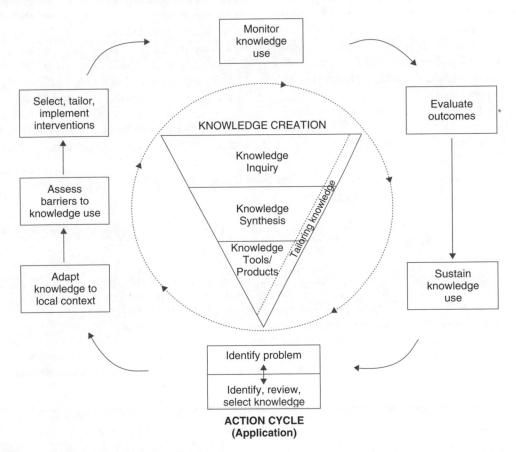

Figure 39.2   The Knowledge-to-Action process

From Graham I *et al.* (2006) Lost in knowledge translation: time for a map. *Journal of Continuing Education in the Health Professions* **26**: 13–24. Reprinted with permission of John Wiley & Sons Inc.

may be targeted and hopefully overcome or diminished by intervention strategies. Attempts should also be made to identify facilitators that can be taken advantage of. This information is used to develop and implement interventions to facilitate and promote awareness and uptake of the knowledge. The next step involves monitoring knowledge use to determine the effectiveness of the intervention strategies in promoting the uptake of knowledge and whether the interventions have brought about the desired change or whether new interventions may be required.

The impact of using the knowledge should be evaluated to determine whether application of the knowledge has actually made a difference in terms of positive outcomes for patients, practitioners or the healthcare system. In recognising that barriers to ongoing knowledge use may be different to the barriers that needed to be addressed when the knowledge was first introduced, a plan should be drawn up to sustain the change over time. Although the action phases in Figure 39.2 are depicted as a cyclical process, in reality they may occur sequentially or simultaneously and the knowledge phases may influence the action phases.

Research Example 39.2 provides an example of knowledge translation, albeit using a different framework to guide the implementation process.

INTERVENTIONS TO PROMOTE BEHAVIOURAL CHANGE

Translating research findings into practice requires practitioners to change their behaviour so that they adopt and use research-based knowledge. However, changing behaviour can be notoriously difficult to achieve. As the Knowledge to Action framework identifies, there is a need to select appropriate interventions to implement change. Interventions may be many and varied and where possible should be evidence-based. Table 39.1 identifies nine of the most common approaches that have been identified by the Effective Practice and Organisation of Care Group (EPOC). This group is part of the Cochrane Collaboration and produces systematic reviews of educational, behavioural, financial, regulatory and organisational interventions designed to improve the practice of healthcare professionals and the organisation of healthcare services.

There are many studies that have examined the effectiveness of different implementation strategies to promote behavioural change and several systematic reviews of these studies have been conducted. Bero *et al.* (1998) undertook an overview of 18 systematic reviews on this topic published between 1989

RESEARCH EXAMPLE

39.2   Knowledge Translation

Graham K, Logan J (2004) Using the Ottawa model of research use to implement a skin care programme. *Journal of Nursing Care Quality* **19**(1): 18–24.

The authors used the Ottawa model of research use to guide the implementation of clinical guidelines on skin care intended to prevent the development of decubitus ulcers in a surgical setting in a large hospital in Canada. Existing clinical guidelines were appraised and adapted for local use. An assessment was made of the knowledge, skills, attitudes and motivation of healthcare practitioners, together with their receptiveness to change. In addition, potential barriers and facilitators to implementation of the guidelines in the practice environment were identified. With the information gleaned, strategies to address the barriers and implement the guidelines were developed. A range of outcome measures was used to evaluate the impact of the guidelines at the level of the patient, practitioner and healthcare system. The authors identified that although the evaluation demonstrated positive results, adoption took longer than anticipated. They concluded that there is a tendency to underestimate the time taken to change practice in complex care environments.

Table 39.1 Interventions to promote behavioural change. Adapted from Cochrane Effective Practice and Organisation of Care Group

Intervention	Description
Audit and feedback	Any written or verbal summary of clinical performance of healthcare professionals over a specified period of time. The summary may also include recommendations for clinical action
Education outreach visits	Use of a trained person who meets with professionals in their practice setting to provide information with the intent of improving practice
Educational materials	Distribution of published or printed recommendations for clinical care, including clinical guidelines, audiovisual materials and electronic publications
Interactive educational meetings	Participation of professionals in workshops that include discussion
Local consensus processes	Inclusion of participating professionals in discussion to ensure that they agree that the chosen clinical problem was important and the approach to managing the problem was appropriate
Local opinion leaders	Use of providers nominated by their colleagues as 'educationally influential'
Multifaceted interventions	A combination that includes two or more of audit and feedback, reminders, local consensus processes and patient-mediated interventions
Reminders	Any intervention, manual or computerised, that prompts professionals to perform a clinical action
Tailoring	An intervention tailored to address prospectively identified barriers to change

Reproduced from O'Brien MA (2008) Closing the gap between nursing research and practice. In: Cullum N, Ciliska D, Haynes RD, Marks S (eds) *Evidence Based Nursing: an introduction*. Oxford, Blackwell Publishing, p 246, with permission from Blackwell Publishing.

and 1995 and identified a number of consistent themes.

- Most reviews reported modest changes in behaviour after interventions.
- Passive dissemination of information was generally ineffective in changing practices, no matter how important the issue or how strong the evidence.
- Multifaceted interventions, a combination of methods including two or more interventions, seemed to be more effective than single interventions.

The authors grouped interventions into three types based on how effective the interventions were in promoting behavioural change.

- *Consistently effective interventions* – these included educational outreach visits; manual or computerised reminders; multifaceted interventions that comprised two or more approaches of audit and feedback, reminders and interactive educational meetings.
- *Interventions of variable effectiveness* – these included audit and feedback; the use of local opinion leaders; local consensus processes; and patient-mediated interventions.
- *Interventions that have little or no effect* – these included the passive dissemination of educational materials; and didactic educational meetings.

The authors concluded that specific implementation strategies are needed to promote changes in practice, and the more concerted the effort the more successful it is likely to be. A follow-up overview of 41 systematic reviews undertaken by Grimshaw *et al.* (2001) confirmed that passive approaches were generally ineffective and unlikely to lead to behavioural change, although they could be useful in raising awareness. Multifaceted interventions that targeted several barriers to change were more likely to be effective than single interventions. Audit and feedback and the use of local opinion leaders were found to be of variable effectiveness, whereas educational outreach and reminders were more likely to be effective. The review concluded that most of the interventions were effective under some circumstances; however, none were effective under all circumstances.

In a more recent study, Grimshaw *et al.* (2004) reviewed 235 studies that examined the effectiveness of different interventions to promote the use of clinical guidelines. The most commonly evaluated single interventions were audit and feedback, dissemination of educational materials and reminders. Modest to moderate improvements in care were produced by the majority of single interventions and there was considerable variation within and across different interventions. In the case of multifaceted interventions, there appeared to be no relationship between the number of components in the interventions and the effects of such interventions. The researchers concluded that there is insufficient evidence to inform decisions about which dissemination and implementation strategies are likely to be most effective in promoting the uptake of clinical guidelines.

ACHIEVING CHANGE

So far this chapter has focused on translating research findings into research products such as clinical guidelines, and considering implementation strategies that can be used to facilitate the uptake of research products into everyday practice. Implementation strategies are intended to lead to a change in how practitioners provide care. In order to select appropriate strategies an understanding of the principles underpinning successful change is necessary.

Any plan for introducing change must seek to overcome barriers to its successful implementation. It is important, therefore, to identify potential barriers to change in the local context. The most common barriers to implementing research-based change are summarised by Pearson *et al.* (2007).

Staff information and skills deficits: includes lack of knowledge regarding current recommendations and guidelines or results of clinical research, and lack of skills in accessing and applying research finding to practice.

Psychosocial barriers include attitudes, beliefs, values and previous experience that affect practice and an individual's willingness to change.

Organisational barriers include systems and processes that may create an organisational culture that is not responsive to change.

Resource barriers include a lack of required tools, equipment, staff and other resources needed to achieve change.

The Knowledge to Action framework presented earlier draws attention to the need to assess barriers to implementing change and plan accordingly. Attempts to overcome or at least reduce some of the barriers should be undertaken before introducing the change. For example, before a nutrition screening tool and accompanying clinical guideline can be introduced it may be necessary to overcome the following potential barriers.

Staff information and skills deficits: nurses may not have sufficient knowledge about nutrition screening and support and may lack the skills to use the screening tool and implement the clinical guideline.

Psychosocial barriers: nurses may feel that existing practice is satisfactory and therefore there is no need to change, or they may be reluctant to take on new responsibilities as it is seen as extra work.

Organisational barriers: other priorities may take precedence over nutrition support, which could lead to a lack of managerial commitment to making the change happen; communication systems may be lacking, which means that dissemination of information about the new initiative may be poor, etc.

Resource barriers: clinical areas may not have appropriate, calibrated, well-maintained equipment to weigh and measure a patient's height accurately; new nursing documentation may need to be introduced to record the results of the screening and care plan; additional staff may be required to facilitate the introduction, etc.

Once barriers have been identified consideration needs to be given to how change might be achieved. There is a wealth of literature accumulated over the past 50 years that describes a wide range of approaches to change management. The evidence is derived from different organisations, not just the healthcare sector, and by using a broad range of methodologies (Cameron *et al.* 2001). It is beyond the scope of this chapter to explore the different theoretical perspectives on change management. The National Institute for Health Research Service Delivery and Organisation research programme (NIHR SDO) has produced a comprehensive review of different models of change management (Iles & Sutherland 2001) to help healthcare practitioners and managers access the literature and consider the evidence available about different approaches to change. Additional related publications provide more practical guidance on developing change management skills based on selected change management theories (Iles & Cranfield 2004) and making informed decisions on change (Cameron *et al.* 2001). These publications can be downloaded from the SDO website free of charge (see information on website at the end of this chapter). NICE also produces generic and guidance-specific implementation tools that support the implementation of all types of NICE guidance but can be useful more broadly. These are available via the NICE website.

CONCLUSIONS

Translating research findings into practice is a complex undertaking that involves identifying and evaluating different sources of evidence, translating evidence into clear guidance for practice, implementing change and finally evaluating the impact of change. It is important that those who want to implement clinical research findings also draw on the evidence base about the effectiveness of implementation strategies to inform their plans. In the same way that a research study should be undertaken in a systematic and rigorous manner, the process of translating research findings into practice should be carefully planned and executed. There are a number of frameworks and tools that can assist at different stages of the process in order to enhance the likelihood of success.

References

AGREE Collaboration (2001) *The Appraisal Guidelines for Research and Evaluation (AGREE) instrument.* London, The AGREE Trust.

Bero L, Grilli R, Grimshaw J, Harvey E, Oxman A, Thomson M (1998) Closing the gap between research and practice: an overview of systematic reviews of interventions to promote the implementation of research findings. *British Medical Journal* **317**: 465–468.

Buchanan M, Harris C, Graham I, Harrison M, Lorimer K, Piercianowski T, Friedberg E (2005) Adapting national and international leg ulcer practice guidelines for local use: the Ontario leg ulcer community care protocol. *Advances in Skin and Wound Care* **18**(6): 307–318.

Cameron M, Cranfield S, Iles V, Stone J (2001) *Making Informed Decisions on Change*. London, London School of Hygiene and Tropical Medicine.

Campbell S, Hancock H, Lloyd H (2006) Implementing evidence-based practice. In: Gerrish K, Lacey A (eds) *The Research Process in Nursing*, 5th edition. Oxford, Blackwell.

Canadian Institutes of Health Research (2005) *About Knowledge Translation*. Ottawa, Canadian Institutes of Health Research. Available at www.cihr-irsc.gc.ca/e/29418.html (accessed 11 June 2009).

Canadian Institutes of Health Research (2007) *Knowledge Translation Strategies for Health Research (Archived)*. Ottawa, Canadian Institutes of Health Research (www.cihr-irsc.gc.ca/e/4342.html).

Fedder G, Eccles M, Grol R, Griffiths C, Grimshaw J (1999) Using clinical guidelines. *British Medical Journal* **318**: 728–730.

Gerrish K, Clayton J (2004) Promoting evidence-based practice: an organisational approach. *Journal of Nursing Management* **12**: 114–123.

Graham I, Harrison M (2008) Appraising and adapting clinical practice guidelines. In: Cullum N, Ciliska D, Haynes RB, Marks S (eds) *Evidence Based Nursing: an introduction*. Oxford, Blackwell, pp 219–230.

Graham I, Harrison M, Brouwers M (2003) Evaluating and adapting practice guidelines for local use: a conceptual framework. In: Pickering S, Thompson J (eds) *Clinical Governance and Best Value: meeting the modernisation agenda*. Edinburgh, Churchill Livingstone, pp 213–229.

Graham I, Logan J, Harrison M, Strauss S, Tetroe J, Caswell W, Robinson N (2006) Lost in knowledge translation: time for a map. *Journal of Continuing Education in the Health Professions* **26**(1): 13–24.

Graham I, Logan J, Tetroe J, Robinson N, Harrison M (2008) Appraising models of implementation in nursing. In: Cullum N, Ciliska D, Haynes RB, Marks S (eds) *Evidence Based Nursing: an introduction*. Oxford, Blackwell, pp 231–243.

Graham K, Logan J (2004) Using the Ottawa model of research use to implement a skin care programme. *Journal of Nursing Care Quality* **19**(1): 18–24.

Greenhalgh T, Robert G, Macfarlane F, Bates P, Kyriakidou O (2004) Diffusion of innovations in service organizations: systematic review and recommendations. *Milbank Quarterly* **82**(4): 581–629.

Grimshaw J, Shirran L, Thomas R, Mowatt G, Fraser C, Bero L (2001) Changing provider behaviour: an overview of systematic reviews of interventions. *Medical Care* **39**(8 Suppl. 2): II2–II25.

Grimshaw J, Thomas R, MacLennan G, Fraser C, Ramsey C, Vale L *et al.* (2004) *Effectiveness and Efficiency of Guideline Dissemination and Implementation Strategies*. Health Technology Assessment **8**(6) (www.ncchta.org/execsumm/summ806.htm).

Grol R (2001) Successes and failures in the implementation of evidence-based guidelines for clinical practice. *Medical Care* **39**(8 Suppl 2): II46–II54.

Hayward R, Wilson M, Tunis S, Bass E, Guyatt G (1995) Users' guides to the medical literature VIII How to use clinical practice guidelines. Are the recommendations valid? *Journal of the American Medical Association* **274**: 570–574.

Iles V, Cranfield S (2004) *Developing Change Management Skills: a resource for health care professionals and managers*. London, London School of Hygiene and Tropical Medicine (www.sdo.nihr.ac.uk/files/adhoc/change-management-developing-skills.pdf).

Iles V, Sutherland K (2001) *Organisational Change: a review for health care managers, professionals and researchers. a resource for health care professionals and managers*. London, London School of Hygiene and Tropical Medicine.

Kitson A, Harvey G, McCormack B (1998) Enabling the implementation of evidence-based practice: a conceptual framework. *Quality in Health Care* **7**: 149–158.

Lohr K, Field M (1992) A provisional instrument for assessing clinical practice guidelines. In: Field MJ, Lohr KN (eds) *Guidelines for Clinical Practice: from development to use*. Washington, DC, Institute of Medicine, National Academy Press.

O'Brien M (2008) Closing the gap between nursing research and practice. In: Cullum N, Ciliska D, Haynes RB, Marks S (eds) *Evidence Based Nursing: an introduction*. Oxford, Blackwell, pp 244–252.

Pearson A, Field J, Jordan Z (2007) *Evidence-based Clinical Practice in Nursing and Health Care: assimilating research, experience and expertise*. Oxford, Blackwell.

Rogers E (2003) *Diffusion of Innovations*, 5th edition. New York, The Free Press.

Rycroft-Malone J (2004) The PARIHS framework: a framework for guiding the implementation of evidence-based practice. *Journal of Nursing Care and Quality* **19**: 297–304.

Sudsawad P (2007) *Knowledge Translation: introduction to models, strategies and measures*. Winsconsin, National Centre for the Dissemination of Disability Research.

Websites

www.agreecollaboration.org – AGREE is an international collaboration of researchers and policy makers who seek to improve the quality and effectiveness of clinical practice guidelines by establishing a shared framework for their development, reporting and assessment.

www.cihr.ca/e/29418.html – the Canadian Institutes of Health Research website provides information on and tools to assist in knowledge translation. There are also knowledge translation learning modules that can be freely accessed (www.cihr.ca/e/39128.html).

www.nice.org.uk – the National Institute for Health and Clinical Excellence (NICE) is an independent organisation responsible for providing national guidance on promoting good health and preventing and treating ill health. It also publishes guidance on implementation strategies (*www.nice.org.uk/usingguidance/implementationtools/implementation_tools.jsp*).

www.sdo.nihr.ac.uk/managingchange.html – National Institute of Health Research Service Delivery and Organisation Programme provides access to a number of downloadable publications on managing change in healthcare settings.

www.sign.ac.uk/about/introduction.html – the Scottish Intercollegiate Guidelines Network (SIGN) undertakes the development and dissemination of national clinical guidelines containing recommendations for effective practice based on current evidence.

40 The Future of Nursing Research

Ann McMahon

Key points

- Healthcare research and development is regarded by the UK Government as strategically important to economic wellbeing as well as health.

- There are five inter-related nursing research policy imperatives, namely: increasing research capacity and capability; developing career pathways in research; creating effective partnerships through research collaboration; and exerting greater influence on the health and social care research and development (R&D) agenda.

- Progressing these policy issues is necessary for nursing research to flourish.

INTRODUCTION

The purpose of nursing research is to develop knowledge to inform nursing decision making and, ultimately, improve patient care, health outcomes and public health. This chapter considers the wider policy context in which research, and nursing research in particular, is carried out. It provides an analysis of the current position of nursing research and considers future direction and potential.

UK HEALTH RESEARCH POLICY

The development of nursing research is heavily influenced within each of the four countries of the UK by national health and social care policy and the associated research and development (R&D) policies in particular. There is a common policy concern to promote the generation and utilisation of research evidence in order to contribute towards improving the health of the population and the quality and cost-effectiveness of healthcare services. This is linked to an overarching government desire to ensure that the UK is an environment where the bioscience sector continues to flourish and contribute towards the long-term economic growth of the country. Consequently, current government policy makes a strong connection between the 'health' and 'wealth' of the country.

Table 40.1 details the departments that manage health (and related) research and development (R&D) across the UK.

Shaped by their specific health and social care priorities, each of the R&D offices is responsible to their respective government health departments for the development and implementation of R&D policy. This manifests in slightly different ways in each of the four countries through:

Table 40.1 UK Government Health Department and R&D Offices

UK Country	Government Health Department	Government Health Department R&D Office
England	Department of Health (DH)	National Institute for Health Research www.nihr.ac.uk
Northern Ireland	Department of Health Social Services and Public Safety (DPSSPS)	DPSSPS Health and Social Care Research and Development (HSC R&D) www.publichealth.hscni.net
Scotland	Scottish Government Health Directorate	Chief Scientists Office (CSO) www.sehd.scot.nhs.uk/cso/
Wales	Welsh Assembly Government	Wales Office of Research and Development for Health and Social Care (WORD) http://wales.gov.uk/topics/health/research/word/?lang=en

- investment in research infrastructure – for example research networks and support facilities such as 'research design centres'
- provision of financial resources to cover the costs to the NHS of supporting externally funded, non-commercial research
- provision of research management support, for example ensuring research governance policies, developed to protect the interests of patients and other research participants, are adhered to
- identification of research priority areas to inform research commissioning policies so that research can, in turn, inform public health and health services policy development
- implementation of schemes to build the research capacity and capability of the healthcare workforce, such as research training support schemes – from early career bursaries through to post-doctoral fellowships
- core funding of research units to undertake specific research programmes
- initiatives to support the translation of research into policy and practice.

In addition to each country having its own strategic arrangements for developing and implementing R&D policy, the UK Clinical Research Collaboration (UKCRC) was established in 2004, to enable the UK to develop a sustainable clinical research environment of international standing. The UKCRC brought together 'the major stakeholders' that were thought to influence clinical research and particularly in the NHS. Membership included representation from the main R&D funding bodies, academic medicine, the NHS and regulatory bodies, along with representatives from industry and patients. The UKCRC initially pursued five work streams:

- building up the infrastructure in the NHS
- building up incentives for research in the NHS
- building up the research workforce
- streamlining the regulatory and governance processes
- co-ordinating clinical research funding.

The nursing profession, as neither a major funder of health research nor a gatekeeper to NHS patients, was not recognised as strategically important enough to be a member of the Board of the UKCRC; however, as will be discussed later, nursing was recognised as essential to the ambition of the UKCRC being realised.

In 2006, the Treasury sought to examine whether it was getting a good enough return on its investment in health research in terms of tangible improvements in public health and better health outcomes. Sir David Cooksey was commissioned to undertake a review of UK Health Research Funding. Cooksey's (2006) recommendations included the following.

- Better coordination of health research was required and this could be achieved through the establishment of an 'Office for Strategic Coordination of Health Research' (OSCHR), under the joint auspices of the Department of Health (DoH) and the Department of Trade and Industry (DTI), with 'strategic input' from the devolved nations.

■ OSCHR should be tasked with:
  ● setting the Government's health research strategy
  ● setting the objectives and the budgets for DoH R&D and Medical Research Council (MRC) and performance managing both organisations
  ● submitting a joint funding bid to the Treasury in each spending review
  ● encouraging stronger partnerships with health industry and with health research charities.

■ Structural developments should include the development of Medical Research Council (MRC) boards to become more representative and streamlined; National Institute for Health Research (NIHR) to be an executive agency of the DoH; DoH and MRC to report to OSCHR quarterly; clarity and delineation of purpose of MRC and NIHR with joint responsibility for translational research.

■ Medicines and therapies that tackle unmet health needs, based on a UK-wide review of impact of disease and illness, should be prioritised and OSCHR should brand high-quality research projects that showed potential to address identified unmet need as a 'UK Priority Health Research Project', thus conferring institutional and procedural advantage.

■ Better coordination of research funders to increase the impact of health research in the context of international development and the establishment of a forum to facilitate collaboration.

■ Measures to strengthen the NHS culture to support research and the diffusion and adoption of new technologies and interventions along with the streamlining of processes and partnership working to bring drugs that address UK health priorities to market faster.

UK NURSING RESEARCH POLICY

Just as each country in the UK has developed its own priorities and strategic direction for R&D, so the nursing profession has also developed R&D policy from a nursing perspective within each of these contexts.

Over a decade ago, the strategy for nursing in England (Department of Health 1999) identified the need to develop a strategy to influence the national research and development agenda, to strengthen the nursing capacity and capability to undertake research, and to use research to support nursing practice. Strictly speaking this statement of intent was never realised, although 12 months after publication recommendations detailing what a nursing R&D strategy needed to contain were published (Department of Health 2000). In addition, concern over the position of the discipline of nursing in the 1996 quadrennial assessment of research activity (the Research Assessment Exercise – RAE) in UK universities led the Higher Education Funding Council for England and the Department of Health to commission research to examine why this might be so and to recommend how it could be addressed (Higher Education Funding Council for England 2001). This report is discussed in the next section.

In Northern Ireland, a study commissioned in 1998 (McKenna & Mason 1998) examined:

■ how the nursing professions could influence the overall R&D agenda
■ how the nursing professions could contribute to the wider R&D programme
■ priorities for research within the nursing professions
■ the R&D needs of the nursing professions
■ how access, dissemination and uptake of research might be improved.

This report provided a baseline assessment. It was evaluated in 2005 and new priorities to further the R&D agenda within nursing in Northern Ireland were identified (McCance & Fitzsimons 2005).

The 2001 strategy for nursing in Scotland sought to develop the highest possible standards in education, research, innovation, accountability and profes-

517

sional practice (Scottish Executive Health Department 2001). The strategy acknowledged achievements to date and recognised that a future strategy for nursing research was a prerequisite to achieving the objective of creating research-aware, research-literate and research-active nurses. Further fuelled by the poor performance of nursing departments in Scottish universities in the RAE, and following extensive consultation, a strategy for nursing research entitled 'Choices and Challenges' (Scottish Executive Health Department 2002) was launched in December 2002.

The 1999 Welsh strategy for nursing clearly articulated the need for the nursing professions to continue to develop a:

> 'sound research base ... to demonstrate conclusively the effectiveness of nursing intervention in improving health' (National Assembly for Wales, 1999, section 97)

The strategy called for the development of more integrated career pathways to enable clinically based nurses to be more research active and academically based nurses to be more clinically engaged. A strategic framework for improving the quality and quantity of R&D carried out by the nursing professions in Wales was published five years later (Welsh Assembly Government 2004).

NURSING RESEARCH: FIVE POLICY IMPERATIVES

In the last edition of this book we demonstrated that there were many similarities between the research policy priorities for nursing across the UK and identified five research policy priorities for research in nursing (McMahon & Lacey 2006). These are illustrated in Figure 40.1. They are as pertinent today as they were in 2006. Each one will be considered in turn.

Capacity and capability building

The necessity to develop higher levels of skill and greater ability to undertake research among more nurses, or develop 'research capacity' (Trostle 1992) within the nursing professions, was universally recognised as a key priority. Nursing's relatively poor performance within the UK Higher Education Funding Council's RAE in 1996 provided the much-needed impetus for the Higher Education Funding Council for England and the Department of Health to commission research to examine why this might be so and to recommend how this could be addressed. Anne Marie Rafferty and colleagues had a major

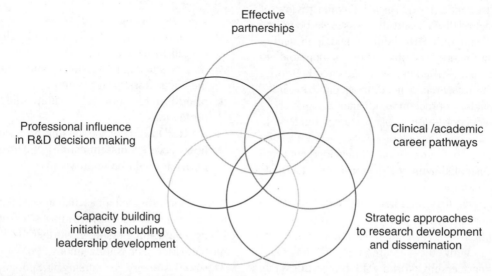

Figure 40.1 UK nursing R&D policy imperatives

influence on policy makers in this regard. Through their considered analysis of the contribution of nursing to health and healthcare and the position of research within the nursing professions, and by drawing comparisons with other applied disciplines, such as education and social work, they developed compelling arguments that persuaded policy makers to invest in the building of research capacity within the nursing professions in England (Higher Education Funding Council for England 2001). The quality and robustness of their arguments were drawn on in subsequent policy developments across the UK (Scottish Executive Health Department 2002; Welsh Assembly Government 2004; McCance & Fitzsimons 2005).

Scotland has perhaps had the greatest amount of ring-fenced investment in nursing, midwifery and allied health professions' (NMAHP) research capacity and capability development across the UK in recent years. Portfolio funding from a range of stakeholders was secured to develop research capability. This included a research training scheme and three regional consortia for NMAHP research. The research training scheme supported full-time PhD studentships and part-time postdoctoral fellowships. The research consortia were charged with the dual roles of producing research of international standing and developing NMAHP research capability within the NHS in Scotland. They were to complement the centrally funded NMAHP research unit, which was established in 1994. The impact of this investment is currently being assessed and next steps considered.

It was also acknowledged that to have the best return on any investment in research capacity building, nurses who develop their research skills should be afforded the opportunity to do so within the context of a clearly defined career pathway, which ideally would integrate both clinical and academic perspectives.

Research career pathways

Traditional views of research careers were based on the assumption that research was carried out by academics based in universities and somewhat divorced from clinical practice, or by nurses known as 'clinical research nurses' who worked in research teams that were typically led by medical doctors. The former

were seen to have a recognised academic career pathway within higher education and the latter to have minimal job security or career development opportunity. There have been significant recent developments to challenge this perceptive.

Kenkre and Foxcroft (2001a,b,c,d,e) mapped out five research career pathways in nursing, which include clinical practice, clinical research, academic, management and pharmaceutical. They sought to illustrate the potential transferability of skills from one context to another and encourage nurses working in research to move across the different pathways. The information described included the typical role, experience, knowledge, training, skills and qualifications expected at each stage along a pathway.

While Kenkre and Foxcroft sought to ease transferability across research career pathways, a more radical move has sought to facilitate a greater integration between research and practice. Indeed, the Scottish Executive stated that clinical/academic career pathways were essential for the future development of nursing and midwifery research in Scotland.

As stated above, 'building up the research workforce' was one of the UKCRC's five work streams at the outset. One of the major drivers for establishing the UKCRC and for the development of this particular work stream arose from concerns within medicine that sustaining a clinical academic medical career was becoming increasingly difficult in a constantly changing NHS. These concerns led to the development and implementation of the recommendations of the 'Walport Report' (UKCRC 2005) as part of a wider agenda to modernise medical careers.

Following publication of the Walport Report, and acknowledging the major contribution nurses make to clinical research, the UKCRC established a subgroup to progress clinical research careers in nursing. Chaired by Professor Janet Finch, the 'Finch Report' recommendations were published in 2007 (UKCRC Subcommittee for Nurses in Clinical Research (Workforce) 2007). In order to contribute meaningfully to the development of a strong evidence base for patient care and public health, the Finch report sought to overcome the barriers which had hitherto limited nurses' potential to sustain both a clinical and a research career without having to choose between the two, and for 'clinical-academic' to become a recognisable career route within the nursing professions (Finch 2009).

At the time of writing this chapter, implementation of this policy intention has varied across the UK. In England, funding has been secured to further build research capacity and capability development at masters, doctoral (PhD) and post-doctoral levels in nursing, midwifery and allied health professions. However, these opportunities have been published ahead of any specific announcements regarding career pathways. In Wales, the situation is reversed, and the profession and other key stakeholders in Wales have recently been consulted on proposals to modernise post-registration nursing careers (Welsh Assembly Government 2008) with a strong emphasis on an integrated clinical-academic career pathway.

Developments in Northern Ireland have been delayed due to a major restructuring of health and social care provision. However, a stakeholder analysis has been conducted and a committee recently established to bring together all relevant parties to explore how a clinical-academic career framework can be progressed in Northern Ireland, demonstrating strong evidence of a commitment to implement the Finch report recommendations.

In Scotland, where a new Chief Nursing Officer has recently been appointed, it is envisaged that the implementation of a clinical-academic career framework called for within *Choices and Challenges* (Scottish Executive Health Department 2002) will be an integral part of the next steps for nursing research in Scotland, as well as the developments discussed in the previous section that are currently being evaluated.

Within the wider context there are infrastructure developments designed to create an environment where clinical research can flourish, which should support the development and sustainability of clinical-academic careers across all disciplines. For example, in England, five Academic Health Science Centres, which are partnerships between NHS teaching hospitals and universities, have been established to undertake world-class research. In addition, the National Institute for Health Research has invested in nine 'Collaborations for Leadership in Applied Health Research and Care' (CLAHRCs). These are collaborative partnerships between universities and

surrounding NHS organisations, which focus on improving patient outcomes through the conduct and application of applied health research (Mawson & Scholefield 2009).

These strategic developments should help to facilitate closer collaboration and a symbiotic relationship between universities and the NHS, which have long been recognised as fundamental to the sustainability of clinical academic careers in nursing (Royal College of Nursing Working Party 2004).

Strategic approaches to R&D

A more strategic approach to the development of research career pathways in nursing would arguably need to be matched by a more strategic approach to the conduct of research itself. Over a decade ago, while the UK funding base for biomedical research was relatively healthy, the balance was shown to be tipping in favour of basic research in areas such as genetics and immunology as opposed to clinical research, which includes nursing (Policy Research Department 1998). Indeed, this was one of the key drivers for the Cooksey review, discussed above. Nursing was therefore not only starting from a relatively low baseline (Higher Education Funding Council for England 2001), but was competing against more established and influential disciplines, such as clinical medicine, for a diminishing resource. It was therefore acknowledged that nursing research needed to become more strategic and focused if it was to flourish in this increasingly competitive environment.

Traditionally, nurses who undertook research did so because they had a concern that they wanted to address. More often than not they undertook their research in full or part fulfilment of a higher education qualification and they covered the costs of their research from their personal resources, i.e. 'own account' (Higher Education Funding Council for England 2001). This situation was seen as neither desirable nor sustainable. It was recognised that if nurses wished to pursue a properly funded research career they would have to carry out research that had already been identified as a priority, and seek out and join a multidisciplinary research team undertaking research within a priority area. This, it was argued, would facilitate the growth of a body of knowledge within a specific field and would significantly increase nurses' potential to secure resources to carry out further research.

One way of making relevant connections and developing such a focus might be through engaging in one of the relatively new clinical research networks across the UK. These networks bring together clinicians and researchers within a field to co-ordinate and support research. Currently there are networks in a range of disease groupings, including cancer, dementias and neurodegenerative diseases, diabetes, medicines for children, mental health, primary care and stroke. In England, there is also a network of 'comprehensive clinical research networks' which aim to mop up all the other areas of disease and clinical need. Ideally, nurses working in clinical practice should be linked into these networks and/or be taking advantage of some of the other research infrastructure developments across the UK. This should ensure that they are working with researchers and clinicians from other disciplines where appropriate, gaining support for their research activity and finding academic collaborators.

The potential downside of taking a more strategic approach to the development of a nursing research career as described here is that the particular concerns of nursing may not be the concerns of the funders of research. That is why professional influence in R&D decision making is also identified as a policy priority in nursing.

Professional influence in strategic R&D decision making

The large amount of nursing research that had been undertaken on 'own account' (Higher Education Funding Council for England 2001) may have resulted from the absence of a dedicated funding stream to address the concerns of nursing practice, such as a research council for nursing, despite repeated calls for such a development over many years (Rafferty *et al.* 2002). Alternatively, the problem may have resulted from the relative paucity of professional influence in multidisciplinary R&D decision-making

arenas. For example, the UKCRC was established to bring together the major stakeholders that influence clinical research in the UK, and nursing was not held in this regard despite numerous attempts from the nursing profession to influence the UKCRC position.

These policy priorities can be seen as part of a vicious circle. To become more strategic and focused in their research endeavours, nurse researchers need to attract significant funding. This requires nurses to develop the capacity and capability to deliver high-quality research, and nursing to a have a strong voice within strategic R&D decision-making arenas where research priorities are agreed and resource allocation decision are made. To achieve this, nurses needed to be more strategic and focused in their research endeavours. The first step for nursing was to examine where it needed to exert greater influence.

As discussed above, it has been acknowledged that a rise in UK R&D investment in basic research was beginning to impact negatively on investment in clinical research, the funding base from which nursing draws its limited resources (Policy Research Department 1998). The Wellcome Trust, which produced this analysis based on citations of funding sources in research publications, identified three main sectors for UK biomedical (basic and clinical) research, namely UK government, private-non-profit and industry. Table 40.2, which draws on data from the PRISM report, provides examples within each of these three main sectors and illustrates the trends in biomedical research funding. The Wellcome Trust reported that within the UK government category, the research councils were the major research funders. The ability of nursing to secure MRC funding had, however, been marginal. Equally, as illustrated in Table 40.2, although the percentage of investment reported in research outputs from this sector had remained stable, there were significant increases in the percentage of investment reported in both the private-non-profit sector and the global industry sector.

To break out of the vicious circle, nursing should analyse the effectiveness of its influence within each of these sectors and develop tailored strategic lobbying strategies based on the results (McMahon & Lacey 2006). The shape of these strategies would

Table 40.2 UK R&D funding sectors

Investment sector	Examples within sector	% UK investment cited in biomedical research outputs 1988	% UK investment cited in biomedical research outputs 1995
UK Government	• Government Health departments • Higher Education Funding Councils • Research Councils	33.9	33.8
Private-non-profit	• Charities • Foundations • Hospital trustees	24.4	31.8
Industry	• Pharmaceutical • Biotechnology • World Bank	13.9	17.4

Table 40.3 Distribution of combined UK health research funding (UKCRC 2006)

Area of research	% distribution
Aetiology	34.5
Underpinning	34.1
Treatment development	8.5
Treatment evaluation	8.1
Detection and diagnosis	5.2
Health services	4.8
Prevention	2.5
Disease management	2.3

Table 40.4 Distribution of research funding from UK medical research charities (UKCRC 2006)

Area of research	% distribution
Aetiology	50.5
Treatment development	13.2
Underpinning	12.2
Treatment evaluation	9.5
Detection and diagnosis	7.2
Disease management	4.5
Prevention	1.6
Health services	1.3

depend, to a large extent, on the direction the profession elected to take in this regard.

Recent work carried out by the UKCRC to secure an optimum return on investment in health research through better co-ordination of research funding may help such lobbying strategies. The UKCRC developed a health research classification system, conducted a comprehensive analysis of UK research funding (UK Clinical Research Collaboration 2006; UK Clinical Research Collaboration & Association of Medical Research Charities 2007) and created a forum for joint funding initiatives. The UKCRC 2006 analysis of UK research funding is presented in Table 40.3.

Although it does not specifically delineate the issues of concern to nursing practice, it clearly demonstrates that the lion's share of research funding

(68.6%) was dedicated to the causes or 'aetiology' of disease and understanding of normal functioning or 'underpinning factors', which, while important, are of less concern to an applied discipline such as nursing. This echoed the earlier findings by Wellcome, cited above. Only 31.4% of UK healthcare research was therefore shared across the applied disciplines, and without a nursing voice within UKCRC, the chances of any influence to shift funding decisions towards the concerns of nursing practice were extremely unlikely. The second report, which looked specifically at the research funding of medical research charities, showed a slightly different picture (Table 40.4), with a much stronger focus on the aetiology of disease. Earlier investigations into the potential of research charities to support nursing research clearly demonstrated that nurses must align themselves to the concerns of the charity and develop a track record of producing high-quality research, if they are to secure research funding from this sector (Crofts & McMahon 2002).

There are essentially two schools of thought regarding how nursing might secure a greater slice of the R&D resource cake. The first is that nursing should swim with the tide, embrace the brave new world and ensure it has a strong voice within the multidisciplinary research arena. The potential benefit of pursuing such a position is that, if successful, nursing may be recognised as an equal player alongside other professional and academic groups. The potential downside of this position is twofold. First, there is a danger that nurses themselves might lose sight of their distinctly nursing values and purpose (Royal College of Nursing 2003). In the worst-case scenario, there may be a nurse at the top table but no way of identifying who she is, as her contribution is indistinguishable from those of her medical colleagues. Second, resources such as those committed to research capacity building, for example, are increasingly offered on an interdisciplinary competitive basis. Without a collective concerted effort to change the culture in nursing, where there is a reported shortfall in the number of applications for R&D resources in a multidisciplinary competitive context (Mead *et al.* 1997) there is a danger that this may lead to a fall in the number of applicants.

The counter argument is that the only way that nursing's distinctive contribution to health and social care research can be fully realised is through the establishment of a Nursing Research Council, with the resources to commission research to inform nursing policy and practice. The benefits of this scenario would lie in the ring-fencing of funding for nursing research and in the capacity to strengthen the distinct voice of research in nursing. The danger would lie in the potential to further marginalise the voice of nursing from the interdisciplinary research arena.

If nursing elects to swim with the tide, it would arguably need to put balances and checks in place to ensure that when at the top table it offered a truly distinct perspective. If the profession chooses to swim against the tide, evidence indicates that these balances and checks would still be required.

In 2008, an article in the *Guardian* online, ran with the headline 'Nursing research takes its place on world stage' (Lipsett 2008). The article reported on the outcome of the UK Higher Education Funding Council's RAE. The RAE is a peer review assessment of research quality that has been conducted four times in the UK, in 1992, 1996, 2001 and 2008. As indicated above, on each of the previous occasions the nursing discipline scored poorly. Indeed, nursing scored lower than any other discipline. There are several reasons why this may have been the case, with nursing's relatively recent engagement in research considered to be a key factor. However, the 2008 RAE showed a marked improvement in nursing's performance. The *Guardian* journalist stated:

'Nursing, for many years medicine's poor relation, has come of age in the 2008 research assessment exercise. Academics in the field can justifiably claim to be world leading in terms of research' (Lipsett 2008)

The 2008 RAE headlines indicate significant progress in nursing research since the previous edition of this book was published. However, although we celebrate nursing's achievements in the nursing unit of assessment in the RAE, we must acknowledge that many notable nursing academics whose contribution was deemed by their university to have a better 'strategic fit' within another subject area were not 'returned' within and scrutinised by the nursing RAE panel. Consequently their contribution and achievements are less accessible. Until further analysis is undertaken across the UK, their important contribution will remain less visible. In addition, many nurses will have made significant contributions to research led by academics within other research disciplines, and perhaps medicine in particular. While their research activities may not obviously inform nursing practice, and thus not be classified as 'nursing research', their contribution to the health research agenda, and ultimately patient and public health, must not go unnoticed. The enormity of the nursing contribution to the UK clinical research endeavour should not be underestimated. Consequently, nursing's potential influence within the UK biomedical research enterprise is yet to be realised.

Effective partnerships

The fifth and final policy imperative to progress nursing research is the development of effective partnerships. This has been touched on already. Resources to develop nursing research capacity have been secured through a mixed portfolio of funding, from the Higher Education Funding Council, the UK health departments and the private-non-profit sector, with the Health Foundation providing the major share. These resources have not only been secured through partnerships, they have also been allocated through partnerships. The individual nurse who applies for a national or local research fellowship must do so in partnership with a university with the full support of their employing organisation.

Clinical-academic career development within nursing will depend on effective partnerships between the university and healthcare sectors. Infrastructure developments may go some way towards facilitating this, but ultimately it will depend on the determination of the people on the front line to work together effectively if these new ways of working are to become the norm. Strategic approaches to research and development require nurses to network extensively, forge alliances with other disciplines with common research concerns and influence decision-making processes. The effectiveness of nursing's professional influence will depend on effective partnership working within nursing as well as across disciplinary boundaries.

Nursing does not have a strong record of drawing on its collective power and speaking with one coherent and strategic voice on research matters, especially when compared to medicine. Such historical resistance has hopefully been overcome recently through the timely development of the Academy of Nursing, Midwifery and Health Visiting Research. The Academy was established in 2009 as a collaborative enterprise by the Royal College of Nursing, CPHVA–UNITE and the Royal College of Midwives in partnership with The Council of Deans for Health, the Nurse Directors group of the Association of UK University Hospitals, the Association for Leaders in Nursing, the Queen's Nursing Institute, Mental Health Nurse Academics UK, the UK Clinical Research Facility Network and Nurses in Primary Care Research. The Academy seeks to provide an expert collaborative voice for all aspects of research involving nursing, midwifery and health visiting in the UK, including policy development, its implementation and evaluation through negotiation and dialogue with other key stakeholders.

Whereas the Academy will function at a policy level, effective partnerships are also required at organisational and individual levels. There are lead nurses in R&D and NHS-based professorial positions throughout the UK. Such post holders often hold a formal joint appointment between an academic institution and a healthcare organisation. It is important that these leadership positions are underpinned by a robust clinical-academic career structure and the firm commitment and support of nurses in executive positions and academic deans is a prerequisite.

There are at least three facets to research leadership roles in healthcare organisations. First, they seek to establish nursing research projects and programmes of research in their respective organisations. Second, they aim to influence the wider R&D agenda to both secure more resources for nursing research and ensure that a nursing perspective is incorporated into collaborative research activities when they are led by other disciplines. And third, such posts often have a strong focus on the development of nursing practice where the aim is to enable research to inform practice and practice to inform research.

CONCLUSIONS

Research is necessary to develop the knowledge base to inform nursing policy and practice, and ultimately improve the quality of patient care, public health and health outcomes. To enhance the nursing contribution to health and social care research there are five policy imperatives that the profession must progress for nurses to stand as equals within the multidisciplinary research arena. The research capacity of the nursing workforce will continue to grow and this is likely to be within the context of a much more integrated clinical-academic career pathway, thus increasing the proximity of the conduct of research to the environments where care is provided and enhancing the relevance of nursing research to practice. Recent trends such as the RAE indicate that nurse researchers will become increasingly more strategic and influential in their research activities and will develop nursing knowledge with a wide range of clinical and academic collaborators. To remain visible, nurses will have to assert their professional identity within this increasingly interdisciplinary context. Should they do so, professional influence will become increasingly evident within policy, organisational and research developments.

References

Cooksey D (2006) *A Review of UK Health Research Funding*. Norwich, The Stationery Office.

Crofts L, McMahon A (2002) Raising the profile of nursing research amongst medical research charities. *NT Research* **7**(5): 378–389.

Department of Health (1999) *Making a Difference: strengthening the nursing, midwifery and health visiting contribution to health and healthcare*. London, Department of Health.

Department of Health (2000) *Towards a Strategy for Nursing Research and Development: proposals for action*. London, Department of Health.

Finch J (2009) The importance of clinical academic careers. *Journal of Research in Nursing* **14**(2): 103–105.

Higher Education Funding Council for England (2001) *Promoting Research in Nursing and the Allied Health Professions*. Research report 01/64. London, Higher Education Funding Council for England.

Kenkre J, Foxcroft D (2001a) Career pathways in research: academic. *Nursing Standard* **16**(7): 40–44.

Kenkre J, Foxcroft D (2001b) Career pathways in research: pharmaceutical. *Nursing Standard* **16**(8): 36–39.

Kenkre J, Foxcroft D (2001c) Career pathways in research: support and management. *Nursing Standard* **16**(6): 33–35.

Kenkre J, Foxcroft D (2001d) Career pathways in research: clinical practice. *Nursing Standard* **16**(4): 40–43.

Kenkre J, Foxcroft D (2001e) Career pathways in research: clinical research. *Nursing Standard* **16**(5): 41–44.

Lipsett A (2008) Nursing research takes its place on world stage. www.guardian.co.uk/education/2008/dec/18/nursing-rae-research.

Mawson S, Scholefield H (2009) The National Institute for Health Research Collaboration for Leadership in Applied Health Research and Care for South Yorkshire. *Journal of Research in Nursing* **14**(2): 169–174.

McCance T, Fitzsimons D (2005) *Using and Doing Research: guiding the future*. Belfast, Northern Ireland Practice and Education Council for Nursing and Midwifery.

McKenna H, Mason C (1998) *Using and Doing Research: a position paper to inform strategy, policy and practice for nursing research in Northern Ireland*. Belfast, DHSS.

McMahon A, Lacey A (2006) The future of nursing research. In: Gerrish K, Lacey A (eds) *The Research Process in Nursing*, 5th edition. Oxford, Blackwell, pp 521–533.

Mead D, Moseley L, Cook R (1997) The performance of nursing in the research stakes: lessons from the field. *NT Research* **2**(5): 335–344.

National Assembly for Wales (1999) *Realising the Potential: a strategic framework for nursing, midwifery and health visiting in Wales into the 21st century*. Cardiff, National Assembly for Wales.

Policy Research Department (PRISM) (1998) *Mapping the Landscape: national biomedical research outputs 1988–95*. London, The Wellcome Trust.

Rafferty AM, Newell R, Traynor M (2002) Nursing and midwifery research in England: working towards establishing a dedicated fund. *Nursing Times Research* **7**: 243–254.

Royal College of Nursing (2003) *Defining Nursing*. Royal College of Nursing, London.

Royal College of Nursing Working Party (2004) *Promoting Excellence in Care Through Research and Development. An RCN Position Statement*. London, Royal College of Nursing.

Scottish Executive Health Department (2001) *Caring for Scotland. The Strategy for Nursing and Midwifery in Scotland*. Edinburgh, NHS Scotland.

Scottish Executive Health Department (2002) *Choices and Challenges. The Strategy for Research and Development in Nursing and Midwifery in Scotland*. Edinburgh, Scottish Executive Health Department.

Trostle J (1992) Research capacity building and international health: definitions, evaluations & strategies for success. *Social Science & Medicine* **35**(11): 1321–1324.

UK Clinical Research Collaboration (2006) *UK Health Research Analysis*. London, UKCRC.

UK Clinical Research Collaboration (2005) *Medically and Dentally Qualified Academic Staff: recommendations for training the researchers and academics of the future* (Walport Report). London, UKCRC Modernising Medical Careers.

UK Clinical Research Collaboration & Association of Medical Research Charities (2007) *From Donation to Innovation: an analysis of health research funded by medium and smaller sized medical research charities.* London, UKCRC/AMRC.

UKCRC Subcommittee for Nurses in Clinical Research (Workforce) (2007) *Developing the Best Research Professionals. Qualified graduate nurses: recommendations for preparing and supporting clinical academic nurses of the future.* London, UKCRC.

Welsh Assembly Government (2008) *Modernising Nursing Careers: a post registration career framework for nurses in Wales.* Cardiff, Welsh Assembly Government.

Welsh Assembly Government (2004) *Realising the Potential. Briefing Paper 6. Achieving the potential through research and development.* Cardiff, Welsh Assembly Government.

Websites

www.rcn.org.uk/development/researchanddevelopment – RCN Research and Development Co-ordinating Centre.

www.rcn.org.uk/development/researchanddevelopment/ career/career – research careers and job profiles.

www.rcn.org.uk/development/researchanddevelopment/ networks – research networks.

www.rcn.org.uk/development/researchanddevelopment/ newsevents – details of the latest developments in R&D. Subscribe to receive the RCN weekly e-bulletin with details of research funding, research policy, publications, conferences, research posts and more.

www.researchacademy.co.uk – Academy of Nursing Midwifery and Health Visiting Research.

Glossary

Abstract A concise summary of a research study, journal article or conference presentation, often limited to 200 words. It is usually found at the beginning of a research article or report, and may be used alone in indexes and conference proceedings.

Action research Research that is characterised by the active participation of the researcher in the study. It may be carried out as part of a change process. It has a strong emphasis on context and the participation of non-researchers. Research methods are often **qualitative**, but can also include **quantitative** data.

Audit A rigorous procedure for measuring and improving the quality of care or clinical outcomes against an agreed standard at local or national level.

Bias The systematic influence of factors other than those being investigated. Bias should be eliminated or minimised, as it reduces the **validity** of the study.

Blended research See **mixed methods**.

Blinding The process, used in **experimental design**, whereby participants are unaware whether they are allocated to the experimental or control group. It may necessitate the use of a **placebo**. Data collectors and professional staff may also be blinded to the experimental group – this is known as **double blinding**, and is used to reduce bias.

Caldicott guardian A person appointed to ensure the confidential, ethical and appropriate use of patient data for research purposes within an NHS organisation in UK. May be a **gatekeeper** for access to patient data.

Care protocol See **clinical guideline**.

Case study The use of a single person, event or context in a research study in order to study a phenomenon in depth. Case study research may use multiple 'cases' to explore a subject area.

Clinical guideline or **care protocol** A document or resource that promotes best practice by incorporating the best available evidence into a written or electronic guide for the clinical care of patients with specific conditions or needs.

Clinical trial A rigorous form of research using experimental methods, usually used to test new drugs and clinical treatments. Clinical trials normally employ **randomised controlled trial** (RCT) methods.

Coding The stage of qualitative data analysis where categories and concepts are identified within the raw data and given individual codes.

Cohort study A form of research within the epidemiological tradition, where a group of research participants is recruited and followed up over time. Common examples are birth cohorts (all children born in a particular time period) and disease cohorts (all patients diagnosed in a particular year).

Conceptual framework An abstract set of concepts and theories that are related to one another and may be used to organise ideas and guide analysis within a study. A conceptual framework may be derived from a particular philosophical position.

Confidence interval A range within which the true value of a parameter (e.g. mean or proportion) is estimated to lie.

Consent form A legal document signed by a research participant who agrees to take part, or have data relating to them included, in a particular research project.

Control group A group of research participants recruited to be compared with an experimental or intervention group. The control group are not given the experimental treatment or condition, but may be given a placebo treatment or condition.

Correlation The extent to which variation in one variable is related to variation in another.

Covert observation A form of participant observation in which those being observed are not aware of the researcher's activity or intentions. Often involves some degree of deception and may therefore be considered unethical.

Cross tabulation A comparison, expressed in a table, of two or more categorical variables to show how they are related to one another, e.g. age group, gender and smoking.

Data cleaning A process of examining data, once collected, to remove error and omissions. Usually applied to quantitative data once it has been entered into computer software for analysis.

Deduction The process of testing theories by the collection of data and analysis. Underlies much **quantitative research**, especially **experimental design**, and is opposed to **induction**.

Delphi technique A research method used to obtain a consensus of opinion of a group of experts by a series (or 'rounds') of intensive questionnaires interspersed with controlled feedback. It is a structured form of data collection that is usually used within a **quantitative research** framework.

Dependent variable The variable that forms the outcome of a study. Experimental studies are designed to explain changes in the dependent variable, possibly caused by an **independent variable**. In studies of nurse-related cross-infection, wound sepsis might be the dependent variable, where hand-washing technique is the independent variable.

Dichotomous variable A variable that can take only one of two values, e.g. yes/no, male/female.

Dissemination The process of informing others about the results of a particular research study. This may be by verbal, written, audiovisual or electronic means.

Emic The view from within a culture or research setting, recognised only by those who participate in that culture – opposed to **etic**.

Empirical That which can be observed, experienced and measured through the human senses, as opposed to theoretical, which is concerned with thought processes.

Emplotment A device used in narrative research to link together diverse events to form a plot which generates a coherent story.

Epidemiology The science of measuring the prevalence and incidence of disease and other phenomena in large populations.

Epistemology The philosophical theory of knowledge. Research approaches are based on differing bodies of knowledge, known as their underlying epistemology.

Ethnicity A multi-faceted biosocial concept that describes social groups in terms of their culture, race, identity, language or other shared characteristics. It can be a marker or proxy for a wide range of factors in a research study.

Ethnography An approach to qualitative research that focuses on culture and subcultures within a society. Ethnographers study behaviour, interaction, customs, rituals, values and institutions, and attempt to interpret them in a narrative account.

Etic The view from outside a research setting or culture, whereby a researcher seeks to interpret the culture to a wider audience – opposed to **emic**.

Evaluation An attempt to assess the worth or value of something.

Evaluation research A type of research that has the purpose of assessing the worth or value of something (e.g. of practice, intervention, innovation or service).

Evidence-based practice The integration of the best available research evidence with expert clinical opinion, while taking into account the preferences of patients.

Experimental design A research design characterised by testing an **hypothesis** under controlled conditions. The method is **quantitative**, and favoured in pure scientific and medical research.

Experimental group A group of research participants who are exposed to an experimental treatment or condition. Often called an **intervention** group. May be compared to a **control** group.

External validity The extent to which a research study can be **generalised** to other populations and contexts. Often called **generalisability**.

Factor analysis A statistical technique to describe variability among items in a questionnaire or measuring tool. The aim of factor analysis is to group together similar items and so reduce the number of variables being described.

Fieldwork Data collection that takes place in the everyday context of the research participants. Commonly used in **qualitative** research using interviews and **participant observation**.

Focus group A group of individuals assembled to take part in a group interview, with the purpose of collecting data and observing the effect of group interaction. Often used in **qualitative** and market research.

Gatekeeper A term used for a person occupying a role that enables the researcher access to a setting or to research participants. May be a head teacher for access to schoolchildren, or a practice manager for access to primary healthcare facilities.

Generalisability The extent to which the findings from a research study can be applied to other populations and contexts. See **external validity**.

Grey literature Literature that has not been published in a formal book or journal (traditional or electronic), but still has value as a source of evidence. Grey literature includes conference proceedings, informal and local publications, and transcripts of verbal communications.

Grounded theory A specific **inductive** methodology in **qualitative** research. Data collection and analysis take place simultaneously, with the ultimate goal of development of new theory.

Hawthorne effect A phenomenon observed in research, whereby the research participants change their behaviour purely as a result of taking part in an experiment. This effect is a threat to the **validity** of the study.

Health services research A broad term used to describe research into healthcare systems, evaluation of healthcare and clinical effectiveness of interventions. Health services research uses a wide range of methodologies and is multidisciplinary in nature, but excludes laboratory and biomedical research.

Hierarchy of evidence A representation of different research methodologies that suggests an order of preference for **evidence-based practice** in terms of rigour and reliability. The hierarchy is controversial, as it sees **randomised controlled trials** as the 'gold standard' against which other methods should be evaluated. Many qualitative researchers challenge the published hierarchy.

Historical research A research methodology that uses historical documents, books, archives and other sources as data to re-examine and interpret the past, as a means of informing present-day policy and practice.

Hypothesis A statement about the relationship between two or more variables, which can be tested **empirically**.

Illness narratives The stories that sick people tell about their experiences.

Independent variable The variable that is thought to cause, or explain in some way, another variable, called the **dependent** variable. In studies of nurse-related cross-infection, wound sepsis might be the dependent variable, where hand washing is the independent variable.

Induction The process of drawing conclusions and building theory from data that have been collected and analysed. Often used in **qualitative research** and opposed to **deduction**.

Inferential statistics Statistical techniques whereby hypotheses are tested and inference made from a sample to a wider population.

Informed consent The process of ensuring that research participants are fully aware of what the study involves, and freely agree to take part. This usually requires a formal signature on a **consent form** after verbal and written information has been given.

In-depth interview An interview technique used in **qualitative** research in which the interviewer imposes minimal structure on the conversation in order to explore the perceptions or experience of the participant. Commonly used in **phenomenology** and **grounded theory** where little is known about the subject of interest.

Intellectual property rights Legal matters concerning the ownership of a new piece of knowledge or a research product such as a validated questionnaire or an item of technology.

Internal consistency A measure of how well items in a **questionnaire** or other data collection tools are related to, and agree with, one another.

Internal validity The extent to which effects observed in a research study are truly caused by the variables under study and not due to any **bias**, **unreliability** or other sources of error.

Interpretivism The belief that human beings continuously interpret and make sense of their environment, and so research into their behaviour and social processes must take the meaning of events into account. This approach underlies **qualitative** research methods and may be opposed to **positivism**.

Intervention group See **experimental group**.

Knowledge translation The process of taking what has been learned through research and applying such knowledge in different practice settings and circumstances.

Likert scale A scale, usually used in **questionnaires**, where the respondent is asked to agree or disagree with a series of statements in order to measure an attitude or other variable.

Mean The statistical measure obtained by adding all scores for a variable together and dividing the sum by the number of items. Often known as a mathematical average.

Median The statistical measure that is the middle value when a range of scores are arranged in ascending or descending order.

Meta-analysis The statistical re-analysis of data from a number of studies to reach an interpretation of their combined data. Often found in **systematic reviews**. May also be attempted in a non-statistical form for **qualitative** studies.

Mixed methods A research study that integrates **quantitative** and **qualitative** methods in order to reflect and account for complexity. Sometimes known as **blended research**.

Mode The numerical value from a **frequency distribution** that occurs most often. This may have no relation to the middle value.

Narrative research A qualitative research approach that relies on the stories of participants about their experiences.

Null hypothesis A **hypothesis** written in negative terms for statistical testing. The null hypothesis usually states that there will be no difference between experimental groups.

Objectivity Observation or measurement that relies on physical reality not amenable to individual interpretation. Examples would include temperature measurement and wound size. It can be argued that even such observations may be open to **subjectivity**.

Overt observation A form of observation where the researcher's intentions and actions are fully open to those being observed.

Paradigm A way of viewing reality, informed by a particular theoretical perspective, belief or set of assumptions.

Participant observation Used in **qualitative research**, the researcher takes part in the research context and may assume a role, e.g. a researcher becomes a nursing assistant in an A&E department in order to observe the interaction of patients and staff. May be **overt** (open) or **covert** (hidden).

Patient Information Sheet (PIS) A document given to research participants which explains to them, in lay language, what participation in the research project will involve. They are then asked to sign a **consent form**.

Peer review A system of assessing the quality of research proposals, conference presentations and journal articles, where respected researchers and other peers of the author are asked to comment critically on the work. Used in the university **Research Assessment Exercise**.

Phenomenon An occurrence, circumstance, experience or fact that is perceptible to the senses.

Phenomenology An inductive approach to **qualitative** research that focuses on understanding the human experience from 'the inside'. Phenomenologists interpret the meaning of the 'lived experience' of study participants through their description.

Pilot study A preliminary study carried out before the full research to test out data collection instruments and other procedures.

Placebo A non-active substance or form of intervention used for the control group in experimental designs to avoid bias. Trial participants may be **blinded** to whether they are taking the active treatment or the placebo.

Population All possible participants or items that could be included in a sample. Might be all qualified nurses in an NHS trust or all patient records in a primary care practice. A **sample** is usually then selected from the population for study.

Positivism A theoretical position derived from 18th-century philosophy, believing that scientific truth can only be derived from that which is observable by the human senses. Positivists would apply the methods of traditional scientific enquiry to the study of human behaviour. **Quantitative** research methods rely on this tradition, rather than **interpretivism**.

Power calculation A statistical calculation that is carried out to determine sample size in a quantitative study, to ensure enough participants or items are included to increase the probability of observing any real effects and reduce the probability of errors.

Practitioner research Any form of research that is conducted by, and for, practitioners in the clinical field.

Primary outcome The most important outcome variable being investigated in a study.

Principal investigator (PI) The lead researcher on a team, and usually the most experienced member. The PI takes overall responsibility for ensuring accountability for the conduct of the research.

Psychometric analysis A statistical process to assess the **validity** and **reliability** of standardised **questionnaires**.

Response rate A measure, usually expressed as a percentage, of how many of the eligible sample members selected for a research study actually took part or completed all the data collection stages. Low response rates can affect the **validity** of the study and introduce **bias**.

Qualitative research The broad term used to denote research designs and methods that yield non-numerical data and are based on an **interpretative** philosophy. Analysis is usually based on narrative and thematic methods.

Quantitative research The broad term used to denote research designs and methods that yield numerical data and are based on a **positivist** philosophy. Analysis is usually based on statistical methods.

Quasi-experimental design A form of experiment where it is not possible or ethical to randomise participants to comparison groups.

Questionnaire A data collection tool, paper or web based, where respondents are asked to complete a series of structured questions or items. Answers are often in 'tick box' format.

Randomised controlled trial (RCT) An experimental design where participants are randomly allocated to comparison groups, sometimes using a **placebo**. Often referred to as the 'gold standard' for evaluating treatment and to form the basis for evidence-based practice. Most clinical trials of treatments use this design.

Random sampling A form of sampling where units are chosen from a population in a systematic but random way to ensure each unit has an equal (and non-zero) chance of being selected.

Realist synthesis A newly emerging form of evidence review that is particularly appropriate for assessing the impact of complex interventions. It emphasises the context of interventions and unpacks how they work in particular settings, enabling theory development.

Reflexivity The process, used in **qualitative research**, whereby the researcher reflects continuously on how their own actions, values and perceptions impact on the research setting and affect the data collection and analysis.

Regression Prediction of one continuous variable from another, using a particular statistical technique.

Reliability A measure of the consistency and accuracy of data collection. A data collection instrument may be said to be unreliable if it generates different readings on repeated measurements at the same time of the same person. Low reliability can cause a research study to lack **validity**, but high **reliability** does not necessarily ensure **validity**.

531

Representative sample A sample that contains a similar proportion of important variables (e.g. age, gender, medical condition) as the population from which it is drawn.

Research The attempt to produce generalisable new knowledge by addressing clearly defined questions with rigorous and systematic methods.

Research Assessment Exercise (RAE) The system used by the funding council for higher education (HEFCE) in the UK to assess the quality of research undertaken in universities. The assessment is related to subject discipline and strength of research output, as measured by publications, external funding grants won and peer esteem.

Research ethics committee (REC) A formal committee at local, national or international level that is charged with ensuring compliance with ethical standards for all research carried out within its geographical, organisational or specialist area.

Research governance A system of regulation of research activity in health and social care organisations introduced in England and Wales in 2001 and updated in 2005.

Research infrastructure The structures and organisations that support research activity, such as research networks, research support and advice centres, information centres, clinical trials units and data processing facilities.

Research proposal A concise document that sets out what is to be done in a proposed piece of research, including aims and objectives, methods, sampling, analysis and costs. A proposal is normally written for funding applications or for permission from regulatory frameworks.

Rigour The strength of a research design in terms of adherence to procedures, accuracy and consistency.

Sample A subset of a **population** drawn for the purpose of research. A sample may be made up of individuals, clinical material such as blood samples, organisations or events.

Sampling The process of selecting a sample. The sampling technique used will affect **validity** of the research.

Sampling frame The list of units, individuals or organisations in a population from which a sample is drawn. Common sampling frames are (for individuals) electoral rolls, GP registration lists, school registers and (for organisations) yearbooks of NHS organisations, mailing lists of university departments of nursing and midwifery in the UK.

Secondary analysis Re-analysis of data collected for another purpose or for a previous research study.

Semi-structured interview An interview technique whereby the interviewer uses pre-determined topics and questions, but retains the flexibility to follow up ideas raised by the participant. Commonly used in **qualitative** research where there is a policy agenda, as in **health services research**.

Sensitivity The percentage of tests or cases where those who have the condition under investigation is correctly identified.

Social desirability The tendency of respondents to a survey or other study to give answers that they consider will meet with social approval.

Specificity The percentage of tests or cases where those who do not have the condition under investigation are correctly identified.

Stakeholder Someone in an organisation or other focus of a study who has an interest (stake) in the evaluation, or other research, and its outcomes. Includes participants, clients, staff and management.

Standard deviation A statistical measure of the spread of data in a sample. It measures dispersion from the **mean**.

Stratification The process of dividing a population into known strata by important variables (e.g. gender) before taking a **sample**.

Structured abstract A form of **abstract** where the information is given under prescribed headings (e.g. aim, method, results, conclusion). Some academic journals and conferences insist on presentation in this style.

Structured interview A form of interview where questions are pre-set both in topic and sequence. Commonly used in **quantitative** research.

Structured observation A form of observation used in **quantitative** research where events or actions being observed are recorded in pre-determined categories, often using checklists or handheld computers as data collection tools.

Subjectivity Observation or measurement that is seen to be influenced by the perception of the individual. Examples would include the experience of pain or gender discrimination. Opposed to **objectivity**.

Survey A research design that collects information from a **sample** or **population** to obtain descriptive and **correlational** data. A whole **population** survey is called a census.

Systematic review A rigorous and systematic literature search using a well-defined question and strict criteria for study inclusion and evaluation. It may also involve amalgamating statistical data from different studies in **meta-analysis**.

Temporality The way that time is used and portrayed in a narrative account.

Thick description Detailed account of cultural behaviours and practices, described in context. Used particularly in **ethnography** and **narrative research**.

Think aloud A technique used for data collection whereby an individual's thinking and decision-making processes are recorded and used as data.

Transcription The process of transferring audio data (usually speech) to written data in narrative form for analysis.

Triangulation The use of two or more data sources, theoretical perspectives or methods in a research study to compare findings and hence achieve greater **validity**.

Trust A healthcare organisation that provides services on behalf of the National Health Service in the UK. A Trust may comprise one hospital or several hospitals or provide primary/community care services as a Primary Care Trust.

Validity The extent to which data, and its interpretation, reflects the phenomenon under investigation without **bias**. Studies and instruments used to collect data are unlikely to be **valid** unless they are also **reliable**. Some qualitative researchers prefer to use terms such as credibility and trustworthiness to describe this concept.

Vignettes Brief scenarios that can be given verbally or in writing to research participants to stimulate a response.

Visual analogue scale (VAS) A line on which a respondent is asked to rate the degree of some subjective variable, usually scored from 0 to 100. Pain is typically measured using a VAS, where 0 represents no pain and 100 represents the worst pain possible.

Index

Page numbers in italic refer to figures or tables.